Nutrition and Cancer Prevention

Nutrition and Cancer Prevention

INVESTIGATING THE ROLE OF MICRONUTRIENTS

edited by

Thomas E. Moon

THE UNIVERSITY OF ARIZONA
HEALTH SCIENCES CENTER
TUCSON, ARIZONA

Marc S. Micozzi

ARMED FORCES INSTITUTE OF PATHOLOGY
WASHINGTON, D.C.

MARCEL DEKKER, INC. New York and Basel

ISBN: 0-8247-7993-2

MARCEL DEKKER, INC.
270 Madison Avenue, New York, New York 10016

Current printing (last digit):
10 9 8 7 6 5 4 3 2 1

PRINTED IN THE UNITED STATES OF AMERICA

Preface

Disease prevention has a history familiar to readers of medical literature. The concept of cancer as a preventable disease has evolved from studies undertaken to identify carcinogens and effect their elimination from the human environment. The broadening of the concept that cancer can be prevented by selectively altering the intake of specific foods or nutrients in the diet has gained scientific credibility and growing importance in the biological literature.

Hypotheses about the possible relation between micronutrients and cancer prevention have come from observational and analytical studies of human dietary intake and cancer rates. To move from the study of complex foods and dietary intake to the testing of specific food constituents (e.g., micronutrients) that might be considered as cancer preventive agents, it is necessary to adopt complementary approaches.

One such approach appears possible through the development of cancer preventive agents by using a program similar to that followed in clinical pharmacology for development of chemotherapeutic agents. However, the many important ways in which development of cancer preventive agents must differ from that of chemotherapeutic agents is an important consideration. The drug development and clinical trials program of clinical pharmacology, so applicable to many areas of modern medical science, may provide a useful model for scientific inquiry into cancer prevention. Clinical drug trials emphasize a process for establishing results by using the products of clinical pharmacology, important to both regulatory affairs and creating a base of scientific knowledge.

In cancer prevention research, whether we are testing a product (such as a micronutrient) as a food or a drug, the process of clinical trials remains important to establishing end results. Randomization in clinical trials accounts for both known and unknown confounding factors in a study, as compared to analytical epidemiology in which only known factors can be controlled. The small relative risks—estimated for most nutritional factors in cancer etiology—also impose the requirement for large-scale clinical trials to obtain definitive, statistically significant results on toxicity and efficacy of proposed cancer preventive agents. The long duration of most clinical trials and great publicity surrounding them allows for the influence of secular trends on both control and treatment groups. Thus, the results of clinical trials must be carefully interpreted.

This book on investigating the role of micronutrients in cancer prevention, leading to clinical trials, is the result of independent ideas that were initiated in 1985 by each of the editors. One of us (MSM) was first contacted by Marcel Dekker, Inc. to prepare an edited volume on the newly developing field of chemoprevention of cancer as a result of a review article that appeared in 1985 in the *Journal of Clinical Pharmacology*. This article had been requested by D. Aviado, then acting editor of the journal, because clinical pharmacologists had not yet heard enough about developing agents for cancer prevention trials. Micozzi and a number of colleagues in the Cancer Prevention Studies Branch (J. Tangrea, P. Taylor, and K. Helzlsouer) and Chemoprevention Branch (C. Boone and G. Kelloff) of the Cancer Prevention Research Program, National Cancer Institute, formed a working group to prepare an appropriate outline for development of cancer prevention agents that would be applicable to clinical pharmacology and clinical trials.

Concurrently, the American Society of Preventive Oncology was planning a session on chemoprevention studies for their March, 1986, annual meeting in Bethesda, Maryland. One of us (TEM) was preparing a presentation for that annual meeting that was based upon his ongoing experiences with the development and conduct of skin and cervical cancer prevention studies using retinoids. He and a number of colleagues at the University of Arizona (D. Alberts, R. Dorr, N. Levine, F. Meyskens, and E. Surwit) had previously made presentations and prepared articles for the February, 1985, meeting in Tucson, entitled Second International Conference on the Modulation and Mediation of Cancer by Vitamins and Micronutrients. Their presentation included a rationale for the use of retinoids as cancer prevention agents, selection of such agents, and considerations for the design of cancer prevention trials.

Upon exploring the possibility of developing a book resulting from the American Society of Preventive Oncology session, Moon was invited by Micozzi to join in the development of this book for Marcel Dekker. Thus, a collaboration for this coedited volume was brought about.

As editors we are aware that this volume provides integrated, in-depth presentations on the multidisciplinary rationale, planning and conduct of cancer prevention research. Through our independent paths to cancer prevention research, including interaction with many different colleagues, we are delighted with the outstanding contributors who have participated. The contributors' expertise covers the areas of biochemistry, biostatistics, clinical oncology, epidemiology, internal medicine, nutrition, pharmacy, pharmacology, physiology, public health, and social science–held together by the common theme of investigating the role of micronutrients in nutrition and cancer prevention. The book will likewise be of interest to those concerned about the causes and prevention of cancer, beyond the role of micronutrients. In addition to nutrition and cancer prevention, this volume provides extensive state-of-the-art information that will be useful in many aspects of human nutritional assessment and nutrient composition analysis, and in the design, implementation, and interpretation of disease prevention trials.

The active voice of our title is "Investigating," chosen to emphasize the orientation of this volume toward *testing* hypotheses utilizing intervention (clinical) trials on nutrition and cancer prevention and *interpreting* the results of trials in this relatively new field. The volume provides a guide to the background, rationale, and selection of cancer prevention agents, as well as the design, implementation, and evaluation of cancer prevention studies. It will offer assistance to many in the conduct of investigations and will be of interest to all in the interpretation of research results in the scientific literature. Likewise, the public is demanding informed, consistent opinions from their physicians and scientists as to the role of nutrition in cancer prevention. Today there remain unique opportunities to conduct cancer investigations based on the patterns of variability in dietary intake and cancer rates in human populations around the United States and the world. Such investigations will contribute important information on the reduction of human cancer incidence. This volume is a handbook for those who seek to enter into, or to understand, the important opportunities for nutrition in cancer prevention that may exist through investigating the role of micronutrients.

Marc S. Micozzi
Thomas E. Moon

Contents

Part Two
METHODOLOGIC ISSUES FOR NUTRITIONAL ASSESSMENT

Part Three
EVIDENCE ON MICRONUTRIENTS AND CANCER PREVENTION

Part Four
PLANNING, CONDUCT, AND INTERPRETATION OF CANCER PREVENTION TRIALS

Contributors

David S. Alberts, M.D. Professor, Section of Hematology/Oncology, The University of Arizona College of Medicine, Tucson, Arizona

John A. Baron, M.D. Associate Professor, Dartmouth Medical School, Hanover, New Hampshire

Gary R. Beecher, Ph.D. Research Leader, Nutrient Composition Laboratory, Beltsville Human Nutrition Research Center, Agricultural Research Service, U. S. Department of Agriculture, Beltsville, Maryland

Hemmige N. Bhagavan, Ph.D. Nutrition Coordinator, Clinical Nutrition Department, Hoffmann-LaRoche Inc., Nutley, New Jersey

Gladys Block, Ph.D. Epidemiologist, Division of Cancer Prevention and Control, National Cancer Institute, National Institutes of Health, Bethesda, Maryland

David P. Byar, M.D. Chief, Biometry Branch, Division of Cancer Prevention and Control, National Cancer Institute, National Institutes of Health, Bethesda, Maryland

Gerald F. Combs, Jr., Ph.D. Associate Professor, Department of Poultry and Avian Sciences, and Division of Nutritional Sciences, Cornell University, Ithaca, New York

Michael W. Connor, D.V.M. Department of Pathology, Boston University School of Medicine, and Assistant Professor, Mallory Institute of Pathology, Boston, Massachusetts

David L. DeMets, Ph.D. Professor and Director, Biostatistics Center, Department of Statistics and Human Oncology, University of Wisconsin, Madison, Wisconsin

E. Robert Greenberg, M.D. Associate Professor, Departments of Community and Family Medicine, Dartmouth Medical School, Hanover, New Hampshire

Anne M. Hartman, M.S. Health Statistician, Division of Cancer Prevention and Control, National Cancer Institute, National Institutes of Health, Bethesda, Maryland

Charles H. Hennekens, M.D., Dr. P.H. Associate Professor, Medicine and Preventive Medicine and Clinical Epidemiology, Channing Laboratory, Brigham Women's Hospital, and Harvard Medical School, Boston, Massachusetts

David J. Hunter, M.B., B.S., M.P.H. Teaching Fellow, Department of Epidemiology, Harvard School of Public Health, and Channing Laboratory, Department of Medicine, Brigham and Women's Hospital and Harvard Medical School, Boston, Massachusetts

Frederick Khachik, Ph.D. Research Chemist, Nutrient Composition Laboratory, Beltsville Human Nutrition Research Center, Agricultural Research Service, U.S. Department of Agriculture, Beltsville, Maryland

Scott M. Lippman, M.D.* Director, Cancer Prevention and Control Clinic, The Arizona Cancer Center, The University of Arizona College of Medicine, Tucson, Arizona

Micheline M. Mathews-Roth, M.D. Associate Professor, Channing Laboratory, Harvard Medical School, and Associate Professor, Department of Medicine, Brigham and Women's Hospital, Boston, Massachusetts

Marilyn Menkes, Ph.D.† Department of Epidemiology, The Johns Hopkins School of Hygiene and Public Health, Baltimore, Maryland

William J. Mergens, Ph.D. Research Leader, Technical and Product Development, Hoffmann-La Roche Inc., Nutley, New Jersey

Curtis J. Mettlin, Ph.D. Director, Department of Cancer Control and Epidemiology, Roswell Park Memorial Institute, Buffalo, New York

Frank L. Meyskens, Jr., M.D. Professor, Arizona Cancer Center, The University of Arizona College of Medicine, Tucson, Arizona

---

**Current affiliation*: Assistant Professor, Department of Medical Oncology, University of Texas System Cancer Center, Houston, Texas.

†Deceased

Marc S. Micozzi, M.D., Ph.D.* Senior Investigator, Cancer Prevention Studies Branch, National Cancer Institute, National Institutes of Health, Bethesda, Maryland

John A. Milner, Ph.D. Director, Division of Nutritional Sciences, and Professor, Department of Food Science, University of Illinois, Urbana, Illinois

Thomas E. Moon, Ph.D. Professor and Chief, Epidemiology and Biometry Section, Family and Community Medicine and the Arizona Cancer Center, The University of Arizona Health Sciences Center, Tucson, Arizona

Paul M. Newberne, D.V.M., Ph.D. Department of Pathology, Boston University School of Medicine, and Professor of Pathology, Mallory Institute of Pathology, Boston, Massachusetts

David W. Nierenberg, M.D. Associate Professor, Division of Clinical Pharmacology, Dartmouth Medical School, Hanover, New Hampshire

Blossom H. Patterson, M.A. Mathematical Statistician, Division of Cancer Prevention and Control, National Cancer Institute, National Institutes of Health, Bethesda, Maryland

Yei-Mei Peng, Ph.D. Research Assistant Professor, Section of Hematology/Oncology, The University of Arizona College of Medicine, Tucson, Arizona

Steven Piantadosi, M.D., Ph.D.† Biometry Branch, National Cancer Institute, National Institutes of Health, Bethesda, Maryland

Ross L. Prentice Director for Division of Public Health Sciences, Fred Hutchinson Cancer Research Center, Seattle, Washington

Thomas F. Schrager, Ph.D. Department of Pathology, Boston University School of Medicine, and Assistant Professor, Mallory Institute of Pathology, Boston, Massachusetts

Steven G. Self, Ph.D. Associate Member, Public Health Sciences, Fred Hutchinson Cancer Research Center, Seattle, Washington

Meir J. Stampfer, M.D., Dr.P.H. Assistant Professor, Department of Medicine, Channing Laboratory, and Department of Medicine, Brigham and Women's Hospital and Harvard Medical School, Boston, Massachusetts

---

**Current affiliation*: Associate Director, Armed Forces Institute of Pathology, Washington, D.C.

†*Current affiliation*: Director of Biostatistics, The Johns Hopkins Oncology Center, Baltimore, Maryland

Marguerite M. Stevens, Ph.D. Research Assistant Professor, Department of Community and Family Medicine, Dartmouth Medical School, National Institutes Hampshire

Joseph A. Tangrea, R.Ph., M.P.H. Pharmaceutical Research Coordinator, Cancer Prevention Studies Branch, National Cancer Institute, National Institutes of Health, Bethesda, Maryland

Michael J. Wargovich, Ph.D. Assistant Professor, Department of Medical Oncology, The University of Texas M. D. Anderson Cancer Center, Houston, Texas

Walter C. Willett, M.D., Dr. P.H. Professor, Department of Epidemiology, Harvard School of Public Health, and Channing Laboratory, Department of Medicine, Brigham and Women's Hospital and Harvard Medical School, Boston, Massachusetts

Nutrition and Cancer Prevention

Part One

RATIONALE FOR NUTRITIONAL PREVENTION OF CANCER

1
General Introduction: Rationale for the Nutritional Prevention of Cancer

MARC S. MICOZZI* and JOSEPH A. TANGREA
National Cancer Institute, National Institutes of Health, Bethesda, Maryland

THE CONCEPT OF NUTRITIONAL PREVENTION OF CANCER

Nutritional prevention of cancer may be defined as the prevention of cancer in human population by dietary agents that inhibit carcinogenesis. This concept is based upon the cancer-inhibiting potential of certain chemical compounds. The characteristics of dietary agents relevant to human cancer prevention include their mechanisms of action, toxicity, and efficacy. A theoretical approach to the selection of dietary agents for human clinical trials will be presented in this volume. Dietary agents currently used in clinical trials include micronutrients and their synthetic analogues. The cancer-preventive activity of this class of agents will be specifically addressed.

Cancer prevention offers considerable opportunities for the improvement of human health. Scientific advances have also led to the recognition that many chronic diseases may be preventable. Cancer is no longer considered an integral component of the aging process. Environmental factors, acting in the presence of possible genetic factors, are now recognized as important determinants of human cancer. These environmental determinants may include dietary habits and lifestyle.

Cancer prevention may focus on several levels in the effort to reduce cancer incidence and mortality in human populations. For example, reduction in exposure to environmental risk factors may reasonably be expected to reduce cancer incidence. Within the United States, it has been estimated that 80-90% of cancers may be attributable to environmental factors and that diet and nutrition may account for approximately 30% of attributable risk. (Doll, 1977;

**Current affiliation*: Armed Forces Institute of Pathology, Washington, D.C.

Doll and Peto, 1981.) Other risks, such as smoking and various occupational exposures to industrial carcinogens, are also recognized. Strategies for recognition of populations at high risk may result in effective allocation of health resources and may also create special opportunities for cancer prevention studies.

Carcinogenesis induced by chemicals involves the separate and independent processes of tumor initiation and tumor promotion (Fig. 1). Initiation causes molecular or cellular alterations, which may lead to cancer or which may remain dormant in the absence of a promoter. A promoter may induce cellular proliferation, leading to expansion of clones of initiated cells (Yuspa, 1982).

There is increasing evidence that chemical carcinogenesis can be reversed if the chemical insult is removed or neutralized. Although mutations in cells caused by initiation appear to be irreversible, the slow process of promotion may be reversed or slowed to the point of never reaching tumor production as the endpoint. The initiation and promotion processes are consistent with a multistage model in which progressive neoplastic enhancement of cells occurs through a series of carcinogenic events in populations of exposed cells. Several such rare events in succession are thought to be necessary in order to transform a population of normal cells into malignant cells. These stages of cell transformation may be observable histopathologically (Rywlin, 1984). Understanding the multistage initiation and promotion processes and their potential for inhibition is a key to cancer prevention.

Identification of agents that may inhibit the multistage process of carcinogenesis and prevent the occurrence of neoplasms is underway. It may be easier or more appropriate in some situations to prescribe preventive agents than to proscribe unhealthy diets and other practices. For example, cancer prevention may be more readily achieved by prescription of a specific micronutrient than by attempting major modifications of the human diet.

Compounds that inhibit carcinogenesis may be used in high-risk groups or in the general population. Appropriate agents may be identified within a broad

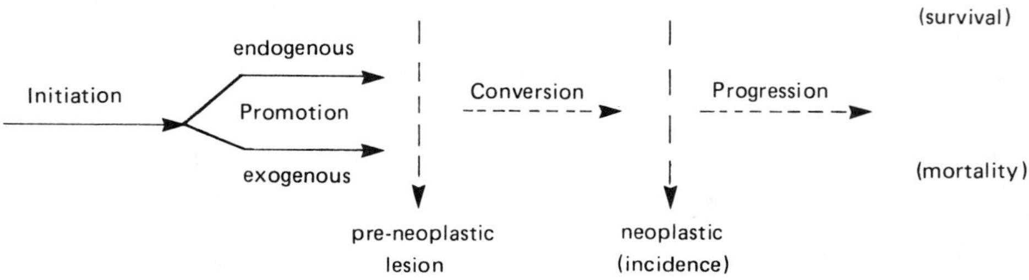

Fig. 1 Processes of tumor initiation and promotion.

Table 1 Actions of Cancer Preventive Agents

1.	Induce detoxification of carcinogens
2.	Scavenge reactive carcinogen species
3.	Induce cellular differentiation
4.	Reverse any other reversible preneoplastic processes

spectrum of dietary compounds that (a) induce detoxification of carcinogens, (b) scavenge reactive carcinogen species, (c) induce cellular differentiation, and (d) reverse any other reversible preneoplastic process (Table 1).

Numerous mechanisms for the inhibition of carcinogenesis have been proposed (Wattenberg, 1978). The mechanisms of action of those agents that inhibit cancer initiation are based upon the proposed metabolic processing of carcinogens, which occurs in a stepwise fashion. Most carcinogens display ultimate reactive forms consisting of a positively charged electrophilic nucleus, which chemically interacts with macromolecules like DNA. Many carcinogens are metabolically activated to this form via oxidation by the microsomal mixed function oxidase system or by other metabolic pathways. Other important carcinogens apparently do not require metabolic activation prior to manifesting an ability to cause initiation at the cellular level (Miller and Miller, 1974).

Because many carcinogens are viewed as environmental chemicals that enter the body, metabolic processing of chemical carcinogens is relevant to cancer prevention (Fig. 2). A *procarcinogen* is a chemical absorbed into the metabolic system from the environment, subsequently transformed into a proximate carcinogen. The *proximate* carcinogen is then metabolically converted into the *ultimate* carcinogen, which displays its final activity at the molecular or cellular level. Preventive compounds may act at different steps in the metabolic processing of a carcinogen. Thus, a dietary agent may (a) prevent formation or absorption; (b) modulate biotransformation; (c) accelerate solubilization and excretion; or (d) block the action of ultimate carcinogens once they are formed.

Other pertinent characteristics of dietary agents include their structure/activity relationships, toxicity, efficacy, dose, and dosage form. Selection of these agents involves in vitro and in vivo screening for efficacy, preclinical toxicity and pharmacokinetic studies, and clinical studies in humans, as well as clinical dosage form development. A wide range of compounds have been noted to manifest cancer-inhibiting potential. These observations indicate that structurally related compounds (or their active moieties) may share cancer-inhibiting potential; they further suggest avenues for development of future preventive agents. Agents that may inhibit later stages in the multistage process of carcinogenesis may be particularly useful for preventing cancer in populations already exposed to carcinogens.

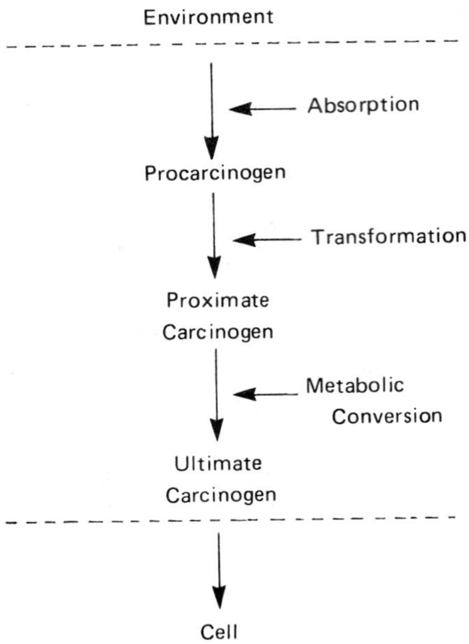

Fig. 2 metabolic processing of chemical carcinogens.

An important characteristic of dietary preventive agents is low toxicity, since the potential target population includes individuals who are not ill, but only at risk of cancer, and may also include individuals with only a "normal" risk of exposure to environmental carcinogens. This requirement for low toxicity is in contrast to the typical features of chemotherapeutic agents for cancer therapy.

It has been recognized that potential chemical inhibitors of carcinogenesis occur in the human diet and include micronutrients, other metabolically active constitutents, or food additives. Micronutrients are present in low concentrations and mediate critical aspects of human biochemistry and metabolism. Synthetic analogues of micronutrients that have greater efficacy (and less toxicity) than the parent compound may be of particular interest for use as cancer-preventive agents.

POTENTIAL FOR NUTRITIONAL INHIBITION OF CARCINOGENESIS

The potential for nutritional inhibition of carcinogenesis has been suggested both by animal experimental and human epidemiologic studies. Early studies in animals were conducted as a result of clinical and epidemiologic observations in humans (Newell, 1980). The dramatic geographic and ecologic variations in cancer patterns, as well as the changing incidence of cancer in migrants, point to differential exposures in human populations. Dietary factors probably play a prominent role in explaining these differing cancer rates. As a result of these and other observations, a full range of investigations are now being conducted. A human clinical trial is seen as the ultimate test of efficacy of a dietary agent. The potential for chemical inhibition of carcinogenesis by dietary agents will be considered in the context of (a) human epidemiologic evidence, interpretation, and limitations; and (b) human intervention studies.

HUMAN EPIDEMIOLOGIC EVIDENCE, INTERPRETATION, AND LIMITATIONS

Observational epidemiology, involving both descriptive and etiologic studies of cancer, helps to suggest dietary factors that may inhibit carcinogenesis. Correlation studies generally estimate the relationship between environmental factors and cancer frequencies. Cross-sectional analyses of international differences in cancer incidence and mortality rates indicate the importance of environmental factors in the etiology of cancer (Armstrong and Doll, 1975; Hems, 1978; Hirayama, 1978; Gaskill et al., 1979; Gray et al., 1979; Kolonel et al., 1981; Micozzi, 1985; 1987). Breast cancer mortality rates, for example, are almost eight times higher in the United States than in Japan. These differences are not explained by genetic factors (Carter and Micozzi, 1986), as epidemiologic studies of Japanese migrants to the United States demonstrate higher rates of some cancers in migrants than in Japanese living in Japan (Buell and Dunn, 1965; Buell, 1973; Dunn, 1977). For example, as migrants undergo progressive acculturation to a Western lifestyle (Marmot and Syme, 1976), breast cancer rates in migrants progress towards those of the host country. It has been suggested that persons who emigrate during childhood and adolescence experience the greatest degree of change in cancer patterns (Buell, 1973). These crude observations on populations are not definitive tests of cancer preventive agents but are useful in generating hypotheses and selecting dietary agents for further testing.

Case-control and cohort studies conducted prospectively are more specific approaches to identifying potential cancer preventive agents. Unlike correlation analyses, which are generally limited to a few variables known only at the population level, case-control and cohort approaches study individuals and usually obtain information on a large number of different variables. In these studies, information on exposure to potential cancer protective factors is determined through dietary assessment (e.g., Colditz et al., 1985) or direct measurement of biologic specimens (e.g., Wald et al., 1980, 1984; Graham et al., 1982). Although several potential dietary preventive agents have been suggested (e.g.,

Kark et al., 1981; Shekelle et al., 1981; Willett et al., 1983), these studies also have limitations.

The human diet is varied and complex and cannot be easily assessed or simply characterized. The precision and accuracy of information collected by dietary interview is limited by the human capacity for recall. Diet records or diaries are laborious to maintain and can only be collected on a limited number of individuals over a brief period of time. In addition, knowledge of their diagnosis among cancer patients in case-control studies may bias dietary recall. The specific nutrient content of the foods reported to be ingested by individuals must also be determined. The accurary of translation from foods to nutrients is dependent upon the availability and reliability of food composition tables. Although these tables are constantly being revised, many of the values reported are out of date, incomplete, or too generalized to be useful in cancer prevention studies.

While biologic samples generally provide objective measurements of nutrient levels, their relevance to nutrient intake is not always clear, and they also have methodologic limitations. Adequate methods for measuring many potential dietary preventive agents are not yet available. The relation between dietary intake and nutrient levels in biologic samples is remote for many micronutrients, such as vitamin A (retinol). Moreover, samples are generally obtained at one point in time for determination of nutrient levels in biologic fluids. For many nutrients, little or no data are available regarding the relationship of a single biologic measurement of one micronutrient level at one point in time to long-term nutrient status or to the multistage process of carcinogenesis. If nutrient intake in early life is relevant to long-term cancer risk (Miller and Bulbrook, 1980), for example, case-control studies on elderly cancer patients may not be sufficient to illustrate the definitive role of nutrient intake in the multistage process of carcinogenesis (Micozzi, 1985; 1987). Biologic measurements of nutrient levels on cancer patients in case-control studies may also be influenced by the effects of disease on the nutrient of interest (Shamberger et al., 1973; Robinson et al., 1979; McConnell et al., 1980). For example, a low measurement for a potential dietary preventive agent in a patient with cancer may reflect an effect of the disease on the agent, rather than a lack of protection.

Furthermore, attention must be paid to the particular chemical form or derivative of the nutrient or other agent, which is measured in biologic specimens (e.g., Shekelle et al., 1981; Peto et al., 1981). Potential dietary preventive agents must be considered as chemical compounds, even though their presence in the human diet has led to their recognition. Definitive tests of dietary preventive agents should be conducted under controlled conditions, where the agent or agents serve as the only variable between the treated and control groups.

Table 2 Human Intervention Studies on Cancer Preventive Agents

1. Need for controlled clinical trials
2. Scope and design of trials
3. Pharmacologic and toxicologic information required

HUMAN INTERVENTION STUDIES

Human intervention studies of potential cancer preventive agents may be considered from three perspectives: (a) the *need* for controlled clinical trials; (b) the scope and design of these trials; and (c) the requirements for pharmacologic and toxicologic information prior to initiating clinical trials (Table 2).

While observational epidemiology has been used to identify dietary compounds that may inhibit carcinogenesis, this approach generally lacks specificity. Intervention research on potential cancer preventive agents is a new and more definitive approach, which provides evidence of efficacy unachievable by observational and analytical epidemiology. It is important both practically and theoretically to test potential cancer-preventive agents in a rigorous fashion in humans. A large, randomized, placebo-controlled trial among individuals with no prior history of the disease is the most reliable test (Hennekens et al., 1984). In a clinical trial of a single micronutrient, randomization techniques are designed to achieve treatment groups that differ only in the specific micronutrient under study. In addition to testing the value of cancer-preventive agents, such studies assist in resolving uncertainty about the relevance of animal models, questions about participant acceptance of the intervention, and the cost/benefit ratio (DeWys and Greenwald, 1983).

The target population for such studies includes individuals who are free of cancer but are at some definable risk of its development. If a trial is to be conducted in essentially healthy individuals, this imposes the requirement of a large sample population to ascertain outcome. In a group at *high* risk of cancer, the expected number of events to be observed will be significantly greater than in a low- or normal-risk group. Studying a high-risk group, therefore, is efficient in that a larger number of cancer cases can be identified within smaller populations over shorter periods of time. Nonetheless, such studies are typically long, usually requiring three to five years in order to show an effect. It should be noted, however, that while the study of a high-risk population is both efficient and advantageous logistically and operationally, caution must be exercised in the application of study results to a broader population.

Intervention studies are controlled in that the study population is divided into two or more treatment groups by random assignment. However, more than one treatment or intervention may be tested in the same trial through a factorial design, in which multiple agents are given in various combinations. This consideration is important, since the optimal cancer preventive regimen may contain several different agents, depending upon their mechanisms of action.

Before a potential cancer-preventive agent can be used in a clinical trial, information must be acquired on its safety and efficacy. Ideally, it is also helpful if some evidence of mechanism of action is available. The efficacy of dietary preventive agents may be initially established in vitro and in animal tumor systems in vivo. In vitro and in vivo screening for efficacy, if positive, is generally followed by specific evaluation of acute, subacute/subchronic, and chronic toxicity in animals. These methods are important components of clinical pharmacology, which may be applied directly in the selection of cancer-preventive agents.

Existing cancer-preventive compounds have a wide range of chemical structures, suggesting by structure-activity relationships that other active compounds may exist within this spectrum (Wattenberg, 1978). Dietary agents with potential cancer-prevention activity may be initially identified through structural homology with agents having known preventive activity or in the development of synthetic analogues of micronutrients. Potential cancer-preventive agents may also be identified by initial experimental findings in the laboratory, observations in the clinical setting, or from descriptive or analytic epidemiologic studies.

Factors relevant to investigating the potential role of micronutrients in cancer prevention are (a) the experimental and epidemiological evidence for the cancer-modifying effects of nutrients; (b) proposed mechanisms for the chemical inhibition of carcinogenesis; (c) methodologic issues in human nutritional assessment and measurement; and (d) issues in the planning, conduct, and interpretation of prevention trials which, when properly designed and executed, provide definitives tests of a cancer-preventive micronutrient or micronutrients. These issues are comprehensively discussed and considered in the remainder of this volume.

REFERENCES

Armstrong, B., Doll, R. (1975). Environmental factors and cancer incidence and mortality in different countries, with special reference to dietary practices. *Int. J. Cancer 15*: 617-631.

Buell, P. (1973). Changing incidence of breast cancer in Japanese-American women. *J. Natl. Cancer Inst. 51*: 1479-1483.

Buell, P., Dunn, J. E. (1986). Cancer mortality of Japanese Isei and Nisei of California. *Cancer 18*: 656-664.

Carter, C. L., Micozzi, M. S. (1986). The genetics of human breast cancer. *Yearbook of Physical Anthropology 29*: 161-180.

Colditz, G. A., Branch, L. G., Lipnick, R. J., Willett, W. C., Rosner, B., Posner, B. M., Hennekens, C. H. (1985). Increased green and yellow vegetable intake and lowered cancer deaths in an elderly population. *Am. J. Clin. Nutr. 4*: 32-36.

DeWys, W. D., Greenwald, P. (1983). Clinical trials: A recent emphasis in the prevention program of the National Cancer Institute. *Semin. Oncol. 10*: 360-364.

Doll, R. (1977). Strategy for detection of cancer hazards to man. *Nature 265*: 589-596.

Doll, R., Peto, R. (1981). The causes of cancer. *J. Natl. Cancer Inst. 66*:1191-1308.

Dunn, J. E. (1977). Breast cancer among American Japanese in the San Francisco Bay area. In *Epidemiology and Cancer Registries in the Pacific Basin*. NCI Monograph, No. 47, pp. 157-160. [DHEW Pub. No. (NIH) 77-1223].

Gaskill, S. P., McGuire, W. L., Osborne, C. K., Stern, M. P. (1979). Breast cancer mortality and diet in the United States. *Cancer Res. 39*:3628-3637.

Graham, S., Marshall, J., Mettlin, C., Rzepka, T., Nemoto, T., Byers, T. (1982). Diet in the epidemiology of breast cancer. *Am. J. Epdiemiol. 116*: 68-75.

Gray, G. E., Pike, M. C., Henderson, B. E. (1979). Breast cancer incidence and mortality rates in different countries in relation to known risk factors and dietary practices. *Br. J. Cancer 39*: 1-7.

Hems, G. (1978). Contributions of diet and childbearing to breast cancer rates. *Br. J. Cancer 37*: 974-982.

Hennekens, C. H., Stampfer, M. J., Willett, W. (1984). Micronutrients and cancer chemoprevention. *Cancer Detection and Prevention 7*: 147–158.

Hirayama, T. (1978). Epidemiology of breast cancer with special reference to the role of diet. *Preventive Medicine 7*: 173–195.

Kark, J. D., Smith, A. H., Switzer, B. R., Hames, C. G. (1981). Serum vitamin A (retinol) and cancer incidence in Evans Country, Georgia. *J. Natl. Cancer Inst. 66*: 7-16.

Kolonel, L. N., Hankin, J. H., Lee, J., Chu, S. Y., Nomura, A. M. Y., Hinds, M. W. (1981). Nutrient intakes in relation to cancer incidence in Hawaii. *Br. J. Cancer 44*: 332-339.

Marmot, M. G., Syme, S. L. (1976). Acculturation and coronary heart disease in Japanese Americans. *Am. J. Epidemiol. 104*: 171-200.

McConnell, K. P., Jayer, R. M., Bland, K. I., Blotcky, A. J. (1980). The relationship of dietary selenium and breast cancer. *J. Surg. Onc. 15*: 67-70.

Micozzi, M. S. (1985). Nutrition, body size and breast cancer. *Yearbook of Physical Anthropology 28*: 175-206.

Micozzi, M. S. (1987). Cross-cultural correlations of childhood growth and adult breast cancer. *American Journal of Physical Anthropology 73*: 525-537.

Miller, A. B., Bulbrook, R. D. (1980). The epidemiology and etiology of breast cancer. *N. Engl. J. Med. 303*: 1246-1248.

Miller, E. C., Miller, J. A. (1974). Biochemical mechanisms of chemical carcinogenesis. In Busch, H. (Ed.), *The Molecular Biology of Cancer*. Academic Press, New York, pp. 377-402.

Newell, G. R. (1980). Overview of cancer prevention. *Cancer Bulletin 32*:128-129.

Peto, R., Doll, R., Buckley, J. D., Sporn, M. B. (1981). Can dietary beta-carotene materially reduce human cancer rates? *Nature 290*: 201-208.

Robinson, M. F., Godfrey, P. J., Thomson, C. D., et al. (1979). Blood selenium and glutathion peroxidase activity in normal subjects and in surgical patients with and without cancer in New Zealand. *Am. J. Clin. Nutr. 32*: 1477-1485.

Rywlin, A. M. (1984). Terminology of premalignant lesions in light of the multistep theory of carcinogenesis. *Human Pathology 15*: 806-807.

Shamberger, R. J., Rukovena, E., Longfield, A. K., et al. (1973). Antioxidants and cancer. I. Selenium in the blood of normal and cancer patients. *J. Natl. Cancer Inst. 50*: 867-870.

Shekelle, R. B., Lepper, M., Liu, S., et al. (1981). Dietary vitamin A and risk of cancer in the Western Electric Study. *Lancet 2*: 1185-1190.

Wald, N. J., Idel, M., Boreham, J., Bailey, A. (1980). Low serum vitamin A and vitamin E levels in relation to the future risk of breast cancer. *Br. J. Cancer 49*: 321-324.

Wald, N. J., Idel, M., Borcham, J., Bailey, A. (1980). Low serum vitamin A and subsequent risk of cancer: Preliminary results of a prospective study. *Lancet 2*: 813-815.

Wattenberg, L. W. (1978). Inhibitors of chemical carcinogenesis. *Adv. Cancer Res. 26*: 197-226.

Willett, W., Polk, B. F., Hames, C., et al. (1983). Prediagnostic serum selenium and the risk of cancer. *Lancet 2*: 130-134.

Yuspa, S. H., Harris, C. C. (1982). Molecular and cellular basis of chemical carcinogenesis. In Schottenfeld, D., Fraumeni, J. F. (Eds.), *Cancer Epidemiology and Prevention*. W. B. Saunders, Philadelphia, pp. 23-43.

2
Mechanisms for Nutritional Inhibition of Carcinogenesis

JOHN A. MILNER
University of Illinois, Urbana, Illinois

ABSTRACT

The existence of an etiologic relationship between dietary practices and human cancer is supported by data obtained from a variety of sources. Dietary practices may increase or decrease cancer risk depending upon intakes of individual nutrients and their interactions. The multitude and complexities of interrelationships that can exist among dietary constituents possibly accounts for reported inconsistencies among human studies. Nevertheless, based upon laboratory, epidemiological, and clinical data, modification in the dietary habits of humans appears to offer a means of reducing cancer risks. Selective dietary factors have long been recognized as influencing the development of tumors in experimental animals. The intake of various micronutrients has been observed to significantly alter cancer incidence and severity in a variety of experimental circumstances by modifying specific phases of carcinogenesis. Dietary constituents can alter the formation and bioactivation of carcinogens, modify the promotion and progression of neoplastic tissue, modulate immunocompetence, and lead to variations in rates of tumor growth. The influence of individual micronutrients on the constituent steps of carcinogenesis, as discussed in this chapter, continues to be an area of active examination. Continued research will likely supply needed information on the particular role of nutrients and nonnutrients in the carcinogenic process, identify critical times for nutritional intervention, and hopefully lead to sound and accurate dietary recommendations for populations at large.

INTRODUCTION

Cancer, the second leading cause of death of Americans, accounts for approximately 20% of all deaths in this country. During the last few decades emphasis has gradually shifted from the assumption that cancer is an inevitable consequence of aging to a recognition that the environment is involved in its development. Changes in cancer death rates over a relatively short period of time point to the importance of environmental rather than genetic factors in cancer susceptibility. As many as 90% of the cancer cases have been correlated with exposure to environmental factors. Among these factors, to which humans are routinely exposed, food is one that probably influences the risk of developing this disease. Wynder and Gori (1977) implicated food factors in the etiology of 60% of cancers in women and more than 40% in men. While many investigators have pointed to abnormal nutrition as a significant factor in cancer in both sexes, the range of risk associated with dietary practices has been from 10 to 70%, depending upon the specific cancer evaluated (Doll and Peto, 1981). Since the relationship between food and cancer is not solely dependent on the presence or absence of carcinogens or cocarcinogens in the food supply, but depends on the influence of the dietary intakes and interactions of nutrients and nonnutrients on the complex and poorly understood cancer process, it is not surprising that such variations in the impact of diet upon cancer risk have been reported.

Some of the best evidence for a role of nutrition in the development of cancer comes from studies of migrant populations (Haeustel and Kurihara, 1968; Phillips, 1975; Enstrom, 1978; Gori, 1979). Generally, cancer incidence patterns of migrants change from that of their native country to that common to the population of the host country. Although these shifts could reflect changes in the environment of lifestyle in different countries, it is thought that the history of general pollution and food contamination is probably not responsible for observed differences in cancer incidence. The other major line of evidence that diet, rather than other environmental or genetic factors, is involved in the development of human cancers comes from studies of homogeneous populations that live and work in the same environment as their cohorts and are exposed to the same environmental pollutants, yet have different rates of cancer incidence. Comparison of the cancer incidence and mortality rates in Seventh Day Adventists living and working in Los Angeles and Mormon versus non-Mormon populations living in Utah and California revealed significant differences in cancer incidences for almost all types of tumors (Phillips, 1975; Enstrom, 1978).

While it has long been known that dietary modifications can alter the course of tumor formation and development, only in recent years have investigators actively examined specific dietary constituents for their impact on the cancer process. Table 1 shows some of the dietary factors known to significantly alter cancinogenesis in experimental animals. During recent years considerable atten-

Table 1 Some Dietary Factors Known to Alter Experimental Carcinogenesis

General	Amino acids	Vitamins	Minerals
Calories	Methionine	Riboflavin	Calcium
Lipids	Cysteine	Folic acid	Zinc
Carbohydrates	Tryptophan	B_{12}	Copper
Proteins	Arginine	A, C	Iron
Fiber		D, E	Selenium
		Choline	

tion has been given to the influence of dietary intakes of the macronutrients, including fiber, as factors in cancer development. While these dietary constituents are likely suspects, much less attention has been given to the components of those classes of nutrients and to the other components of the diet that are consumed in much smaller quantities. Although knowledge concerning the precise role of individual foods and food constituents in carcinogenesis is limited, the Committee on Diet, Nutrition, and Cancer of the National Research Council was able to draw some major conclusions and develop interim dietary guidelines (1982). Continued examination of dietary constituents will likely result in more specific dietary recommendations for the general population and indicate critical times when nutritional intervention may be most beneficial.

This chapter will not attempt to cover major dietary constituents but will focus on the mechanism(s) for nutritional modulation of carcinogenesis by nutrients and nonnutrients that are ingested in microgram quantities from a typical diet. While this chapter is limited to these dietary constituents, it must be emphasized that purified microconstitutents are not consumed alone, and relevant data that are reviewed are a reflection of the interactions of the specified micronutrients with the other constituents of the diet. It is unfortuante that many investigators continue to focus on intakes of macroconstituents without considering the impact of the microconstituents. Nutritionists have long recognized that quantity of a dietary constituent does not dictate relative importance in either disease prevention or treatment. The consumption of micronutrients and nonnutrients likely has profound importance in explaining some of the variation in cancer incidence observed in human beings.

THE CARCINOGENESIS PROCESS

Cancers represent populations of cells that have acquired the ability to multiply and spread without normal restraints. Two major hypotheses of the process of carcinogenesis are (a) the initiation-promotion hypothesis (Boutwell, 1975) and (b) the electrophilic hypothesis (Miller, 1978). The former basically proposes that carcinogenesis occurs in two or more discrete and distinct phases. These phases have been defined as (a) initiation and (b) promotion. The initiation phase is described as an early, rapid, and largely irreversible change resulting in a permanently altered cell. Promotion of carcinogenesis is a more gradual process(es) by which an initiated cell is converted or transformed into a tumor cell. The electrophilic hypothesis of carcinogenesis is that metabolic activation of most carcinogens occurs through reactive, electrophilic intermediates, which, by altering critical cell nucleophilic targets, such as DNA, are directly responsible for the carcinogenic activity of a compound. Evidence for the involvement of free radicals in carcinogenesis is also available (Mason, 1982). It is generally accepted that the immune system also plays an important role in host resistance to cancer, both in a prophylactic sense of an efficient immunosurveillance system destroying neoplastic cells at an early stage of carcinogenesis,and in the protective sense by retarding the growth of established tumors.

The schematic representation of the process of carcinogenesis presented in Fig. 1 is a simplistic overview of the incompletely understood process by which normal cells are transformed into neoplastic cells. The process of carcinogenesis may be separated both mechanistically and temporally. Normally, the first phase of this process is the metabolic activation of the parent carcinogens to chemically reactive products or ultimate carcinogens, which react with a critical factor(s) within the cell. This process, occurring usually within a few hours after exposure, can be repaired by many cells, thereby presumably leaving the normal cell unaltered. However, cells unable to remove this damage either die or become initiated cells. For nutrients to impact the initiation phase of carcinogenesis, they must modify the biological behavior of the cell prior to or at the time of exposure to the carcinogen.

In contrast to the short duration of the initiation phase, promotion is a prolonged process that is considered to last decades in human beings. This phase of carcinogenesis is extremely complex, with a variety of cellular changes occurring. As discussed below, nutrients can have an influence during the early or late stages of the promotion phase. The final phase of carcinogenesis is progression. This phase results in the conversion of the premalignant cell to a malignant cell of increased virulence. During some circumstances the early pathological changes occurring in these cells appear to be reversed by known dietary constituents, such as ascorbic acid and the retinoids. However, it is unknown if this represents a complete reversibility to the normal cell. To date little information is available on the effect of specific nutrients on the progres-

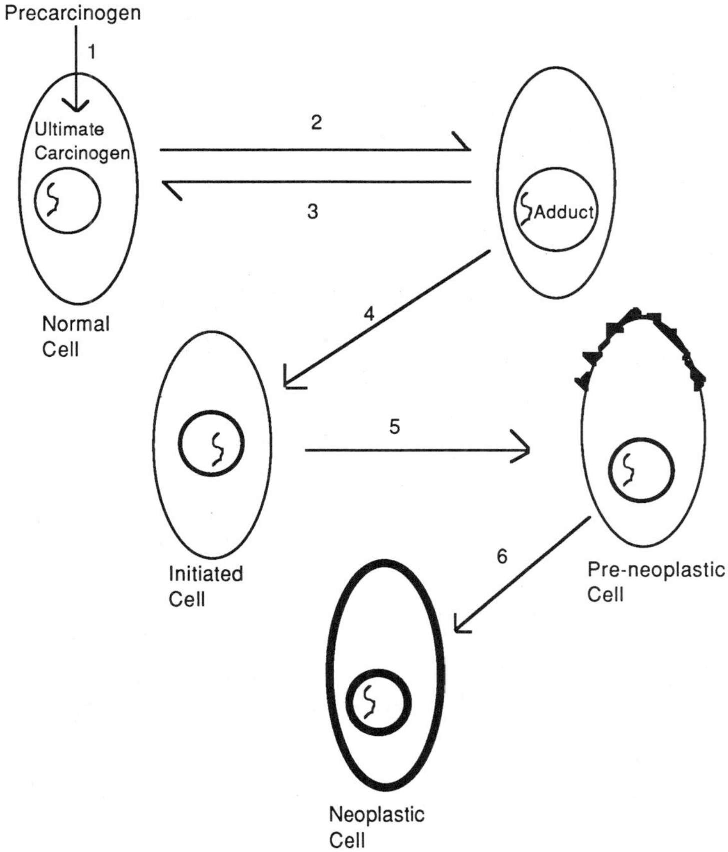

Fig. 1 Steps in the chemical induction of carcinogenesis. Step 1 refers to the bioactivation of the parent carcinogen to the ultimate carcinogen. Steps 2 and 3 refer to the reversible reaction of the ultimate carcinogen with cellular macromolecules. DNA is the presumed important macromolecule. Step 4 is the replication phase of carcinogenesis. Step 5 refers to the promotion of the initiated cell. Step 6 refers to the progression of the preneoplastic cell into the neoplastic cell.

little information is available on the effect of specific nutrients on the progression of malignant cells to cells with increasing invasive or metastatic properties.

It is not possible to conclusively extrapolate from data obtained with animal models of carcinogenesis to assess human risk because of problems in evaluating the influence of dosages, metabolism, physiology, etc. Nevertheless, there is overwhelming evidence that human cancers develop at the cellular level with considerable similarity to that observed in experimental animals. In fact, these similarities first became evident when agents known to cause cancer in humans were found to also lead to tumor development in animals (Doll and Peto, 1981; Krantiris, 1983). Furthermore, the similarities in the process of cancer are evident by similar classes of oncogenes being present in tumors of rodents and of human beings (Weinberg, 1985).

CARCINOGENIC EXPOSURE AND METABOLIC ACTIVATION

In the course of living, humans will inevitably be exposed to compounds that are not essential for life or "natural" from the standpoint of evolution. Such agents may be acutely toxic, potentially toxic following activation, or exhibit long-term effects such as cancer development. The ability of a dietary constituent to modify the formation of a potential carcinogenic agent is best exemplified by studies showing that vitamin C can reduce the formation of N-nitrosamines (Mirrish et al., 1972) as discussed below. Most N-nitrosamines are very strong carcinogenic compounds and induce tumors in various species of animals (Schmaehl and Habs, 1980). While ascorbic acid may be a significant factor in reducing in vivo formation of this carcinogen (Reed et al., 1983), other dietary consittuents may have the opposite effect. The intake of some phenols, such as those present in vegetables, or thiocyanate and iodide may enhance cancer development by stimulation nitrosation and thus, the formation of these carcinogenic compounds (Mirrish et al., 1975).

As previously indicated, chemical initiators of carcinogenesis are by definition very reactive and are usually unstable and, therefore, do not usually persist within the environment for extended periods. Thus, the usual carcinogenic sequence is exposure to a stable but toxic chemical that during the detoxification process is transformed into a highly reactive derivative(s) that interacts with cellular macromolecules. Due largely to the pioneering work of Miller and Miller (1966), substantial evidence exists about the essential role of drug-metabolizing enzymes in the bioactivation of the parent carcinogen into the biologically reactive carcinogenic intermediates. The major reactions are hydroxylation and subsequent conjugation. Some dietary nutrients may modify the development of cancer by modifying the formation of specific carcinogens, altering the metabolic activation of carcinogens, or possibly changing the occurrence of cocarcinogens or anticarcinogens. The ability of selective micronutrients, such as vitamin A and selenium, to modify the metabolic activation of carcinogens is well appreciated and discussed further in this review. Similarly, a shift in metabolism of benzo(a)pyrene by a nonnutrient such as butylated hydroxytoluene (BHT) has the effect of reducing the carcinogenicity of this compound (Wattenberg, 1972; Wilson et al., 1981).

Various investigators have shown that certain minor constituents of commonly consumed plant foods, such as flavones, isothiocyanates, phenols, and indoles, have the ability of altering the metabolic activation of carcinogens (Wilson et al., 1981; Wattenberg, 1983; Slaga and Digiovanni, 1984; Wattenberg, 1985). The inverse association between the risk of cancer of the gastrointestinal tract and the consumption of selected vegetables, particularly the cruciferae, suggests a possible role of some of these nonnutrient dietary constituents in the bioactivation of carcinogens and ultimately the risk of human beings to cancer.

The effects of several micronutrients that are known to modify the process of carcinogenesis are briefly discussed in this chapter and will be covered in greater detail in subsequent chapters. This discussion is limited to those nutrients and nonnutrients for which sufficient information is available to verify an effect upon the process of carcinogenesis and generally to those dietary constituents for which possible mechanisms can be explored. While considerable information exists for some nutrients, the complex interrelationships that exist between nutrients in more practical diets remains poorly understood.

MECHANISMS OF ACTION OF SELECTIVE NUTRIENTS

Vitamin A

Vitamin A functions as a constituent of visual pigments, allows for normal reproductive capacity in both males and females, and allows for normal cellular growth and differentiation. Only retinaldehyde and retinol and its esters can serve all of these functions. Recent intense interest in retinol has stemmed from several epidemiologic investigations noting an inverse relationship between vitamin A intake and the risk of developing cancer. A deficiency of this vitamin has been recognized for over 60 years to increase the susceptibility of experimental animals to some chemically induced tumors and, more recently, the incidence associated with viral induction (Mori, 1922; Meyskens and Prasad, 1983; Sporn and Roberts, 1983; Moon and Itri, 1983; Olson, 1986). Treatment with some carcinogens or inducing agents results in a marked reduction in the liver stores of this vitamin. Thus, marginal deficiencies may become evident following exposure to some carcinogens and allow for the expression of chemical transformation. The ability of vitamin A to modify cellular differentiation has often been cited as the mechanism by which this vitamin modifies the susceptibility of experimental animals to cancer. Neoplastic cells are inherently characterized by a defect or change in the process of differentiation. The importance of this observation in human cancer risk is emphasized by the fact that most primary cancers in humans arise in epithelial tissues that depend upon vitamin A for normal cellular differentiation.

Retinoids is a term coined to refer to both natural and synthetic analogues of retinol. These compounds possess varying amounts of vitamin A activity depending on their specific structural characteristics. Supplementation of various retinoids has been shown to be effective inhibitors of chemical carcinogenesis in the skin, mammary gland, esophagus, respiratory tract, pancreas, and urinary bladder of experimental animals (Sporn and Roberts, 1983; Moon and Itri, 1984; Olson, 1986). Continuous retinoid administration is required for the continued inhibitory effects of this nutrient (Thompson, 1979). While the retinoids are generally most effective when administered shortly after the carcinogenic insult, even when treatment is delayed, these compounds are often effective cancer chemopreventive agents (McCormick and Moon, 1982). However, there is a critical period in which retinoid supplementation is no longer effective in inhibiting tumor development. Such data suggest the retinoids may have an important function in inhibiting the early stages of carcinogenesis and that, with time, critical events occur within the cell that prevent the benefits of dietary supplementation (McCormick and Moon, 1982). These studies suggest that retinoids can inhibit cancer by suppressing the progression of early cellular lesions. Inconsistent data between laboratories of effects of retinoids may be a consequence of the use of inappropriate retinoids for examination, the dose used, the species tested, or the initiating carcinogen.

Recent laboratory evidence (Santamaria et al., 1983) supports the suggestion of Peto et al. (1981) that dietary β-carotene may be as important in cancer prevention as preformed retinol. At present it is not clear if vitamin A activity or the presence of constituent groups similar to that found in retinol, such as unsaturated double bonds or the aromatic characteristic, is the most important determinant of the efficacy of the retinoids. Nevertheless, it is known that at least one retinoid without vitamin A activity is able to reduce UV-induced skin cancer in experimental animals (Matthews-Roth, 1982). It should be noted that some retinoids can enhance carcinogenesis, at least during some experimental circumstances (Birt et al., 1984). Thus, it is difficult to make generalizations about the dietary benefits of vitamin A and the retinoids until more definitive data are available.

The mechanism(s) by which retinoids inhibit experimental carcinogenesis is largely unknown. While vitamin A deficiency enhances carcinogenesis, and vitamin A excess inhibits this process, there is little evidence that a continuum exists between the deficiency and excess states. Thus, the increased risk of animals to cancer during a deficiency state are likely mechanistically and physiologically different from the prophylactic and therapeutic effects of near toxic dosages of retinoids.

Several vitamin A compounds and analogs are known to inhibit the in vitro microsomal mixed function oxidases that are capable of metabolizing carcinogenic compounds (Hill and Shih, 1974). Thus, during some circumstances the beneficial effects of supplemental retinoids may be related to alterations in the initiation phase of carcinogenesis. However, the greatest effect of retinoids appears to be involved primarily in the promotional phase of tumor growth (Verma and Boutwell, 1977; McCormick and Moon, 1982; Bertram, 1983; Olson, 1986). Vitamin A and the retinoids in general may modify preneoplastic and/or neoplastic cells by stimulating cellular differentiation, blocking cellular division, or enhancing the destruction of cells. None of the possible mechanisms would be mutually exclusive. In some tissues retinoids can inhibit differentiation and proliferation and DNA synthesis (Mehta and Moon, 1981; Bertram, 1983). Of the various theories accounting for the effects of retinoids upon cancer promotion, the following have received the greatest attention: (a) retinoids participate in sugar transfer reactions by means of the intermediate retinyl phosphate mannose, which plays a critical role in the control of differentiation and carcinogenesis, (b) retinoids control gene expression by interacting with cyclic AMP-dependent and -independent protein kinase, (c) retinoids control of gene expression is mediated by specific intracellular binding proteins in a manner analogous to that observed with the steroid hormones. Data are available that both support and refute each of these hypotheses, as recently reviewed by Roberts and Sporn (1984).

Vitamin A has long been associated with the immunologic system (Dennert, 1984) by altering both humoral and cell-mediated immunity. In cell-mediated immunity, retinoids not only influence the total T-cell population but also appear to stimulate cellular lysis and growth inhibition. During the early processing of the antigen by macrophages during humoral immunity, retinoids may directly interact with the B cell or activate the B cell by way of an increased number of T helper cells (Dennert, 1984).

Vitamin C

Vitamin C, an essential nutrient for man, has been proposed as protective against cancer for over 50 years. In 1936, Eufinger and Gaehtgens proposed that vitamin C influenced the pattern of pathologically modified white blood cells and described the successful treatment of a patient with myeloid leukemia. Since this early observation, vitamin C has been implicated in human cancer prevention largely upon the basis of several epidemiologic studies showing that consumption of foods containing high concentrations of this vitamin was associated with a reduction in cancer incidence, especially cancer of the stomach and esophagus (Weisburger, 1980; Glatthaar et al., 1986). Results from several clinical studies have provided inconclusive evidence about the specific role of vitamin C in human carcinogenesis.

Experimental data from animals and cell culture systems suggest several mechanism by which vitamin C might interfere with the cancer process. An important mechanism by which vitamin C may interfere with cancer development is by inhibiting N-nitrosamine formation. N-nitrosamines and their potential hazards have been recognized for many years. Vitamin C effectively competes with nitrite, thereby inhibiting its reaction with amines or amides to form carcinogenic nitroso compounds (Mirvish et al., 1972; Mirvish et al., 1975). Reed and coworkers (1983) demonstrated that vitamin C treatment reduced N-nitroso compound formation in a selected group of human subjects at risk for gastric cancer. Supplementation of the diet with ascorbic acid and α-tocopherol (400 mg each) were also found to result in a significant reduction in the mutagenic compounds excreted in human feces, suggesting that antioxidants in the diet may lower the body's exposure to endogenously formed mutagens (Dion et al., 1982).

Glatthaar et al. (1986) reviewed the proposed mechanism of vitamin C involvement in cancer development. The potential for bioactivation of carcinogens by microsomal hydroxylation and demethylation systems and the associated electron transport protein components, such as cytochrome P-450, have been observed in animal studies to be decreased during condition of ascorbic acid depletion (Cameron et al., 1979). Guinea pigs not exhibiting signs of scurvy, but with liver ascorbate reduced 30% of that in liver of control animals, had only 50% of the hepatic microsomal hydroxylation and demethylation capacity of controls (Cameron et al., 1979). Nevertheless, overall, the protective effects of ascorbic acid on the development of neoplasia by carcinogens are not impressive, except for experiments where nitroso compound formation is inhibited.

The ability of vitamin C to modify tumor cells has been documented through studies examining synergism with various drugs, inhibition of the action of cytotoxic drugs and interference with tumor cell metabolism (Prasad, 1980; Benedict et al., 1982; Glatthaar et al., 1986). Ascorbate may react with free copper ions, thereby leading to enhanced peroxide formation. While such metabolic effects may account for the inhibition of some tumor cells, the effectiveness of vitamin C is likely dependent upon cellular catalase and peroxidase activities (Glatthaar et al., 1986). Under some conditions it is possible to cause a reverse of chemically transformed cells to normal appearing morphological phenotypes by adding ascorbic acid (Benedict et al., 1982). The exact mechanism by which vitamin C leads to this inhibition and reversion is unknown.

Disturbances of homeostasis generally trigger cellular and humoral defense reactions in the host, causing an acute inflammatory response during which sophisticated mechanisms respond to protect host tissues against endogenous oxidative and hydrolytic agents. Recent studies suggest that vitamin C enhances the immune function, thereby reducing the risk of certain types of cancer (Schmidt and Moser, 1985). As a biologic redox reagent, vitamin C can interfere with oxidative processes during the functional stimulation of polymorphonuclear leukocytes and macrophages involving, among other function, chemotaxis and phagocytosis (Schmidt and Moser, 1985).

Vitamin D and Calcium

Recently, 1,25-dihydroxyvitamin D_3 has been shown to inhibit the proliferation of some neoplastic cells including the differentiation of murine and human myeloid leukemia cells in vitro (Abe et al., 1981; Tanaka et al., 1982; Dokoh et al., 1984). Suppression of growth of these malignant cells appears to depend upon a receptor-mediated process. Such results point to a previous unsuspected involvement of vitamin D in cell proliferation and differentiation and suggest that analogs of the vitamin D hormone may be of interest as possible therapeutic agents in the treatment of malignancy. The mechanism of action of vitamin D hormone in induction of differentiation of the neoplastic cells remains largely unknown. Ornithine decarboxylase induction by vitamin D in intestinal cells may indicate the involvement of this vitamin-hormone in the polyamine biosynthesis pathways (Shinki et al., 1981). However, studies by Wood et al. (1983) suggest that vitamin D is effective in inhibiting papillomas induced by methylcholanthrene either before or after treatment with phorbol esters, suggesting some mechanism other than polyamine regulation is involved in explaining the action of this vitamin.

The function of vitamin D in differentiation may relate to its action on intracellular calcium metabolism. Several studies provide indirect evidence of a possible involvement of calcium in carcinogenesis based on the effects of this mineral on the activity and pharmacokinetics of carcinogens and promoters and on the ability of carcinogen or tumor proliferation to induce disturbances in calcium homeostasis (Jaffe, 1982; MacManus, 1982). Whatever the mechanism, calcium seems to have an active role in the promotion, rather than the initiation, of carcinogenesis (Jaffe, 1982). The association of calcium-activated oxygen release and the expression of tumor promoters is of considerable interest (Green et al., 1983). Normal epithelial cells cease to proliferate or differentiate in calcium-deprived medium, however, under the influence of carcinogens or promoters, cells may become resistant to the regulatory calcium signals and proliferate.

Vitamin E

Vitamin E (α-tocopherol) is the major radical trap in lipid membranes. Few studies have adequately evaluated the role of the lipid phase antioxidants in experimental carcinogenesis. However, their potential role is supported by the hypothesis that cellular damage produced by active oxygen contributes to the promotional phase of carcinogenesis (Mason, 1982) and that antioxidants such as α-tocopherol can, at times, protect against this damage. Consumption of a diet devoid of vitamin E for extended periods has been shown to alter the mixed function oxidase system that is required for carcinogen activation (Galrola and Chen, 1982). Also, α-tocopherol has been shown to inhibit endogenous nitrosation reactions leading to the formation of carcinogenic nitrosamines, implying that if nitrosation is a determinant of human cancer, then α-tocopherol should be protective. Support for this hypothesis comes from the observation that administration of vitamin E and ascorbic acid to volunteers on Western diets causes dramatic reduction in fecal mutagenicity (Dion et al., 1982). The anticarcinogenic effects of vitamin E have largely been observed with extremely high and nonphysiological concentrations of this vitamin (Harber and Wissler, 1962; Harman, 1969). While the observed effects may relate to reduced lipid peroxidation, other studies suggest that vitamin E may also be involved in cellular mitosis and DNA production (Konings and Trieling, 1977). Data by Ip and Horvath (1983) suggest that vitamin E may potentiate the inhibitory effects of selenium on the promotion or proliferative phases of carcinogenesis.

Choline and Other B Vitamins

Choline deficiency produces various pathologic lesions in virtually every organ of the body. A vast body of literature describes the consequences of a dietary choline deficiency upon hepatic tissue growth and development. The majority of carcinogen studies conducted have been limited to observations in the liver. A deficiency of choline enhances the initiating potency of several carcinogens (Rogers and Newberne, 1982; Poirier et al., 1984; Shinozuka et al., 1986). While a dietary deficiency exerts strong promoting effects, it can also lead directly to tumor formation (Shinozuka et al., 1986). It is possible that the effects of a choline-deficient diet are only promotional and that the development of hepatocellular carcinomas after chronic feeding of a deficient diet result from the promotion of naturally occurring preneoplastic lesions. Considerable evidence shows that choline deficiency leads to enhanced liver cell proliferation, an inadequate supply of methyl groups for cell proliferation, and hypomethylation of DNA (Ghoshal and Farber, 1983; Poirier et al., 1984; Shinozuka et al., 1986). Enzymatic methylation of DNA is recognized as a mechanism for genetic control and likely has a role in oncogene activation (Riggs and Jones, 1983). The reduction in hypomethylation caused by choline deficiency possibly leads to the expression of oncogenes preexisting within the liver. Cellular alterations, either individually or in combination, may play a critical role in the ability of this nutrient to modify the process of carcinogenesis. Continued research with this nutrient is likely to supply valuable information on the mechanism of carcinogenesis.

Since the B vitamins are essential components of any adequate diet and are necessary for the continued maintenance of cellular integrity and metabolic function, severe deficiencies generally reduce the growth rate of tumor cells and interfere with the normal functioning of the organism. Few, yet sometimes contradictory, studies are available in the literature to adequately evaluate the impact of B vitamins intake upon the process of carcinogenesis. The effects of B vitamins on carcinogenesis cannot be easily ascribed to specific effects on initiation and promotion. Thus, the B vitamins in general may function in carcinogenesis by modulating cellular processes including growth and immunosurveillance. However, at least two B vitamins appear to significantly modify the process of carcinogenesis. A significant amount of data suggest that a deficiency of either vitamin B_{12} or folic acid enhances the activity of various chemical carcinogens in various organs, suggesting a cocarcinogenic effect of inadequate intake of these vitamins (Miller et al., 1952; Bennett et al., 1956; Eto and Krumdieck, 1986). A deficiency of either may result in a hypomethylation, as is the case during choline deficiency, and therefore lead to the subsequent activation of oncogenes. Failure of the immune system to defend the host may also account for the increased tumor development that is typically observed in cases of deficiencies of these vitamins (Nauss and Newberne, 1981).

Iron, Zinc, and Copper

Iron deficiency has been correlated with cancer of the upper alimentary tract. Iron deficiency in experimental animals is associated with a fatty liver and with a decreased delay in the time of onset of liver tumors (Vitale et al., 1978). Such results may indicate that iron can, under some circumstances, serve as a modifier of carcinogenesis. Insufficient information is available to adequately evaluate the importance of dietary iron intakes in the cancer risk.

Copper is an essential nutrient implicated as a positive factor in cancer susceptibility. Although some clinical and epidemiological studies concerning exposure to copper have suggested a direct relationship with cancer risk, little evidence is available relating dietary intakes to cancer development. Experimental studies in animals indicate that large dosages of copper protect against chemically induced tumors (Brada and Altman, 1978), yet the influence of more normal intakes of copper does not appear to have been examined.

Zinc, an essential constituent of numerous enzymes, functions in cell replication and tissue repair. The data on effects of excess zinc on chemically induced tumors have been mixed, some showing increased, others decreased tumor development (Duncan and Dreosti, 1975; Fong et al., 1978). Zinc deficiency is also known to modify the growth of neoplasms (Fenton et al., 1980). Whether these effects on the growth of established tumors are a result of alterations in the immune system or on cell proliferation is not completely resolved.

Selenium

The inhibitory effect of selenium on experimentally induced tumors is well documented (Shamberger, 1970, Whanger et al., 1982; Medina, 1986; Milner,

1986). Dietary supplementation has been shown to be effective in inhibiting the formation of chemically induced tumors in the gastrointestinal tract, liver, breast, skin, and pancreas. Generally, selenium as sodium selenite is effective in inhibiting chemically induced, virally induced, and transplantable tumors. Selenomethionine or other organic selenium compounds present in foods have not been as extensively examined but appear to be less effective in inhibiting carcinogenesis than selenite supplementation (Thompson et al., 1984). The ability of this trace element to exhibit such dramatic effects across such a variety of experimental conditions suggests a generalized mechanism rather than a tissue or cell specific reaction (Shamberger 1970; Milner, 1986). The protection offered by selenium is generally observed at concentrations far greater than those known to saturate the requirements for growth and glutathione peroxidase activity. As observed with vitamin A, the continuous intake of selenium is necessary for maximum inhibition of carcinogenesis (Ip, 1981). As indicated for the retinoids, during at least one experimental condition selenium supplementation enhances tumor development (Birt et al., 1984).

The mechanism of selenium inhibition of carcinogenesis appears complex and is poorly understood. Studies have shown that selenium inhibits the initiation phase of carcinogenesis (Ip, 1981). In studies with 7,12-dimethylbenz(a)-anthracene, at least part of the protection appears to relate to the inhibition of an enzyme(s) responsible for the formation of antidihydrodiol epoxide adducts (Milner et al., 1985). Other studies have clearly demonstrated effects of this trace element when given following carcinogen administration (Shamberger, 1970; Thompson and Becci, 1980; Milner, 1986). Such results suggest that selenium owes at least part of its effects to a decrease in proliferation phase of carcinogenesis. The active form of selenium within these cells leading to cancer inhibition is unknown but may be selenodiglutathione or some closely related intermediate (Milner, 1986).

A variety of studies show the interactive nature of selenium with other dietary constituents. Two of the most promising candidates for chemoprevention, vitamin A and selenium, have been shown to act additively in the inhibition of chemically induced mammary cancer (Thompson et al., 1981). Likewise, vitamin E apparently provides a more favorable environment against oxidative stress, thereby potentiating the action of selenium (Ip, 1986). Other nutrients may have the opposite influence on the beneficial action of selenium. Vitamin C appears to be one such nutrient, since it has been reported to nullify the preventive action of selenite (Ip, 1986).

Other Agents

Considerable evidence indicates that the liberation or generation of activated oxygen species (hydrogen peroxide, superoxide anions, hydroxyl radicals, etc.)

within the cell is highly damaging and may directly or indirectly contribute to carcinogenesis (Cerutti, 1985). Agents, such as synthetic antioxidant, including BHA and BHT, dietary antioxidants such as β-carotene, ascorbic acid, or α-tocopherol, can experientially reduce cancer incidence. Nevertheless, the experimental and epidemiological evidence for the role of antioxidants per se in the prevention of cancer show numerous inconsistencies, making it difficult to draw firm conclusions for their potential benefit. Nevertheless, there is a strong rationale for their potential protective effect. Various investigators have suggested that phenolic antioxidants (BHT, BHA) possibly inhibit carcinogenesis by an alteration in metabolic activation and not by their antioxidant properties (Wattenberg, 1985). β-Carotene, as indicated previously, could likewise owe its anticarcinogenic effects to properties other than its property as an antioxidant.

SUMMARY AND CONCLUSIONS

Unquestionably, nutrition is not the sole determinant of the observed patterns of cancer. Furthermore, adjustment of dietary practices to conform to the recommended dietary goals may not be necessary, or even appropriate, for all segments of the population. Sophisticated techniques and procedures are needed to adequately assess the potential merit of nutritional intervention in each individual in relationship to cancer risk. However, it is clear that a variety of essential nutrient can significantly modify the carcinogenic process at specific sites including carcinogen formation and metabolism; initiation, promotion and tumor progression; cellular and host defenses; cellular differentiation; and tumor growth. Much research remains to be conducted before we can fully appreciate or understand exactly how dietary components contribute to carcinogenesis. However, the accumulated epidemiologic and laboratory findings that correlate dietary components with the incidence of cancer are rather convincing. Hopefully continued research will lead to recognition of the critical sites where nutrition intervention in the cancer process would be appropriate and lead to sound, realistic recommendations for dietary practices.

REFERENCES

Abe, E., Miyaura, C., Sakagai, H., et al. (1981). Differentiation of mouse myeloid leukemia cells induced by α-25-dihydroxyvitamin D_3. *Proc. Natl. Acad. Sci. USA 78*: 4990.

Benedict, W. F., Wheatley, W. L., and Jones, P. A. (1982). Differences in anchorage-dependent growth and tumorigenicities between transformed C3H/10T1/2 cells with morphologies that are or are not reverted to a normal phenotype by ascorbic acid. *Cancer Res. 42*: 1041.

Bennett, M. A., Ramsey, J., Donnelly, A. J. (1956). Retardation of induction of *p*-dimethylaminoazobenzene liver tumors by vitamine B_{12}. *Int. Z. Vitaminforsch. 26*: 417.

Bertram, J. S. (1983). Inhibition of neoplastic transformation in vitro by retinoids. *Cancer Surv. 2*: 243.

Birt, D., Davies, M. H. , Pour, P. M., et al. (1984). Lack of inhibitions by retinoids of bis(2-oxypropyl)nitrosamine-induced carcinogenesis in Syrian hamsters. *Carcinogenesis 4*: 1215.

Birt, D. F., Julius, A. D., Pour, P. M. (1984). Increased pancreatic carcinogenesis in syrian hamsters fed high selenium diets. *Proc. Am. Assoc. Cancer Res. 25*: 133.

Boutwell, R. K. (1974). The function and mechanism of promoters of carcinogenesis. *Crit. Rev. Toxicol. 2*; 419.

Brada, Z., Altman, N. H. (1978). The inhibitory effect of copper on ethionine carcinogenesis. *Adv. Exp. Med. Biol. 91*: 193.

Cameron, E., Pauling, E., and Leibovitz, B. (1979). Ascorbic acid and cancer. A review. *Cancer Res. 39*: 663.

Cerutti, P. A. (1985). Prooxidant states and tumor promotion. *Science* (Washington, DC) *227*: 375.

Committee on Diet, Nutrition and Cancer, Assembly of Life Sciences, National Research Council (1982). *Diet, Nutrition, and Cancer.* National Academy Press, Washington, D.C.

Dennert, G. (1984). Retinoids and the immune system: Immunostimulation by vitamin A. In *Retinoids*, Sporn, M. B., Roberts, A. B. and Goodman, D. S., (Eds.), vol. 2, p. 373. Academic Press, New York.

Dion, P. W., Bright-See, E. B., Smith, C. C., et al. (1982). The effect of dietary ascorbic acid and a-tocopherol on fecal mutagenicity. *Mutat. Res. 102*: 27.

Doll, R., Peto, R. (1981). The causes of cancer; quantitative estimates of avoidable risks of cancer in the United States today. *J. Natl. Cancer Inst. 66*: 1192.

Dokoh, S., Donaldson, C. A., Haussler, M. R. (1984). Influence of 1,25-dihydroxyvitamin D_3 on cultured osteogenic sarcoma cells: Correlation with the 1,25-dihydroxyvitamin D_3 receptor. *Cancer Res. 44*: 2103.

Duncan, J. R., Dreosti, I. E. (1975). Zinc intake, neoplastic DNA synthesis, and chemical carcinogenesis in rats and mice. *J. Natl. Cancer Inst. 55*: 195.

Enstrom, J. E. (1978). Cancer and total mortality among active Mormons. *Cancer 42*: 1943.

Eto, I., Krumdieck, C. L. (1986). Role of vitamin B_{12} and folate deficiencies in carcinogenesis. In *Essential Nutrients in Carcinogenesis*, Poirer, L. A., Newberne, P. M. and Pariza, M. W. (Eds.), p. 313. Plenum Press, New York.

Eufinger, H., Gaehtgens, G. (1936). Über die Einwirkung des Vitamin C auf das pathologisch veränderte weisse Blutbild. *Klin. Wochenschr. 15*: 150.

Fenton, M. R., Burke, J. P., Tursi, F. D., Arena, F. P. (1980). Effect of a zinc-deficient diet on the growth of an IgM-secreting plasmacytoma (TEPC-183). *J. Natl. Cancer Inst. 65*: 1271.

Fong, L. Y. Y., Sivak, A., Newberne, P. M. (1978). Zinc deficiency and methylbenzylnitrosamine-induced esophageal cancer in rats. *J. Natl. Cancer Inst. 61*: 145.

Gairola, C., Chen, L. H. (1982). Effect of dietary vitamin E on the aryl hydrocarbon hydroxylase activity of various tissues in rat. *Int. J. Vitam. Nutr. Res. 52*: 398.

Ghoshal, A. K., Farber, E. (1983). The induction of resistant hepatocytes during initiation of liver carcinogenesis with chemicals in rats fed a choline deficient methionine low diet. *Carcinogenesis 7*: 801.

Glatthaar, B. E., Hornig, D. H., Moser, U. (1986). The role of ascorbic acid in carcinogenesis. In *Essential Nutrients in Carcinogenesis*. Poirier, L. A., Newberne, P. M. and Pariza, M. W. (Eds.), p. 357, Plenum Press, New York.

Gori, G. B. (1979). Dietary and nutritional implications in the multifactorial etiology of certain prevalent human cancers. *Cancer 43*: 2151.

Green, T. R., Wu, D. E., Wirtz, M. K. (1983). The oxygen-generating oxidoreductase of human neutrophils: Evidence of an obligatory requirement for calcium and magnesium for expression of catalytic activity. *Biochem. Biophys. Res. Commun. 122*: 734.

Haenszel, W., Kurihara, M. (1968). Studies of Japanese Migrants. I. Mortality from cancer and other diseases among Japanese in the United States. *J. Natl. Cancer Inst. 40*: 43.

Harber, S. L., Wissler, R. W. (1962). Effect of vitamin E on carcinogenicity of methylcholanthrene. *Proc. Soc. Exp. Biol. Med. 111*: 774.

Harman, D. (1969). Dibenzanthracene induced cancer. Inhibiting effect of vitamin E. *Clin. Res. 17*: 125.

Hill, D. L., Shih, T. W. (1974). Vitamin A compounds and analogues as inhibitors of mixed-function oxidases that metabolize carcinogenic polycyclic hydrocarbons and other compounds. *Cancer Res. 34*: 564.

Ip, C. (1981). Prophylaxis of mammary neoplasia by selenium supplementation in the initiation and promotion phases of chemical carcinogenesis. *Cancer Res. 41*: 4386.

Ip, C. (1986). The chemopreventive role of selenium in carcinogenesis. In *Essential Nutrients in Carcinogenesis*, Poirier, L. A., Newberne, P. M., Pariza, M. W. (Eds.), p. 431, Plenum Press, New York.

Ip, C., Horvath, P. (1983). Synergistic effect of vitamin E and selenium in the chemoprevention of mammary carcinogenesis in rats. *Proc. Am. Assoc. Cancer Res. 24*: 382.

Jaffe, L. F. (1982). Eggs are activated by a calcium explosion; Carcinogenesis may involve calcium adaptation and habituation. In *Ions, Cell Proliferation and Cancer*, Boynton, A. L., McKeehan, W. L., and Whitfield, J. F. (Eds.), Academic Press, New York.

Konings, A. W. T., Trieling, W. B. (1977). The inhibition of DNA synthesis in vitamin E-depleted lymphosarcoma cells by x-rays and cytostatics. *Int. J. Radiat. Biol. 31*: 397.

Krontiris, T. G. (1983). The emerging genetics of human cancer. *N. Engl. J. Med. 309*: 404.

MacManus, J. P. (1982). Calcium-binding proteins and cell proliferation. In *Ions, Cell Proliferation and Cancer*, Boynton, A. L., McKeehan, W. L. and Whitfield, J. F. (Eds.), Academic Press, New York.

Mason, R. P. (1982). In *Free Radical in Biology*, vol. 5, p. 161, W. A. Pryor, (Ed.). Academic Press, New York.

Matthews-Roth, M. M. (1982). Antitumor activity of β-carotene, canthaxanthin and phytoene. *Oncology* (Basel) *39*: 33.
McCormick, D. L., Moon, R. C. (1982). Influence of delayed administration of retinyl acetate on mammary carcinogenesis. *Cancer Res. 42*: 2639.
Medina, D. (1986). Selenium and murine mammary tumorigenesis. In *Diet, Nutrition and Cancer: A Critical Evaluation*, Reddy, B., Cohen, L. (Eds.). CRC Press, Boca Raton, Fla.
Mehta, R. G., Moon, R. C. (1981). Inhibition of DNA synthesis by retinyl acetate during chemically induced mammary carcinogenesis. *Cancer Res. 40*: 1109.
Meyskens, F. L., Prasad, K., Eds. (1983). *The Modulation and Mediation of Cancer by Retinoids*. S. Karger, Basel.
Miller, E. C. (1978). Some current perspectives on chemical carcinogenesis in humans and experimental animals: Presidential address. *Cancer Res. 38*: 1479.
Miller, E. C., Miller, J. A. (1966). Mechanisms of chemical carcinogenesis: the nature of proximate carcinogens and reaction with DNA. *Pharmacol. Rev. 18*: 805.
Miller, E. C., Plescia, A. M., Miller, J. A., et al. (1952). The metabolism of methylated aminoazo dyes. I. The demethylation of 3′-methyl-4-dimethyl-C^{14}-aminoazobenzene in vivo. *J. Biol. Chem. 196*: 863.
Milner, J. A. (1986). Inhibition of chemical carcinogenesis and tumorigenesis by selenium. In *Essential Nutrients in Carcinogenesis*, Poirier, L. A., Newberne, P. M. and Pariza, M. W. (Eds.), p. 449. Plenum Press, New York.
Milner, J. A., Dipple, A., Pigott, M. A. (1985). Selective effects of sodium selenite on 7,12-dimethylbenz(a)anthracene-DNA binding in fetal mouse cell cultures. *Cancer Res. 45*: 6347.
Mirvish, S. S., Cardesa, A., Wallcave, L., and Shubik, P. (1975). Induction of mouse lung adenomas by amines or ureas plus nitrite and by N-nitroso compounds: Effect of ascorbate, gallic acid, thocyanate, and caffeine. *J. Natl. Cancer Inst. 55*: 633.
Mirvish, S. S., Wallacave, L., Eagen, M., Shubik, P. (1972). Ascorbate-nitrite reaction: Possible means of blocking the formation of carcinogenic N-nitroso compounds. *Science 177*: 65.
Moon, R. C., Itri, L. M. (1984). Retinoids and cancer. In *The Retinoids*, vol. 2, p. 327. M. B. Sporn, A. B. Roberts, D. S. Goodman (Eds.). Academic Press, New York.
Mori, S. (1922). The changes in the paraocular glands which follow the administration of diets low in fat-soluble A with notes of the effect of the dame diets on the salivary glands and the mucosa of the larynx and trachea. *John Hopkins Hosp. Bull. 33*: 357.
Nauss, K. M., Newberne, P. M. (1981). Effects of dietary folate, vitamin B_{12} and methionine/choline deficiency on immune fucntion. *Adv. Exp. Med. Biol. 135*: 63.
Olson, J. A. (1986). Some thoughts on the relationship between vitamin A and cancer. In *Essential Nutrients in Carcinogenesis*. Poirier, L. A., Newberne, P. M. and Pariza, M. W. (Eds.), p. 379. Plenum Press, New York.

Peto, R., Doll, R., Buckley, J. D., Sporn, M. B. (1981). Can dietary β-carotene materially reduce human cancer rates? *Nature 290*: 201.
Phillips, R. L. (1975). Role of lifestyle and dietary habits in risk of cancer among Seventh Day Adventists. *Cancer Res. 35*: 3513-3522.
Poirier, L. A., Mikol, Y. B., Hoover, K., et al. (1984). The inhibition of methionine and choline of liver carcinoma formation in male C3H mice fed phenobarbital. *Proc. Am. Assoc. Cancer Res. 25*: 132.
Prasad, K. N. (1980). Modulation of the effects of tumor therapeutic agents by vitamin C. *Life Sci. 27*: 275.
Reed, P. I., Summers, K., Smith, P. L. R., et al. (1983). Effect of ascorbic acid treatment on gastric juice nitrite and N-nitroso compound concentrations in achlorhydric subjects. *Gut 24*: 492
Riggs, A. D., Jones, P. A. (1983). 5-Methylcytosine, gene regulation and cancer. *Adv. Cancer Res. 40*: 1.
Roberts, A. B., Sporn, M. B. (1984). Cellular biology and biochemistry of the retinoids. In *Retinoids*, Sporn, M. B., Roberts, A. B., Goodman, D. S. (Eds.), vol. 2, p. 210. Academic Press, New York.
Rogers, A. E., Newberne, P. M. (1982). Lipotrope deficiency in experimental carcinogenesis. *Nutr. Cancer 2*: 104.
Santamaria, L., Bianchi, A., Annaboldi, A., Anderoni, L., Bermond, P. (1983). Dietary carotnoids block photocarcinogenic enhancement of benzo(a)pyrene and inhibit its carcinogenesis in the dark. *Experientia* (Basel) *39*: 1043.
Schmaehl, D., and Habs, M. (1980). Carcinogenicity of N-nitroso compounds in human nutrition. *Oncology 37*: 237.
Schmidt, K., Moser, U. (1985). Vitamin C—a modulator of host defense mechanism: An overview. *Int. J. Vitam. Nutr. Res. 27*(Suppl.): 363.
Shamberger, R. J. (1970). Relationship of selenium to cancer: I. Inhibitory effect of selenium on carcinogenesis. *J. Natl. Cancer Inst. 44*: 931.
Shinki, T., Takahashi, N., Miyaura, C. (1981). Ornithin decarboxylase activity in chick duodenum induced by 1-25-dihydroxycholecalciferol. *Biochem. J. 195*: 685.
Shinozuka, H., Katyal, S. L., Perera, M. I. R. (1986). Choline deficiency and chemical carcinogenesis. In *Essential Nutrients in Carcinogenesis*, Poirier, L. A., Newberne, P. M. and Pariza, M. W. (Eds.), p. 253. Plenum Press, New York.
Slaga, T. J., Digiovanni, J. (1984). Inhibition of chemical carcinogenesis. In *Chemical Carcinogens*, C. E. Searle (Ed.), vol. 2, p. 1279. American Chemical Society, Washington, D.C.
Sporn, M. B., Roberts, A. B. (1983). Role of retinoids in differentiation and carcinogenesis. *Cancer Res. 43*: 3034.
Tanaka, H., Abe, E., Miyaura, C., et al. (1982). 1α,25-dihydrocholecalciferol and a human myeloid leukemia cell line (HL-60). The presence of a cytosol receptor and induction of differentiation. *Biochem. J. 204*: 713.
Thompson, H. J., Becci, P. J. (1980). Selenium inhibition of N-methyl-N-nitrosourea induced mammary carcinogenesis in the rat. *J. Natl. Cancer Inst. 65*: 1299.

Thompson, H. J., Becci, P. J., Brown, C. C., Moon, R. C. (1979). Effect of the duration of retinyl acetate feeding on inhibition of 1-methyl-1-nitrosourea-induced mammary cardinogenesis in the rat. *Cancer Res. 39*: 3977.

Thompson, A. J., Meeker, L. D., Becci, P. (1981). Effect of combined selenium and retinyl acetate treatment on mammary carcinogenesis. *Cancer Res. 41*: 1413.

Thompson, H. J. Meeker, L. D., Kokoska, S. (1984). Effect of inorganic and organic forms of dietary selenium on the promotional stage of mammary carccinogenesis in the rat. *Cancer Res. 44*: 2803.

Verma, A. K., Boutwell, R. K. (1977). Vitamin A acid (retinoid acid) a potent inhibitor of 12-O-tetradecanoyl-phorbol-13-acetate-induced ornithine decarboxylase activity in mouse epidermis. *Cancer Res. 37*: 2196

Vitale, J. J., Broitman, S. A., Vavrousek-Jakuba, E., Roddy, P. W., Gottlieb, L. S. (1978). The effects of iron deficiency and the quality and quantity of fat on chemically induced cancer. *Adv. Exp. Med. Biol. 91*: 229.

Wattenberg, L. W. (1972). Inhibition of carcinogenic and toxic effects of polycyclic hydrocarbons by phenolic antioxidants and ethoxyquin. *J. Natl. Cancer Inst. 48*: 1425.

Wattenberg, L. W. (1983). Inhibition of neoplasia by minor dietary constituents. *Cancer Res.* (Suppl) *43*: 2448s.

Wattenberg, L. W. (1985). Chemoprevention of cancer. *Cancer Res. 45*: 1.

Weinberg, R. A. (1985). The action of oncogenes in the cytoplasm and nucleus. *Science* (Wash. DC) *230*: 770.

Weisburger, J. H., Harquardt, H., Mower, H. F., et al. (1980). Inhibition of carcinogenesis: Vitamin C and the prevention of cancer. *Prev. Med. 9*: 352.

Whanger, P., Schmitz, J.A., Exon, J. H. (1982). Influence of diet on the effects of selenium in the genesis of mammary tumors. *Nutr. Cancer 3*: 240.

Wilson, A. G. E., Kung, H. C., Boroujerdi, M., Anderson, M. W. (1981). Inhibition in vivo of the formation of adducts between metabolites of benzo-(a)pyrene and DNA by aryl hydrocarbon hydroxylase inducers. *Cancer Res. 41*: 3453.

Wood, A. W., Chang, R. L., Huang, M.-T., et al. (1983). 1α-25-Dihydroxyvitamin D_3 inhibits phorbol ester-dependent chemical carcinogenesis in mouse skin. *Biochem. Biophys. Res. Commun. 116*: 605.

Wynder, E. L., Gori, G. B. (1977). Contribution of the environment to cancer incidence: an epidemiologic exercise. *J. Natl. Cancer Inst. 58*: 825.

3

Experimental Evidence on the Nutritional Prevention of Cancer

PAUL M. NEWBERNE, THOMAS F. SCHRAGER, and
MICHAEL W. CONNER
Boston University School of Medicine and Mallory Institute of Pathology, Boston, Massachusetts

Dietary factors have not as yet had their roles clearly defined with respect to the development of human cancer. However, the proportion of human cancers in which diet may play a role can now be estimated with some degree of precision (Doll and Peto, 1981). Despite the fact that diet and nutrition represent the most complex mixture of chemicals to which the biological systems of humans and animals are exposed, we now have evidence for a role for nutrients in cancer causation (Poirier et al., 1986). Diet is made up of groups of foods, classified broadly into the two major categories of macronutrients and micronutrients, each of which contains numerous individual components of significance to cancer prevention. There are also many significant interactions among the various nutrients, the outcome of which determines the degree of susceptibility to cancer, but these have not been extensively investigated as yet.

The complexities of studying nutrition and its relation to tumor development are significant; overt human cancers usually take many years to develop, often with a lag time of 20 to 40 years. Experimental animal models evolve through a multistage process, and there is reason to believe that this is the case with human cancer. More than one factor may be involved in most cancers, and it is difficult to establish links between single or multiple dietary factors (Greenwald, 1984). Despite these difficulties, such links do exist. However imprecise our understanding about them may be, strong suggestions clearly point to a need to examine in detail those leads that imply that changes in the diet can influence susceptibility to human cancer. Many of these leads are under intense investigation by human cancer prevention programs. Integrated, bold, and innovative programs now in progress include the Chemoprevention

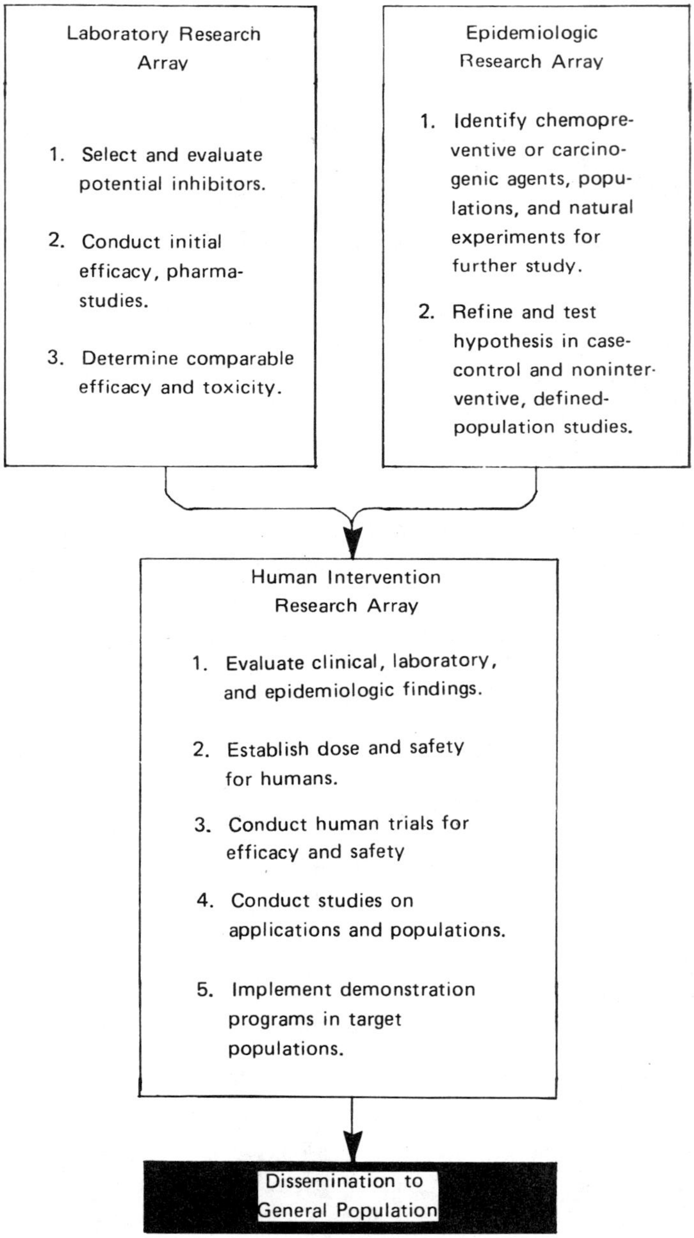

Fig. 1 National Cancer Institute Chemoprevention Program.

Program (see Fig. 1) and the Diet, Nutrition and Cancer Program of the National Cancer Institute.

The task of identifying important nutritional factors with respect to cancer causation requires the integrated skills and input of scientists from many different disciplines. This is now taking place in fundamental research laboratories and in epidemiological studies in this and other countries. Results of these studies will be of great value in prevention efforts.

Unfortunately, there have been some important public displays of disagreement among dedicated individuals in the last few years regarding the role of nutrition in cancer causation and prevention (Marshall, 1986). A number of problems involved in this area of research surfaced in the News and Comments section of *Science* early in 1986, when it was pointed out that not all of the administrators and nutritionists at the National Cancer Institute are in agreement on the potential or importance of diet with respect to cancer prevention. In addition, the National Academy of Science refused to publish the results of five years of effort by members of the Food and Nutrition Board (Marshall, 1985). These individuals had labored long and hard on the development of the revised recommended daily allowances (RDA) of nutrients. These two instances serve to illuminate the many problems in the area of nutrition and cancer prevention. Attempting to change food habits in human populations is fraught with many pitfalls, particularly when recommendations originate in federal agencies.

Some critics complain that the enthusiasm has moved ahead of the data, while others correctly point out that if we wait until all data are in, we will never initiate potentially useful programs.

This chapter will review the data relative to putative risk factors associated with macro- and micronutrients. Reference will be made to human studies to indicate leads and suggestions but with primary emphasis on animal studies. The emerging evidence suggests that manipulation of some of our dietary nutrients may be a major tool toward prevention of some forms of cancer. Equally important may be the addition of small amounts of other factors (i.e., carotene, selenium). A major question has been raised which cannot be answered at this time: Can an impatient public, anxious for some early results, and a reluctant bureaucracy, which provides the funding, have the stamina and discipline to stay with the efforts required to achieve success? Only time will tell.

CALORIES

Much of the epidemiologic data relating calories to risk for cancer do not permit quantitation of total dietary intake, and thus total calories. Many of the dietary studies in human populations are routinely based on preselected food lists. It was the international distribution of hormone-dependent cancers that first generated the suspicion several years ago that these types of tumors may be related to affluence and, in this way, associated with an increase in overall total coloric intake (Berg, 1975). It was suggested that diets consumed by affluent populations from early life through old age might have a tendency to overstimulate the endocrine system and, in this manner, lead to metabolic aberrations which, in turn, might increase the risk for certain types of cancer of the endocrine system. This of course remains to be confirmed by epidemilogy and experimental animal work.

Hill et al. (1979) reported that an advantaged socioeconomic group in Hong Kong had more than twice the mortality from colorectal cancer when compared to the lowest affluent group. The estimated daily caloric intake was 2700 in the lowest socioeconomic group and 3900 in the highest. In another study it was concluded that mortality rates from gastric cancer decreases as the per capita food intake increases; however, large bowel cancer rates rise (Gregor et al., 1969). One can propose a number of reasons for this, one of which may be a longer life span in the populations with increased per capita food intake, associated with decreased gastric cancer. This could allow more time for large bowel tumors to develop.

Gaskill et al. (1979) and Doll and Peto (1981) have reported significant correlations for total calories in breast cancer in women. On the other hand, the American Cancer Society (ACS), in long term prospective studies, have shown that mortality from cancer was significantly elevated only in those individuals who were 40% or more overweight (Low and Garfinkel, 1979). This was reconfirmed in 1987 by the ACS. The data referred to breast cancer in women, but men under similar weight excesses were at greater risk for cancer of the colon and rectum. Women appeared to be at higher risk for endometrial cancer as well when they were as much as 40% overweight.

The earliest indications for a role for caloric intake in animal tumor risk were data of Tannenbaum, who showed that tumors induced by benzo(a)pyrene in mice were inhibited by caloric restriction (Tannenbaum, 1942a, 1944, 1945a,b). The level of dietary fat has a profound effect on the growth of skin tumors and of induced breast tumors. Mice with a daily dietary intake of 11.7 kilocalories had about 25% more spontaneous tumors than mice with a daily intake of 9.6 kilocalories. Furthermore, calories from dietary fat had a greater enhancing effect than calories from carbohydrate. Others have found that a low fat, low calorie diet resulted in fewer tumors than a high saturated fat diet where the level of fat was elevated (Lavik and Baumann, 1943).

Studies in animals conducted in our own laboratories have also shown an effect of calories on risk for induced and spontaneous cancer. Some groups of rats were allowed to consume a balanced diet ad libitum and others were given 75% of the amount consumed by the ad libitum groups. Both groups were then administered a liver carcinogen, aflatoxin B_1, 15 μg per day for a total dose of 375 μg. Food intake was measured daily, and paired feeding principles were

Table 1 Liver Tumor Incidence in Control ad lib and 75% Restricted Groups

	12 Months		24 Months		Total	
Treatment	M	F	M	F	M	F
Control, ad lib	0/80	0/77	0/48	0/54	0/80	0/77
Control, ad lib + AFB_1	3/79	1/78	41/53[a]	28/60[a]	44/79[a]	29/78[a]
75% Restricted	0/80	0/80	0/64	0/72	0/80	0/80
75% Restricted + AFB_1	0/80	0/79	19/60[a]	12/67[a]	19/80[a]	12/79[a]

[a]Statistically significant ($p < 0.01$).
Source: Newberne and Conner, 1986.

Table 2 Proliferative Lesions Other than Hepatocellular

Proliferation site type	Control ad lib		Ad lib + AFB_1		75% of ad lib		75% of ad lib + AFB_1	
	M	F	M	F	M	F	M	F
Pituitary								
Hyperplasia	8	15	10	19	7	3	6	2
Adenoma	19	37	15	32	3	8	2	3
Thyroid								
Follicular								
Hyperplasia	2	3	1	2	3	1	0	1
Adenoma	3	2	3	2	0	1	0	0
Adrenal								
Cortical								
Hyperplasia	2	1	2	2	1	2	2	0
Adenoma	0	2	2	1	0	1	0	0
Medullary								
Hyperplasia	2	2	1	2	2	1	1	2
Adenoma	1	0	1	1	0	1	0	0
Mammary								
Adenoma	2	11	1	10	1	2	0	1
Carcinoma	1	8	0	12	0[a]	1[a]	0[a]	2[a]

Source: Newberne and Conner, 1986.

followed. At the end of 24 months all survivors were sacrificed and subjected to a complete gross and microscopic examination. The results are shown in Tables 1 and 2. There was significantly increased survival of the restricted groups, whether or not they received the carcinogen. Liver tumor incidence was also significantly decreased in both sexes (Table 1). An equally interesting observation was the marked reduction in tumors associated with the endocrine system, including proliferative alterations and neoplasms of the pituitary, thyroid, adrenal, and mammary glands (Table 2). We have found similar effects on induced colon cancer in rats. Figure 2 illustrates that higher caloric intake, irrespective of the fat content of the diet, results in a greater risk for colon cancer in Sprague Dawley rats. This was not the case however, with Fischer 344 rats, pointing out an interesting strain difference (Newberne and Nauss, 1986). These few examples of epidemiologic and experimental animal results serve to indicate that caloric intake is an important factor to be considered in risk for cancer and, given the excessive food consumption in North America where some cancer rates are also high, this seems to be an obvious choice for further intensive investigations.

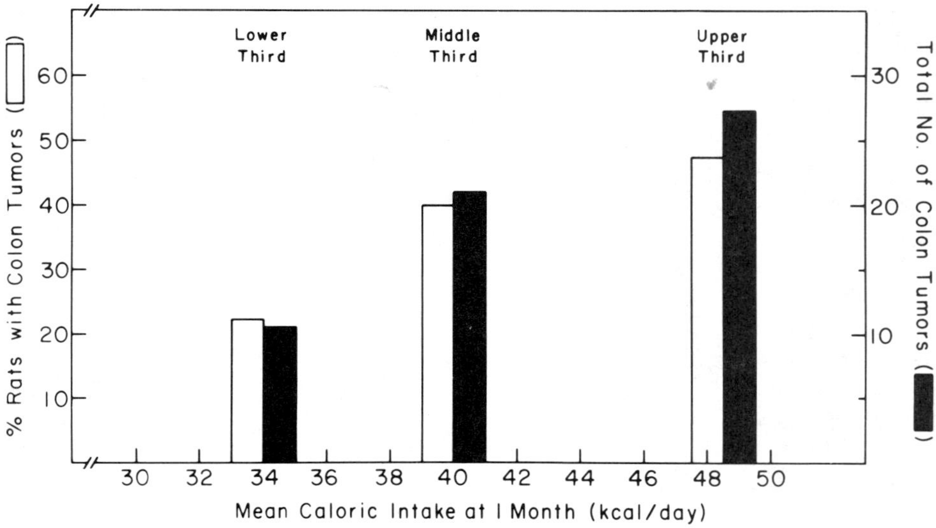

Fig. 2 Effect of caloric intake on DMH-induced colon tumorigenesis in Sprague-Dawley rats.

PROTEIN

Cancer of the kidney, pancreas, colorectum, prostate, endometrium, and breast in human populations have been associated with above-average levels of dietary protein intake (Diet, Nutrition and Cancer, 1982). It is difficult if not impossible, however, to correctly interpret the data provided in many of these studies, since in almost all cases protein is accompanied by other dietary nutrients, particularly fat. If protein is in fact associated with cancers of the various sites, the influence must be more indirect than direct.

In analyzing the diet histories of more than 4000 subjects, Kolonel et al. (1981) observed a correlation of 0.7 for total protein and total fat consumption. Armstrong and Doll (1975), in a larger study, observed a correlation between total protein and total fat with the incidence rates for 27 types of cancer in 23 countries and the mortality rates for 14 types of cancer in 32 countries. These correlations turned out to be 0.7 for total protein and 0.93 for total fat. Total protein and animal protein were significantly correlated with the incidence and mortality from breast cancer.

The mortality rates for breast cancer in 41 countries was correlated with per capita food intake by Hems (1978, 1980), who found that there was a direct relationship between breast cancer and the intake of protein, calories, and total fat from animal products, independent of other dietary components.

There are correlations between international mortality rates for colon cancer and meat consumption, particularly beef. The strongest correlations for cancer of the large intestine has been recorded for consumption of eggs followed by beef and pork. However, the time-trend data for per capita beef intake and colorectal cancer incidence showed no clear association in studies done in the United States. Tables 3 and 4 illustrate clearly that beef consumption per se

Table 3 Colorectal Cancer and Beef Consumption

Year	Beef consumption (lb/capita/wk)	Cancer mortality[a] (rate/100,000)
1940	1.06	20
1945	–	21
1950	1.20	20
1955	–	19
1960	1.64	19
1965	1.92	19
1970	2.25	19

[a]From Drasar and Irving, 1973.

Table 4 Beef Eating and Colon Cancer

Frequency (per week)	Cases (%) (No. 295)	Controls (%) (No. 632)
0-<1	10.8	8.7
2	15.4	17.4
3	30.2	25.0
4	20.0	22.5
5+	23.6	26.4

Source: Graham et al., 1978.

cannot be accorded a significant role in colon cancer (Drasar and Irving, 1973; Graham et al., 1978). One must be cautious in attempting to assign a significant aspect of human cancer to beef consumption; the consumption of beef during the last four decades has increased 2½ times; during this same period the incidence rate of colon cancer, a primary target organ for putative effects of protein, has remained stable. This should not infer, however, that other types of cancer may not be associated with increased intake of beef and other sources of protein.

There is some evidence for a correlation between protein intake and cancer in animal studies. These studies have been much better controlled (i.e., diet, exercise, and other environmental exposures) than the observational epidemiologic studies. The work of Ross and Bras (1965; 1973) has clearly served to point out the effects of protein on the development of spontaneous tumors in experimental animals. However, the total incidence of various types of tumors in their studies was related directly to caloric intake, but tumors appeared sooner when the caloric intake from protein was high.

The rats used in the studies of Ross et al. developed so many different types of tumors that one cannot easily delineate the effect of diet on specific types. The highest number of any tumor type for any one diet occurred as fibrosarcomas in animals fed a 30% protein diet. The authors were particularly interested in the effects of protein and noted that bladder tumor incidence was highest in the group with the highest percentage of calories from protein. These observations preceded the current interest in amino acids, particularly tryptophan, and their mutagenic metabolites and the possible relation of these substances to bladder and other types of cancer. There are data (Jagerstad et al. 1986) showing that the manner in which meat is cooked determines to some extent the presence of some types of mutagenic amino acid metabolites; boiling, broiling, or even caramelizing beef can result in pyrolytic products, which are mutagenic.

There have been a number of studies with animals in which protein correlated well with the incidence of induced tumors (Walters and Roe, 1964; Madhavan and Gopalan, 1968; Wells et al., 1976; Temcharoen et al., 1978; Clinton et al., 1979). One of the first of these was that of Madhaven and Gopalan (1968), who observed that about a third of the rats fed a high protein diet and exposed to aflatoxin developed tumors of the liver, whereas those fed a low protein diet had none. Weils et al. (1976) and Temcharoen et al. (1978) have essentially confirmed the work of Madhaven an Gopalan, showing that high protein diets enhance the induction of the liver tumors in animals exposed to aflatoxin.

In recent studies from our laboratories, we have found an interesting linear decrease in aflatoxin-induced liver cancer in rats as the dietary protein concentration was reduced from 20% to 6% (Table 5). Mechanistically, this may be related to the influence of protein on the metabolism of carcinogens; dietary protein modulates the microscomal enzyme systems concerned with the metabolic activation or deactivation of some types of chemicals. Mgbodile and Campbell (1972) observed an increase in activity in the microsomal components of the liver cell associated with the chemical activation of carcinogens in rats fed higher protein diets. Our own results agree with theirs (Table 6) in terms of protein effects on carcinogen metabolism. It seems reasonable to assume that protein may, in fact, influence cancer, particularly if exposure is to chemicals that require metabolic activation or deactivation.

Table 5 Influence of Dietary Protein Concentration on Response to Aflatoxin B_1

Group no.	Dietary treatment (% protein)	Tumor incidence at 24 months: No.	%
1	20	21/26	80.7
2	20[a]	17/28	60.7
3	15[a]	10/29	34.4
4	10[a]	4/30	13.3
5	6	2/27	7.4

[a]Pair-fed to the 20% protein group. from Newberne and Rogers, 1986.

Table 6 Influence of Dietary Protein on Liver Microsomal Characteristics and AFB_1-Adduct Formation

	Dietary Protein		
	6%	20% pr. fed to 6%	20% ad. lib
Microsomal protein, mg/g liver	6.8 (±0.49)	10.9 (±0.3)	12.2 (±0.10)
CYT-P-450, nmol/mg protein	0.11 (±0.02)	0.43 (±0.08)	0.40 (±0.03)
P-450 reductase, nmol P-450 reduced	6.7 (±0.09)	16.8 (±0.09)	17.1 (±1.1)
Covalent AFB^1 adducts ng/mg/DNA	6.7 (±0.09)	16.8 (±0.09)	17.1 (±1.1)

6-10 rats per group, assayed in duplicate; for AFB_1 adduct studies, ^3H-AFB_1 and cold AFB_1 to S.A. 7 μCi/μmol at dose of 1 mg/kg, killed six hours later for assay.

CARBOHYDRATES (EXCLUDING FIBER)

If carbohydrates are considered separately from fiber, there is very little in the literature about the effects of this class of nutrients on cancer. Armstrong and Doll (1975) found a correlation between sugar intake and pancreatic cancer mortality in women and a weak association between liver cancer incidence and the intake of sugar. However, Hems (1980) reported that a high intake of refined sugar was associated more with an increased incidence of breast cancer. These reports are in direct opposition to the findings of the same investigators, who reported an inverse relationship between breast cancer and starch. Drasar and Irving (1973) observed a correlation between consumption of several sugars and an increased risk for breast cancer in a study involving 37 countries. Moreover, starchy foods, including bread and potatoes, have been reported to correlate with both esophageal and gastric cancer.

Direct evidence for an effect of carbohydrates per se, however, is lacking. It would be particularly important to relate carbohydrates quality and quantity to the activity of the microflora of the gut; this in turn might be involved with the ingesta passing through the lumen and its harmful potential through metabolic activation or deactivation of gut chemicals in the contents, or by deconjugation of carcinogens. This should prove to be a fruitful area for research, but to date very little effort has been directed toward elucidating effects of microflora of the digestive tract on risk for cancer (Goldin, 1986).

FIBER

Crude, nonabsorbable fiber is a form of carbohydrate but should be set apart from the more refined carbohydrates (i.e., sugars) as part of the diet with respect to risk for cancer and other chronic diseases. This is particularly the case when considering refined carbohydrates, such as sucrose, dextrose, high fructose corn syrups, and starches, because the latter are absorbable and many fiber substances are not or are only poorly absorbed.

Strictly speaking, there are many different types of fiber, and these must be considered separately because they vary as to degree of solubility. These include cellulose, hemicellulose, pectins, and gums, which differ in the complexity of their composition and thus in their capacity to absorb and hold water, to dilute intestinal tract carcinogens, and to bind bile acids. They also vary in capacity to decrease intestinal transit time and to influence the metabolic activity of the microflora of the large bowel (Newberne, 1985). However, by whatever mechanism fiber may act, a major characteristic common to all types of fiber is the capacity to form bulk in the gastrointestinal tract.

During the past several decades western populations have decreased their consumption of fiber (Diet, Nutrition and Cancer, 1982). Burkitt and Trowell (1975) suggested that chronic diseases of the bowel, including colon cancer, are significantly associated with a low intake of dietary fiber in Western populations. This hypothesis has been examined by many investigators both in epidemiology and in laboratory studies. The epidemiologic studies have provided conflicting results; Table 7 illustrates the results of many of the international studies, and Table 8 lists results of intracountry observations. Overall, more studies report an inverse relationship.

The data from relatively large numbers of studies in human populations clearly indicate that fiber is an important aspect of the diet, that its quality and consumption rate varies from one area of the world to the other, and that, presently, there seems to be a greater risk for colon tumors when nondigestible fiber is low in the diet.

The campaign by commercial companies to capitalize on the current fiber promotion by the National Cancer Institute has created some degree of controversy (Science, 1986), and this is regrettable. The significance of adequate dietary fiber to a healthy gastrointestinal tract cannot be doubted, and this is brought to the attention of the public.

In terms of experimental animal studies, bran and other types of nondigestible carbohydrates (fiber) have been reported to have positive or negative effects on induced colon cancer (Newberne, 1985). A summary (Table 9) of rodent studies using induced colon cancer (Greenwald, 1986) as an endpoint lists results of effects of various fibers in experimental animals. A specific study (Table 10) serves to illustrate effects of bran, corn oil, and beef fat on induced colon cancer.

Table 7 International Correlational Studies of Fiber and Colon Cancer

			Associations		
Authors	Year	Site	Inverse	None	Direct
Drasar, Irving	1973	37 countries	–	x	–
Irving, Drasar	1973	37 countries	x (cereals)	–	–
Armstrong, Doll	1975	32 countries	x (cereals)	–	–
Howell	1975	37 countries	x (cereals, pulses)	–	–
Knox	1977	20 countries	x (fruit, vec., wheat)	–	–
Liu et al.	1979	20 countries	x (crude fiber)	–	–
McKeown-Eyssen, Bright-see	1984	38 countries	x (dietary fiber)	–	–

When adjustments for other food components are made, the association no longer holds. However, these adjustments may not be totally appropriate.

Table 8 Intracountry Correlational Studies of Fiber and Colon Cancer

			Associations		
Authors	Year	Site	inverse	none	direct
Bingham et al.	1979	UK	x (cellulose, pectins)	–	–
Bingham et al.					
Lyon, Sorenson	1978	US			
Enstrom	1980	Mormons	x (fruits, vegetables)	–	–
Malhotra	1977	India	x (fiber-rich diet)	–	–
Rozen et al.	1981	Israel	x (crude fiber)	–	–
Maisto, Bremner	1981	S. Africa	x (fiber-rich diet)	–	–
Jensen	1983	Denmark			
		SDA's	x (vegetarian diet)	–	–

Not statistically significant or no test for significance shown.

Table 9 Summary of Reports of the Effects of Various Fibers in Experimentally Induced Colorectal Tumors in Rodents[a]

Tumorigenic effect	Fiber sources and number of studies					
	cellulose	wheat bran	pectin	corn bran	marine[b] fiber	other[c]
Protective	6	10	1	0	0	2
No effect	0	2	1	0	0	0
Enhancement	0	2	2	3	3	1

[a]Summarizes 27 reports of effects of fibers fed to rodents with experimentally induced colon tumors (some reports included multiple fiber types).
[b]Marine- and algal-origin polysaccharides used as additives to certain foods during processing.
[c]Includes soy bran, crude fiber, lignin, and undefined rodent diets.

Table 10 Fiber, Dimethylhdrazine, and Colon Tumors in Rats

Treatment	% Colon tumors	Tumors per tumor-bearing rat
4 Doses DMH	68	1.9
Beef fat, no bran		
Beef fat, plus bran	38	1.1
Corn oil, no bran	65	1.5
Corn oil, plus bran	43	1.6
8 Doses DMH		
Beef fat, no bran		
Beef fat, plus bran	63	3.1
Corn oil, no bran	90	2.8
Corn oil, plus bran	66	3.4

Source: Abridged from Wilson et al., 1977, with permission.

Table 11 Effects of soluble and Insoluble Fiber on Induced Colon Tumors in Rats

Treatment	Tumor Incidence (%)	Tumors/tumor-bearing rat
Pectin 5%	91	2.0 ± 0.2
Pectin 10%	74	2.4 ± 0.4
Pectin 20%	41	2.4 ± 0.4
Guar gum 5%	65	1.7 ± 0.3
Guar gum 10%	50	1.3 ± 0.1
Guar gum 20%	42	1.3 ± 0.2
Cellulose, powdered 5%	75	2.8 ± 0.5
Cellulose, powdered 10%	92	5.1 ± 0.5
Cellulose, powdered 20%	100	6.5 ± 0.6
Fiber free	65	1.3 ± 0.3

Source: From Klurfeld et al., 1986, abridged, with permission.

On the other hand, Klurfeld has reported some recent data (1986) where soluble fibers (pectin and guar gum) decreased colon tumors but cellulose (insoluble) increased risk for induced colon cancer (Table 11) in a dose-response fashion. Thus, the type of fiber has a profound effect on risk for developing cancer in animals and, apparently, in humans. There is still a distinct possibility that colon cancer is caused by dietary or other carcinogens, unrelated to fiber or other dietary constituents (Eastwood, 1987). Some degree of caution should be exercised in modifying our diets with respect to fiber.

FAT

The quality and quantity of dietary fats have been examined both epidemiologiacally and in experimental animals with regard to risk for specific tumor types, perhaps more than any other single dietary nutrient (Armstrong and Doll, 1975; Gaskill et al., 1979; Nauss et al., 1983, 1987; Reddy, 1986).

Breast cancer is the number one ranking cancer in women around the world. Epidemiological studies have shown a direct association between per capita intake of fat and breast cancer (Parkin et al., 1984; Miller, 1986). Most of the studies have shown correlations higher for total fat than for any of the other dietary factors considered at the same time. The overall consumption of fat in intercountry studies is more closely related to breast cancer than to any of the other dietary nutrients (Newberne, 1985). However, intracountry studies are not as convincing as results of those between countries (Miller, 1986).

Inter- and intracountry studies have been used to compare the fat consumed with the incidence of breast cancer. A study by Gaskill et al. (1979) indicated a significant correlation within the United States of fat intake and breast cancer mortality rates, if all states were combined. However, other factors influence these figures, including the age of first marriage, geographic location, and the age of the individual at first successful pregnancy.

Kolonel et al. (1981) examined the consumption of fat and correlated it with breast cancer incidence in Hawaii (1983). They found a significant association between breast cancer and total fat consumption, particularly with animal fat and with both saturated and unsaturated fats.

Epidemiologic studies have also indicated an association between dietary fat and prostate cancer in men (Hirayama, 1977, Schuman et al., 1982; Kolonel et al., 1983; Armstrong and Doll, 1985). Thus, epidemiologic evidence supports the suggestion that dietary fat is related to risk for breast cancer in women and to prostate cancer in men.

Rat models for breast cancer studies are sufficiently well standardized to have produced a body of useful information. The tumors induced by these methods are often benign, however, or of borderline malignancy, particularly when the carcinogens are given in low doses. Further development and analysis of the models are needed to resolve conflicts in the experimental data and increase correspondence between the rat mammary gland tumors and human breast cancer. Much useful data have been assembled using this model, some of which are described here.

The fat content of the diet has highly significant, reproducible effects on chemically induced mammary gland tumorigenesis in female rats. The effective fats reduce tumor latency and may increase final tumor incidence and frequency. The enhancement of tumorigenesis by fat can be reduced by the addition of selenium to the diet by treatment with indomethacin and by hormonal manipulations. The mechanism of the fat effect is not known; it may be due in part to enhanced growth from highly efficient utilization of calories from fat, to oxidative damage to cell constituents, or to other as yet unidentified factors or mechanisms. Subtle endocrine alterations or abnormal metabolism of carcinogens and promoting agents are probably also involved. These and other potential factors have been reviewed (Welsch, 1985). The effect of fat can be demonstrated if it is fed throughout the rat's lifetime or if it is fed only before or only after carcinogen exposure. This suggests that fat influences mammary tumorigenesis by more than one mechanism (i.e., during initiation, promotion, etc.).

Although, as noted above, the mechanisms of the high fat effect are not known, numerous hypotheses have been proposed and tested. These fall into two groups: (a) mechanisms specific for the mammary gland and (b) mechanisms that may be generally applicable to the various organs in which high fat diets appear to enhance carcinogenesis. Specific mechanisms examined in the mammary gland include effects of high fat diets on circulating hormones, mammary gland tissue hormone receptors, mammary gland growth and differentiation, and mammary gland metabolism and binding of DMBA. More generalized hypotheses include effects of the high fat diets on caloric balance; carcinogen kinetics; tissue peroxide content; cellular immunological responses; prostaglandin secretion, balance, and distribution; cell membrane composition; and response to growth factors. These proposed mechanisms have resulted in the accumulation of a large amount of useful information about interactions of dietary fat and mammary tumorigenesis, even if the mechanisms of the interactions have not been documented.

The availability of single-dose models for mammary tumorigenesis has made possible investigations into the timing and duration of the enhancing effect of high dietary fat. The predominant effect is exerted after carcinogen exposure; it is directly correlated to duration of feeding of the high fat diet and inversely correlated to the time between carcinogen exposure and introduction of the high fat diet.

The polyunsaturated vegetable oils appear to act primarily during the post-exposure period, although data have been reported that show that this is partially due to the longer feeding period (Dao and Chan, 1983). Recent reports using a low dose of DMBA shown an enhancing effect of corn oil fed only before DMBA exposure (Clinton et al., 1986). Lard (pig fat), which is a mixed, predominantly monounsaturated fat, enhances tumorigenesis when fed only before carcinogen exposure (Rogers et al., 1982, 1985, 1986; Sylvester et al., 1983, 1986a). Beef tallow, a highly saturated fat, may have an effect at or before exposure to the carcinogen, but the determinants of the effect at initiation are not yet known.

Contributions of fatty acid composition, of the antioxidants butylated hydroxyanisole (BHA) and butylated hydroxy toluene (BHT), to the effect of lard, which is somewhat variable, or evidence of contaminating estrogenic or toxic or carcinogenic compounds were not observed in an extensive series of experiments examining time of the activity of lard (Rogers et al., 1986).

Tables 12, 13, and 14 list only a small fraction of the many hundreds of studies that have been reported. A majority of the studies about dietary fat and mammary tumorigenesis have used dimethylbenzanthracene (DMBA), while fewer investigators have used N-methylnitrosourea (MNU) and methylcholanthrene (MCA), among others. The tables list the carcinogen that was used in the individual studies.

Tables 13 and 14 list results obtained in Sprague Dawley rats, using varying doses of DMBA (Rogers and Lee, 1986), different routes of administration, and variation in the duration of the studies. The ability to use a single dose of carcinogen has permitted investigators to delineate, with some degree of precision, effects of dietary fat on the initiation or promotion stages, or on both. Table 14 lists results of studies using semi-purified diets, compared to those fed crude "chow-type" diets, as shown in Table 13. Also, routes of administration of the carcinogen were varied.

Table 12 lists the results of administering a single dose of DMBA or MNU to rats fed 4-5% dietary fat. There did not appear to be any appreciable difference between the groups fed the two types of diet. This is somewhat different from other tumor target sites where the crude ingredient type diets usually protect against carcinogenesis (Newberne et al., 1985).

Mammary tumors induced in rats by a single dose of DMBA are comprised of a spectrum of morphologic characteristics ranging from benign fibroadenomas to adenomas, and to papillomas with hyperplastic, atypical or dysplastic epithelium. There are also significant stromal and myoepithelial components as well, in those tumors which are cytologically malignant or which invade surrounding tissues. Russo et al. (1983) have described the histological characteristics of these tumors in detail.

Carcinogenesis, toxicokinetics, metabolic activation of DMBA, as well as specific aspects of these mammary carcinogens is given by Rogers and Lee (1986). There are a number of factors in addition to fat that can influence ex-

Table 12 Mammary Gland Tumor Histology in Rats Given a Single Dose of DMBA or MNU at 50-60 Days and Fed Diets Containing 4-5% Fat

Carcinogen	Dose (mg)	Weeks carcinogen to necropsy	Mammary tumors No./Rat	Mammary tumors % Malignant	Reference
DMBA	20	32	3.8	81	McCormick et al., 1982
DMBA	16	2	6.4	74	McCormick et al., 1985
DMBA	8	30	3.2	34	
DMBA	8	30	2.2	26	McCormick et al., 1984
DMBA	20	28	2.5		Isaas, 1985
	15	28	1.5		
	10	28	0.7		
	5	28	0.2		
	2.5	28	0.04		
DMBA	7.5	19	1.2	100	Sylvester et al., 1986a
DMBA	2.5	10-12	0.5	17	Rogers et al., 1986
MNU	50	3.	3.2	82	Grubbs et al., 1983a
MNU	50	26	3.5	78	Grubbs et al., 1983b
MNU	35	–	2.3	79	McCormick et al., 1983

Table 13 Mammary Tumors Induced by DMBA in 50-60-day-old, Female Sprague-Dawley Rats Fed Natural Ingreedient Diets

			Mammary tumors			
Dose (mg)	Route	Weeks DMBA-Necropsy	Latency[a] (wks)	Incidence	No./Rat at Risk	Reference
20	ig	28	20	60	0.7	Minton et al., 1983
20	ig	17	7	85	2.6	Thompson et al., 1982
15	ig	40	16	89	1.0	
20	ig	11	–	100	3.9	Welsch and Dehogg, 1983
5	ig	26	–	85	2.0	
15	ig	30	–	75	1.6	Moon et al., 1976
5	ig	30	–	46	0.6	
8	ig	30	14	88	8.6	McCormick et al., 1984
5	ig	28	22	63	2.4	Welsch et al., 1981a
5	iv	16	11	72	2.7	Sylvester et al., 1983
1	sc[b]	–	9	100	1.0	Sinho and Dao, 1980
0.5	sc[b]	19	12	63	0.63	Jabara and Anderson, 1972
0.1	sc[b]	19	17	30	0.30	Jabara and Anderson, 1972

[a]DMBA to first palpable tumor.
[b]Applied locally to the surgically exposed gland.

Table 14 Mammary Tumors Induced by DMBA Given to 50-55-day-old Female Sprague-Dawley Rats Fed Purified Control Diets Containing 3.5% Fat[a]

DMBA		Weeks DMBA to Necropsy	Mammary Tumors		No./Rats at risk	Reference
Dose (mg)	Route		Latency[b]	Incidence		
5	ig	17	–	70	2.3	Hopkins and Carroll, 1979
		17	11	77	2.3	Carroll and Khor, 1981
5	ig	20-22	–	46	1.3	Ip and Ip, 1981
		22	17	44	1.0	Carter et al., 1983
2.5	ig	35	16	68	1.4	Rogers et al., 1986
		35	22	83	1.7	Lee and Rogers, 1983
		10-12	9	78	2.9	Rogers et al., 1986
5	iv	16	10	88	5.4	Alysworth et al., 1984a
2.5	iv	19	13	83	1.7	Rogers et al., 1986
1	sc	19	6	84	1.8	Rogers et al.,1986
0.5	sc	25	15	79	1.3	Rogers et al., 1986
0.25	sc	17	11	80	1.3	Rogers et al., 1986

[a]Fat included polyunsaturated vegetable oils and mixed or largely saturated animal fats.
[b]DMBA to first palpable tumor: some values read from graphs.

perimental mammary cancer. These include protein (which appears to have only limited influence), alcohol, selenium and retinoids, antioxidants and cruciferous vegetables, among others, which reduce risk; however, the results are variable. Overall, unsaturated fat has the most profound, consistent effect in these models. The intervention studies now underway in women at high risk of breast cancer should provide the evidence needed to determine if adjusting our fat intake downward will decrease risk for mammary cancer (Clifford et al., 1986).

Perhaps the next most studied aspect of fat in relation to cancer risk, aside from the breast, is that of the gastrointestinal tract, particularly the large bowel. In these investigations dietary fat has been associated with cancer at a number of sites along the gastrointestinal tract, including the stomach and the large bowel, but major emphasis has been placed on the latter.

A correlation between mortality and cancer of the large intestine and per capita total fat intake was reported by Knox (1977). Others have reported varying results from epidemiologic studies in relation to cancer of the large bowel and fat intake, but the correlations have been largely based on international studies. Studies from individual countries have been less convincing and, generally, have not shown a significant correlation between total fat intake and large bowel cancer (Lyon and Sorenson, 1978; Bingham et al., 1979; Enig et al., 1979; Kolonel and Marchand, 1986).

The diets of Danish residents are associated with a high risk and that of the Finns with a low risk for colon cancer based on food fat content. Consumption of total fat is similar for both groups, but the differences in fiber may account for part of the variation of large bowel cancer. Phillips (1975) has also reported a direct association between colon cancer and the frequent consumption of high fat food in studies about Seventh Day Adventists in the United States. Dales et al. (197) observed a direct association between colon cancer and frequent consumption of foods high in saturated fat, the association stronger for those who consumed the diets not only high in saturated fat but also low in fiber content. Numerous investigations clearly point to a suggestion for fat and colon cancer interactions, but many of the data are conflicting and difficult to interpret (Haenszel et al., 1973, 1980; Bjelke, 1975; Howell, 1975; Graham et al., 1978). The data of Enstrom (1980) points out that trends in beef intake (and thus fat intake) in the United States do not correlate with trends in the incidence of colorectal cancer, either from incidence or from mortality.

As noted by Kolonel and Marchand (1986), the epidemiologic evidence for dietary fat as a risk factor for colon cancer is inconsistent. Moreover, the metabolic studies are equally divided and are of no help in attempting to inerpret epidemiologic data. Based on current evidence, one cannot conclude that dietary fat either promotes colon carcinogenesis or, in fact, has a significant role in human colon cancer. This seems clear despite the continued reports by some (Reddy, 1986), supporting at best a weak association between dietary fat and colon cancer in humans and rodents.

As noted above, human data on dietary fat and colon cancer are at best inconsistent and inconslusive. The data on animal studies are even less convincing; there is no good conclusive evidence for a positive effect of fat on colon cancer induced by chemicals. Some of these studies are described here.

One of the earlier demonstrations that dietary fat might have an effect on colon carcinogenesis was a report by Nigro et al. (1975). These investigators demonstrated that rats, under the conditions their study, treated with AOM, developed more intestinal tumors when fed a diet containing 35% beef fat, compared to those fed a regular "chow-type" control diet that contained considerably less fat. These data are difficult to interpret because the laboratory chow used in these studies was an ill-defined diet with varied components, and one cannot effectively sort out the influence of calories and other factors from fat on tumorigenesis.

Reddy et al. (1977, 1981, 1986) have produced a number of reports regarding large bowel carcinogenesis induced by DMH or AOM and the effects of quality and quantity of fat on incidence and multiplicity of tumors. These investigators have reported that rats fed 20% beef fat had a significant increase in the incidence of colon tumors compared to those fed 5% fat. In some of these studies it didn't appear to matter whether the fat was saturated or unsaturated; it was associated with about the same tumor incidence. It appeared from these studies that the animals ate the same quantity of diet but since the caloric density of low and high fat diet differed, those eating the high fat diets received more calories. Other investigators have also reported on the effects of dietary fat on carcinogenesis in rodents; the data are equivocal; when examined in detail as to the dietary composition, the effect of fats on colon carcinogenesis is inconclusive (Broitman, 1981).

Experiments in our laboratory using both DMH (which requires metabolic activation) and NMU (a direct-acting carcinogen) to induce colon tumors in rats have failed to support the hypothesis that quality and quantity of fat in our experimental systems influence carcinogenesis (Nauss et al., 1983). We have observed no effect on tumor incidence by either the quality (corn oil, beef fat, or Crisco) or the quantity (5%, 20%, or 24%) of fat on tumor induction (Table 15). More recently, we have published a report comparing two strains of rats (Sprague-Dawley and Fischer 344) and two levels of dietary fat. When compared as to fat-treatment groups, there was no difference in tumor incidence or frequency among the groups fed low or high fat concentration in the diet. However, when each rat was placed in a group with similar caloric intake, those of the Sprague-Dawley strain developed colon cancer in a dose-related fashion that correlated with caloric intake (Table 16). The Fischer strain did not exhibit such an effect (Newberne and Nauss, 1986). These data are similar to those reported by Clinton and Visek (1986) with DMBA-induced mammary cancer.

Table 15 Three Studies Demonstrating No Effect of Dietary Fat on Chemically Induced Colon Cancer in Rats

	Study 1 DMH (ig)[a]		Study 2 NMU (ir)[b]		Study 3[c] DMH(ig vs. sc) ig		sc	
Dietary fat ( )	Incidence[d]	Frequency[e]	Incidence	Frequency	Incidence	Frequency	Incidence	Frequency
Mixed fat (5)	77	1.6	55	1.6	—	—	—	—
Corn oil (5)	—	—	—	—	63	1.4	58	1.3
Beef oil (24)	63	1.5	63	1.4	—	—	—	—
Corn oil (24)	63	1.4	55	1.2	68	1.3	48	1.6
Crisco (24)	55	1.5	38	1.1	—	—	—	—

Abbreviations: DMH, 1,2-dimethylhydrazine; NMU, N-methylnitrosourea; ig, intragastric; sc, subcutaneous; ir, intrarectal.
[a]Nauss et al., 1983; total dose = 75 mg DMH, 2HCl/kg body wt.
[b]Nauss et al., 1984; total dose NMU, 6 mg/rat.
[c]Locniskar et al., 1985; total dose 15 mg DMH, 2HCl/kg body wt.
[d]Incidence = No. of animals in a group bearing colon tumors (n = 40).
[e]Frequency = No. of tumors per tumor-bearing rat.

Table 16 Effect of Caloric Intake on Colon Tumor Incidence and Frequency[a]

	Food intake interval		
	Lower third	Middle third	Upper third
SPRAGUE-DAWLEY			
Tumor incidence (%)	23	30	58
Total No. of colon tumors	12	15	33
Mean caloric intake (k cal/day)	45 ± 3	53 ± 2	64 ± 5
Mean body wt. (g)	401 ± 40	424 ± 30	461 ± 63
FISCHER 344			
Tumor incidence 9(%)	33	20	38
Total No. of colon tumors	17	12	17
Mean caloric intake (kcal/day)	30 ± 3	36 ± 1	42 ± 3
Mean body wt. (g)	253 ± 30	252 ± 34	283 ± 42

[a]Measured after three months on experimental diets. Animals divided into three intervals according to food consumption (n + 40 rats/interval).
Results expressed as mean + S.D.

There are a number of reports in the literature relative to the influence of cholesterol on human and animal cancer (Liu et al., 1979; Broitman, 1981). Pearce and Dayton (1971) clearly indicated, in a study using groups of over 400 men in each trial treatment, that those fed high levels of polyunsaturated fats as a means of lowering serum cholesterol had a much higher incidence of cancer deaths than those fed a conventional diet. Other studies have suggested a similar effect (Miettinen et al., 1972). However, Ederer et al. (1971), in examining five control trials of cholesterol-lowering diets, failed to find any significant difference in relative risks between those fed the diet affecting serum cholesterol concentrations and those that did not receive cholesterol-lowering diets. There are numerous other epidemiologic reports in the literature to which the reader may turn for further information (Bjelke, 1974; Rose and Shipley, 1980; Rose et al., 1981).

Results of studies referred to above are conflicting and inconsistent. Nevertheless, cholesterol as well as other lipids may have an influence on certain types of carcinogenesis and certain types of cancer, in part by way of its influence on cell membranes. This must yet be established, however.

A brief word regarding the relationship of fecal steroid excretion and bowel carcinogenesis is in order at this point. It has been pointed out by a number of investigators that the metabolites of fats in the colon of individuals at risk might provide a carcinogenic effect with evidence to confirm or deny an influence of dietary fat on colon cancer. The amounts of neutral and acidic fecal steroids correspond quite well to the level of dietary fat intake. Studies of the ratios of primary to secondary bile acids or the ratio of cholesterol to its metabolic products reveal no differences among populations at risk or those that are not at risk for large bowel cancer (Ederer, 1971; Moskowitz et al., 1979; Mower et al., 1979; Miller et al., 1981). A number of other investigators have alluded to evidence for and against the influence of dietary fat on potential carcinogens produced from bile acids, but the evidence is at best equivocal.

VITAMINS

Vitamin A (Retinoids)

Of all vitamins considered to date with respect to lowering risk for some forms of cancer, the family of retinoids have been given greatest emphasis. This class of substances is comprised broadly of naturally occurring forms of vitamin A, of synthetic analogues, and of selected carotenoids, particularly alpha- and beta-carotene. Some studies have yielded encouraging results (Kummet and Meyskens, 1983; Meyskens, 1984; Sporn and Roberts, 1986), particularly with the synthetic compounds (13-*cis* retinoic acid and others), while others of this class, as well as preformed vitamin A, have been disappointing (Willett, 1986).

Vitamin A is a generic term for a family of substances possessing vitamin A activity. To these naturally occurring materials have been added a number of synthetic analogues, all of which are now categorized under the generic term "retinoids." While vitamin A was the first vitamin isolated and identified as one of the nutrients of significance to human health, most knowledge about its use and biological effects centers only on its relation to vision. Despite this, there has been an accumulating data base indicating that vitamins A (the retinoids) are very much involved with regulation of cell proliferation and in this way may relate to the neoplastic process (Sporn and Roberts, 1986).

A number of epidemiological investigations have indicated an inverse relationship between "vitamin A" and a variety of cancers of various organ sites, primarily those of the epithelial surfaces (respitatory, urinary, skin), which require vitamin A for their integrity. In the epidemiologic studies the estimates of vitamin A intake have been based primarily on the frequency of ingestion of the group of foods known to be rich in vitamin A, beta-carotene, and certain other members of this family of nutrients The green and yellow vegetables are those most often associated with provitamin A (carotene) in the diet.

For this reason the studies have usually measured an indirect effect of vitamin A or of beta-carotene. However, not all studies with diet or from serum analyses have shown a beneficial effect (Wald et al., 1984; Willett et al., 1984, 1986).

One of the first investigators to report the correlation between vitamin A and lung cancer was Bjelke (1975). This investigator studied Norwegian men and observed lower values for lung cancer cases compared to nonsmokers. Additional studies by Gregor et al. (1980) and MacLennan et al. (1977), while varying somewhat in their assessment, have indicated that those with lung cancer had consumed less vitamin A. Others have also pointed out that lung cancer incidence has varied inversely with carotene intake and with foods that contain higher concentrations of vitamin A (Smith and Jick, 1978, Mettlin et al., 1979; Shekelle et al., 1981).

Mettlin (1979) has pointed to a relationship between vitamin A consumption and urinary bladder cancer. This has also been indicated in cancer of the larynx (Graham et al., 1981), esophagus, (Cook-Mozaffari et al., 1979; Mettlin et al., 1981) and stomach (Higginson, 1966; Sokula, 1976; Hirayama, 1977). More recent cohort studies in the United Kingdom and in the United States have suggested an inverse relationship between serum levels of vitamin A and cancer risk in general (Cambien et al., 1980; Wald et al., 1980, 1984). The latter studies are difficult to interpret because serum levels are usually buffered by liver stores of vitamin A, and these reports have been about populations not generally considered to be deficient in vitamin A. It should be emphasized here, however, that vitamin A deficiency does occur without clinical evidence in the United States and, thus, some subpopulations of our society are potentially at greater risk for cancer because of this deficiency.

There are a number of lines of evidence based on experimental animal models that indicate that vitamin A and other members of the retinoid family have a marked influence on the induction of cancer. These reports include a large number of studies done with the synthetic retinoids, including 13-*cis* retinoic acid (Newberne and McConnell, 1980).

Some of the earlier studies in regard to vitamin A and its influence on neoplasia or on neoplasticlike lesions were actually done in cultures (Crocker and Sander, 1970).There are a number of features in common between early neoplastic lesions in the respiratory tract and those associated with uncomplicated vitamin A deficiency. Squamous metaplasia of the tracheal or bronchial epithelium is associated with both carcinogen-induced changes and with vitamin A deficiency. Crocker and Sander (1970) demonstrated that vitamin A inhibited the induced squamous cell metaplasia and proliferation of the epithelium of the respiratory tract in vitro caused by benzo(a)pyrene. Nettesheim and Williams (1976) found that vitamin A deficiency enhanced the induction of respiratory lesions by 3-methylcholanthrene (MCA); however, the interpretation of these data is difficult. The early lesions have as yet not been established as definitive precursors of cancer, although they are associated with it. It should be reemphasized here that the lesions referred to as "preneoplastic" cannot be take as a priori evidence for exposure to cancer-inducing agents or conditions, or that cancer will develop as a result of these observed tissue alterations.

There are conflicting reports regarding vitamin A effects on cancer induction, some of which derive from studies in our own laboratory. For example, we reported (Smith et al., 1975) that an excess of vitamin A had no inhibitory effect on lung tumors induced by benzo(a)pyrene in hamsters. This is in contrast to the report of Saffiotti et al. (1967), who observed that a high intake of vitamin A appeared to protect against squamous metaplasia and respiratory neoplasms in hamsters induced by benzo(a)pyrene. These data are also difficult to interpret, because it is not clear how the results from different groups of animals and of different experiments were compiled.

Some studies have indicated that certain types of experimental tumors are enhanced by vitamin A. For example, retinyl acetate has been shown to enhance hormone-induced mammary tumorigenesis in mice (Welsch et al., 1981). Rogers et al. (1973) reported that a high intake of vitamin A increased the frequency and incidence of large bowel tumor in rats exposed to DMH.

A number of studies regarding vitamin A and, in particular, the synthetic retinoids have been reported by Sporn et al. (1976, 1979, 1986). This area of research has a great deal of promise because many of the synthetic retinoids have unquestioned inhibitory effects on experimentally induced tumors of many sites in animal models. We have observed a portective effect on lung tumors in hamsters by 13-cis retinoic acid (Newberne and McConnell, 1980). It is still too early to know whether or not these or other animal studies can be extrapolated to human populations. Some very interesting clinical studies are now in progress, which should provide some answers within a few years, relative to the inhibitory effects of retinoids on cancer in subsets of human populations at high risk (Meyskens, 1984; Butrum, 1986; Clifford et al., 1986).

In addition to vitamin A and synthetic retinoids, a major interest has focused recently on the carotenoids, particularly beta-carotene. These are the precursors of vitamin A in mammalian systems; carotenoids can be converted into vitamin A in vivo. In addition, in humans and in some animal species, they are absorbed unchanged from the gastrointestinal tract and are stored in tissues throughout the body, particularly in the fat storage depots. Peto et al. (1981) have put forth the hypothesis that beta-carotene, rather than vitamin A, may be the beneficial factor in tumor inhibition when carotenoids are consumed.

Matthews-Roth et al. (1977) reported that beta-carotene and phytoene exert a significant protective effect against the development of ultraviolet-induced skin tumors in hairless mice. Phytoene does not have vitamin A activity; thus, any protective effect that is exerted must reside in the carotenoid structure per se rather than in its being converted to vitamin A and acting through this mechanism. In addition, Shamberger (1971), in some earlier studies, reported a relationship between carotene and carcinogenesis. This investigator conducted studies in which beta-carotene was applied to the skin of mice along with croton oil; it was observed that this treatment increased the incidence of epidermal tumors initiated by DMBA. Thus, more research is required into the actions of vitamin A and the carotenoids in relation to carcinogenesis before it can be said with certainty that vitamin A and the retinoids, including carotenes and carotenoids, are effective in inhibiting or reducing the incidence or frequency of certain types of cancer in animals and in human populations.

It should be noted here that there are at least two major studies now in progress (Butrum et al.,1986) designed to learn more about carotenoids and retinoids in humans. One deals with food analysis and the other with the metabolism and physiology of these important substances in humans.

Vitamin C (Ascorbic Acid)

Reports appeared in the literature in 1960 noting that consuming foods rich in ascorbic acid was inversely related to the appearance of certain types of cancer (Meinsma, 1964; Higginson, 1966). Shortly thereafter there were other reports that suggested that vitamin C protected against gastric cancer, perhaps by blocking the reaction of secondary amines with nitrite to form N-nitroso compounds, some of which are gastric carcinogens (Kolonel et al., 1981).

Some of the epidemiologic studies conducted early in the 1970s were concerned with human populations along the Caspian littoral of Iran. In these studies there was an inverse association between esophageal cancer and the consumption of fresh fruits that contain ascorbic acid (Cook-Mozaffari et al., 1975, 1979; Hormozdiari et al., 1975; Cook-Mozaffari, 1979). More recently, another report has appeared (Wassertheil-Smoller et al., 1981), which indicates an inverse relationship between vitamin C consumption and uterine cervical dysplasia in women in New York. On the other hand, Jain et al. (1980) failed to find an association between ascorbic acid consumption and colon cancer in a case control study. There is additional evidence suggesting a role for ascorbic acid from animal studies. It has been shown conclusively that ascorbic acid can prevent nitrosation of amines, which in turn prevents the formation of nitrosamines, some of which are gastric carcinogens (Mirvish et al., 1972, 1981).

Vitamin E

To date there is no epidemiologic evidence to suggest that vitamin E has an influence on risk for cancer in humans. The only seemingly possible correlation may be through studies related to the consumption of certain foods that contain vitamin E. These, however, are still speculative and will not be covered in this report.

Data in the literature indicate that vitamin E or alpha-tocopherol can have an influence on tumors induced in experimental animals. There is some indication that vitamin E acts similarly to ascorbic acid in blocking the formation of nitrosamines. Vitamin E is fat-soluble, and nitric oxide nitrosation takes place most easily in lipophilic solvents. Thus, inhibition of nitrosation through this mechanism can occur in a lipid milieu; blocking of nitrosation by ascorbate occurs in the gastrointestinal tract, an aqueous environment.

Several investigators have studied the effects of alpha-tocopherol on DMBA-induced mammary tumors in animals (Newberne, 1985) and other types of experimental cancer. The well-known effect of vitamin E as a blocking agent in nitrosation confirms a role as a protective agent in the environment, however. Segregating the effects of ascorbic acid from alpha-tocopherol on blocking nitrosation is yet to be done but, as noted above, one (vitamin C) is hydrophilic while the other (vitamin E) is lipophilic.

Choline and Other B Vitamins

A number of the B vitamins have been investigated in relation to their effects on experimental cancer. Much earlier work was complicated by failure to control for the intake of other dietary nutrients, particularly protein and total calories. Some of the data are in fact conflicting or negative in terms of the protective effects of B vitamins on cancer (Kensler, 1941; Boutwell et al., 1949). In other cases some of the B vitamins have been shown to have a protective effect, primarily through the influence on metabolic pathways of carcinogens. Kensler et al. (1941) demonstrated that riboflavin offered some protection against live liver cancer caused by azo dyes in rats because it enhanced the detoxification of the carcinogen by a flavin-dependent enzyme system. On the other hand, instead of a protective effect, one can envision that riboflavin might also be an enhancer under some conditions, particularly if it is required for activation of the parent compound to the ultimate carcinogen.

The complex interrelationships between the B vitamins choline, methionine, folic acid, and B_{12} have been examined in detail with reference to effects on tumor induction by N-nitroso compounds, mycotoxins, and polycyclic aromatic hydrocarbons. The most consistent results obtained with animals fed diets low in the lipotropic factors choline and methionine are an enhancement of cancer of the liver, the pancreas, and, to a lesser extent, the colon. The diets used by Newberne and Rogers (1986) do not have a consistent effect on tumor induction in target organs other than the liver and the colon. The effects of lipotropic agents on carcinogenesis appear to be mediated through effects on metabolism, but other possible mechanisms are under investigation. Based on observations in human populations and in laboratory animals, sources of methyl groups (choline, methionine, protein) and of transfer factors (folate, B_{12}) are highly important in risk for liver cancer and perhaps for cancer at other sites (Newberne et al., 1983).

A concerted effort has been applied in recent years to determine whether or not the metabolism and transport of B-complex vitamins or of the binding of the appropriate coenzyme forms to apoenzymes are altered in tumor cells (Bell et al., 1972; Thanassi et al., 1981; Tryfiates, 1981). In some cases the transport and binding of the coenzyme forms have been reported but it is not known whether these alterations have any influence on the induction of or protection from carcinogenesis.

Thus the B vitamins require considerably more investigation to determine whether or not they are related to human cancer and to further elucidate their real or potential role in experimental animal models. At this point there are no valid conclusions on B vitamins except in the case of experimental models consuming diets low in lipotropic factors where it has been clearly shown that they do play a role in susceptibility to chemical carcinogenesis. The lipotropes appear to be associated with methylation or hypomethylation of nucleic acids and by this mechanisms may influence control of cell replication. This issue is receiving significant attention in a number of laboratories in regard to control mechanisms to cell proliferation.

MINERALS

There are very few studies reported in the literature relative to the effects of oral ingestion of minerals on carcinogenesis. Only in recent years has there emerged an interest in regard to some of the trace elements; the macroelements (Ca, P, Mg) have been largely ignored. Many of the studies reported in experimental systems have been associated with parenteral administration of essential and of toxic agents. These studies have been reviewed in some detail and will not be covered further in this review (Sunderman, 1977). While the results of these studies are interesting, insofar as target organ toxicity is concerned they have done little to elucidate the risk or protective effects of trace minerals in the amounts that occur naturally in the diet or in the environment of humans.

Selenium

In the 1930s an association was clearly identified between selenium deficiency or excess and important livestock diseases. The discovery that selenosis (an excess) and selenium deficiency occurred in some animal species was reponsible for mapping the distribution of selenium in the soils and in plant foods in animal and human tissues in the United States and other countries. It is important to know what is in the soil because, of all of the elements that are dependent upon the soil concentration for transport into plants and animal tissues, selenium is the most prominent member of the trace elements directly related to soil content. When there is an excess, some plants tend to concentrate selenium, and when the deficiency is moderate to severe the plants contain very little of it. Because of this, food products grown on such soils are directly affected by the selenium content of the soil.

The National Academy of Sciences issued a report in 1971 (Selenium in Nutrition, 1971) on epidemiological correlations of diseases in humans and in animals and pointed the way for investigators to further develop knowledge regarding selenium.

Shamberger and colleagues (Shamberger and Frost, 1969; Shamberger, 1970; Shamberger and Willis, 1971; Shamberger et al., 1973, 1976) have reported in numerous publications on the relationship between selenium and cancer. They reported an inverse relationship for cancer of the gastrointestinal and genitourinary tracts with the selenium content of staple foods. Shamberger and colleagues (1973) examined the selenium levels in the blood of 100 cancer patients and compaed these with the selenium content in the blood of 48 normal subjects. The analyses revealed that patients with gastrointestinal cancer and Hodgkin's disease had significantly lower levels of selenium than normal subjects, but there were no differences between normal individuals and patients with cancer at other sites.

Results of experimental animals studies with selenium have been controversial and inconsistent as to the evidence for a carcinogenic or protective role for this important element. Studies conducted at the FDA during the 1940s indicated that high levels of selenium induced or enhanced liver tumor formation (Nelson et al., 1943). In addition, results of studies from Russia (Volgarev and Tscherkes, 1967), reported two decades later, suggested that animals given high selenium supplements in the diet developed liver cirrhosis as well as heptocellular carcinoma.

There are a number of major defects in both of these studies; the Food and Drug Administration investigators used diets that were low in protein or with protein of poor quality, both of which can adversely affect the liver. In addition, the natural products were suspected of contamination with the natural heaptocarcinogen, aflatoxin. The Russian studies did not use a selenium-free control group.

There is an accumulation of data that clearly indicates a protective role, in animal models, for selenium against certain types of tumors. For example, Schrauzer et al. (1978) reported that breast tumors in female C3H mice were reduced from 82% in controls to 10% in selenium-supplemented mice. Harr et al. (1972) and Ip and Sinha (1981) demonstrated beneificial effects of supplementation of selenium at dietary concentrations hardly above those exhibiting physiological effects. An interesting aspect of the studies by Ip and Sanha related to their finding that the incidence of mammary tumors, induced by DMBA, was enhanced by diets high in polyunsaturated fats and by a dietary deficiency of selenium. Supplementation at a level of 0.1 μg/g, barely above the nutritional requirements, resulted in protection against tumor formation.

Numerous other investigators have reported an effect of selenium on tumor incidence in animal models; generally it has reduced the incidence or frequency of tumor of various sites (Shamberger, 1970, Griffin, 1979; Medina, 1980; Thompson and Becci, 1984; Ip, 1985).

We have examined the acute and chronic effects of selenium on aflatoxin-induced tissue damage, which clearly indicated an effect of selenium within the range of safety concentrations for animals (Newberne and Conner, 1974). For example, the acute effects of aflatoxin are enhanced by either a deficiency or an excess of selenium; these observations carry over into the chronic effects (Newberne and McConnell, 1980), where it is clear that a protective effect is exerted by levels somewhat higher than nutritional needs. When a toxic level and above is reached, however, the carcinogenic effect is enhanced (Newberne et al., 1987).

Further studies in our laboratory (unpublished) have shown that selenium, interacting with various fats, does indeed have an effect on biological response but that this does not appear to be through its influence on modulating tissue peroxidation. These data point to a potentially very important aspect of the biological activity of selenium. It appears that the in vivo and in vitro effects of selenium may be to decrease the activity of hydroxylating enzymes that activate parent chemical, such as aflatoxin B, to their reactive carcinogenic metabolites. This appears to be one of the mechanisms of action of selenium, in this case acting through glucuronyltransferase (GSH-TX) (Bansel et al., 1978). However, additional effects may be through the selenium-dependant enzyme glutathione peroxidase (GSH-PZ).

The report of the National Academy of Sciences (1971) alluded to the effects of selenium on certain biological systems. It was reported that while the mechanism of action is not clear, selenium does protect against acute and chronic toxicity of some of the heavy metals, and this protection does not appear to be through an increased elimination of the toxic elements. Rather, it appears that there is an increased accumulation of nontoxic forms of the heavy metal.

The animal data regarding selenium and cancer strongly suggest an effect of this trace element on the induction of cancer in animal models, but the limited evidence does not permit firm conclusions. There are suggestions for an effect of selenium on the rate of DNA repair and on its influence on activating enzymes. In addition it appears to influence the cell cycle by extending the time for the G_2/M phase (Medina and Shepherd, 1980). It is clear that increasing selenium to a point just below the toxic level protects against certain types of tumors in animals; in other cases the results are equivocal or negative. This area of nutrition and cancer is open for some fruitful further investigations (Petering et al., 1967; Dewys and Pories, 1972; Duncan and Dreosti, 1975; Fong et al., 1978; Gabrial et al., 1982; Newberne and Rogers, 1986).

Zinc

The question of whether or not zinc is involved in cancer risk has been raised only recently. An hypothesis has been based on assumptions made from a few studies in human populations (Gyorkey et al., 1967; Strain et al., 1972; Lin et al., 1977; Van Rensburg, 1981) and a number of animal experiments (Petering et al., 1967; DeWys and Pories, 1972; Fong et al., 1978).

Zinc is essential to more than 100 enzyme systems; furthermore, it has been demonstrated to be effective in reversing certain types of diseases in human populations and its role in animal nutrition has been established for many decades. It is also accepted that severe zinc deficiency does occur in humans and that more moderate forms of deficiency are not uncommon (Prasad, 1978).

Zinc deficiency in humans and in animals results in depressed immune function in both the cell-mediated and humoral arms of the system (Golden et al., 1978; Gross and Newberne, 1980; Beisel, 1982). The levels of zinc in blood and other body issues have been examined in cancer patients and compared to controls by a number of investigators. Schrauzer et al. (1977a,b) demonstrated that the mean zinc concentration in food and in blood correlated inversely with mortality rates from cancer of the large bowel, breast, ovary, lung, bladder, and oral cavity. Strain et al. (1972), in patients with bronchogenic carcinoma, observed that zinc levels differed between the cancer patient and age-matched controls. Furthermore, copper levels were lower in controls resulting in high ratios of zinc to copper in cancer patients. Davies et al. (1968) had reported earlier that the level of zinc in the plasma of bronchogenic carcinoma patients was lower than that for other patients with other types of cancer and was also lower than normal laboratory values.

We have reported levels of zinc in serum, hair, and from the diseased but noncancerous esophageal tissue from esophageal cancer patients significantly lower than levels from patients with other types of cancer, with patients with other types of disease, or in normal subject (Lin et al., 1977). The concentration of zinc in the hair, serum, and soft tissues was lower in all cancer patients than in normal subjects. Furthermore, the serum of such patients had much lower iron levels than normal subjects.

The studies of Petering et al. (1967), working with transplanted Walker 256 carcinoma in rats, showed that zinc deficiency inhibited the growth of transplanted tumors in animals and also prolonged survival time. These data were confirmed by DeWys and Poires (1972). The effects of zinc were extended to leukemia, lung carcinoma, and plasmacytoma TEPC-183 (Fenton et al., 1980).

While these observations are not surprising in view of the fact that rapidly growing tissues require zinc for cell proliferation, they are in contrast to animal studies conducted in our own laboratory using the esophagus as the tumor target organ (Gabrial et al., 1982; Newberne et al., 1985). We have consistently observed an enhancing effect of zinc deficiency on nitrosamine-induced esophageal cancer. In our model the enhancing effect by zinc deficiency is further enhanced by administration of ethanol.

A major research need is to determine why the esophagus epithelium in zinc deficiency increases DNA synthesis and cell proliferation, whereas this slows down in all other tissues of the same animal.

Zinc supplementation over and above the nutritional requirements has not, in our hands, had any effect on tumor inhibition. Poswillo and Cohen (1971), on the other hand, have reported that a high level of dietary zinc, greatly exceeding the nutritional requirements, suppressed the carcinogenic effect of DMBA in hamsters. Additional evidence for an effect of excess zinc was reported also by Duncan and Dreosti (1975).

Conflicting reports from our laboratory and other laboratories in regards to zinc deficiency can be explained largely on the basis of the target tissue. As noted above, zinc deficiency inhibits the growth of all tissues in mammals so far examined, with the exception of esophagus. In this case a zinc deficiency actually enhances the proliferative activity of esophageal epithelium, permitting more cells to be exposed to the carcinogenic process. This very likely provides the explanation for the conflicting results reported from several laboratories.

From the foregoing conclusions it seems clear that the epidemiologic evidence, while suggestive, is not yet available to make specific comments on the effects of zinc and human cancer, but in experimental animal models it does have a profound effect; the results of the studies depend on the tissue examined and the animal model used in the investigation.

SUMMARY AND CONCLUSION

The field of research into the relationship of nutrients to many different types of cancer has received considerable emphasis during the past several years. The National Academy of Sciences report on Diet, Nutrition and Cancer (1982) served as a focal point for generating scientific interest and stimulating research in a science that heretofore has been considered by many scientists as too "soft" to bother with. This has changed radically during the last few years, and prominent scientists from other areas of biology have taken up the challenge and are now conducting intensive studies into the role of specific macro- and micronutrients in modulating risk for cancer. As a result, the complexity and significance of nutrition to human health has become more apparent and the level of appreciation for what we eat has been raised in the minds of both the scientific and lay communities.

Total calories, from whatever source, appears to be of considerable significance in some studies but not in others. The animal data for effects of calories are stronger than epidemiologic data, but studies into calorie/cancer interrelationships are sparse.

The available evidence suggests that dietary protein consumed in excess quantities over long periods of time may raise the level of risk for certain types of cancers. While only suggestive from epidemiological studies, data from controlled animal studies support the hypothesis that protein modifies risk, probably through the influence of protein on enzyme systems responsible for activating or deactivating carcinogens. There is no convincing evidence, however, that beef should be singled out as special risk, as some have proposed, because the incidence of colon cancer, with which it has been associated, has remained about constant over the past 50 years, while beef consumption has more than doubled during the same period. Nevertheless, some modest reduction in total red meat consumption and substitution of chicken and fish is appropriate in terms of overall health.

The case for fiber effects on colon cancer does not appear to be as strong as the original hypothesis suggested when Burkitt first proposed it. He suggested that dietary fiber prevents colon cancer after comparing the available evidence from economically developed countries, where colon cancer is common, to developing countries, where colon cancer is uncommon. Since that time, numerous epidemiologic and experimental investigations have been conducted, none of which has provided a weight of evidence that permits a conclusion that fiber does, in fact, prevent or reduce risk for colon cancer. There are about as many negative as there are positive studies. In sum total, however, this investigator believes that some increase in fiber consumption by Western populations is justified. Sources of fiber recommended include wheat, as a source of bran, and suitable fruits and vegetables.

The suggestion that an African diet protects against colon cancer fails to take into consideration that fiber is not the only difference between African and Western diets; protein, starch, and fat are different also. Moreover, endemic diseases of the gastrointestinal tract differ between the two populations.

It would seem from available data that to dilute the stool, and thus any real or potential carcinogenic chemical or condition in the colon, would not be a bad idea. This can be achieved by consuming bran, particularly wheat bran. To properly nourish the colonic mucosa and maintain an appropriate cell turnover, volatile fatty acids may be important, and these can be derived from cellulose, hemicellulose, and pectins present in fruits and vegetables.

The fat content of the diet has perhaps come in for more consideration with respect to cancer risk than any other component. Much of the data derive from the disappearance rate of fat from countries and these compared to populations where breast cancer is in high or low incidence. Intercountry data are convincing in that a high rate of disappearance of fat correlates well with a high incidence of breast cancer. Intracountry comparisons are much less sound. Intervention studies are in progress but the conjectures about the potential value of decreasing fat consumption in high risk populations are just that—conjecture. The enthusiasm has outrun the data, and we must await results of well-controlled studies before broad sweeping recommendations to the public should be made.

The case for dietary fat and its effect on colon cancer is much less sound than for fat and breast cancer. While the postulations are logical that fat increases bile acid secretion and this in turn affects colon mucosal cell turnover, along with providing putative procarcinogens, the linkage is lacking. As pointed out by Kolonel (1986), the data from human studies leave much to be desired with about as many negative as positive epidemiologic studies and with little if any support as yet from metabolic epidemiologic observations.

The studies in animals purporting to show a positive effect of high fat diets on induced colon cancer are equivocal at best. If one examines the data critically, it will be concluded that there is no evidence for either quality or quantity of dietary fat affecting incidence or frequency of colon cancer in rodents.

At this point, the vitamins that appear to be of significance to human cancer are the retinoids, the family of natural and synthetic vitamin A-active substances, and the carotenoids. Much of the data are from animal studies, but the results of well-controlled investigations are so interesting and significant that human intervention trials have been initiated and results are eagerly awaited. The epidemiologic data suggesting that green and yellow vegetables have protective properties for some types of human tumors probably reflect a feeling for their content of carotenoids.

Minerals have received much less attention with regard to cancer risk than the nutrients listed above. However, some epidemiologic data and a significant amount of animal information strongly suggest a protective role for zinc and selenium. There are numerous examples where these two important essential nutrients may be in short supply or biologically unavailable in some human subpopulations.

Until more specific data become available from well-designed studies, overall, the recommendations for a well-rounded, balanced diet, consumed in moderation, may be our best approach to lowering risk for cancer. These were suggested by grade school teachers and public health personnel as early as 40 years ago and more recently have been recommended by the National Academy of Sciences and the National Cancer Institute. Foods from the four basic food groups should be consumed on a routine basis; refrain from excessive alcohol consumption; maintain reasonable body weight; and do not use tobacco. Some of the advice being freely offered (i.e., cut fat consumption in half and eat wheat bran to prevent colon cancer) by those who should know better will likely not achieve the proposed goals. Results of ongoing prospective observational and intervention studies will provide the basis for sound recommendations to the public regarding dietary guidelines. Animal research will likely provide the mechanisms whereby nutrients influence risk.

We can be cautiously encouraged by the manner in which nutrition and cancer research is proceeding. If food faddism, natural food enthusiasts, and economically oriented charlatans can be contained, the public should have within a few years access to sound advice based on acceptable data as to how to best feed themselves in order to resist cancer and other chronic diseases. This, of course, assumes that the National Cancer Institute and other funding agencies continue to support the research now in progress or planned.

REFERENCES

Armstrong, B., Doll, R. (1975). Environmental factors and cancer incidence and mortality in different countries with special reference to dietary practices. *Intl. J. Cancer 15*: 617.

Aylsworth, C. F., Van Vugt, D. A., Sylvester, W., Meites, J. (1984a). Role of estrogen and prolactin in stimulation of carcinogen-induced mammary tumor development by a high-fat diet. *Cancer Res. 44*: 2835.

Aylsworth, C. F., Jones, C., Trosko, J. E., Meites, J., Welsch, C. W. (1984b). Promotion of 7,12-dimethylbenz[a] anthracene-induced mammary tumorigenesis by high dietary fat in the rat: Possible role of intercellular communication. *J. Natl. Cancer Inst. 72*: 637.

American Cancer Society Cancer Statistics (1986). New York.

Bansal, B. R., Rhoads, J. E., Jr., Bansal, S. E. (1978). Effects of diet on colon carcinogenesis and the immune system in rats treated with 1,2-dimethylhydrazine. *Cancer Res. 38*: 3293.

Beisel, W. R. (1982). Single nutrients and immunity. *Am. J. Clin. Nutr. 35*: 417.

Bell, E. D., Tong, D., Mainwaring, W. I. P., Hayward, J. L., Bulbrook, R. D. (1972). Tryptophan metabolism and recurrence rates after mastectomy in patients with breast cancer. *Clin. Chim. Acta 42*: 445.

Benson, A. M., Batzinger, R. P., Os, S. L., et al. (1978). Elevation of hepatic glutathione S-transferase activities. *Cancer Res. 38*: 4486.

Berg, J.W., Howell, M. A. (1973). The geographic pathology of bowel cancer. *Cancer 34*: 805.

Berg, J. W. (1975). Can nutrition explain the pattern of international epidemiology of hormone-dependent cancer? *Cancer Res. 35*: 3345.

Bingham, S., Williams, D. R. R., Cole, T. J., James, W. P. T. (1979). Dietary fiber and regional large-bowel cancer mortality in Britain. *Br. J. Cancer 40*: 456.

Bjelke, E. (1974). Letter to the editor: colon cancer and blood-cholesterol. *Lancet 1*: 1116.

Bjelke, E. (1975). Dietary vitamin A and human lung cancer. *Intl. J. Cancer 15*: 561.

Bjelke, E. (1978). Dietary factors and the epidemiology of cancer of the stomach and large bowel. *Akt. Ernahrungs. Klin. Prax.* Suppl. 2: 10.

Boutwell, R. K., Brush, M. K., Rusch, H. P. (1949). The influence of vitamins of the B complex on the induction of epithelial tumors in mice. *Cancer Res. 9*: 747.

Broitman, S. A. (1981). Cholesterol excretion and colon cancer. *Cancer Res. 41*: 3738.

Burkitt, D. P., Trowell, H. C. (1975). Refined carbohydrate foods and disease. In *Some Implications of Dietary Fibre*. Academic Press, New York.

Butrum, R. R., Lanza, E., Clifford, C. K. (1986). The diet and cancer branch NCI: current projects and future research directions. In *Dietary Fat and Cancer*, C. Ip et al. (Eds.). Alan R. Liss, New York, p. 773.

Cambien, F. Ducimetiere, P., Richard J. (1980). Total serum cholesterol and cancer mortality in a middle-aged population. *Am. J. Epidemiol. 112*: 388.

Carroll, K. K., Khor, H. T. (1981). Effects of level and type of deitary fat on incidence of mammary tumors induced in female Sprague-Dawley rats by 7,12-dimethylbenz(a)anthracene. *Lipids 6*: 415.

Carter, C. A., Milholland, R. J., Shea, W., Ip, M. M. (1983). Effect of the prostaglandin synthetase inhibitor indomethacin on 7,12-dimethylbenz(a) anthracene-induced mammary tumorigenesis in rats fed different levels of fat. *Cancer Res. 43*: 3559.

Chen, W. F., Patchefsky, A. S., Goldsmith, H. S. (1978). Colonic protection from dimethylhydrazine by a high fiber diet. *Surg. Gynecol. Obstet. 147*: 503.

Clifford, C. K., Butrum, R. R., Greenwald, P., Yates, J. N. (1986). Clinical trials of low fat diets and breast cancer prevention. In *Dietary Fat and Cancer*, C. Ip et al. (Eds.). Alan R. Liss, New York, p. 93.

Clinton, S. K., Truex, C. G., Visek, W. J. (1979). Dietary protein aryl hydrocarbon hydroxylase and chemical carcinogenesis in rats. *J. Nutr. 109*: 55.

Clinton, S. K., Visek, W. (1986). The macronutrients in experimental carcinogenesis of the breast, colon and In *Dietary Fat and Cancer*, C. Ip et al. (Eds.). Alan R. Liss, New York, p. 377.

Cook-Mozaffari, P. (1979). The epidemiology of cancer of the esophagus. *Nutr. Cancer 1*: 51.

Cook-Mozaffari, P. J., Azordegan, F., Day, N. E., Ressicand, A., Sabal, C., Aramesh, B. (1979). Oesophageal cancer studies in the Caspian littoral of Iran: results of a case-control study. *Br. J. Cancer 39*: 293.

Crocker, T. T., Sander, L. L. (1970). Influence of vitamin A and 3,7-dimethyl-2, 6-octadienal (citral) on the effect of benzo(a)pyrene on hamster trachea in organ culture. *Cancer Res. 30*: 1312.

Dales, L. G., Friedman, G. D., Ury, H. K., Grossman, S., Williams, S. R. (1978). A case-control study of relationships of diet and other traits to colorectal cancer in American blacks. *Am. J. Epidemiol. 109*: 132.

Dao, T. L., Chan, P. C. (1983). Effect of duration of high fat intake on enhancement of mammary carcinogenesis in rats. *J. Natl. Cancer Inst. 71*: 201.

Davies, I. J., Musa, M., Dormandy, T. L. (1968). Measurement of plasma zinc, II. In malignant disease. *J. Clin. Pathol. 21*: 363.

DeWys, W., Proies, W. (1972). Inhibition of a spectrum of animal tumors by dietary zinc deficiency. *J. Natl. Cancer Inst. 48*: 375.

Diet, Nutrition and Cancer. National Academy of Sciences, Washington, D.C., 1982.

Doll, R., Peto, R. (1981). The causes of cancer: quantitative estimates of avoidable risks of cancer in the United States today. *J. Natl. Cancer Inst. 66*: 1191.

Drasar, B., Irving D. (1973). Environmental factors and cancers of the colon and breast. *Br. J. Cancer 27*: 167.

Duncan, J. R., Dreosti, I. E. (1975). Zinc intake, neoplastic DNA synthesis, and chemical carcinogenesis in rats and mice. *J. Natl. Cancer Inst. 55*: 195.

Dyer, A. R., Stamler, J., Paul, O., Shekelle, R. B., Schoenberger, J. A., Berkson, D. M., Lepper, M., Collette, P., Shekelle, S., Lindberg, H. A. (1981). Serum cholesterol and risk of death from cancer and other causes in three Chicago epidemiological studies. *J. Chronic Dis. 34*: 249.

Eastwood, M. (1987). Dietary fiber and the risk for cancer. *Nutrition Reviews 45*: 193.

Ederer, F., Leren, P., Turpeinen, O., Frantz, I. D., Jr. (1971). Cancer among men on cholesterol-lowering diets: experience from five clinical trials. *Lancet 2*: 203.

Engel, R. W., Copeland, D. H. (1952). The influence of dietary casein level on tumor induction with 2-acetylaminofluorene. *Cancer Res. 12*: 905.

Enig, M. G., Munn, R. J., Keeney, M. (1979). Response to letters. *Fed. Proc. Fed. Am. Soc. Exp. Biol. 38*: 2437.

Enstrom, J. E. (1975). Colorectal cancer and consumption of beef and of fat. *Br. J. Cancer 32*: 432.

Enstrom, J. E. (1980). Health and dietary practices in cancer mortality among California Mormons. In *Cancer Incidence in Defined Populations*, airns, J., Lyon, J. L., and Skolnick, M. (Eds.). Cold Spring Harbor Laboratory, New York, p. 69.

Fenton, M. R. Burke, J. P., Tursi, F. D., Arena, F. P. (1980). Effect of a zinc-deficient diet on the growth of an IgM-secreting plasmacytoma (TEPC-183). *J. Natl. Cancer Inst. 65*: 1271.

Fong, L. Y. Y., Sivak, A., Newberne, P. M. (1978). Zinc deficiency and methylnitrosamine-induced esophageal cancer in rats. *J. Natl. Cancer Inst. 61*: 145.

Gabrial, G., Schrager, T., Newberne, P. M. (1982). Zinc deficiency, alcohol and a retinoid: association with esophageal cancer in rats. *J. Natl. Cancer Inst. 68*: 785.

Gaskill, S. P., McGuire, W. L., Osborne, C. K., Stern, M. P. (1979). Breast cancer mortality and diet in the United States. *Cancer Res. 39*: 3628.

Golden, M. H. N., Golden, B. E., Harland, P. S. E., and Jackson, A. A. (1978). Zinc and immunocompetence in protein-energy malnutrition. *Lancet 1*: 1226.

Goldin, Barry R. (1986). The metabolism of the intestinal microflora and its relationship to dietary fat, colon and breast cancer. In *Dietary Fat and Cancer*, C. Ip et al. (Eds.). Alan R. Liss, Inc., New York, p.p. 655-685.

Graham, S., Schotz, W., Martino, P. (1972). Alimentary factors in the epidemiology of gastric cancer. *Cancer 30*: 927.

Graham, S., Dayal, H., Swanson, M., Mittelman, A., Wilkinson, G. (1978). Diet in the epidemiology of cancer of the colon and rectum. *J. Natl. Cancer Inst. 61*: 709.

Graham, S., Mettlin, C., Marshall, J., Priore, R., Rzepka, T., Shedd, D. (1981). Dietary factors in the epidemiology of cancer of the larynx. *Am. J. Epidemiol. 113*: 675.

Greenwald, P. (1984). Manipulation of nutrients to prevent cancer. Hospital Practice, May, pp. 119-134.

Greenwald, P. (1986). Dietary fiber and colon cancer risks, Food Research Institute, Madison, Wisconsin, "Emerging prospectives on colorectal cancer," Oct. 15-16.

Gregor, A., Lee, P. N., Roe, F. J. C., Wilson, M. J., Melton, A. (1980). Comparison of dietary histories in lung cancer cases and controls with special reference to vitamin A. *Nutr. Cancer 2*: 93.

Gregor, O., Toman, R., Prusova, F. (1969). Gastrointestinal cancer and nutrition. *Gut 10*: 1031.

Griffin, A. C. (1979). Role of selenium in the chemoprevention of cancer. *Adv. Cancer Res. 29*: 419.

Gross, R. L., Newberne, P. M. (1980). Role of nutrition in immunologic function. *Physiol. Rev. 60*: 188.

Grubbs, C. J., Peckham, J. C., McDonough, K. D. (1983a). Effect of ovarian hormones on the induction of 1-methyl-1-nitrosourea-induced mammary cancer. *Carcinogenesis 4*: 495.

Grubbs, C. J., Peckham, J. C., Cato, K. D. (1983b). Mammary carcinogenesis in rats in relation to age at time of N-nitroso-N-methylurea administration. *J. Natl. Cancer Inst.*

Gyorkey, F., Min, K. W., Huff, J. A., Gyorkey, F. (1967). Zinc and magnesium in human prostate gland: normal hyperplastic and neoplastic. *Cancer Res. 27*: 1348.

Haenszel, W., Berg, J. W., Segi, M., Kurihara, M., Locke, F. B. (1973). Large-bowel cancer in Hawaiian Japanese. *J. Natl. Cancer Inst. 51*: 1765.

Haenszel, W., Locke, F. B., Segi, M. (1980). A case-control study of large bowel cancer in Japan. *J. Natl. Cancer Inst. 64*: 17.

Harr, J. R., Exon, J. H., Whanger, P. D., Weswig, P. H. (1972). Effect of dietary selenium on N-2-fluorenyl-acetamide (FAA)-induced cancer in vitamin E supplemented, selenium depleted rats. *Clin. Toxicol. 5*: 187.

Hems, G., Stuart, A. (1975). Breast cancer rate in populations of single women. *Br. J. Cancer 31*: 118.

Hems, G. (1978). The contributions of diet and childbearing to breast-cancer rates. *Br. J. Cancer 37*: 974.

Hems, G. (1980). Associations between breast-cancer mortality rates, child bearing and diet in the United Kingdom. *Br. J. Cancer 41*: 429.

Higginson, J. (1966). Etiological factors in gastrointestinal cancer in man. *J. Natl. Cancer Inst. 37*:527.

Hill, M., MacLennan, R., Newcombe, K. (1979). Letter to the editor: Diet and large bowel cancer in three socioeconomic groups in Hong Kong. *Lancet 1*: 436.

Hirayama, T. (1977). Changing patterns of cancer in Japan with special reference to the decrease in stomach cancer mortality. In *Origins of Human Cancer, Book A: Incidence of Cancer in Humans*, Hiatt, H. H., Watson, J. D., and Winsten, J. A. (Eds.). Cold Spring Harbor Laboratory, New York, p. 55.

Hopkins, G. J., Carroll, K. K. (1979). Relationship between amount and type of dietary fat in promotion of mammary carcinogenesis induced by 7,12-dimethylbenzanthracene. *J. Natl. Cancer Inst. 62*: 1009-1012.

Hormozdiari, N., Day, N. E., Aramesh, B., Mahboudi, F. (1975). Dietary factors and esophageal cancer in the Caspian littoral of Iran. *Cancer Res. 35*: 3493.

Howell, M. A. (1975). Diet as an etiological factor in the development of cancers of the colon and rectum. *J. Chronic Dis. 28*: 67.

Ip, C., Ip, M. (1981). Serum estrogens and estrogen responsiveness in 7,12-dimethylbenz(a)anthracene-induced mammary tumors as influenced by dietary fat. *J. Natl. Cancer Inst. 66*: 291.

Ip, C, Sinha, D. K. (1981). Enhancement of mammary tumorigenesis by dietary selenium deficiency in rats with a high polyunsaturated fat intake. *Cancer Res. 41*: 31.

Ip, C. (1985). Selenium inhibition of chemical carcinogenesis. *Fed. Proc. 44*: 2573.

Isaacs, J. T. (1985). Determintion of the number of events required for mammary carcinogenesis in the Sprague-Dawley female rat. *Cancer Res. 45*: 4827.

Jabara, A. G., Anderson, P. S. (1982). Effects of progesterone on mammary carcinogenesis when various doses of DMBA were applied directly to rat mammae. *Pathology 14*:313-316.

Jagerstad, M., Reutersward, A. L., Gruivas, S., et al. (1986). Effects of meat composition and cooking on the formation of mutagenic derivations. In *Diet Nutrition and Cancer*, H. Hayashi et al., (Eds.). Japan Scientific Societies Press, Tokyo, pp. 87-96.

Jain, M., Cook, G. M., Davis, F. G., Grace, M. G., Howe, G. R., Miller, A. B. (1980). A case-control study of diet and colorectal cancer. *Intl. J. Cancer 26*: 757.

Kark, J. D., Smith, A. H., James, C. G. (1980). The relationship of serum cholesterol to the incidence of cancer in Evans County, Georgia. *J. Chronic Dis. 33*: 311.

Kensler, C. J., Suguira, N., Young, N. F., Halter, C. R., Rhoads, C. P. (1941). Partial protection of rats by riboflavin with casein. *Science 93*: 308.

Klurfeld, D. M., Weber, M. M., Buck, C. L., Kritchensky, D. (1986). Dose response of colonic carcinogenesis to different amount and types of cellulose. *Fed. Proc. 45*: 1076.

Knox, E. G. (1977). Foods and diseases. *Br. J. Prev. Soc. Med. 31*: 71.

Kolonel, L. N., Hankin, J. H., Lee, J., Chu, S. Y., Nomura, A. M. Y., Hinds, M. W. (1981). Nutrient intakes in relation to cancer incidence in Hawaii. *Br. J. Cancer 44*: 332.

Kolonel, L. N., Nomura, A. M., Hinds, M. W., Hirohata, T., Hankin, J. H., Lee J. (1983). Role of diet in cancer incidence in Hawaii. *Cancer Res. 43*: 2397s.

Kolonel, L. N., Marchand, L. L. (1986). The epidemiology of colon cancer and dietary fat. In *Dietary Fat and Cancer*, C. Ip et al. (Eds.). Alan R. Liss, New York, p. 6.

Kummet, T., Meyskens, F. L., Jr. (1983). Vitamin A: a natural inhibitor of human malignancy. *Nutr. Cancer 5*: 281.

Lavik, P. S., Baumann, C. A. (1943). Further studies on the tumor promoting action of fat. *Cancer Res. 3*: 749.

Lee, S. Y., Rogers, A. E. (1983). Dimethylbenzathracene mammary tumorigenesis in Sprague-Dawley rats fed diets differing in content of beef tallow or rapeseed oil. *Nutr. Res. 3*: 361-371.

Lew, E. A., Garfinkel, L. (1979). Variations in mortality by weight among 750,000 men and women. *J. Chronic Dis. 32*: 563.

Lin, H. J., Chan, W. C., Fong, Y. Y., Newberne, P. M. (1977). Zinc levels in serum, hair and tumors from patients with esophageal cancer. *Nutr. Rep. Intl. 15*: 635.

Liu, K., Stamler, J., Moss, D., Garside, D., Persky, V., Soltero, I. (1979). Dietary cholesterol, fat and fibre and colon-cancer mortality. *Lancet 2*: 782.

Locniskar, M., Nauss, K. M., Kaufman, P., Newberne, P. M. (1985). Interaction of dietary fat and route of administration on DMH induced colon tumorigenesis in rats. *Carcinogenesis 6*: 349.

Lyon, J. L., Sorenson, A. W. (1978). Colon cancer in a low-risk population. *Am. J. Clin. Nutr. 31*: S227.

MacLennan, R., DaCosta, J., Day, N. E., Law, C. H., Ng, Y. K., Shanmugaratnan, K. (1977). Risk factors for lung cancer in Singapore Chinese, a population with high female incidence rates. *Intl. J. Cancer 20*: 854.

Madhavan, T. V., Gopalan, C. (1968). The effect of dietary protein on carcinogenesis of aflatoxin. *Arch. Pathol. 85*: 133.

Marshall, E. (1985). Nutrition report and the Academy of Science. *230*: 1324.

Marshall, E. (1986). Dietary advice, with a grain of salt and a large helping of pepper. *Science 231*: 537.

Matthews-Roth, M. M., Pathak, M. A., Fitzpatrick, T. B., Harber, L. H., Kass, E. H. (1977). Beta carotene therapy for erythropoietic protoporphyria and photosensitivity diseases. *Arch. Dermatol. 113*: 1229.

McCormick, D. L., Mehta, R. G., Thompson, C. A., Dinger, N., Caldwell, J. A., Moon, R. C. (1982). Enhanced inhibition of mammary carcinogenesis by combined treatment with N-4-hydroxyphenyl retinamide and ovariectomy. *Cancer Res. 42*: 508.

McCormick, D. L., Sowell, Z. L., Thompson, C. A., Moon, R. C. (1983). Inhibition by retinoid and ovariectomy of additional primary malignancies in rats following surgical removal of the first mammary cancer. *Cancer 51*: 594.

McCormick, D. L., Major, N., Moon, R. C. (1984). Inhibition of 7,12-dimethylbenz(a)anthracene-induced rat mammary carcinogenesis by concomitant or postcarcinogen antioxidant exposure. *Cancer Res. 44*: 2858.

McCormick, D. L., Madigan, M. J., Moon, R. C. (1985). Modulation of rat mammary carcinogenesis by indomethacin. *Cancer Res. 45*: 1803.

Medina, D., Shepherd, F. (1980). Selenium-mediated inhibition of mouse mammary tumorigenesis. *Cancer Lett. 8*: 241.

Meinsma, L. (in Dutch: English summary) (1964). Nutrition and cancer. *Voeding 25*: 357.

Mettlin, C., Graham, S., Swanson, M. (1979), Vitamin A and lung cancer. *J. Natl. Cancer Inst. 62*: 1435.

Mettlin, C., Graham, S., Priore, R., Marshall, J., Swanson, M. (1981). Diet and cancer of the esophagus. *Nutr. Cancer 2*: 143.

Meyskens, F. L., Jr. (1984). Prevention and treatment of cancer with vitamin A and the retinoids. In *Vitamins, Nutrition and Cancer*, Prasad, K. N. (Ed.). Karger, Basel, p. 266.

Mgbodile, M. U. K., Campbell, T. C. (1972). Effect of protein deprivation of male weanling rats on the kinetics of hepatic microsomal enzyme activity. *J. Nutr. 102*: 53.

Miettinen, M., Turpeinen, O., Karvonen, M. J., Elosuo, R., Paanilainen, E. (1972). Effect of cholesterol-lowering diet on mortality from coronary heart disease and other causes: a twelve-year clinical trial in men and women. *Lancet 2*: 835.

Miller, A. B. (1986). Dietary fat and the epidemiology of breast cancer. In *Dietary Fat and Cancer*, Ip, C. et al. (Eds.). Alan R. Liss, New York, p. 17.

Miller, J. A., Miller, E. C. (1953). The carcinogenic aminoazo dyes. *Adv. Cancer Res. 1*: 339.

Miller, S. R., Tartter, P., Papatistas, A., Slater, G., Aufses, Jr. (1981). Serum cholesterol and human colon cancer. *J. Natl. Cancer Inst. 67*: 297.

Minton, J. P., Abou-Issa, H., Foecking, M. K., Sriram, M. G. (1983). Caffeine and unsaturated fat diet significantly promotes DMBA-induced breast cancer in rats. *Cancer 51*: 1249.

Mirvish, S. S., Wallcave, L., Eagen, M., Shubik, P. (1972). Ascorbate-nitrite reaction: possible means of blocking the formation of carcinogenic N-nitroso compounds. *Science 177*: 65.

Mirvish, S. S. (1981). Inhibition of the formation of carcinogenic N-nitroso compounds by ascorbic acid and other compounds. In *Cancer: Achievements, Challenges, and Prospects for the 1980s*, Vol. 1, Burchenal, J. H. and Oettgen, H. F., (Eds.). Grune and Stratton, New York, p. 557.

Moon, R. C., Grubbs, C. J., Sporn, M. B. (1976). Inhibition of 7,12-dimethylbenz(a) anthracene-induced mammary carcinogenesis by retinyl acetate. *Cancer Res. 36*: 2626.

Moskowitz, M., White, C., Barnett, R. N., Stevens, S., Russell, E., Vargo, D., Floch, M. H. (1979). Diet, fecal bile acids and neutral sterols in carcinoma of the colon. *Dig. Dis. Sci. 24*: 746.

Mower, H. F., Ray, R. M., Shoff, R., Stemmermann, G. N., Nomura, A., Glober, G. A., Kamiyama, S., Shimada, A., Yamakawa, H. (1979). Fecal bile acids in two Japanese populations with different colon cancer risks. *Cancer Res. 39*: 328.

National Academy of Sciences (1980). *Recommended Dietary Allowances*, 9th ed. Committee on Dietary Allowances. Food and Nutrition Board, National Academy of Sciences, Washington, D.C.

Nauss, K. M., Locniskar, M., Newberne, P. M. (1983). Alternations in quality and quantity of dietary fat on 1,2-dimethylhydrazine-induced colon tumorigenesis in rats. *Cancer Res.*

Nauss, K. M., Locniskar, M., Sondergaard, D., Newberne, P. M. (1984). Lack of effect of dietary fat on NMY-induced colon tumorigenesis in rats. *Carcinogenesis 5*: 225.

Nauss, K. M., Bueche, D., Newberne, P. M. (1987). Effect of vitamin nutriture on experimental esophageal carcinogenesis. *J. Natl. Cancer Inst. 79*: 145-157.

Nelson, A. A., Fitzhugh, O. G., Calvery, H. O. (1943). Liver tumors following cirrhosis caused by selenium in rats. *Cancer Res. 3*: 230.

Nettesheim, P., Williams, M. L. (1976). The influence of vitamin A on the susceptibility of the rat lung to 3-methylcholanthrene. *Intl. J. Cancer 17*: 351.

Newberne, P. M., Conner, M. (1974). Acute studies with selenium and aflatoxin B_1 liver injury. Trace Sub. Conf. VIII, University of Missouri, 323.

Newberne, P. M., McConnell, R. G. (1980). Dietary nutrients and contaminants in laboratory animal experimentaion. Proc. 4th Int. Symp. Lab Animals, Boston, Mass. October 28-31, *J. Environ. Pathol. Toxicol. 4*: 105.

Newberne, P. M., McConnell, R. G. (1980). Nutrient deficiencies in cancer causation. *J. Environ. Pathol. Toxicol. 3*: 323.

Newberne, P. M. (1983). Influence of selenium on response to toxins. *The Toxicol. 3*: 140.

Newberne, P. M., Rogers, A. E., and Nauss, K. M. (1983). Choline, methionine and related factors in oncogenesis. In *Nutritional Factors in the Induction and Maintenance of Malignancy*, C. Butterworth and M. Hutchinson (Eds.). Academic Press, New York, pp. 247-241.

Newberne, P. M., Schrager, T. F., Conner, M. W. (1985). Nutrients and other risk factors associated with cancer. In *Vitamins and Cancer: Human Cancer Prevention by Vitamins and Micronutrients*. F. Meyskens and K. Prasad (Eds.). Humana Press, pp. 113-138.

Newberne, P. M. (1985). The influence of nutrition, immunologic status and other factors on the development of cancer. In *Toxicological Risks*, Vol. II, D. Clayson, R. Krewski, and I. Munro (Eds.). CRC Press, Boca Raton, Fla., pp. 43-87.

Newberne, P. M., Nauss, K. M. (1986). Dietary fat and colon cancer: Variable results in animals. In *Dietary Fat and Cancer*, C. Ip, D. Birt, A. Rogers, and C. Mettlin (Eds.). Alan R. Liss, New York, pp. 311-330.

Newberne, P. M., Rogers, A. E. (1986). Labile methyl groups and the promotion of cancer. *Ann. Rev. Nutr. 6*: 407.

Newberne, P. M., Conner, M. W. (1987). The role of diet and nutrition in safety evaluations of drugs and other chemicals. In *Human Risk Assessment: The Role of Animal Selection and Extrapolation*, M. V. Roloff (Ed.). Taylor and Frances Ltd., London, pp. 65-79.

Newberne, P. M., Punyarit, P., de Camargo, J., Suphakarn, V. (1987). The role of necrosis in hepatocellular proliferation in liver tumors. In *Mouse Liver Tumors*, Arch. Toxicol. Supp. 10, p. 54.

Nigro, N. D., Singh, D. V., Campbell, R. L., Pak, M. S. (1975). Effect of dietary beef fat on intestinal tumor formation by azoxymethane in rats. *J. Natl. Cancer Inst. 54*: 439.

Parkin, D. M., St. Jernsward, J., Muir, C. S. (1984). Estimates of the worldwide frequency of twelve major cancers. *Bull. World Hlth. Org. 62*: 163.

Pearce, M. L., Dayton, S. (1971). Incidence of cancer in men on a diet high in polyunsaturated fat. *Lancet 1*: 464.

Petering, H. G., Buskirk, H. H., Crim, J. A. (1967). The effect of dietary mineral supplements of the rat on the antitumor activity of 3-ethoxy-2-oxobutyraldehyde bis (thiosemicarbazone). *Cancer Res. 27*: 1115.

Peterson, B., Trell, E., Sternby, N. H. (1981). Low cholesterol level as risk factor for noncompany death in middle-aged men. *J. Am. Med. Assoc. 245*: 2056.

Peto, R., Doll, R., Buckley, J. D., Sporn, M. B. (1981). Can dietary beta-carotene materially reduce human cancer rates? *Nature* (London) *290*: 201.

Phillips, R. L. (1975). Role of lifestyle in dietary habits in risk of cancer among Seventh Day Adventists. *Cancer Res. 35*: 3513.

Poirier, Lionel A., Newberne, Paul M., Pariza, Michael W. (Eds.) (1986). *Essential Nutrients in Carcinogenesis*. Plenum Press, New York.

Poswillo, D. E., Cohen, B. (1971). Inhibition of carcinogenesis by dietary zinc. *Nature* (London) *231*: 447.

Prasad, A. S. (1978). *Trace Elements and Iron in Human Metabolism*. Plenum Publishing Corp., New York.

Reddy, B. S., Watanabe, K., Weisburger, J. H. (1977). Effect of high-fat diet on colon carcinogenesis in F344 rats treated with 1,2-dimethylhydrazine, methylazoxymethanol acetate, or methylnitrosourea. *Cancer Res. 37*: 4156.

Reddy, B. S., Cohen, L. A., McCoy, G. D., Hill, P., Weisburger, J. H., Wynder, E. L. (1981). Nutrition and its relationship to cancer. *Adv. Cancer Res. 41*: 888.

Reddy, B. S. (1986). Amount and type of dietary fat and colon cancer in animal model studies. In *Dietary Fat and Cancer*, C. Ip et al. (Eds.). Alan R. Liss, New York, pp. 295-309.

Rogers, A. E., Fernstrom, J. D., GE, K., McConnell, R. G. Leavitt, W. W. Wetsel, W. C., Yang, S. O., Camelio, E. A. (1982). Endocrine interactions in the nutritional modulation of mammary carcinogenesis in rats. In *Molecular Interrelations of Nutrition and Cancer*, Arnott, M. S., Van Eys, J., Wang, Y. M. (Eds.). Raven, New York, pp. 381-399.

Rogers, A. E., Conner, B. H., Boulanger, C. L., Lee, S. Y., Carr, F. A., Dumouchel, W. H. (1985). Enhancement of 7,12-dimethylbenz(a)anthracene mammary carcinogenesis by a high lard diet. In *Dietary Fiber*, Vahouny G. V., Kirtchevsky, D. (Eds.). Plenum, New York, pp. 444-455.

Rogers, A. E., Conner, B., Boulanger, C., Lee, S. (1986). Mammary tumorigenesis in rats fed diets high in lard. *Lipids* (in press).

Rogers, A. E., Herndon, B. J., Newberne, P. M. (1900). Induction by dimethylhydrazine of intestinal carcinoma in normal rats and rats fed high or low levels of vitamin A. *Cancer Res. 33*: 1003.

Rose, G., Shipley, M. J. (1980). Plasma lipids and mortality: a source of error. *Lancet 1*: 523.

Rose, G. Blackburn, H., Keys, A., Taylor, H. L., Kannel, W. B., Paul, O., Reid, D. D., Stamler, J. (1981). Colon cancer and blood-cholesterol. *Lancet 1*: 181.

Ross, M. H., Bras, G. (1965). Tumor incidence patterns and nutrition in the rat. *J. Nutr. 87*; 245.

Ross, M. H., Bras, G. (1973). Influence of protein under- and overnutruition on spontaneous tumor prevalence in the rat. *J. Nutr. 103*: 944.

Russo, J., Tay, L. K., Ciocca, D. R., Russo, I. H. (1983). Molecular and cellular basis of the mammary gland susceptibility to carcinogenesis. *Environmental Health Perspectives 49*: 185.

Saffiotti, U., Montesano, R., Sellakumar, A. R., Borg, S. A. (1967). Experimental cancer of the lung: inhibition by vitamin A of the induction of tracheobronchial squamous metaplasia and squamous cell tumors. *Cancer 20*: 857.

Schrauzer, G. N. (1976). Selenium and cancer: a review. *Bioinorg. Chem. 5*: 275.

Schrauzer, G. N., White, D. A., Schnieder, C. J. (1977a). Cancer mortality correlation studies. III. Statistical associations with dietary selenium intakes. *Bioinorg. Chem.* 7: 23.

Schrauzer, G. N., White, D. A., Schneider, C. J. (1977b). Cancer mortality correlation studies. IV. Associations with dietary intakes and blood levels of certain trace elements, notably Se-antagonists. *Bioinorg. Chem.* 7: 35.

Schrauzer, G. N., White, D. A., Schneider, C. J. (1978). Selenium and cancer effects of selenium and of the diet on the genesis of spontaneous mammary tumors in virgin inbred female C_3H/St mice. *Bioinorg. Chem. 8*: 387.

Schuman, L. M., Mandell, J. S., Radke, A., Seal, V., Halberg, F. (1982). Some selected cases of the epidemiology of prostatic cancer 1976-1979. In *Trends in Cancer Incidence*, K. Magnus (Ed.). Hemisphere Corp., New York, pp. 345-354.

Science (1986). News and Comments *231*: 537.

Selenium in Nutrition (1971). Rep. Subcommittee on Selenium, Committee on Animal Nutrition. National Academy of Sciences, Washington, D.C.

Shamberger, R. J., Frost, D. V. (1969). Letter to the editor: possible protective effect of selenium against human cancer. *Cancer Med. Assoc. J. 100*: 682.

Shamberger, R. J. (1970). Relation of selenium to cancer. I. Inhibitory effect of selenium on carcinogenesis. *J. Natl. Cancer Inst. 44*: 931.

Shamberger, R. J. (1971). Inhibitory effect of vitamin A on carcinogenesis. *J. Natl. Cancer Inst. 47*: 667.

Shamberger, R. J., Willis, C. E. (1971). Selenium distribution and human cancer mortality. *CRC Crit. Rev. Clin. Lab. Sci. 2*: 211.

Shamberger, R. J., Rukovena, E., Longfield, A. K., Tytko, S. A., Deodhar, S., Willis, C. E. (1973). Antioxidants and cancer. I. Selenium in the blood of normals and cancer patients. *J. Natl. Cancer Inst. 50*: 863.

Shamberger, R. J., Tytko, S. A., Willis, C.E. (1976). Antioxidants and cancer. VI. Selenium and age adjusted human cancer mortality. *Arch. Environ. Health 31*: 231.

Shekelle, R. B., Liu, S., Raynor, W. J., Jr., Lepper, M., Maliza, C., Rossoff, A. H. (1981). Dietary vitamin A and risk of cancer in the Western Electric study. *Lancet 2*: 1185.

Sinha, D. K., Dao, T. L. (1980). Induction of mammary tumors in aging rats by 7,12-dimethylbenz(a) anthracene: role of DNA synthesis during carcinogenesis. *J. Natl. Cancer Inst. 64*: 519.

Smith, D. M., Rogers, A. E., Herndon, B. J., Newberne, P. M. (1975). Vitamin A (retinyl acetate) and benzo(a)pyrene-induced respiratory tract carcinogenesis in hamsters fed a commercial diet. *Cancer Res. 35*: 11.

Smith, P. G., Jick, H. (1978). Cancers among users of preparations containing vitamin A. *Cancer 42*: 808.

Sokula, A. (1976). Letter to the editor: vitamin A and lung cancer. *Br. Med. J. 2*: 298.

Sparnins, V. L., Chuan, J., Wattenberg, L. W. (1982). Enhancement of glutathione S-transferase activity of the esophagus by phenols, and benzyl iosthiolyanate. *Cancer Res. 42*: 205.

Sporn, M. B., Dunlop, N. M., Newton, D. L., Smith, J. M. (1976). Prevention of chemical carcinogenesis by vitamin A and its synthetic analogs (retinoids). *Fed. Proc. Fed. Am. Soc. Exp. Biol. 35*: 1332.

Sporn, M. B., Newton, D. L. (1979). Chemoprevention of cancer with retinoids. *Fed. Proc. Fed. Am. Soc. Exp. Biol. 38*: 2528.

Sporn, M. B., Roberts, A. B. (1986). Suppression of carcinogenesis by retinoids: Interactions with peptide growth factors and their receptors as a key mechanism. In *Diet, Nutrition and Cancer*, Y. Hayashi et al. (Eds.). Japan Sci. Press, Tokyo, pp. 149-158.

Strain, W. H., Mansour, E. G., Flynn, A., Pories, W. J., Tomaro, A. J., Hill, O. A., Jr. (1972). Letter to the editor: plasma-zinc concentration in patients with bronchogenic cancer. *Lancet 1*: 1021.

Sunderman, F. W., Jr. (1977). Metal carcinogenesis. In *Toxicology of Trace Elements*, Goyer, R. A., and Mehlman, M. A. (Eds.). Hemisphere Publishing Corporation, Washington, D.C., p. 257.

Sylvester, P. W., Aylsworth, C. F., Van Vugt, D. A., Meites, J. (1983). Effects of alterations in early hormonal environment on development and hormone dependency of carcinogen-induced mammary tumors in rats. *Cancer Res. 43*: 5342.

Sylvester, P. W., Ip, C., Ip, M. (1986a). Effects of high deitary fat on the growth and development of ovarian-independent carcinogen-induced mammary tumors in rats. *Cancer Res. 46*: 763.

Sylvester, P. W., Russell, M., Ip, M. M., Ip, C. (1986b). Comparative effects of different animal and vegetable fats fed before and during carcinogen administration on mammary tumorigenesis, sexual maturation and endocrine function in rats. *Cancer Res. 45*: 757.

Tannenbaum, A. (1942a). The genesis and growth of tumors II. Effects of caloric restriction per se. *Cancer Res. 2*: 460.

Tannenbaum, A. (1942b). The genesis and growth of tumors III. Effects of a high fat diet. *Cancer Res. 2*: 468.

Tannenbaum, A. (1944). The dependence of the genesis of induced skin tumors on the calorie intake during different states of carcinogenesis. *Cancer Res. 4*: 673.

Tannenbaum, A. (1045a). A dependence of tumor formation on the composition of the calorie-restriction. *Cancer Res. 5*: 609.

Tannenbaum, A. (1945b). The dependence of tumor formation on the composition of the calorie-restricted diet as well as on the degree of restriction. *Cancer Res. 5*: 616.

Temcharoen, P., Anukarahanonta, T., Bhamarapravati, N. (1978). Influence of dietary protein and vitamin B12 on the toxicity and carcinogenicity of aflatoxins in rat liver. *Cancer Res. 38*: 2185.

Thanassi, J. W., Nutter, L. M., Meisler, N. T., Commers, P., Chiu, J. F. (1981). Vitamin B_6 metabolism in Morris hepatomas. *J. Biol. Chem. 256*: 3370.

Thompson, H. J., Meeker, L. D., Tagliaferro, A. R., Becci, P. J. (1982). Effect of retinyl acetate on the occurrence of ovarian hormone-responsive and non-responsive mammary cancers in the rat. *Cancer Res. 42*: 903.

Thompson, H. J., Becci, P. J. (1984). Selenium inhibition of NMU-induced mammary carcinogenesis in the rat. *J. Natl. Cancer Inst. 65*: 1299.

Tryfiates, G. P. (1981). Effects of pyridoxine on serum protein expression in hepatoma-bearing rats. *J. Natl. Cancer Inst. 66*: 339.

Van Rensburg, S. J. (1981). Epidemiologic and dietary evidence for a specific nutritional predisposition to esophageal cancer. *J. Natl. Cancer Inst. 67*: 243.

Volgarev, M. N., Tscherkes, L. A. (1967). Further studies in tissue changes associated with sodium selenate. *Symp. Selenium in Biomedicine*, 1st Int. Symp., AVI Publishing Co., Westport, Conn., p. 179.

Wald, N., Idle, M., Boreham, J., Bailey, A. (1980). Low serum vitamin A and subsequent risk of cancer-preliminary results of a prospective study. *Lancet 2*: 813.

Wald, N. J., Boreham, J., Hayward, J. L., Bulbrook, R. D. (1984). Plasma retinol, B-carotene and vitamin E levels in relation to the future risk of breast cancer. *Br. J. Cancer 49*: 321.

Walters, M. A., Roe, F. J. C. (1964). The effect of dietary casein on the induction of lung tumors by the injection of 9,10-dimethyl-1,2-benzanthracene (DMBA) into newborn mice. *Br. J. Cancer 18*: 312.

Wassertheil-Smoller, S., Romney, S. L., Wylie-Rosett, J., Slagle, S., Miller, G., Lucido, D., Dutagupta, C., Palan, P. R. (1981). Dietary vitamin C and uterine cervical dysplasia. *Am. J. Epidemiol. 114*: 714.

Weils, P., Alftergood, L., Alfin-Slater, R. B. (1976). Effect of varying levels of dietary protein on tumor development and lipid metabolism in rats exposed to aflatoxin. *J. Am. Oil Chem. Soc. 53*: 559.

Welsch, C. W., Goodrich-Smith, M., Brown, C. K., Crowe, N. (1981). Enhancement by retinyl acetate of hormone-induced mammary tumorigenesis in female GR/A mice. *J. Natl. Cancer Inst. 67*: 935.

Welsch, C. W., Goodrich-Smith, M., Brown, C. K., Greene, H. D., Hamel, E. (1981). Selenium and the genesis of murine mammary tumors. *Carcinogenesis 2*: 519.

Welsch, C. W., DeHoog, J. V. (1983). Retinoid feeding, hormone inhibition, and/or immune stimulation and the genesis of carcinogen-induced rat mammary carcinomas. *Cancer Res. 43*: 585.

Welsch, C. W. (1985). Host factors affecting the growth of carcinogen-induced rat mammary carcinomas: A review and tribute to Charles Brenton Huggins. *Cancer Res. 45*: 3415.

Willett, W. C., Polk, B. F., Underwood, B. A., et al. (1984). Relation of serum vitamins A and E and carotenoids to the risk of cancer. *N. Engl. J. Med. 310*: 430-434.

Willett, W. (1986). Vitamin A and selenium intake in relation to human cancer risk. In *Diet, Nutrition and Cancer*, Y. Hayashi et al. (Eds.), Japan Sci. Soc. Press, Tokyo, pp. 237-245.

Williams, R. R., Sorlie, P. D., Feinleib, M., McNamara, P. M., Kannel, W. B., Dawber, T. R. (1981). Cancer incidence by levels of cholesterol. *J. Am. Med. Assoc. 245*: 247.

4

Human Epidemiological Evidence on the Nutritional Prevention of Cancer

DAVID J. HUNTER and WALTER C. WILLETT
Brigham and Women's Hospital and Harvard Medical School, Boston, Massachusetts

INTRODUCTION

The perception that the causes of cancer may be largely environmental in origin has led to great interest in the role of diet in cancer etiology. In their review of possible environmental determinants of cancer, Doll and Peto have estimated that 35% of cancers in the United States (with an estimated range of 10 to 70%) may be due to dietary factors (Doll and Peto, 1981). Most diet-cancer hypotheses propose either that a dietary component acts as a carcinogen or cocarcinogen so that excess amounts of the component increase cancer risk, or that a dietary constituent acts as an anticarcinogen such that high levels in the diet reduce cancer risk. In its simplest form, this dichotomy suggests two broad strategies for the nutritional prevention of cancer: (a) reduction or removal of exposure to dietary factors demonstrated to increase risk, (b) increased intake of dietary constituents with an apparent preventive action. The first strategy has already received wide, often controversial, application in the control of known or suspected carcinogenic food additives (International Agency for Research on Cancer, 1980). These carcinogens are principally non-nutrient additives, however. Although attractive hypotheses exist, successful application of the first strategy to foods and nutrients has yet to be clearly demonstrated. Similarly, there is growing evidence that cancer incidence may be reduced by increasing intake of certain foods and nutrients. It has been suggested that this strategy is the more promising of the two as addition of nutrients to the diet may be more easily achieved on a large scale than reduction of exposure—"prescription" may be more readily practiced than "proscription" (Peto et al., 1981). There is certainly ample precendent for the elimination of widely prevalent diseases by the relatively simple fortification of foods with vitamins (e.g., vitamin D and ricketts) or minerals (e.g., iodine and goiter).

Before firm dietary recommendations can be made, however, diet-cancer hypotheses must be generated and tested, and proposed interventions must be assessed. These activities involve scientists from many disciplines, ranging from molecular biologists to sociologists. Among the relevant disciplines, epidemiology plays a central role. Epidemiologic principles and practice are fundamental to the whole process, from hypothesis generation to eventual application. Since the epidemiologic evidence for the most important specific diet-cancer hypotheses is reviewed elsewhere in this volume, we will concentrate on the general contribution that epidemiologic methods can make to the ultimate goal of the nutritional prevention of cancer. We will review the strengths and limitations of the principal epidemiologic study designs and the place of each design in the overall strategy of achieving cancer control; the main methods used in the measurement of dietary exposures; and the scope and limits of interpretation of epidemiologic evidence in the assessment of causality in diet-cancer relationships.

EPIDEMIOLOGIC STUDY DESIGNS

Epidemiologic studies are essentially either *observational* studies or *intervention* studies. As the nomenclature suggests, in an observational study an epidemiologist observes human experience and attempts to reach valid conclusions about the nature of the relations between exposures and diseases among the individuals or populations under study. While an epidemiologist may select for reasons of efficiency to conduct a study among individuals at high risk of a particular exposure or disease, the epidemiologist's role is to merely ascertain exposure status, not alter it. The principal observational study designs are descriptive studies in populations, the cohort study, and the case-control study. In an intervention study, the scientist intervenes in the "natural" progression of events and assigns exposure to individuals in the study. The most widespread intervention design is the randomized trial. This is the study design that most closely emulates the rigor of a laboratory experiment, and indeed has been called the "paradigm" for observational study designs (Miettinen, 1985). For ethical and practical reasons, however, it is not possible to conduct randomized trials to evaluate many hypotheses. Exposing human subjects to a suspected carcinogen, for instance, is clearly not ethical. Fortunately or unfortunately, humans exist who have knowingly or unknowingly been exposed to many such potential carcinogens, and in these persons the effects can usually be ethically observed. MacMahon (1979) has summarized the other main advantages of observational study designs: they can be cost-effective ("humans . . . house and feed themselves and keep themselves clean at no expense to the investigator"), they allow assessment of exposures with potentially long latent effects, and they allow assessment of "a broad range of dosages of a variety of potentially toxic substances."

Observational Studies

Descriptive Studies in Populations

The first level of hypothesis generation and refinement in the epidemiologic process is frequently the inspection of descriptive data. These data describe population characteristics, rather than the characteristics of individuals. The underlying principle is that observed differences in disease rates between populations are probably due to underlying differences in the prevalence of causal exposures. Comparison of exposure prevalences may thus provide clues as to which exposures may be causal.

Geographic correlation studies, sometimes called ecologic studies, usually compare the prevalence or frequency of an exposure in a number of geographic areas, with the incidence of cancer in those areas. Each geographic area contributes one data point; the areas used as units of analysis may be counties, cities, states, or entire nations. Age-adjusted rates of breast and colon cancer in the United States, for instance, are more than five times the rates found in many other countries (Armstrong and Doll, 1975). These large international differences in cancer incidence are among the principal observations that support a major role for environmental factors in cancer causation. In general, a positive correlation betweeen increasing exposure and increasing cancer incidence suggests that the exposure of interest may be a risk factor for that cancer. An inverse relationship between exposure and cancer incidence suggests that the exposure may be protective. Two well-known examples of positive correlations are those between total fat intake per capita and national age-adjusted breast cancer mortality rates among women ($p = 0.89$), and between total fat intake per capita and mortality from colon cancer ($r = 0.85$ for men and 0.81 for women) (Armstrong and Doll, 1975; Carroll, 1975). The negative correlations observed between dietary selenium intakes and the international rates of several cancers, in particular breast cancer ($r = 0.8$), and colon cancer ($r = 0.7$) (Schrauzer, 1977), similarly suggest that dietary selenium may protect against these cancers.

Several lines of evidence indicate that genetic predisposition cannot account for most of these international differences in cancer incidence. Studies of migrant populations have shown that, for most of the common cancers, migrants acquire the cancer incidence profile of their new country, usually within one generation (Haenszel et al., 1972; Buell, 1973). In addition, major secular trends in cancer incidence have been observed within genetically stable populations. The continuing decrease in stomach cancer in the United States (Howson, Hiyama, and Wynder, 1986), and the substantial increase in the incidence of breast cancer in Iceland (Bjarnason et al., 1974), both suggest that concurrent changes in environmental exposures have occurred.

Populations with special exposure characteristics within a country may provide a useful unit for comparison. Religious groups, for instance, are frequently of interest because of unique lifestyle characteristics. All-site age-adjusted cancer incidence among Mormons in Utah is approximately two-thirds the rate of Utah's non-Mormons (Lyon, Gardner, and West, 1980). Most of this difference is accounted for by a much lower incidence among Mormons of smoking- and alcohol-related cancers, consistent with the Church teaching of abstinence from alcohol and tobacco. Lower incidences of cancer at other sites, e.g., breast, ovary, and colon, may be attributable to other aspects of the Mormon lifestyle. A similar deficit in smoking- and alcohol-related cancers has been reported for Seventh Day Adventists (Phillips et al., 1980), as well as lower mortality from colon cancer. A high proportion of Seventh Day Adventists are lacto-vegetarians, giving rise to several hypotheses relating meat eating to risk of cancer at this site.

The essential problem with descriptive studies of dietary factors is that diet, as a socially and economically determined exposure, is also strongly correlated with many factors that may independently influence disease risk. This is a particular difficulty for international studies where the range of socioeconomic and cultural factors between countries is large. With a few exceptions, such as Japan, countries with low breast and colon cancer rates also tend to be less economically developed. Thus, any correlate of economic development will correlate with breast and colon cancer rates; indeed, the correlation between gross national product and breast cancer mortality rates is 0.72 (Amstrong and Doll, 1975). As levels of television set or auto ownership also correlate strongly with gross national product, they will also be related to breast cancer mortality rate. The fact that nonsensical associations with patently noncausal variables can be generated by international correlation studies is a warning that causal inference should not be attempted from them. The underlying limitation is that controlling for alternative causes, both known and unknown, is particularly difficult. For a limited number of variables, standardization may be used to reduce or eliminate their ability to confound the relationship under study. Thus, almost all geographic comparisons are age-standardized, and a study of nutrient intake and lung cancer, for instance, could feasibly be standardized by the national prevalence of cigarette smoking or the per capita tobacco consumption. However, geographic comparisons cannot be standardized by many different alternative causes simultaneously, when information on these alternative causes is inadequate or when the alternative causes are unsuspected. It has been traditionally accepted that geographic correlation studies are useful for hypothesis generation but that the assignment of causal status to exposure variables requires additional experience from other study designs.

Cohort Studies

In a cohort (or follow-up) study, a group of persons whose exposure status has been ascertained is followed over time with respect to disease incidence. When a sufficient number of cases of the disease of interest have occurred in the cohort, then the incidence of disease in exposed persons can be compared with the incidence in the unexposed. If the exposure is not a simple dichotomy, then levels of exposure may be compared to look for dose-response effects. A cohort may be *fixed*—with its members enrolled over a short period and then no new members entered, or *dynamic*—in which losses due to death or migration may be replaced by persons meeting the eligibility criteria. If a cohort enrolled by an investigator or group of investigators is followed forward over time, it is usually referred to as a *prospective* cohort. Occasionally, information about a cohort can be reconstructed from records (e.g., military service or industrial employment records) after both exposure and disease have occurred. As the cohort is formally assembled for study purposes after the relevant population experience has occurred, this is termed a *retrospective* cohort.

Cohort studies offer many advantages over other study designs in the evaluation of diet-cancer hypotheses. The advent of dietary assessment methods suitable for application to large numbers of persons (see below) has enabled investigators to obtain dietary exposure informaton from cohorts of thousands or even tens of thousands of people. Large cohorts usually contain large numbers of persons whose dietary patterns reflect the common, prevailing patterns present in the communities they are enrolled from, thus increasing the generalizability of the study results. Large cohorts also often include persons with unusual dietary habits, which may also be informative. Because exposure information in cohort studies can be collected close to the time that exposure occurs, it should be more accurate and is potentially much more detailed than information collected years, or even decades later. As diet is a complex mixture of exposures, this superior quality of exposure information is a highly desirable feature for diet-cancer research. Periodic resurvey of the cohort allows exposure of the cohort to be reassessed and the exposure profile of each individual in the cohort to be updated if appropriate. This permits classification of study participants by categories of exposure with respect to time, as well as dose. Relatively complex hypotheses incorporating concepts of latency of effects and duration of exposure can thus be evaluated. A further advantage of this approach is the potential to collect accurate information about exposure to alternative causes of the cancer of interest. This makes possible control of confounding by permitting accurate cross-classification of two or more variables, and thus enhances the likelihood of reaching valid conclusions with respect to the dietary exposure of interest.

A feature of cohort design that is becoming increasingly important in the formulation of dietary recommendations is the ability to evaluate multiple disease endpoints. The most efficient way of detecting incident cases of a particular cancer in a cohort is frequently to detect *all* cases of cancer, especially if information is being derived from a cancer registry or death certificates. For cohorts that are periodically resurveyed and in which initial diagnostic information is provided by the cohort members themselves, self-report of almost all disease deemed worthy of study by the investigators is feasible. The ability to evaluate the full range of effects of a given exposure allows a complete assessment of the likely impact on overall health of a change in exposure status. This also permits several hypotheses to be evaluated simultaneously, resulting in more cost-effective research. Large studies that combine detailed exposure and disease information may allow investigators to uncover hitherto unsuspected diet-cancer associations, and thus function as efficient data bases for hypothesis generation.

The main limitation of cohort studies is the time they take to conduct. By definition, incident cases of a cancer are the outcome of interest, and thus prevalent cases are usually excluded from cohort membership. Fortunately, cancer is still a relatively rare phenomenon; a U.S. woman's lifetime risk of breast cancer for instance, is approximately 10% (American Cancer Society, 1987). To collect enough cases of breast cancer for a statistically powerful analysis will thus require the investigator to follow the cohort for many years, if not decades. The larger the cohort, the more cases of disease will occur, so the follow-up period may be reduced by enrollment of a larger initial cohort. The incidence of most cancers increases sharply at older ages, so enrollment of a relatively older cohort will yield more cases sooner than a younger one. Other strategies for maximizing efficiency include the deliberate oversampling of high-risk individuals. The generalizability of results to unselected populations becomes increasingly problematic the more highly selected the cohort becomes.

Another limitation of a cohort (as well as a case-control study) is that the range of exposures that can be investigated is limited by the experience of members in the study population. Concern has been expressed by many that it may be impossible to find associations with dietary factors in studies within one country because the diets are homogeneous. This is a legitimate consideration; and it is true that the full range of dietary intake that would often be of interest can seldom be found within one population. It seems unlikely that a simple conclusion can be reached with respect to this issue, since the between-person intake can vary substantially from nutrient to nutrient. For example, individuals appear to differ substantially more in their beta-carotene than in their selenium blood levels (although both reflect dietary intake) (Menkes et al., 1986). In general, it does appear that sufficient dietary heterogeneity does exist within the United States to evaluate most current hypotheses. Evidence that dietary questionnaire estimates of nutrient intake correlate with biochemical measures of nutrient intake, or with detailed food diaries, indicates both that variation does exist and that it is measurable (Willett et al., 1983a). Moreover, the capacity to predict coronary heart disease using dietary assessment methods (Shekelle, Shryock, and Paul, 1982; Kushi et al., 1985) indirectly suggests that dietary associations with cancer should also be observable if they truly exist.

A typical use of a cohort design to evaluate a hypothesis relating intake of a micronutrient to cancer incidence is the evaluation of dietary vitamin A and risk of cancer in the Western Electric Study (Shekelle et al., 1981). Among a cohort of 1954 men enrolled in the study in 1957-1958 and for whom follow-up information was available in 1978, carotene and retinol consumption indexes were constructed from responses to a dietary interview and questionnaire administered at enrollment and one year later. The 19-year cumulative incidence of death from lung cancer and other cancers was calculated for each quartile of carotene and retinol intake. For lung cancer, the level of the carotene index was inversely related to the 19-year mortality from lung cancer, with the relative risk of men in the lowest quartile being 7.0 times that of men in the highest. No significant relationships were seen between carotene and the group of combined other cancers, or between retinol and either lung or other cancers. In a proportional hazards (Cox-type) regression analysis adjusting for age and cigarette smoking, the carotene index was still significantly associated with lung cancer mortality, providing some assurance that the carotene effect was not caused by a difference in smoking habit between high and low carotene consumers. The single most desirable feature of the cohort design that this study demonstrates is the evaluation of dietary and other exposures before onset of disease. The single least favorable feature (from the standpoint of someone contemplating a new investigation) is the two-decade duration of the study.

Cohort studies that seek to enroll large numbers of subjects without prior ascertainment of exposure status have been criticized on efficiency grounds (Miettinen, 1985). Most exposures are distributed either normally or log-normally in the general population, and unselected sampling will thus result in a small number of subjects at the extremes of exposure (who are usually of particular interest) relative to large numbers in the middle range. The principles of experimental design suggest that sampling of the extremes of exposure, and possibly some fraction of the middle range, will provide a study population that can be efficiently used to evaluate an exposure–disease hypothesis, without collecting large amounts of relatively uninformative information. While this design is more efficient in the context of a single exposure-disease relation, it ignores one of the fundamental strengths of the cohort design—the ability to evaluate simultaneously many exposure-disease hypotheses. Diet is a complex mixture of exposures, and a population selected to optimally assess the effect of fat consumption, for instance, may be inadequate for the assessment of some other dietary constituent, say, vitamin A. The ability to evaluate many hypotheses more than compensates for the apparent inefficiency compared to an experimental design testing a single hypothesis. Another frequent criticism of cohort studies is their cost relative to case-control studies. Again, a cohort study designed to assess many exposure-disease relations may be a cost-effective alternative to many single-disease case-control studies.

Case-Control Studies

Much of the available data relating diet to cancer risk has been derived from case-control studies. These are generally less time-consuming and less expensive than cohort studies. In a case-control study a group of cases of the cancer under study is compared to a group of controls with respect to prior exposure to the dietary factor of interest. MacLennan and coworkers (1977), for instance, identified all cases of lung cancer diagnosed during an 18-month period in three Singapore hospitals. Controls were selected from other hospital patients without smoking-related diseases. Information about frequency of consumption of various foods was collected from 233 cases and 300 controls, and low consumption of dark green leafy vegetables was found in this study to be associated with increased risk of lung cancer. Incidence rates cannot usually be calculated from case-control studies; the measure obtained is the exposure odds—(the probability of exposure)/(1 – the probability of exposure). The measure of association in case-control studies—the *exposure odds ratio*—is the odds of exposure in cases, divided by the odds of exposure in controls. It can be shown that if controls are selected independently of exposure status (Rothman, 1986), the exposure odds ratio is an unbiased estimate of the incidence rate ratio that would have been calculated in an underlying cohort study. The central condition to assure the unbiasedness of this estimate is that the controls are representative with respect to exposure status of the population that gave rise to the cases. The main operational difficulty in case-control studies is the definition of this underlying population, and thus the selection of appropriate controls.

Even if these conditions are met, there are other potential sources of bias in case-control studies to which nutritional studies may be particularly prone. The most important problem is the measurement of exposure. Diet is a complex and varied mixture of exposures. Due to the latency period of most cancers, the time during which causal exposures may have occurred precedes the development of cancer by years, perhaps decades. Thus, a case-control study will most appropriately seek to measure diet years, or decades, in the past. The imperfection of human memory alone ensures that few people will be able to accurately describe their past diet. This will lead to misclassification of exposure to foods and nutrients, as subjects describe a past diet that differs from their actual past diet. More serious with respect to a case-control analysis, this inability to accurately depict past diet may differ between cases as a group, and controls as a group. Cases differ, after all, from typical controls by having been diagnosed as having a serious, possibly fatal, disease. This fact alone means that their psychological state as they attempt to describe their past dietary intake will be different from that of the controls. This may lead them, consciously or unconsciously, to alter the answers they would otherwise have given, particularly if they are aware of prevailing diet-cancer hypotheses. As more such hypotheses are made, and as more dietary recommendations are made on the basis of accumulated evidence, this form of bias—*recall bias*—may become more pervasive in case-control studies. A further problem with this design is that the diet of cancer cases frequently changes, often quite radically, in the months preceding, and immediately after, diagnosis. Preclinical disease may change dietary patterns, as may the stress of diagnostic procedures, chemotherapy, and surgery. The consistent finding that responses to questions about remote dietary intake are biased by recent intake (Jensen et al., 1984; Rohan and Potter, 1984) is further reason to be concerned for the validity of historical data obtained from cancer cases.

Several techniques have been developed to minimize the impact of recall bias. Interviewers may be blinded to the case-control status of each interview (not always feasible in hospital situations); cases may be interviewed before diagnostic tests are performed (i.e., before they know their diagnosis) or as soon as possible after the diagnosis is made. It is nevertheless very difficult to be assured that a small (e.g., 5%) systematic error due to recall has not occurred. Differences of 5-10% in the means of nutrient intakes between cases and controls translate into potentially important relative risks (Jain et al., 1982), thus some uncertainty will always attend a case-control study. In all study designs, of course, one will usually be more confident that an apparent effect is not due to chance or bias if the apparent effect is large. Unfortunately, for most dietary exposures to an individual food or nutrient, realistic relative risks are frequently in the range of 0.5 to 2.0, risks that are susceptible to small systematic biases.

The case-control study has several advantages, however, which assure its place in the epidemiologic armamentarium. In contrast to cohort studies, they provide a relatively rapid test of diet-cancer hypotheses. A case-control study of a common cancer will typically take two or three years to conduct and analyze. Even very large cohort studies may never accumulate enough cases of an uncommon cancer for adequate analysis, whereas a case-control study based in one or more cancer referral centers may do so in a year or two. For these reasons alone, and also because they typically require much less data collection, case-control studies are usually less expensive than cohort studies. This ensures that case-control studies will continue to play a role in cancer control strategies.

Nested Case-Control Studies

An increasingly popular study design, particularly when biologic specimens are used as measures of exposure, is the nested case-control study. This design is particularly efficient when biologic specimens have been collected from the entire cohort prospectively, but it would be very expensive to analyze all specimens. Cases of cancer arising in the cohort are compared, not to the entire cohort, but to selected controls, minimizing the number of laboratory analyses necessary. Willett and colleagues used a nested case-control design in their study of serum selenium and cancer (Willett et al., 1983b). Serum had been collected from participants in the Hypertension Detection and Follow-up Program and stored since entry to the study in 1973. One hundred and eleven subjects who had developed cancer in a five-year follow-up period were identified, and two controls were selected for almost all cases. Thus 321 serum samples were retrieved from storage and analyzed for their selenium concentration. The risk of cancer for subjects in the lowest quintile of serum selenium was twice that of subjects in the highest. Low serum levels of vitamins A and E compounded the effect of low selenium; relative risks for the lowest tertile of selenium were 3.9 and 2.4 in the lowest tertiles of vitamins A and E, respectively.

Intervention Studies

In many situations, intervention studies (described at greater length elsewhere in this volume) may provide the ultimate test of specific micronutrient-cancer hypotheses. The potential to control confounding by randomization is the single most desirable feature of this study design. It is worth considering some of the limitations of randomized trials.

The major limitation has already been referred to—the inability to test hypotheses that may place subjects at risk. This automatically excludes the use of trials to investigate exposures that are possible risk factors for disease. Trials involving major lifestyle changes or substantial commitments of time will usually have difficulties enrolling subjects and ensuring compliance. Trials are thus restricted to the assessment of therapies or the assessment of nontoxic putative preventive agents. A further practical limitation is that the feasible duration of most trials may be less than the time required to test hypotheses incorporating concepts of latency in which the relevant exposures may be postulated to act many years, or even several decades, before the onset of disease.

The generalizability of trials may pose further problems of interpretation. Observational studies are usually based on heterogeneous populations, however, trials are frequently restricted to relatively homogeneous subgroups. Many micronutrient-cancer hypotheses for instance, propose that persons with a relatively low intake of certain micronutrients are at higher risk. Trials that do not deliberately screen and select populations with a large proportion of low-intake subjects may not have the power to test these hypotheses. It is important to realize that intervention studies are merely one of the options in epidemiologic study design and are not a panacea for the weaknesses of observational data.

While it may be tempting to plunge into an intervention study at an early stage of the development of micronutrient-cancer hypothesis, extensive observational data is usually required to achieve optimal selection of the study population and to provide the necessary background for correct interpretation and generalizability of the results.

MEASURING DIETARY EXPOSURE

Assessment of Micronutrient Intake

Diet and cancer is a relatively new area of epidemiologic research, largely because dietary assessment instruments suitable for use in large epidemiologic studies have only recently been developed, tested, and validated. The human diet is a varied and complex mixture of exposures and presents formidable challenge to those who attempt to quantify it. The usually agreed-upon "gold standard" method of dietary assessment is the food diary, in which subjects accurately record all foods consumed on a meal-by-meal basis. This method often requires subjects to weigh or otherwise measure each piece of food eaten, to record exact recipes used in mixed dishes, and name exact brand names of commercially produced foods. The major drawback of this approach is that it is very time-consuming and laborious for the subjects, and this is largely limited to small groups of highly motivated persons over short periods of time. It also requires a relatively large time commitment by trained nutritionists to convert the diary information into machine-readable form. Food diaries are still useful in validation studies, however, as the yardstick by which other methods are evaluated.

To measure long-term dietary intake, several other methods are available which do not require such prohibitive subject commitment. Short-term recall methods, particularly 24-hour recall, have been commonly used. Subjects write down, or are interviewed about, everything they ate in the previous 24-hour period, and this is assumed to be typical of each subject's usual intake. Unfortunately, day-to-day variation in individual intake of foods and nutrients is large (Beaton, Milner, and Corey, 1976), and thus a single day's intake is unlikely to be representative of long-term dietary habits.

The most practical approach to usual dietary assessment is the food-frequency method. Questions relate to usual intake over an extended period of time, such as a year. This longer time interval is more likely to be representative of long-term diet patterns than shorter periods of days or weeks, the periods assessed by most other methods. A food-frequency questionnaire consists of two parts: a list of foods and a set of frequency response options to indicate how often each food is consumed during the specified time period. Quantitative estimates of food and nutrient consumption may be obtained by either the investigator or the respondent, specifying a "usual" portion size for each food in terms of which frequency is to be estimated. At the first level of analysis, the relationship between cancer and individual foods or groups of foods may be examined. Going further, nutrient intakes can be calculated for each individual by multiplying the amount of each food consumed by the concentration of each nutrient of interest in that food and then summing the contribution of each food to intake of the nutrient. Results obtained with food-frequency questionnaires are reproducible and correlate with intakes determined by more detailed dietary methods (Willett et al., 1985, 1987) as well as with biochemical indices of nutrient intake (Willett et al., 1983a).

The precision of nutrient intake measures derived from diet assessments varies widely, and for some nutrients they may be meaningless. Cholesterol intake, for example, can be reasonably assessed, as cholesterol is present in a reasonably small number of foods with a relatively constant cholesterol composition. Many trace elements, on the other hand, are widespread among foods, and their concentration in these foods varies. Selenium concentration in foods, for example, depends largely on the selenium concentration of the soils in which the food was grown. Differences approach tenfold in the selenium content of cereals grown in low- and high-selenium soils have been reported (Arthur, 1972). Application of a single composition estimate to a food grown in different geographic areas may thus lead to considerable misclassification. The diversity of the food distribution network and the fact that most people are unaware of the exact source of production of their foods means that estimates of nutrients such as selenium are likely to be unreliable, except in studies conducted in defined geographic areas with well-documented sources of food supply. Methods of food preservation may alter nutrient composition. Fifty percent or more of the vitamin C initially present in fruits and vegetables may be lost during freezing or canning, for instance (Schroeder, 1971). The alternative method of nutrient intake estimation, to collect duplicate meals (each subject collects a second portion of all foods consumed, and this food is subjected to direct chemical analysis) is, however, too unwieldy and expensive to consider in large studies.

A further difficulty in the measurement of exposure is that even if the actual amount of a micronutrient in the diet can be accurately estimated, differences in bioavailability may mean that the effect of equal ingested amounts of a micronutrient may vary among subjects. Bioavailability has been defined as "the degree to which a nutrient becomes available to the target tissue after ingestion" (Sauberlich, 1985), and thus incorporates not only the concept of gut absorption, but subsequent metabolic processes that may facilitate, or hinder, delivery of the nutrient to the relevant site of biochemical action. Intestinal absorption of many micronutrients (e.g., vitamin C) is efficient at low doses, however, saturation of absorption may occur at higher intakes. Slight differences in chemical structure may also translate into large differences in absorption. In a study of selenium supplementation in a group of nursing mothers, selenium given as a selenium-yeast compound was apparently better absorbed than sodium selenite (Kumpulainen et al., 1985). As food composition tables usually reflect total micronutrient concentration and do not contain information on specific chemical form or complexes with other species, it is not currently possible to adjust for these differences. Interactions with other foods and nutrients can further affect the bioavailability of micronutrients. Absorption of a standard dose of radiolabeled selenite in water was reduced by 8% when it was given with orange juice and by 14% when given with a meal (Solomons et al., 1985). The physiological importance of many of these interactions is largely unknown. As our level of understanding of the nature and extent of these interactions improves, it may be possible to adjust intake estimates of a particular nutrient by concurrently obtained estimates of other components of diet with which it interacts. Meanwhile, the effect of these problems in the estimation of micronutrient intake is to introduce misclassification of the exposure measure. One result is that small effects of a nutrient are difficult to detect. A further implication is that estimates of the size of a consistently detected micronutrient-cancer relationship probably underestimates the true magnitude of the underlying association.

The problem of controlling for caloric intake is an important issue in the analysis of nutrient data. Because total caloric intake may be a risk factor for certain cancers and intakes of most nutrients tend to be positively correlated with caloric intake (Jain et al., 1980), then nutrients may be associated with disease simply due to their correlation with caloric intake. The conventional approach to control for total caloric intake has been to compute "nutrient densities" (by dividing nutrient values by caloric intake for each individual). This approach, however, does not necessarily control for the effect of caloric intake, because if caloric intake is associated with cancer, dividing nutrient values by this caloric intake creates a variable which will be associated with disease in the opposite direction to caloric intake (Willett and Stampfer, 1986). Willett and Stampfer suggest the use of "calorie-adjusted" nutrient intakes, calculated as the residuals from the regression model, with absolute nutrient intake as the dependent variable and caloric intake as the independent variable. Provided the usual regression assumptions are met, these "calorie-adjusted" nutrient intakes will be uncorrelated with energy intake, and thus provide a measure of nutrient exposure that is independent of the effect of caloric intake.

Biochemical Indicators of Nutrient Intake

For some nutrients, biologic specimens may provide a better means of assessing dietary intake than questionnaires. Serum levels of carotene and vitamin E, for instance, are sensitive to dietary intake and can thus be used to study the relationship between intakes of these nutrients and cancer. Morris, Stampfer, and Willett (1983) demonstrated that toenail clippings represent a measure of selenium intake integrated over an extended period. Many nutrients, however, are under tight homeostatic control, such that serum or tissue levels may not vary until the extremes of intake are reached. Serum retinol, for instance, is relatively invariant to short-term changes in intake, because the liver is an efficient storage organ for retinol and buffers serum levels over a wide range of intakes. Although the technical means exist to measure many micronutrients in either blood or tissues, the nature of the relation between intake and blood or tissue level has been determined for relatively few. This validation step is essential before micronutrient levels in biologic specimens are used to make inference about dietary exposure and cancer associations. Even when an association is found, interpretation should be cautious, as relations between biochemical indicators and disease are no less susceptible to confounding than other exposure-disease associations. An apparent effect of plasma carotenoids could, for instance, be due to other substances in green and yellow vegetables.

A further important limitation of biochemical measurements is the possibility that prevalent disease may affect the measurements. This is a particular problem in case-control studies, in which blood or other tissues from the cases are, by definition, obtained after disease has occurred. In this situation, changes in metabolism, nutrient intake, or absorption caused by the disease, and possibly the treatment, may lead to the detection of effects of disease, rather than antecedent diet. Even if biologic specimens are collected before the diagnosis of disease, the possibility exists that preclinical disease may affect biochemical measurements. Thus, in preliminary results reported by Wald and colleagues from a case-control study nested in a cohort of 16,000 men, the 86 subjects who developed cancer after 1 to 3.75 years of follow-up had a lower mean serum vitamin A than controls. Further follow-up, however, revealed no such difference for 116 cancer cases diagnosed 3 or more years after the blood was drawn (Wald, Boreham, and Bailey, 1986). Since even late-stage promotional events are thought to occur several years prior to the diagnosis of most cancers, the lower levels of retinol observed in the blood of men shortly before diagnosis are more likely to be a consequence, not a cause, of disease. Similarly, serum cholesterol among cases of cancer arising in the Multiple Risk Factor Intervention Trial was significantly lower in those diagnosed with cancer within two years of blood drawing. This difference attenuated in a dose-response manner with increasing duration of follow-up (Sherwin et al., 1987). Thus, the possibility that disease may affect biological measurements should always be considered, even in "prospective" studies.

INTERPRETATION OF EPIDEMIOLOGIC DATA

We have discussed the relative strengths and weaknesses of the principal study designs; the question remains how to synthesize the results from the available studies to summarize the evidence for particular hypotheses in order to decide on future research directions or preventive action. While the statistical principles and practice of appropriate data analysis are relatively well defined in the context of a single study, formal rules for the aggregation of results from many studies are less developed. Studies vary widely in both generalizability, depending mainly on the choice of study population, and "quality," depending on aspects of design, technical methods, and control of confounding. When reviewing a body of epidemiologic evidence it is appropriate to weight studies according to some assessment of "quality" (with "better" studies being more heavily weighted), however, in the absence of uniform definitions of what constitutes this "quality," there is considerable room for subjectivity in the assignment of weights. In general, for instance, biochemical results from bloods stored prospectively as part of a cohort study would be preferred to results from blood collected as part of a case-control study on which onset of disease may have affected blood levels. If, however, storage conditions were suboptimal for the cohort bloods, or specimens from cases were handled in a different manner from those of controls, then confidence in the study results would be reduced. The danger is, of course, that in the absence of objective criteria for assessment of study quality, evaluation of available data will be colored by the assessor's prior beliefs about the likelihood of the hypothesis. A further weakness of the "literature review" approach is that studies with "positive" findings may be more likely to be published than those with "negative" or "null" results. Over time this may lead to an accumulation of evidence in favor of the prevailing hypotheses in the published literature, which may not accurately reflect the results of the larger body of data actually gathered (Simes, 1986).

Given these reservations, how then do we proceed to reach conclusions from the available data? The role of geographic correlation studies in a formal assessment of the evidence is a matter of controversy. Despite their inherent weaknesses, their superficial ease of interpretation tends to overwhelm reservations, and they often weigh more heavily in the overall assessment than they should. Descriptive studies may be particularly useful when no association is observed; this can provide considerable evidence that a causal relation does not exist. For instance, the finding that breast cancer rates are similar in Seventh Day Adventist women compared with non-Seventh Day Adventist women of similar socioeconomic status suggests that mean consumption per se is not causally related to breast cancer. Evidence from case-control and cohort studies should be considered in the light of the appropriateness of the study design, the rigor of its conduct, and the probability of the presence of bias. No single observational study can be definitive, thus a number of studies with consistent results is the minimum required before a real association may be inferred with some confidence. The attribution of causality to an observed association is yet a further step, usually made more confidently when a plausible biological mechanism exists. Intervention studies provide the best evidence for the direction and magnitude of the effect of specific interventions. As these studies are frequently focused on highly selected "at-risk" populations for efficiency reasons, care should be taken in making inference to more general populations.

The evidence that particular micronutrients may prevent certain cancers is comprehensively explored elsewhere in this volume. In the light of the above criteria, however, what general statements can be made about the current strength of the epidemiologic evidence? Although a number of promising leads (e.g., beta-carotene, selenium) are being explored, sparse and at times contradictory evidence means that no micronutrient-cancer hypothesis currently enjoys the status of fact. For several of these hypotheses, observational and intervention studies already in place should clarify their plausibility and likely contribution to cancer prevention. A consistent association observed between low intake of green and yellow vegetables and cancer, in particular lung cancer, is probably the diet-cancer relation for which current epidemiologic evidence is strongest. Although this finding is highly suggestive of an underlying micronutrient-cancer relation, a specific micronutrient remains to be definitively identified. The exploration of existing micronutrient-cancer hypotheses and future hypotheses that will doubtless appear will require judicious selection from the range of epidemiologic study designs, the use of up-to-date methods to minimize bias, and a continued effort to validate and refine these methods.

REFERENCES

American Cancer Society (1987). In *Cancer Facts and Figures–1987.* American Cancer Society. New York, p. 10.

Armstrong, B., Doll, R. (1975). Environmental factors and cancer incidence and mortality in different countries with special reference to dietary practices. *Int. J. Cancer 15*: 617-631.

Arthur D. (1972). Selenium content of Canadian foods. *Can. Inst. Food Sci. Technol. 5*: 165-169.

Beaton, G. N., Milner, J., Corey, P. (1976). Sources of variance in 24-hour dietary recall data: implications for nutrition study design and interpretation. *Am. J. Clin. Nutr. 32*: 2546-2559.

Bjarnason, O., Day, N., Snaedal, G., Tulinius, N. (1974). The effect of year of birth on the breast cancer age-incidence curve in Iceland. *Int. J. Cancer. 13*: 689-696.

Buell, P. (1973). Changing incidence of breast cancer in Japanese-American women. *J.N.C.I. 51*: 1479-1483.

Carroll, K. K. (1975). Experimental evidence of dietary factors and hormone-dependent cancers. *Cancer Res. 35*: 3374-3383.

Doll, R., Peto, R. (1981). The causes of cancer: quantitative estimates of avoidable risks of cancer in the United States today. *J.N.C.I. 66*: 1191-1308.

Haenszel, W., Kurihara, M., Segi, M., Lee, R. K. C. (1972). Stomach cancer among Japanese in Hawaii. *J.N.C.I. 49*: 969-988.

Howson, C. P., Hiyama, T., Wynder, E. L. (1986). The decline in gastric cancer: Epidemiology of an unplanned triumph. *Epidemiol. Rev. 8*: 1-27.

International Agency for Research on Cancer (1980). IARC Monographs on the evaluation of the carcinogenic risk of chemicals to humans. Volume 22, Some non-nutritive sweetening agents. International Agency for Research on Cancer, Lyon, France 208 pp.

Jain, M., Cook, G. M., Davis, F. G., Grace, M. G., Howe, O. R., Miller, A. B. (1980). A case-control study of diet and colo-rectal cancer. *Int. J. Cancer. 26*: 757-768.

Jain, M. G., Harrison, L., Howe, G. R., Miller, A. B. (1982). Evaluation of a self-administered dietary questionnaire for use in a cohort study. *Am. J. Clin. Nutr. 36*: 931-935.

Jensen, D. M., Wahrendorf, J., Rosenquist, A., Geser, A. (1984). The reliability of questionnaire derived historical dietary information and temporal stability of food habits in individuals. *Am. J. Epidemiol. 120*: 281-290.

Kumpulainen, J., Salmenpera, L., Siimes, M. A., Koivistoinen, P., Perheentupa, J. (1985). Selenium status of exclusively breast-fed infants as influenced by maternal organic or inorganic selenium supplementation. *Am. J. Clin. Nutr. 42*: 829-835.

Kushi, L. H., Lew, R. A., Stare, F. J., Ellison, C. R., el Lozy, M., Bourke, G., Daley, L., Graham, I., Hickey, N., Mulcahy, R., Kevaney, J. (1985). Diet and 20-year mortality from coronary heart disease. *N. Engl. J. Med. 312*: 811-818.

Lyon, J. L., Gardner, J. W., West, D. W. (1980). Cancer incidence in Mormons and non-Mormons in Utah during 1967-75. *J.N.C.I. 5*: 1055-1061.

MacLennan, R., DaCosta, J., Day, N. E., Law, C. H., Ng, Y. K., Shanmugaratnan K. (1977). Risk factors for lung cancer in Singapore Chinese, a population with high female incidence rates. *Int. J. Cancer. 20*: 854-860.

MacMahon, B. (1979). Strengths and Limitations of Epidemiology. *Current Issues and Studies*. National Academy of Sciences, Washington, D.C., pp. 91-104.

Menkes, M. S., Comstock, G. W., Vuilleumier, J. P., Helsins, K. J., Rider, A. A., Brookmeyer, R. (1986). Serum beta-carotene, vitamins A and E, selenium, and the risk of lung cancer. *N. Engl. J. Med. 315*: 1250-1254.

Miettinen, O. S. (1985). In *Theoretical Epidemiology*. John Wiley and Sons, New York, p. 30.

Morris, J. S., Stampfer, M. J., Willett, W. (1983). Toenails as an indicator of dietary selenium. *Biol. Trace Element Res. 5*: 529-537.

Peto, R., Doll, R., Buckley, J. D., Sporn, M. D. (1981). Can dietary beta-carotene materially reduce human cancer rates? *Nature 290*: 201-208.

Phillips, R. C., Garfinkel, L., Kuzma, J. W., Beeson, W. L., Lotz, T., Brin, B. (1980). Mortality among California Seventh-Day Adventists for selected sites. *J.N.C.I. 5*: 1097-1107.

Rohan, J. E., Potter, J. O. (1984). Retrospective assessment of dietary intake. *Am. J. Epidemiol. 120*: 876-887.

Rothman, K. J. (1980). In *Modern Epidemiology*. Little, Brown and Company, Boston, p. 63.

Sauberlich, H. E. (1985). Bioavailability of vitamins. *Prog. Food Nutr. Sci. 4*: 1-33.

Schrauzer, G. N., White, D. A., Schneider, C. J. (1977). Cancer mortality correlation studies.. III. Statistical associations with dietary selenium intakes. *Bioinorgan. Chem. 7*: 23-31.

Schroeder, H. A. (1971). Losses of vitamins and trace minerals resulting from processing and preservation of foods. *Am. J. Clin. Nutr. 24*: 562-573.

Shekelle, R. B., Lepper, M., Liu, S., Maliza, C., Raynor, W. J., Rossof, A. N. (1981). Dietary vitamin A and risk of cancer in the Western Electric Study. *Lancet ii*: 1185-1190.

Shekelle, R. B., Shryock, A. M., Paul, O. (1982). Diet, serum cholesterol and death from coronary heart disease. *N. Engl. J. Med. 304*: 65-70.

Sherwin, R. W., Wentworth, D. N., Cutter, J. A., Hulley, S. B., Kuller, L. M., Stamler, J. (1987). Serum cholesterol levels and cancer mortality in 361 662 men screened for the Multiple Risk Factor Intervention Trial. *J.A.M.A. 257*: 943-948.

Simes, R. J. (1986). Publication bias: The case for an international registry of clinical trials. *J. Clin. Oncol. 4*: 1529-1541.

Solomons, N. W., Christensen, M. J., Janghorbani, M., Young, V. R. (1985). Absorption of selenium from single meals using an extrinsic, stable-isotope tracer, ^{74}Se. *Trace Elem. in Med. 2*: 59-63.

Wald, N., Boreham, J., Bailey, A. (1986). Serum retinol and subsequent risk of cancer. *Br. J. Cancer 54*: 957-961.

Willett, W. C., Stampfer, M. J., Underwood, B A., Speizer, F. E., Rosner, B., Hennekens, C. H. (1983a). Validation of a dietary questionnaire with plasma carotenoid and l-tocopherol levels. *Am. J. Clin. Nutr. 38*: 631-639.

Willett, W. C., Polk, B. F., Morris, J. S., Stampfer, M. J., Pressel, S., Schneider, K., Hames, C. G. (1983b). Prediagnostic serum selenium and risk of cancer. *Lancet ii*: 130-134.

Willett, W. C., Sampson, L., Stampfer, M. J., Rosner, B., Bain, C., Witschi, J., Hennekens, C. H., Speizer, F. E. (1985). Reproducibility and validity of a semiquantitative food frequency questionnaire. *Am. J. Epidemiol. 122*: 51-55.

Willett, W. C., Stampfer, M. J., (1986). Total energy intake: Implications for epidemiologic analyses. *Am. J. Epidemiol. 124*: 17–27.

Willett, W. C., Reynolds, R. D., Citrell-Hoehner, S., Sampson, L., Browne, M. L. (1987). Validation of a semi-quantitative food frequency questionnaire: Comparison with a 1-year diet record. *J.A.D.A. 87*: 43-47.

Part Two
METHODOLOGIC ISSUES FOR NUTRITIONAL ASSESSMENT

5

Analysis of Micronutrients in Foods

GARY R. BEECHER and FREDERICK KHACHIK
Human Nutrition Research Center, U. S. Department of Agriculture, Beltsville, Maryland

INTRODUCTION

Several micronutrients common in the diets of human have been suggested to be associated with a reduction in the incidence of cancer or inhibition of carcinogen-induced neoplasia. These dietary components include retinoids, carotenoids, tocopherols, ascorbic acid, selenium, and several other minor constituents known to occur in specific classes of foods, e.g., indoles, phenols, and aromatic isothiocyanates in green, leafy vegetables. Possible mechanisms of action for several of the micronutrients are discussed in Part 3 of this volume.

The ability to establish a statistically sound relationship between dietary micronutrients and incidence of cancer requires accurate and precise food composition data. Several of the micronutrients associated with cancer prevention appear to have more than one biological activity. For example, dietary β-carotene is largely converted to retinol in the intestinal mucosa and thereby contributes to "vitamin A activity." However, a small amount of β-carotene as well as other carotenoids are absorbed intact, can be easily quantified in serum or plasma, and may act as antioxidants (Burton and Ingold, 1984). Heretofore, food composition tables have tabulated the levels of micronutrients in foods in formats that correspond to vitamin activities as outlined in the Recommended Dietary Allowances (RDAs). Thus, only total vitamin A or total vitamin E activity may be reported, and the contribution of each chemical form of the vitamin to the total activity cannot be ascertained from the food tables. In the case of selenium, only recently has a range of dietary intakes been recommended (Food and Nutrition Board, 1980). As a result, few food tables report levels of this nutrient.

Technological advances in chemical instrumentation during the past two decades have provided analysts with powerful new tools to quantify low levels and various forms of nutrients in foods. Improvements in high performance liquid chromatography (HPLC) and particularly in column technology have been especially important in the development of new analytical techniques for several micronutrients (Macrae, 1982). Thus, many carotenoids in a green vegetable can be separated and quantified during a single HPLC run using reversed phase columns. Procedures for analyzing several micronutrients in foods employing HPLC techniques will be discussed in this chapter.

The micronutrients considered in this chapter have been limited to carotenoids, retinoids, vitamin E, all of which may be important in cancer prevention. Analytical procedures for carotenoids are discussed in detail since many carotenoid-containing foods have been associated with a reduction in the incidence of cancer in several epidemiologic studies (see Chapter 8). In addition, a dearth of analytic techniques and data are available for this complex group of micronutrients. Recently, rugged HPLC techniques have been developed for retinoids and vitamin E, which will also be reviewed.

CAROTENOIDS

In the simplest form of carotenoid analysis, these pigments are extracted from natural sources, purified by alkaline treatment (saponification) and/or chromatography, and finally carotenoid content is estimated by direct absorptivity measurements. For example, the carotenoid content of grapefruit (Lime et al., 1954; Ting and Deszyck, 1958) and tomato products (MacGillivray, 1935; Vogele, 1937; Davis, 1949) have been determined spectrophotometrically. However, since extracts from natural sources usually contain a variety of carotenoids that exhibit different absorption properties, the spectrophotometric measurement does not provide an accurate measure of the levels of these compounds. In addition, interference from noncarotenoid pigments often found in food extracts also contributes to analytic errors. The generation of analytic data on carotenoids in various food tables according to these methods will be evaluated later in this chapter.

In the past decade, although the methods of isolation and extraction procedures for carotenoids have not significantly changed, the detection techniques for these compounds have been greatly improved. This is primarily due to advances in high performance liquid chromatography (HPLC), which allows the separation of the various components of a mixture and can provide an accurate measurement of the levels of each constituent. The general extraction and isolation procedures for carotenoids will be described. Attempts have been made to emphasize separation and detection of carotenoids by providing some of the most recent examples of the HPLC analyses of these pigments in various food extracts.

Analysis of Carotenoids by High Performance Liquid Chromatography

High performance liquid chromatography (HPLC) has been shown to be the most efficient technique for the analysis of carotenoids in complex food extracts. The reproducibility, high sensitivity, and reasonably short analysis time in separation of carotenoids by HPLC provides reliable analytical data and minimizes the isomerization and decomposition of these sensitive compounds by light, heat, and air. Various HPLC conditions have been developed by different workers to separate the carotenoids in the extracts of natural products. The choice of the column (i.e., column dimension, adsorbent and particle size), the eluting solvents and their composition, and the column flow rate is very critical in developing optimum separation conditions for carotenoids. Wright and Shearer (1984) have separated the carotenes, xanthophylls, and chlorophylls of photosynthetic pigments from phytoplankton by HPLC on an octadecyl silane (ODS, 5-μm particle size) column employing a linear gradient from 90% acetonitrile to ethyl acetate over 20 min with a flow rate of 2 ml/min. Under these conditions HPLC separations of 44 pigments from representatives of the *Bacilliarophyceae, Dinophyceae, Cryptophyceae*, and *Cyanophyceae* were accomplished. A comprehensive review on the HPLC of plant pigments has been published by Schwartz et al. (1981). Separation of *cis*-isomers of β-carotene are best achieved on an HPLC Lime column as reported by Tsukida et al. (1982). Although this column separates various *cis*-isomers of β-carotene, it is not known if separation of other classes of carotenoids that are encountered in food extracts can also be simultaneously accomplished on this column. This is primarily owing to the lack of commercial availability of the Lime HPLC column. Meanwhile, the C-18 reversed phase HPLC columns of different brands remain the column of choice, as their application in separation of carotenoids in complex food extracts have become increasingly important. Recently the separation and quantification of the major carotenoid and chlorophyll constituents in extracts of several green vegetables (broccoli, cabbage, spinach, Brussels sprouts, kale) by HPLC on a C-18 reversed phase column employing a combination of isocratic and gradient chromatography (eluent A, Table 1) has been accomplished (Khachik et al., 1986). The major constituents of these green vegetables were shown to belong to three classes of compounds, in order of elution on a C-18 reversed phase column these were: oxygenated carotenoids (xanthophylls), chlorophylls and their derivatives, and the hydrocarbon carotenoids. A typical HPLC profile of raw broccoli extract is shown in Fig. 1. The general chromatographic profiles of the other raw green vegetables were shown to be very similar to that of the broccoli. The extract of several other green vegetables (lima beans, green peas, green beans) examined by HPLC recently have also shown to consist of the same components; however, minor differences seems to exist among some of these vegetables. For

Table 1 Chromatographic Conditions for Separation of Various Carotenoids

Eluent A, gradient, at a column flow rate of 0.5 ml/min					
at time 0	acetonitrile	75%	at time 12	acetonitrile	40.0%
	hexane	5%	during 15 min	hexane	22.5%
	methylene chloride	5%		methylene chloride	22.5%
	methanol	15%		methanol	15.0%
Eluent B, gradient, at a column flow rate of 0.7 ml/min					
at time 0	acetonitrile	65%	at time 23	acetonitrile	40.0%
	hexane	10%	during 10 min	hexane	22.5%
	methylene chloride	10%		methylene chloride	22.5%
	methanol	15%		methanol	15.0%
Eluent C, gradient, at a column flow rate of 0.70 ml/min					
at time 0	acetonitrile	85.0%	at time 10	acetonitrile	45.0%
	hexane	2.5%	during 30 min	hexane	22.5%
	methylene chloride	2.5%		methylene chloride	22.5%
	methanol	10.0%		methanol	10.0%
Eluent D, isocratic, at a column flow rate of 0.70 ml/min					
	acetonitrile	55%			
	methylene chloride	20%			
	methanol	25%			
Eluent E, gradient, at a column flow rate of 0.70 ml/min					
at time 0	acetonitrile	85.0%	at time 15	acetonitrile	50.0%
	hexane	2.5%	during 15 min	hexane	20.0%
	methylene chloride	2.5%		methylene chloride	20.0%
	methanol	10.0%		methanol	10.0%
Eluent F, isocratic, at a column flow rate of 1.0 ml/min					
	acetonitrile	55%			
	methylene chloride	23%			
	methanol	22%			
Eluent G, gradient, at a column flow rate of 0.5 ml/min					
at time 0	5% formic acid in water	98%	at time 10	5% formic acid in water	20%
	methanol	2%	in 45 min	methanol	80%

Separations carried out on a Microsorb (25 cm × 4.6 mm i.d.) C-18 (5-μm particle size) reversed phase column, protected with a Brownlee guard cartridge (3 cm × 4.6 mm i.d.) and packed with spheri-5 C-18 (5-μm particle size).

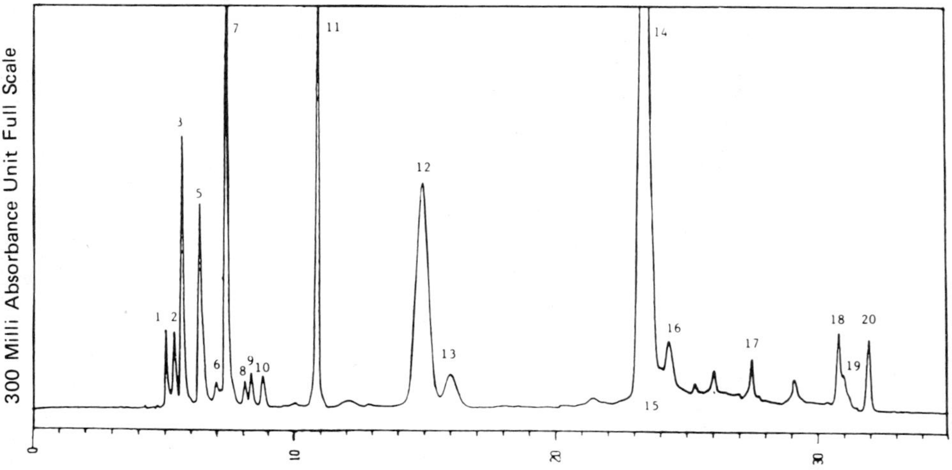

Fig. 1 HPLC profile of raw broccoli extract. Chromatographic conditions (eluent A, Table 1) and peak identification (Table 2) are described in the tables. (Used with permission from Khachik et al., 1986.)

example the HPLC profile (eluent A) of lima bean extract (Fig. 2) in addition to the components found in green vegetables shows the presence of α-carotene, which has been shown to be absent in most of the green vegetables examined (Khachik and Beecher, unpublished results). Peak identification of the various components of the green vegetable extracts in the order of elution on a C-18 reversed phase column separated by HPLC are shown in Table 2. The chemical structures of some of the abundant xanthophylls in green vegetables and β-apo-8′-carotenal, an internal standard employed for quantification of these carotenoids, are shown in Fig. 3. For convenience, various HPLC conditions employed in separation of carotenoids from food extracts that have been described in detail in this chapter have been tabulated in Table 1.

HPLC Separation of Carotenol Fatty Acid Esters

There are numerous reports on separation of various classes of carotenoids either isolated from natural sources or employed in a mixture of reference samples by HPLC. However, in these reports the development of the HPLC techniques for carotenol fatty acid esters, one of the classes of carotenoids often isolated from natural sources, has not yet received much attention. One of the very rare examples of the separation of carotenol fatty acid esters by HPLC has been reported

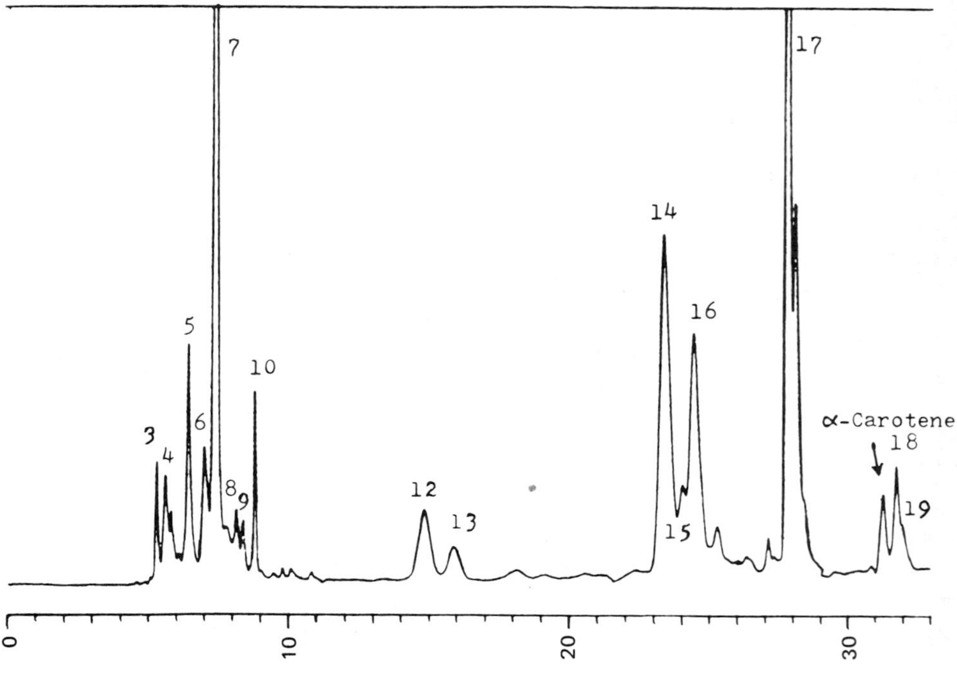

Fig. 2 HPLC profile of cooked lima bean extract. Chromatographic conditions (eluent A, Table 1) and peak identification (Table 2) are described in the tables.

by Gregory et al. (1986), who employed this technique to separate and quantify the fatty acid esters of lutein, isolated from Marigold flowers. The carotenoid extracts isolated from natural sources that are suspected to contain carotenol fatty acid esters are customarily saponified to remove the fatty acids and regenerate the hydroxycarotenoids (Noga and Lenz, 1983). Depending on the nature of carotenoids present, the saponification and extraction of carotenoids in these extracts may result in destruction or structural transformation of these compounds. Therefore the development of a rapid HPLC method that can separate carotenol fatty acid esters within a reasonable time in most cases may eliminate the saponification step. In addition, such HPLC methods can be applied to the simultaneous chromatographic separation of the various classes of carotenoids and provide valuable information on the identity and levels of these compounds in foods as they normally occur. Recently, HPLC conditions have been developed for separation and quantification of the abundant carotenoids and

Table 2 Peak Identification of the Various Components of the Green Vegetable Extracts Separated by HPLC

Chemical class	Peak	Components	λ monitored (nm)
Xanthophylls	1	all-*trans*-neoxanthin	445
	2	9′-*cis*-neoxanthin	445
	3	violaxanthin	445
	4	neochrome	445
	5	all-*trans*-lutein epoxide	445
	6	neolutein epoxide A (13- or 13′-*cis*-lutein epoxide)	445
	7	all-*trans*-lutein	445
	8	neolutein B (9- or 9′-*cis*-lutein)	445
	9	neolutein B′ (9′- or 9-*cis*-lutein)	445
	10	neolutein A	445
Apocarotenoid	11	β-apo-8′-carotenal (int std)	455
Chlorophylls	12	chlorophyll b	455
	13	chlorophyll b′	455
	14	chlorophyll a	430
	15	chlorophyll a′	430
	16	pheophytin b	430
	17	pheophytin a	410
Hydrocarbon carotenoids	18	all-*trans*-β-carotene	450
	19	15,15′-*cis*-β-carotene	450
	20	decapreno-β-carotene (int std)	500

carotenol fatty acid esters in the extracts from several varieties of squash (Khachik and Beecher, 1988). As many as 25 carotenoids as well as several of their stereoisomers were separated on a C-18 reversed phase column, which were assigned to four classes of compounds: xanthophylls, carotenol mono-fatty acid esters, hydrocarbon carotenoids, and carotenol di-fatty acid esters. The separations were achieved by employing a combination of isocratic and gradient chromatography and a solvent system that consisted of acetonitrile, methanol, methylene chloride, and hexane (eluent B, Table 1). The general chromatographic profiles of carotenoids in the unsaponified and saponified extracts from samples of baby food squash (*Cucurbita maxima*) of Northrup King and strained Butternut

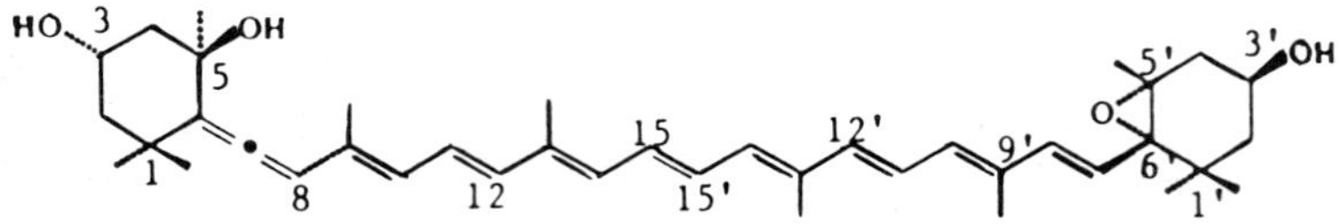

NEOXANTHIN

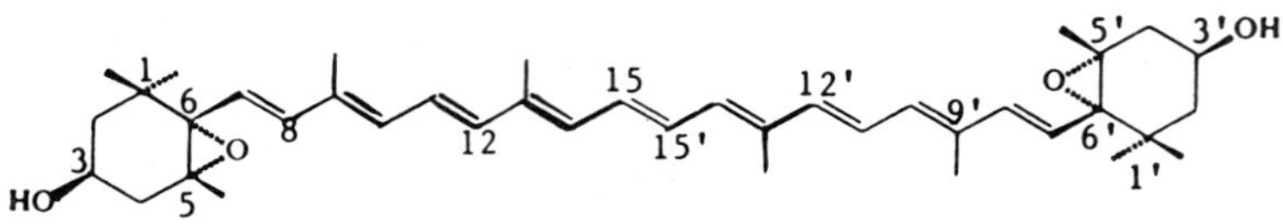

VIOLAXANTHIN

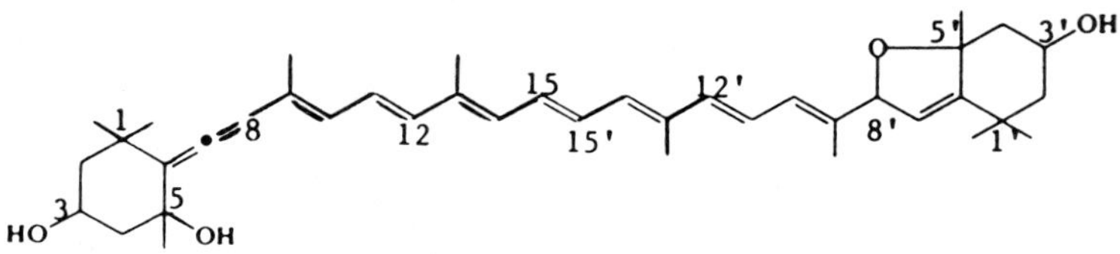

NEOCHROME

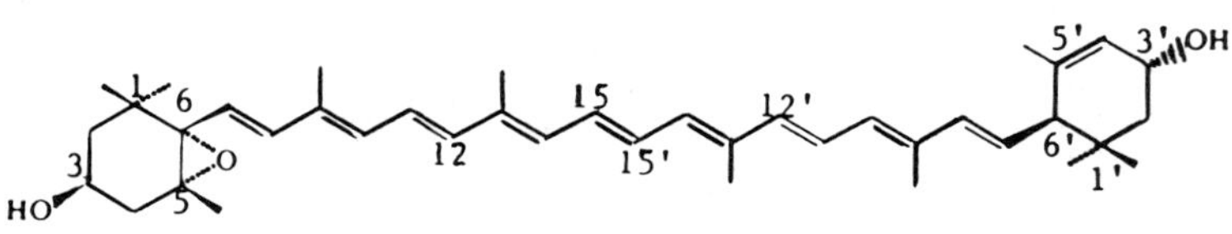

LUTEIN EPOXIDE

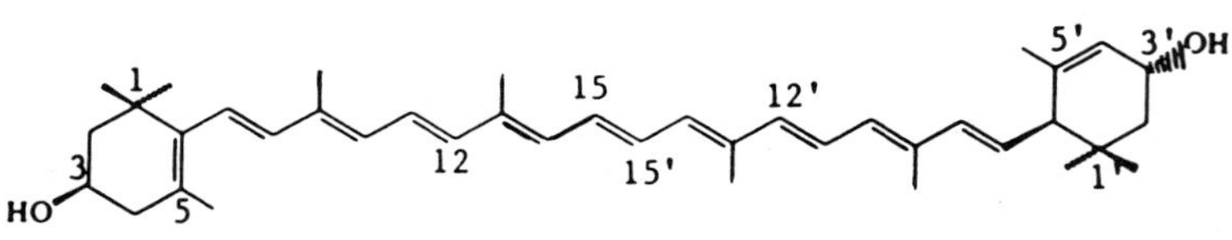

LUTEIN

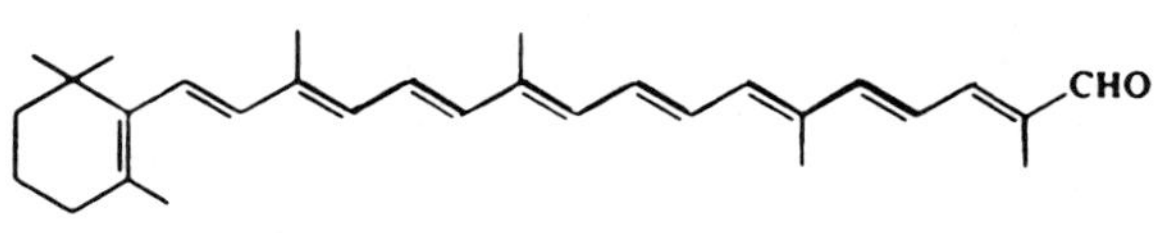

β-Apo-8'-Carotenal (INTERNAL STANDARD)

Fig. 3 Chemical structures of β-apo-8′-carotenal (internal standard) and some of the major carotenoid constituents found in the extracts of green vegetables.

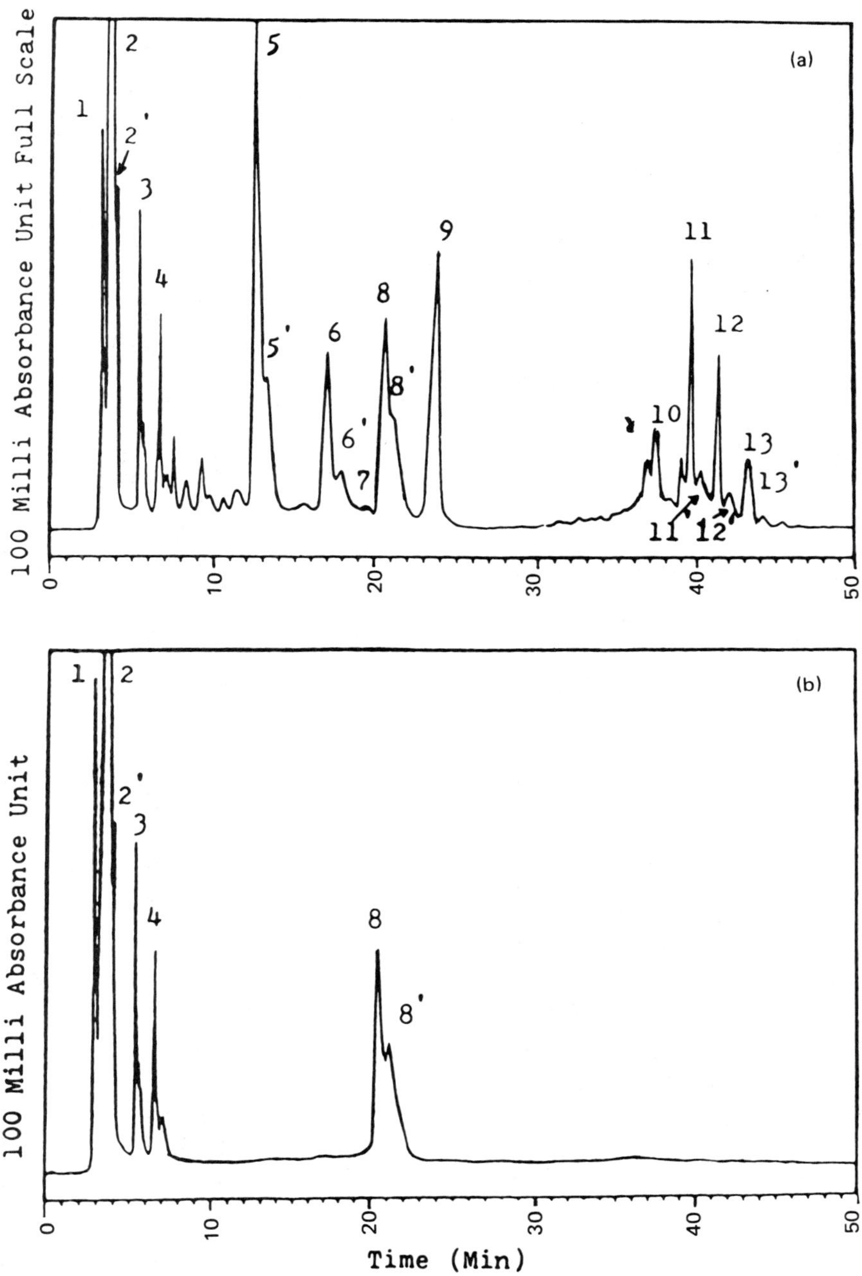

Fig. 4 HPLC profiles of baby food squash extract of Northrup King variety, (a) upper trace, before saponification; (b) lower trace, after saponification. Chromatographic conditions (eluent B, Table 1) and peak identification (Table 3) are described in the tables. (Used with permission from Khachik and Beecher, 1988.)

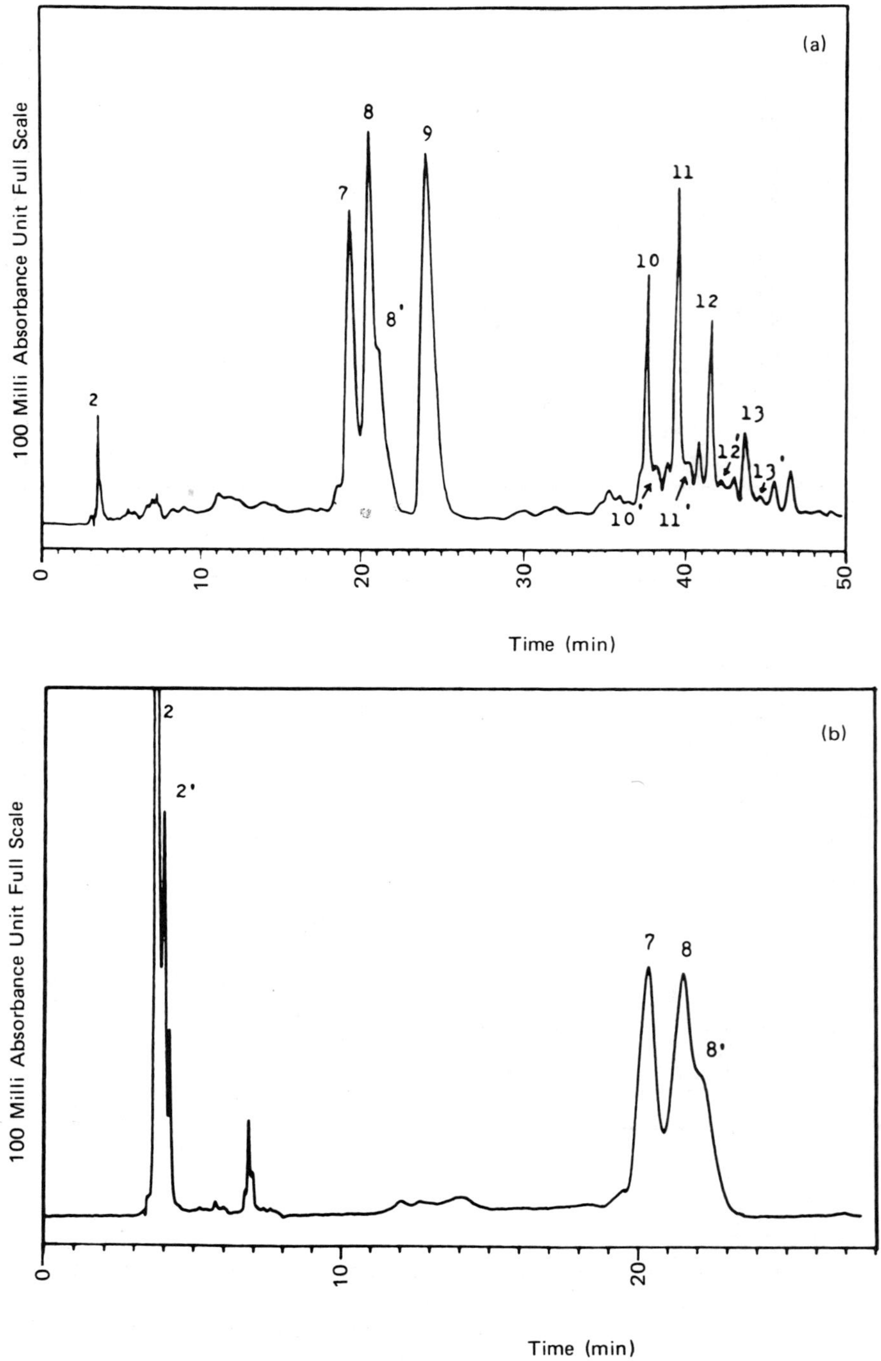
(a)
100 Milli Absorbance Unit Full Scale
2
7
8
8'
9
10
11
12
13
10'
11'
12'
13'
0
10
20
30
40
50
Time (min)
(b)
100 Milli Absorbance Unit Full Scale
2
2'
7
8
8'
0
10
20
Time (min)

Table 3 HPLC Peak Identification of the Abundant Carotenoids and Carotenol Fatty Acid Esters in Several Varieties of Baby Food Squash (Brand G and H)

Chemical class	Peak	Components	RT (min)[a]
Xanthophylls	1	flavoxanthin	3.12
	2	all-*trans*-luteen	3.52
	2′	neolutein A or A′ (13- or 13′-*cis*-lutein)	4.00
	3	3-hydroxy-2′,3′-dehydro-β,ε-carotene	5.52
	4	9- or 9′-*cis*-β-cryptoxanthin	6.72
Carotenol mono-fatty	5	all-*trans*-lutein monomyristate (β,ε-carotene-3-monol monomyristate-3′-monol)	12.64
acid esters	5′	neolutein monomyristate A or A′	13.20
	6	all-*trans*-lutein monopalmitate (β,ε-carotene-3-monol monopalmitate-3′-monol)	17.04
	6′	neolutein monopalmitate A or A′	17.99
Hydrocarton carotenoids	7	all-*trans*-α-carotene	19.64
	8	all-*trans*-β-carotene	20.64
	8′	15,15′-*cis*-β-carotene	21.30
Carotenol di-fatty	9	isozeaxanthin dipelargonate (int std)	23.72
acid esters	10	all-*trans*-lutein dilaurate	37.72
	10′	neolutein dilaurate A or A′	38.50
	11	all-*trans*-lutein dimyristate	39.62
	11′	neolutein dimyristate A or A′	40.40
	12	all-*trans*-lutein myristate/palmitate	41.60
	12′	neolutein myristate/palmitate A or A′	42.40
	13	all-*trans*-lutein dipalmitate	43.60
	13′	neolutein dipalmitate A or A′	44.40

[a]Retention times of the various components under chromatographic conditions (eluent B) described in text.

Fig. 5 HPLC profiles of strained baby food squash extract of Butternut variety, (a) upper trace, before saponification; (b) lower trace, after saponification. Chromatographic conditions (eluent B, Table 1) and peak identification (Table 3) are described in the tables. (Used with permission from Khachik and Beecher, 1988.)

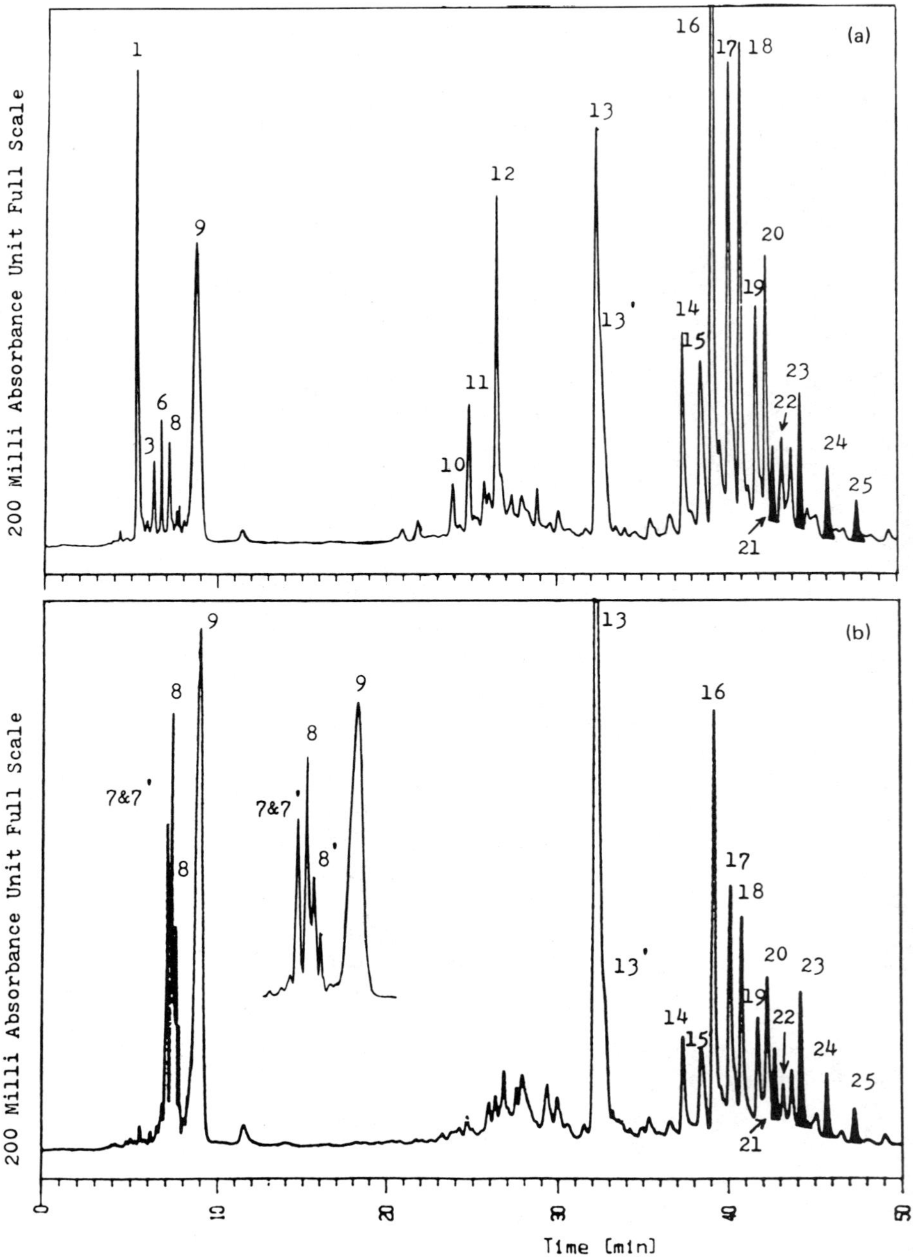

Fig. 6 HPLC profiles of extracts from raw, (a), upper trace, and cooked, (b), lower trace, acorn squash (*Cucurbita pepo*). Chromatographic conditions (eluent C, Table 1) and peak identification (Table 4) are described in the tables. Shaded peaks are lutein di-fatty acid esters. (Used with permission from Khachik and Beecher, 1988.)

Table 4 HPLC Peak Identification of the Abundant Carotenoids and Carotenol Fatty Acid Esters of Acorn Squash in the Order of Chromatographic Elution on a C-18 Reversed Phase Column

Chemical class	Peak	Components	RT (min)[a]
Xanthophylls	1	all-*trans*-violaxanthin	5.43
	2	15,15′ or 13-*cis*-violaxanthin	5.73
	3	all-*trans*-luteoxanthin	6.00
	4	9-*cis*-violaxanthin (violeoxanthin)	6.34
	5	all-*trans*-auroxanthin	6.69
	6	13- or 15,15′-*cis*-violaxanthin	6.70
	7	di-*cis*-violaxanthin	6.87
	7′	di-*cis*-violaxanthin	7.07
	8	all-*trans*-lutein	7.19
	8′	neolutein A or A′ (13 or 13′-*cis*-lutein)	7.45
Apocarotenoid	9	β-apo-8′-carotenol (int std)	8.48
Carotenol mono-fatty acid esters	10	9 or 9′-*cis*-violaxanthin monomyristate	23.90
	11	all-*trans*-violaxanthin monomyristate	24.78
	12	9′ or 9-*cis*-violaxanthin monomyristate	26.46
Hydrocarbon carotenoids	13	all-*trans*-β-carotene	32.38
	13′	15,15′-*cis*-β-carotene	32.60
Carotenol di-fatty	14	all-*trans*-violaxanthin dilaurate	37.50
	15	9-*cis*-violaxanthin dilaurate (violeoxanthin dilaurate)	38.54
	16	all-*trans*-violaxanthin dimyristate	39.26
	17	9-*cis*-violaxanthin dimyristate (violeoxanthin dimyristate)	40.30
	18	all-*trans*-violaxanthin myristate/palmitate	40.94
	19	9-*cis*-violaxanthin myristate/palmitate (violeoxanthin myristate/palmitate)	41.90
	20	all-*trans*-violaxanthin dipalmitate	42.54
	21	all-*trans*-lutein dilaurate	42.86
	22	9-*cis*-violaxanthin dipalmitate (violeoxanthin dipalmitate)	43.50
	23	all-*trans*-lutein dimyristate	44.46
	24	all-*trans*-lutein myristate/palmitate	46.06
	25	all-*trans*-lutein dipalmitate	47.70

[a]Retention times of the various component under chromatographic conditions (eluent C) described in text.

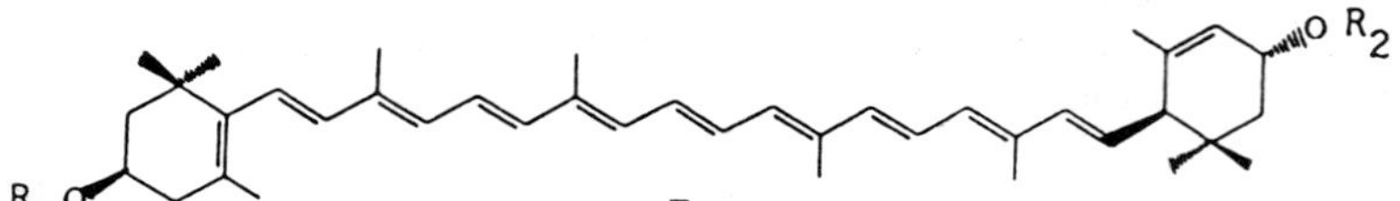

I

(a) $R_1 = R_2 = H$

(b) $R_1 = CH_3(CH_2)_n\overset{O}{\overset{\|}{C}}-$ (n = 12, 14) $R_2 = H$

(c) [R_1 or $R_2 = CH_3(CH_2)_n\overset{O}{\overset{\|}{C}}-$, n = 12], [$R_2$ or $R_1 = CH_3(CH_2)_n\overset{O}{\overset{\|}{C}}-$, n = 14]

(d) $R_1 = R_2 = CH_3(CH_2)_n\overset{O}{\overset{\|}{C}}-$ (n = 10, 12, 14)

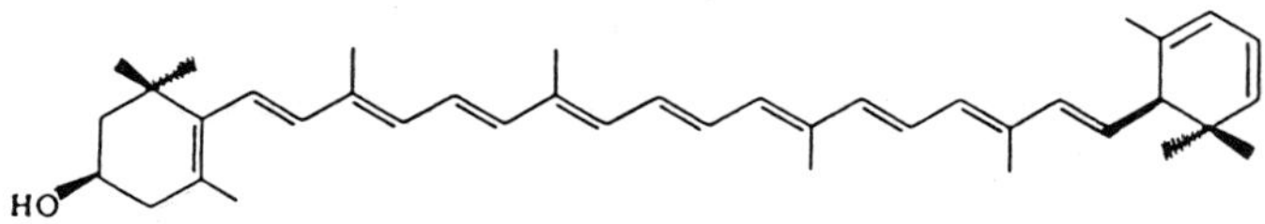

II

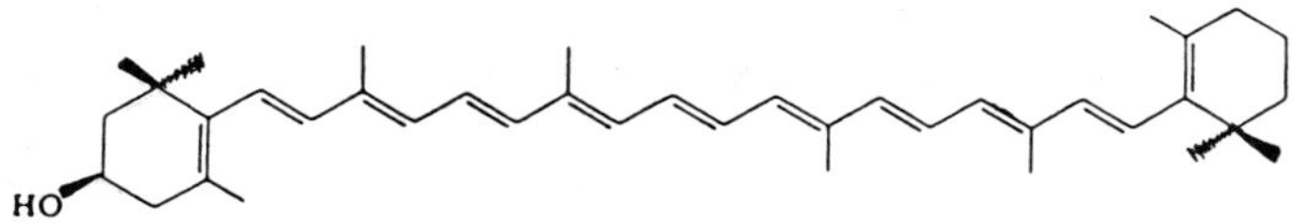

III

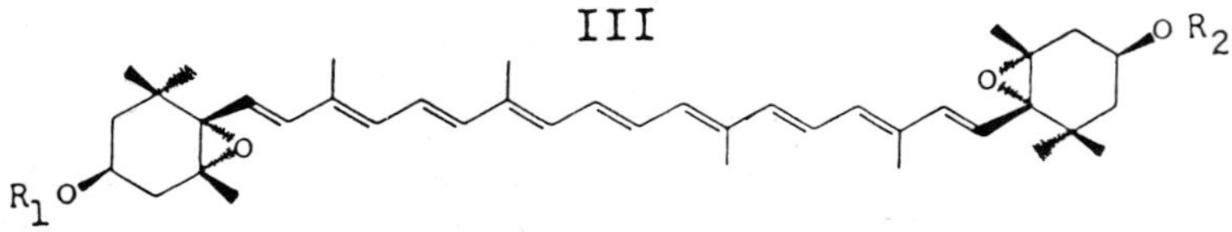

IV

(a) $R_1 = R_2 = H$

(b) $R_1 = CH_3(CH_2)_{12}\overset{O}{\overset{\|}{C}}-$ $R_2 = H$

(c) [R_1 or $R_2 = CH_3(CH_2)_n\overset{O}{\overset{\|}{C}}-$, n = 12], [$R_2$ or $R_1 = CH_3(CH_2)_n\overset{O}{\overset{\|}{C}}-$, n = 14]

(d) $R_1 = R_2 = CH_3(CH_2)_n\overset{O}{\overset{\|}{C}}-$ (n = 10, 12, 14)

Fig. 7 The chemical structures of some of the abundant carotenoids and carotenol fatty acid esters in squash varieties. Only the all-*trans*-isomers are shown. I(a) = lutein, I(b) = natural lutein mono-fatty acid esters, I(c) = mixed lutein di-fatty acid esters, I(d) = lutein di-fatty acid esters; II = 3-hydroxy-2′,3′-dehydro-β,ε-carotene; III = β-cryptoxanthin; IV(a) = violaxanthin, IV(b) = violaxanthin monomyristate, IV(c) = mixed violaxanthin di-fatty acid esters; IV(d) = violaxanthin di-fatty acid esters.

squash varieties grown and processed by two leading food processing companies in the United States under controlled conditions are shown in Figs. 4 and 5. Peak identification of the abundant carotenoids and carotenol fatty acid esters from the extracts of baby food squash of Northrup King and strained Butternut varieties in the order of elution on a C-18 column is shown in Table 3. The chromatographic profiles (eluent C, Table 1) of extracts from raw and cooked acorn squash (*Cucurbita pepo*) grown in New Jersey are shown in Fig. 6. The effect of cooking and processing on qualitative and quantitative distribution of carotenoids will be described later in this chapter. Peak identification of the carotenoids in acorn squash (*Cucurbita pepo*) in the order of elution on a C-18 reversed phase column is shown in Table 4. The chemical structures of some of the squash carotenoids and their corresponding esters are shown in Fig. 7. The detailed identification of these compounds by spectroscopy, partial synthesis, and chromatography has been described elsewhere (Khachik et al., 1988a).

Varietal Differences

The chromatographic profiles of the varieties of squash described above demonstrate significant differences in qualitative distribution of carotenoids and the related fatty acid esters in different cultivars of this vegetable. Particularly noticeable is the presence of lutein and lutein mono-fatty acid esters (lutein monomyristate and lutein monopalmitate) and the absence of α-carotene in baby food squash of Northrup King variety and the absence of lutein mono-fatty acid esters and the presence of α-carotene in strained baby food squash of Butternut variety. These cultivar differences can be better understood if the photosynthetic mechanisms leading to the formation of these compounds are considered. Since the hydroxylation of α-carotene is known to be responsible for the formation of lutein in plant photosynthesis (Goodwin, 1980a), it seems more likely that the mono- and di-fatty acid esters of lutein in squash are formed from lutein. However, the actual photosynthetic mechanism leading to the formation of these compounds is not known at the present time. From extensive NMR studies of the native lutein monomyristate and monopalmitate isolated from the extracts of baby food squash of Northrup King variety and from NMR data obtained from several synthetic model compounds, it has been demonstrated that the site of the ester moiety in the mono-esters of lutein is on the β- rather than α-ionone ring (Khachik et al., 1988a). The preferential esterification of the β-ionone ring, which results in the formation of the lutein mono-fatty acid esters is not clearly understood. The chromatographic profiles of the extracts from baby food squash of Northrup King variety grown in two different locations in the United States (Fremont, Michigan, and Asheville, North Carolina) show no significant difference (Khachik and Beecher, 1988). However, the concentration of the carotenoids and related esters in baby food squash grown in Michigan is much lower than that of the same brand grown in North Carolina. This may be related to environmental factors affecting the biosynthesis of carotenoids (i.e., light, temperature, nitrogen metabolism, and soil nutrients). The effect of environment on the synthesis of carotenoids in seed-bearing plants has been reviewed by Goodwin (1980b).

Correlation Between HPLC Retention Times and the Equivalent Chain Lengths of Di-Fatty Acid Esters of Carotenoids

In gas liquid chromatography (GLC), the correlation between the number of carbons in saturated fatty acids and related esters has been extensively used to predict the elution sequence of these compounds from a gas liquid chromatographic column (Jamieson, 1970). Under identical chromatographic conditions, a parameter known as equivalent chain length (ECL) for a number of known saturated monocarboxylic methyl esters is obtained by plotting the logarithms of the retention times of these compounds against the number of carbon atoms in their corresponding acids. ECL values of unknown esters, chromatographed under identical conditions, are then determined from the reference curve using the observed retention times. Similar correlations at first appear to exist between the HPLC retention times of the various classes of carotenol fatty acid esters separated from squash extracts and the number of carbon atoms in their fatty acids' side chains. For example, under the chromatographic conditions (eluents B) employed for the separation of the squash carotenoids in baby foods, there is a steady increase of about 3.90-4.00 minutes in the HPLC retention times of lutein dimyristate (Table 3), as the total number of carbon atoms in the fatty acid side chains in this compound is increased by four to lutein dipalmitate. However, this correlation does not hold for lutein dilaurate. Recently, the retention times of a number of synthetic (C-10, C-12, C-12/C-14, C-14, C-14/C-16, C-16) esters of carotenoids such as lutein, zeaxanthin, isozeaxanthin, violaxanthin, auroxanthin, and β-cryptoxanthin separated under various isocratic and gradient chromatography conditions have also revealed that an exact increase in retention times of these carotenol esters is not reproducible (Khachik and Beecher, 1988c). This is probably related to the parameters affecting intermolecular interactions between sample and solvent molecules in liquid chromatography (i.e., dispersion, dipole, and hydrogen bonding). As the number of carbons in straight chain fatty acids is increased by two some noticeable changes in the physical properties (melting point and solubility behavior) of these compounds are observed. It therefore seems more likely that the chromatographic and the solubility behavior of carotenol fatty acid esters are influenced by chromatographic and solubility behavior of the fatty acid side chains, which in turn may reflect in a nonsteady increase in retention times for some of these carotenol esters. From the retention times of various caretenol esters separated by HPLC it appears that within a series of carotenol esters of a given carotenoids as the number of carbon atoms on the fatty acids' side chains are increased, the HPLC retention times of carotenol fatty acid esters on a reversed phase column are also increased.

Artifacts in Carotenoid Analysis by HPLC

In separation of carotenoids by HPLC, the interaction between solute (carotenoids) molecules, injecting solvent, and mobile phase can result in production of HPLC artifacts that may indicate the presence of impurities or *cis*-carotenoids. The effect of this sample-solvent interaction on the resolution of the HPLC peaks for several carotenoids (α- and β-carotene, nonapreno-β-carotene, lycopene, β-apo-8′-carotenal, canthaxanthin, zeaxanthin) injected in various solvents and chromatographed under various isocratic and gradient HPLC conditions has recently been extensively studied (Khachik et al., 1988b). The separations were carried out on a C-18 reversed phase column employing various compositions of eluents such as methanol, acetonitrile, methylene chloride, hexane, and tetrahydrofuran (THF). These studies have revealed that, depending on the solubility of the carotenoids in the HPLC mobile phase and the nature of the injecting solvent, single, double, and in some cases multiple HPLC peaks can be reproducibly generated. Chromatographic profiles of carotenoids injected in solvents such as hexane, acetone, methanol, petroleum ether, and acetonitrile contain single symmetrical HPLC peaks for each carotenoid, while carotenoids injected in solvents such as THF, methylene chloride, chloroform, benzene, and toluene produce additional HPLC peaks. For example, the chromatographic profile of all-*trans*-β-carotene injected in the HPLC solvents (eluent D, see Table 1), as shown in Fig. 8a, results in a single symmetrical HPLC peak. However, if the injecting HPLC solvents are replaced with methylene chloride and β-carotene is then injected in this solvent, the resulting chromatogram shows the presence of an additional peak (peak A′, Fig. 8b). Isolation of these two peaks by preparative HPLC and structural elucidation by NMR and UV/visible absorption spectroscopy has indicated that both peaks A and A′ are all-*trans*-β-carotene and no *cis-trans* isomerization was shown to have taken place. This multiple HPLC peak formation is thought to be dependent on the relative solubility of the carotenoids in the injection and eluting solvents as the sample bolus first interacts with the column. This is based on the observation that as the injection volume is increased, a more pronounced HPLC peak distortion resulted. This effect is clearly demonstrated in the chromatograms (eluent D) obtained

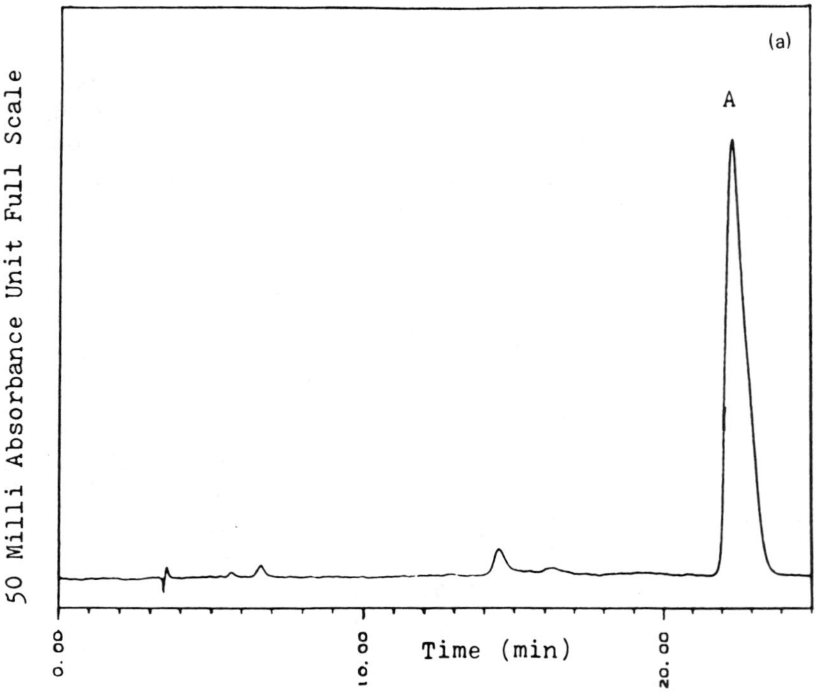
(a)
A
50 Milli Absorbance Unit Full Scale
0.00
10.00
Time (min)
20.00

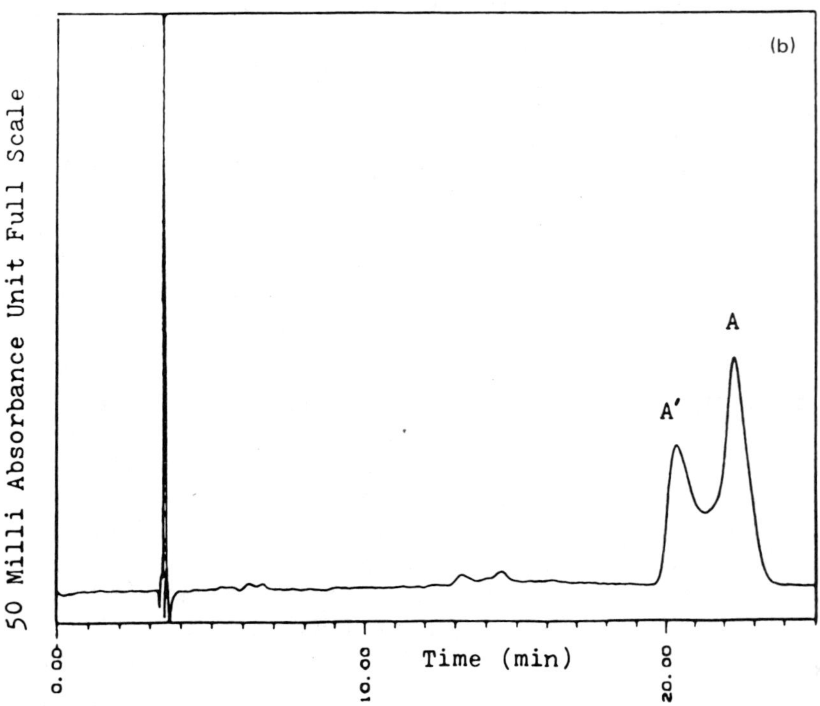
(b)
A'
A
50 Milli Absorbance Unit Full Scale
0.00
10.00
Time (min)
20.00

from 50- and 100-μl injection of a solution of all-*trans*-β-carotene in THF, as shown in Figs. 9a and 9b, respectively. The chromatographic profiles (eluent E) of a mixture of carotenoids (i.e., α- and β-carotene, nonapreno-β-carotene, lycopene, β-apo-8′-carotenal, canthaxanthin, zeaxanthin) injected in acetone (Fig. 10a) and methylene chloride (Fig. 10b) clearly demonstrate that these HPLC artifacts are not unique to β-carotene. Therefore, the choice of the injecting solvent in the HPLC of carotenoids is very critical. Idealy, in common HPLC practice, the sample should be injected in the HPLC eluent, which by minimizing strong interaction between solute, injecting solvent, and the mobile phase should eliminate such artifacts. However, in cases where carotenoids extracted from biological samples are more conveniently solubilized in a solvent other than the HPLC mobile phase, these HPLC artifacts may be eliminated by lowering the concentration of the sample or by reducing the injection volume. Examples of such artifacts have also been reported in reversed phase chromatography of triglycerides (Tsimidou and Macrae, 1985). For a review on other separation artifacts, the reader is referred to the publication of Snyder and Kirkland (1979).

Selection of Internal Standard in HPLC of Carotenoids

Since the preparation of carotenoid samples for HPLC analysis requires extensive extraction and work-up procedures that can be accompanied by various analytical errors, the use of an internal standard is essential. The general requirements of an internal standard can be summarized as follows:

1. It must produce a well-resolved HPLC peak with no interference with the compounds of interest.
2. It must elute relatively close to the compounds of interest.
3. The solubility and chromatographic response of the internal standard in the mobile phase must be similar to those of the compounds of interest (this is normally the case when the internal standard is structurally related to the compounds of interest).
4. For analyses of multicomponent mixtures, more than one internal standard may be required to achieve highest precision.
5. It must be added at a concentration that will produce a peak area or peak height of about unity with compounds of interest.

Fig. 8 Chromatograms of all-*trans*-β-carotene. (a) Upper trace, sample injected in the HPLC solvents (eluent D, Table 1); (b) lower trace, sample injected in methylene chloride (eluent D, Table 1). Peaks A and A′ = all-*trans*-β-carotene. (Used with permission from Khachik et al., 1988b.)

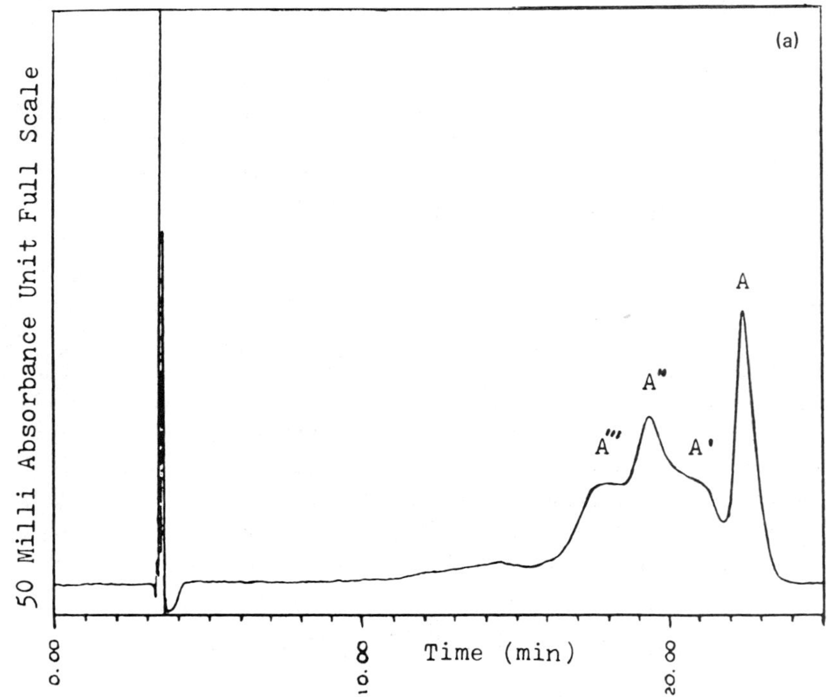
(a)
50 Milli Absorbance Unit Full Scale
A
A"
A'''
A'
0.00
10.00
Time (min)
20.00

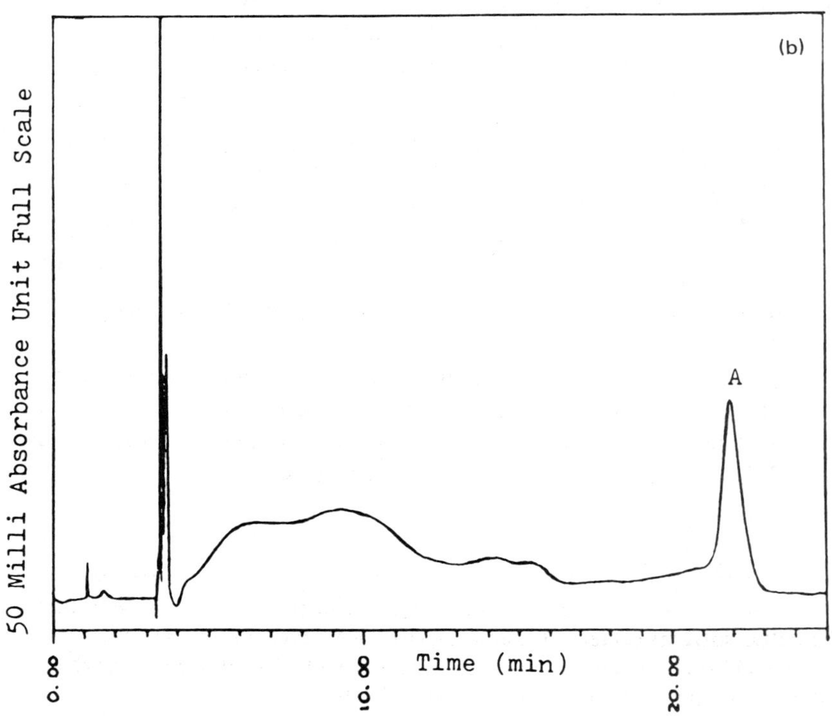
(b)
50 Milli Absorbance Unit Full Scale
A
0.00
10.00
Time (min)
20.00

6. It must not be present in the original sample (i.e., preferably not a naturally occurring carotenoid).
7. It must have similar stability to those of the compounds of interest and it must not react with sample components, column packing, or mobile phase.
8. It is desirable for it to be commercially available in high purity.

Many examples have appeared in the literature of the separation and quantification of plant carotenoids; however, few of these have employed an internal standard. Stancher and Zonta (1982) have employed azobenzene as an internal standard for quantitative determination of β-carotene and vitamin A in Taleggio cheese extract by HPLC. The light absorption of azobenzene and its HPLC retention time on a normal phase silica column are compatible with that of β-carotene. However, on a C-18 reversed phase column, azobenzene elutes much faster than α- and β-carotene and is therefore not suitable as an internal standard. Furthermore, azobenzene is not structurally close to carotenoids and is expected to have different solubility and chromatographic behavior, which may result in its limited application as an internal standard. β-Apo-8′-carotenal has been used as an internal standard in the separation and quantification of citrus carotenoids by reversed phase HPLC (Noga and Lenz, 1983). This compound has also been shown to be a suitable internal standard for quantitative determination of naturally occurring oxygenated carotenoids (xanthophylls), separated from the extracts of several green vegetables by HPLC (see Fig. 1) (Khachik et al., 1986). However, since under several different chromatographic conditions, β-apo-8′-carotenal has been consistently shown to elute much faster than α- and β-carotene on a C-18 reversed phase column, this compound may be found of limited application as an internal standard in the HPLC of carotenoids (Khachik and Beecher, unpublished results). (2R,2R′)-2,2′-Dimethyl-β-carotene has been successfully employed as an internal standard in quantitative determination of β-carotene in human serum (Driskell et al., 1983). Although dimethyl-β-carotene has many attractive features as an internal standard, it is not stable more than two weeks at −70°C, as reported by the authors (Driskell et al., 1983). The preparation of small quantities of this compound requires elaborate synthesis, which contributes to its lack of commercial availability and application (Eugster et al., 1955; Andrews et al., 1974). Decapreno-β-carotene, a C-50-β-carotene, has been employed as an internal standard for quantification of the

---

Fig. 9 Chromatograms of a constant concentration of all-*trans*-β-carotene injected at two different volumes in THF. (a) Upper trace, sample injected in 50 μl THF; (b) Lower trace, sample injected in 100 μl THF. HPLC conditions (eluent D) have been described in Table 1. Peaks A, A′, A″, and A‴ = all-*trans*-β-carotene. (Used with permission from Khachik et al., 1988b.)

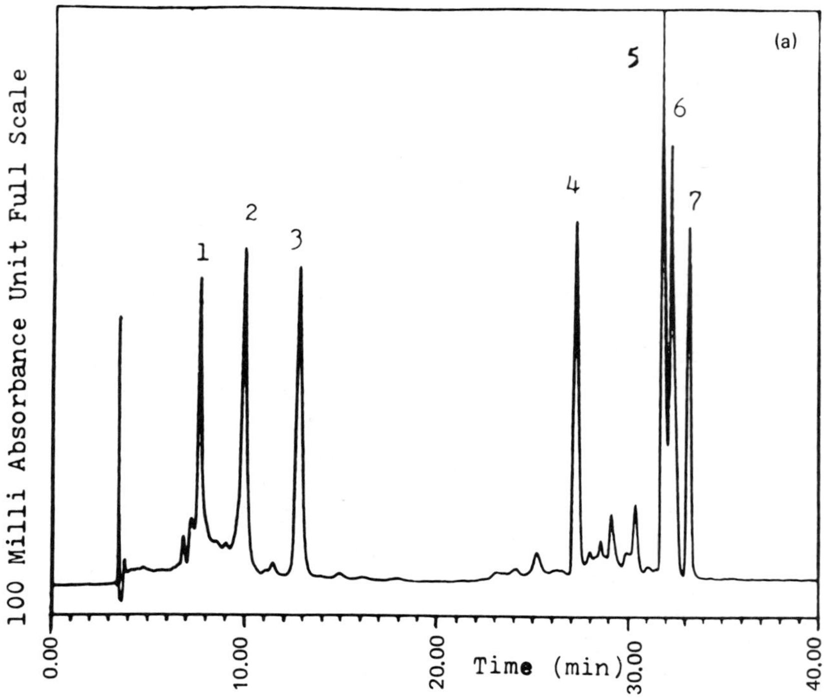
(a)
100 Milli Absorbance Unit Full Scale
1
2
3
4
5
6
7
0.00
10.00
20.00
30.00
40.00
Time (min)

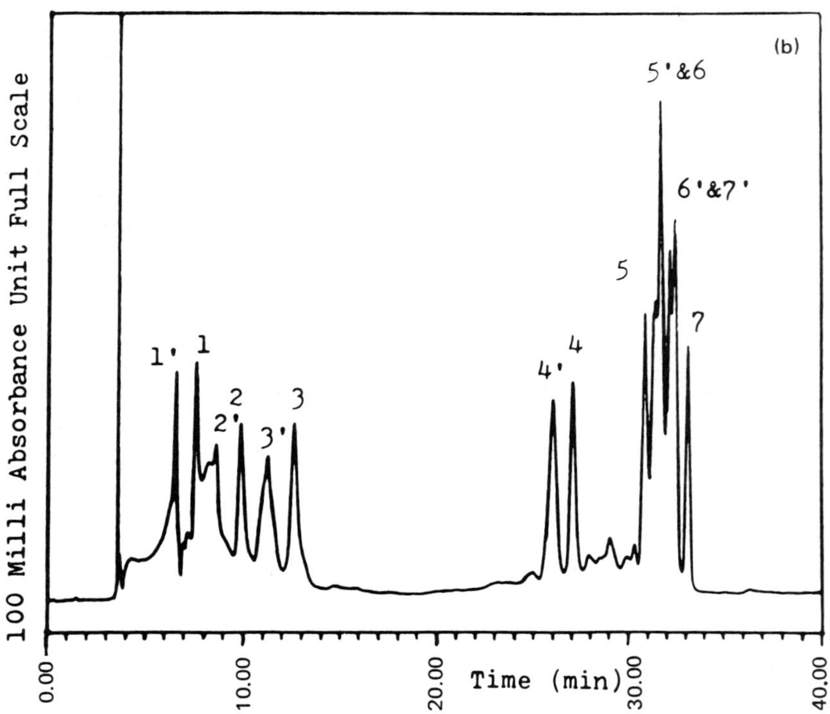
(b)
100 Milli Absorbance Unit Full Scale
1'
1
2'
2
3'
3
4'
4
5
5'&6
6'&7'
7
0.00
10.00
20.00
30.00
40.00
Time (min)

hydrocarbon carotenoids extracted from carrots and several green leafy vegetables (see Fig. 1) (Khachik and Beecher, 1985; Khachik et al., 1986). This internal standard has two more isoprene units than β-carotene and can be readily synthesized according to the method of Surmatis and Ofner (1961). Although decapreno-β-carotene has been shown to serve as a good internal standard, it has several disadvantages that have limited its application in the quantitative determination of hydrocarbon carotenoids. Owing to the length of the polyene chain in decapreno-β-carotene, the low solubility and unique chromatographic properties of this compound requires specific HPLC conditions to elute this compound relatively close to α- and β-carotene. The much higher absorption maxima of decapreno-β-carotene (λ_{max} = 502) relative to α- and β-carotene (λ_{max} = 446, and 454 nm, respectively) in the mixture of HPLC solvents (acetonitrile, methanol, heane, methylene chloride) requires the detection of these compounds at two different wavelengths. In addition, on standing, solutions of decapreno-β-carotene in common HPLC solvents undergo a much more rapid degradation than those of α- and β-carotene. Although the synthesis of this compound is fairly straightforward, it involves a number of synthetic steps, which may also limits its commercial availability. Recently, a C-45-β-carotene, namely, nonapreno-β-carotene, which has one isoprene unit more than α- and β-carotene and one isoprene unit less than decapreno-β-carotene, has been synthesized and employed as an internal standard for quantification of α- and β-carotene by HPLC (Khachik and Beecher, 1986). The chemical structures of β-carotene, C-50-β-carotene, and C-45-β-carotene are shown in Fig. 11. Nonapreno-β-carotene (V) was synthesized in 70% yield from condensation of the Wittig salt of vinyl-β-ionol (III) with β-apo-8′-carotenal (IV), as shown in Fig. 12. Vinyl-β-ionol (II) was prepared from the Grignard reaction between vinyl magnesium bromide and β-ionone (I) in 90% yield. The application of C-45-β-carotene as an internal standard for quantitative determination of the hydrocarbon carotenoids extracted from several yellow-orange vegetables (i.e., carrots, sweet potato, pumpkin, and red palm oil) by HPLC has been thoroughly investigated (Khachik and Beecher, 1987). A typical chromatographic profile (eluent F) of an extract from pumpkin that contains nonapreno-β-carotene as an internal standard is

---

Fig. 10 Chromatographic profiles of a constant concentration of mixture of carotenoid reference samples injected in acetone, (a), upper trace, and methylene chloride, (b), lower trace. Chromatographic conditions (eluent E) have been described in Table 1. 1 = 1′ = all-*trans*-zeaxanthin, 2 = 2′ = all-*trans*-canthaxanthin, 3 = 3′ = all-*trans*-β-apo-8′-carotenal, 4 = 4′ = all-*trans*-lycopene, 5 = 5′ = all-*trans*-α-carotene, 6 = 6′ = all-*trans*-β-carotene, 7 = 7′ = all-*trans*-nonapreno-β-carotene. (Used with permission from Khachik et al., 1988b.)

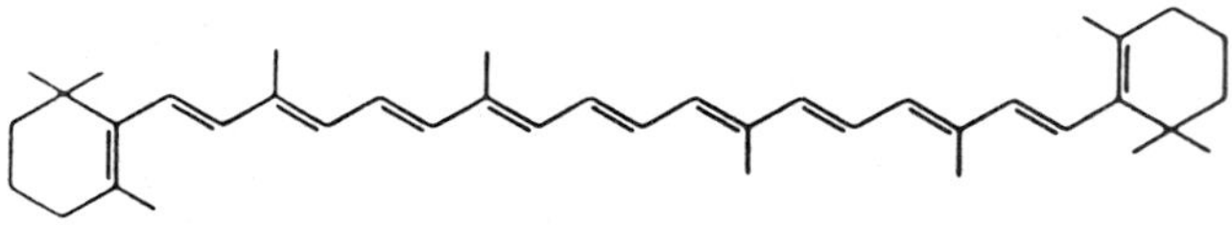

β-carotene

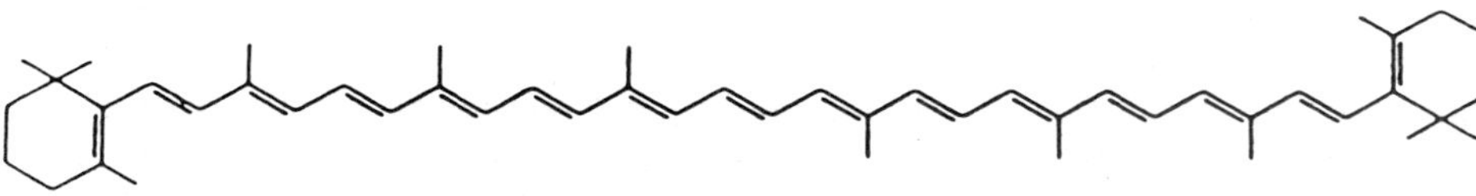

C-50-β-carotene (decapreno-β-carotene)

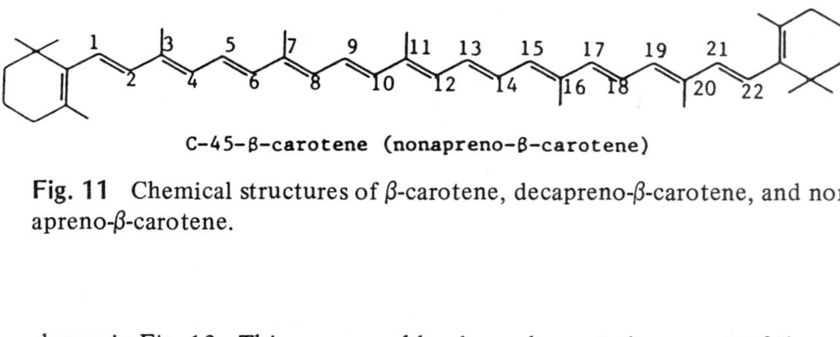

C-45-β-carotene (nonapreno-β-carotene)

Fig. 11 Chemical structures of β-carotene, decapreno-β-carotene, and nonapreno-β-carotene.

shown in Fig. 13. This compound has been shown to have most of the requirements of an internal standard for analysis of the hydrocarbon carotenoids by HPLC. Although C-45-β-carotene serves as a good internal standard for some of the yellow-orange vegetables, development of other internal standards for quantification of various classes of carotenoids in foods with a more complex chromatographic profile may be necessary.

A practical problem in selection of an internal standard is that it not only should satisfy most of the requirements described earlier, but it must be located in a "vacant" region in the chromatogram. For most simple HPLC separations that are derived from the extraction of foods that contain only a few carotenoids, this is usually not difficult. However, for complex food samples that contain a variety of carotenoids with different adsorption affinity towards the HPLC adsorbent, the selection of the internal standard can be tedious and time-consuming. An example of this is the development of an appropriate internal standard for the quantification of squash carotenoids. The chromatographic

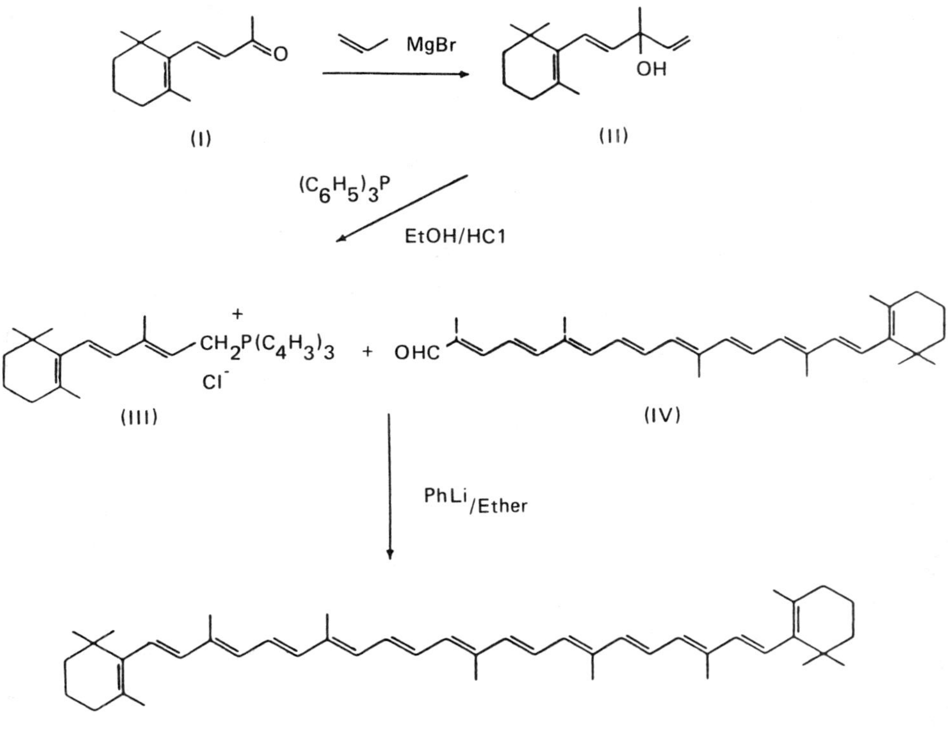

(V)

Fig. 12 Chemical synthesis of nonapreno-β-carotene. (Used with permission from Khachik and Beecher, 1986.)

profiles of the two varieties of strained baby food squash (Figs. 4 and 5) show the presence of four classes of compounds, which have been identified as oxygenated carotenoids, carotenol mono-fatty acid esters, hydrocarbon carotenoids, and carotenol di-fatty acid esters (see Table 3) (Khachik and Beecher, 1988a). As is apparent from these chromatograms, each of these classes of compounds shows a different adsorption affinity towards the C-18 reversed phase column under the conditions employed. An appropriate internal standard for these separations must therefore elute between hydrocarbon carotenoids and carotenol di-fatty acid esters to prevent HPLC peak interference. Although nonapreno-β-carotene elutes after β-carotene under the chromatographic conditions employed, its HPLC peak partially overlaps with β-carotene and therefore it cannot be employed as a suitable internal standard for these separations. A satisfactory internal standard for these separations may then be selected from a close homologue of the naturally occurring carotenol di-fatty acid esters in

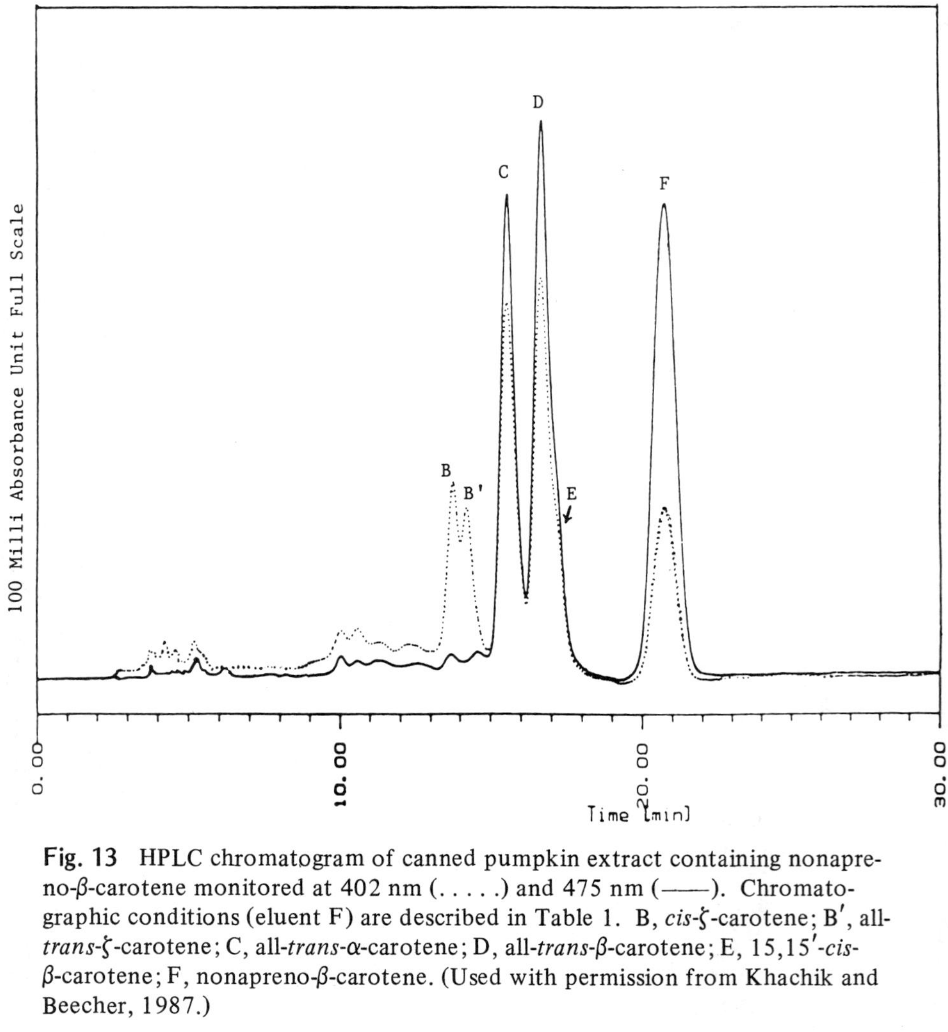

Fig. 13 HPLC chromatogram of canned pumpkin extract containing nonapreno-β-carotene monitored at 402 nm (. . . . .) and 475 nm (——). Chromatographic conditions (eluent F) are described in Table 1. B, *cis*-ζ-carotene; B′, all-*trans*-ζ-carotene; C, all-*trans*-α-carotene; D, all-*trans*-β-carotene; E, 15,15′-*cis*-β-carotene; F, nonapreno-β-carotene. (Used with permission from Khachik and Beecher, 1987.)

the squash varieties. This could be a lutein di-fatty acid ester that preferably is not naturally occurring (i.e., lutein dioctanoate, lutein dipelargonate, lutein didecanoate). Although these carotenol esters can be readily prepared by partial synthesis from the reaction between lutein and the corresponding fatty acid chlorides, the lack of the commerical availability of lutein is a major setback for the application of lutein di-fatty acid esters as internal standard. An alternative to lutein is isozeaxanthin (4,4′-dihydroxy-β-carotene), which among the dihydroxycarotenes has been shown to be the most accessible (Petracek and Zechmeister, 1956; Entschel and Karrer, 1958). This compound can be readily prepared from either reduction of commercially available canthaxanthin with lithium aluminum hydride or from β-carotene and N-bromosuccinimide according to the modified procedures (Petracek and Zechmeister, 1956; Entschel and Karrer, 1958). On the basis of the chromatographic profile and the HPLC retention times of several of the synthetic straight chain (C-6 to C-12) di-fatty acid esters of isozeaxanthin, isozeaxanthin dipelargonate seems to serve as the most appropriate internal standard for squash carotenoids (Khachik and Beecher, 1988). As may well be anticipated, as the number of the carbon atoms in the fatty acids' straight chain of the carotenol esters are increased, the HPLC retention times of these compounds on a C-18 reversed phase column also increase. Therefore, depending on the occurrence of carotenol esters and the chromatographic profile of the extracts from natural sources, a similar approach can be used to modify the length of the fatty acid side chain in isozeaxanthin dipelargonate to arrive at the appropriate internal standard for other HPLC separations. The limitation of this internal standard is in the extraction and work-up procedures that involve saponification. The basic hydrolysis converts isozeaxanthin dipelargonate to isozeaxanthin; therefore, it results in its close elution and HPLC peak interference with xanthophylls such as lutein and zeaxanthin on a C-18 reversed phase column. Since the saponification of food extracts that may contain carotenol fatty acid esters converts these compounds to the parent hydroxycarotenoids (xanthophylls), the internal standard that is selected for such applications should not be sensitive to basic hydrolysis and its HPLC peak must not interfere with those of the regenerated xanthophylls. For example, in the case of acorn squash, the abundant carotenoids have been quantified in the saponified extract employing β-apo-8′-carotenol (see Fig. 6). Although this compound is not structurally similar to the oxygenated carotenoids found in acorn squash, its suitable HPLC retention time (see Fig. 6) as well as its convenient synthesis from commercially available starting materials contribute to its selection as an internal standard.

Quantification of Carotenoids by HPLC Employing Internal Standard

In quantification of carotenoids employing an internal standard, a known compound at a fixed concentration is added to the foods at the beginning of the extraction and the mixture is homogenized, partitioned, and the resulting extract is examined by HPLC. The HPLC peak of this known compound is then used as an internal marker to compensate for the effect of minor variations in separation parameters on peak size as a result of sample-size fluctuation. However, since the injection of sample volumes employing microsampling valves can be achieved at high precision, the benefit of employing the internal standard technique for analysis of carotenoids lies in the homogenization, extraction, and partitioning steps, where variable recoveries of carotenoids may occur. The use of an internal standard actually increases the analysis precision error by $\sqrt{2}$

times, compared to the external calibration method with frequent calibrations. This is owing to the uncertainty of two peak size measurements rather than one. This increase in analytical precision is not greatly appreciated by some carotenoid chemists.

By the addition of a known concentration of an internal standard at the beginning of the extraction, it is hoped that any loss in carotenoid components as a result of sample preparation would also be accompanied by the loss of an equivalent fraction of internal standard. The accuracy of this approach is therefore dependent on the structural equivalence of the internal standards and the carotenoids of interest.

Preparation of the Internal-Standard Calibration Curves

Stock solutions of internal standard and reference samples of carotenoids of known concentrations are prepared, and the HPLC response factor of each solution is determined at various concentrations. A known amount of the internal standard is then added to each solution of carotenoid standards at various concentrations, and the ratio of the peak areas or peak heights of each reference sample to that of the internal standard is plotted versus the concentration of each carotenoid. If calibration mixtures have been prepared properly, the calibration plot for each carotenoid should be linear and intercept the origin. The concentrations of carotenoids in the extract are then determined by relating the area ratio of each carotenoid and the internal standard to those of the calibration curves. In generation of accurate analytical data, the recovery of the internal standard after each extraction and the chromatographic reproducibility in preparation of the calibration curves must be monitored very carefully.

Isolation of Carotenoids from Food Extracts

Isolation of carotenoids from natural sources requires extraction of these pigments employing an appropriate organic solvent. The choice of the organic solvent for extraction depends on the nature of the foods and the solubility behavior of the abundant carotenoids. Organic solvents such as acetone, ether, petroleum ether, methanol, and tetrahydrofuran are among the solvents that have been used for extraction of carotenoids from biological materials. In foods that contain a fairly large amount of water, it is desirable to use an organic solvent that is miscible with water in an attempt to facilitate the denaturing of caroteno-protein complexes and prevent the formation of emulsions. Acetone and tetrahydrofuran (THF) can both be successfully employed as extracting solvents; however, it is advisable to stabilize the extracting solvent with an antioxidant such as butylated hydroxytoluene (BHT) to prevent the promotion of peroxides. In cases where dried fruits and vegetables are to be extracted, the extraction and removal of carotenoids can be facilitated if food samples are kept in water for several hours prior to extraction. This also allows the removal of sugars from some dried and canned fruits and vegetables (i.e., apricots, peaches, sweet potato), which by forming emulsions may result in prolonged extraction and incomplete removal of carotenoids from these foods. In a general homogenization procedure, foods are mixed with the extracting solvent in the presence of sodium or magnesium carbonate in a blender, and the resulting mixture is homogenized at a moderate speed. The function of sodium or magnesium carbonate is to neutralize the traces of organic acids that are commonly present in some foods and can cause destruction and structural transformation of carotenoids. The resulting carotenoid extract is then filtered off and the homogenization of the residue is repeated until the filtrate is no longer colored. The combined filtrate is concentrated, and it is then partitioned in an organic solvent (i.e., petroleum ether or petroleum ether-85% methanol) and water. The organic layer is then removed, dried, and concentrated into the appropriate volume of a solvent suitable for HPLC analysis. During this operation, attempts must be made to avoid heating the carotenoid extracts above 40°C, and preferably to conduct the extraction in an inert atmosphere (i.e., nitrogen or helium) away from air and under subdued light. The carotenoid extracts of foods in most cases must be centrifuged and filtered through microfilters to ensure the removal of small particles, which may create difficulties with HPLC analysis. For detailed instructions on isolation and extraction procedures for carotenoids from natural sources, the reader is referred to the publication by Liaaen-Jensen (1971).

Saponification

The saponification of carotenoid extracts can provide valuable information as to the nature of the carotenoids present in a specific food. The majority of carotenoids are stable towards alkaline treatment; therefore, this method can be effectively used to remove the unwanted chlorophylls and lipids from food extracts. For most of the fruits and vegetables, moderate saponification conditions can be employed successfully. This involves treatment of the extracts with methanolic potassium hydroxide for several hours at room temperature. However, for high fat foods that contain a large concentration of lipids and sterols, more severe treatments may be required. In cases where carotenoids sensitive to saponification may be present (i.e., astaxanthin and fucoxanthin) this step should be omitted. There is some evidence to suggest that some of the epoxycarotenoids may also be sensitive to saponification (Khachik et al., 1986); therefore, in removal of chlorophylls from green plants in which the epoxycarotenoids are present in a fairly high concentration, this treatment should be carried out with great care. Saponification also converts carotenol fatty acid esters into their corresponding hydroxycarotenoids. The recently developed HPLC conditions for separation of several of the naturally occurring straight chain mono- and di-fatty acid esters of carotenoids (i.e., lutein, violaxanthin, violeoxanthin), allow the detection of these compounds in foods as they normally occur. A comparison between the chromatographic profiles of the saponified and unsaponified food extracts should be a common practice in any carotenoid analysis of foods. For a better understanding of the relationship of nutrition in cancer prevention in regard to carotenoids, it is desirable to generate qualitative and quantitative data on carotenoids in various foods as they normally occur. However, in some high fat foods and some fruits with complicated carotenoid profiles (i.e., citrus fruits), saponification may be a more practical approach.

Chromatography

Various chromatographic techniques for separation of carotenoids have been reviewed by Liaaen-Jensen (1971). More recently, the separation of carotenoids and chlorophylls in the extracts of several green leafy vegetables has been accomplished by thin layer chromatography (TLC) employing C-18 reversed phase plates (Khachik et al., 1986). In cases where the individually isolated carotenoids are found to be contaminated with noncarotenoid impurities, each fraction may be rechromatographed on normal phase silica gel adsorbent to remove the impurities. The abundant carotenoids in the extracts of several squash varieties have recently been separated employing both reversed and normal phase TLC plates (Khachik et al., 1988a). The advantage of employing C-18 reversed phase adsorbent in isolation of carotenoids is its wide range of adsorption affinity towards the different classes of carotenoids, which in some cases can result in excellent separations.

Structural Elucidation of Carotenoids in Foods

Structural elucidation of the carotenoids subsequent to their isolation from food extracts is often accompanied by numerous difficulties. Most of the carotenoid-containing foods, in addition to these pigments, contain other organic compounds that may contaminate the isolated carotenoid fractions. The general approach described below is recommended in step-by-step structural determination of carotenoids in extracts from natural products.

In selecting an appropriate chromatographic method for isolation and identification of the carotenoid components of natural products, the development of HPLC conditions, under which the carotenoid constituents of an extract are well resolved, is a very important initial step. With advancements in HPLC instrumentation, columns, and new detection techniques, this can usually be accomplished with great success. The HPLC conditions are then optimized by monitoring each carotenoid at the wavelength of its absorption maximum. At the same time, chromatographic conditions must be optimized to detect other organic constituents that may coelute with carotenoids. In most of the fruits and vegetables, these are UV-absorbing compounds that may create problems in separation and purification of carotenoids.

Employing the HPLC conditions as a starting point, separation conditions for carotenoid constituents of the extract by various chromatographic techniques (thin layer, flash column, conventional gravity column, or medium pressure liquid chromatography) are established. Depending on the chromatographic technique selected for isolation of carotenoids, the separation conditions may be duplicated from the earlier-established HPLC conditions or may require slight modification. Each fraction is then monitored by HPLC to determine the purity of the isolated carotenoid. In cases where carotenoids are found to contain stereoisomers or are contaminated with other fractions and impurities, further purification by preparative HPLC may be necessary. In purity assessment of each fraction by HPLC, it is desirable to monitor the absorption spectra of carotenoids employing a rapid-scanning UV/visible HPLC detector. Since in this technique a number of absorption spectra are obtained as each carotenoid fraction is eluted from the HPLC column, the presence of coeluting carotenoids and impurities can be readily detected. The absorption spectrum of the carotenoid fractions in the HPLC solvents can also provide some preliminary grounds for the nature of the chromophore of the unknown fractions. Finally, an attempt should be made to crystallize the isolated carotenoid. However, if crystallization of carotenoids is to be carried out on a micro scale, this happy event is not always readily accomplished.

The UV/visible absorption spectra of each of the pure fractions are then obtained in various solvents and compared with the absorption spectra of known carotenoids, published in the literature. The most recent data on absorption properties of carotenoids have been tabulated by Ritter and Purcell (1981). For each fraction a possible list of known carotenoids that have light absorption properties similar to the unknown fraction is obtained. As the number of the naturally occurring carotenoids isolated from natural sources are rapidly increasing [this number is approaching 600 (Straub, 1987)], it is quite possible that the carotenoid chemist finds a long list of possible carotenoids that exhibit similar UV/visible absorption properties as those of the isolated fractions. Such a list would sometimes contain as many as 30 carotenoids that have the same chromophore as that of the unknown. This is assuming that the unknown fraction isolated from a specific food is not a new carotenoid and has previously been isolated and characterized. Therefore, the possibility that the isolated fraction may be a new carotenoid with a similar chromophore as those of the known carotenoids must also be considered. The next step is to examine each fraction by mass spectrometry and determine the molecular mass and fragmentation pattern of the unknown carotenoids, which can provide valuable information about the nature of the carotenoid end-groups involved. Several comprehensive reviews on mass spectrometry of carotenoids and their fragmentation patterns have been published (Enzell et al., 1969; Budzikiewicz et al., 1970; Vetter et al., 1971; Enzell and Wahlberg, 1980). Evaluation of the mass spectral data as well as chromatographic behavior of each unknown fraction, in some simple cases, allows the identification of the unknown carotenoid. However, in more difficult cases, nuclear magnetic resonance (NMR) is required to accomplish the structural elucidation of carotenoids. This is particulary necessary when the regio- and stereoisomeric carotenoids are involved. Extensive NMR data on synthetic and naturally occurring carotenoids and more recently on stereoisomeric carotenoids have been published (Vetter et al., 1971; Englert, 1982, Tsukida and Saiki, 1983). In cases where carotenoids with one or more assymetric center(s) are involved, in addition to NMR data, optical activity measurements [i.e., Optical Rotatory Dispersion (ORD), Circular Dichroism (CD)], X-ray crystallography, as well as chemical oxidative degradation of carotenoids of interest may become necessary in determining absolute configuration (Weedon, 1971; Eugster, 1982). The group reactions of carotenoids also provide additional information about the nature of the end-groups in the unknown carotenoids and assist in narrowing down the list of possible carotenoids that may exhibit similar UV/visible absorption properties to those of unknown carotenoids. For a review on these group reactions, the reader is referred to the publication by Liaaen-Jensen (1971). Alternatively, carotenoids that are suspected to be present in an extract from a natural product may be prepared by partial or total chemical synthesis, and their chromatographic (HPLC retention times, R_f values) properties may then be compared with those of the unknown. A comprehensive review on total chemical synthesis of carotenoids has been published by Mayer and Isler (1971).

Structural Transformation of Food Carotenoids as a Result of Cooking

Owing to the sensitivity of carotenoids to heat, light, and oxygen, in generation of analytical data on carotenoid-containing foods, one has to be concerned about the effect of cooking and processing on both qualitative and quantitative distribution of these pigments. As a result of heat treatment, carotenoids may undergo oxidative degradation, structural transformation, and/or *cis-trans* isomerization. The effect of processing on *cis-trans* isomerization and carotene content of vegetables have been reported by Sweeney and Marsh (1971) and Panalaks and Murray (1970). It is reasonable to assume that various carotenoids that have been classified into various groups of compounds according to their chemical structures (i.e., hydroxycarotenoids, epoxycarotenoids, hydrocarbons, etc.) would be expected to exhibit different stability towards heat treatment. In fact, most of the existing data to date is in agreement with such an assumption.

Recently, a study of the effects of cooking and processing on a number of yellow-orange vegetables (carrot, sweet potato, pumpkin) has demonstrated that the destruction of the hydrocarbon carotenoids such as α- and β-carotene as a result of heat treatment is about 8-10% (Khachik and Beecher, 1987). It is often very difficult to compare various analytical data on the effects of cooking and processing on carotenoid levels in fruits and vegetables that have been reported by different sources. In most cases, this is owing to the lack of extensive data on the history of the samples (i.e., cultivar, growing season, location), the length of cooking, and the method of preparation (i.e., frying, steaming, boiling, baking, microwave cooking) of cooked foods which can result in variabilities in analytical data. In determining changes in the carotenoid content in a cooked food, the food must be analyzed in raw, as well as cooked, form. Measures for correction of the weight as a result of evaporation of water and volatiles during cooking must be reflected in generation of analytical data in such studies.

Examination of the raw and cooked extracts from several green vegetables (kale, Brussels sprouts, broccoli, cabbage, spinach) has recently demonstrated that some of the major chlorophyll and carotenoid constituents of these vegetables undergo some interesting structural transformation, once subjected to heat (Khachik et al., 1986). A typical HPLC profile of the major carotenoids and chlorophyll constituents of an extract from Brussels sprouts cooked in a microwave oven for six minutes is shown in Fig. 14. A comparison between this chromatogram and that of raw Brussels sprouts (which is similar to that of raw broccoli shown in Fig. 1) indicates that a number of xanthophylls are destroyed as a result of the cooking process. The only surviving xanthophyll in the cooked vegetable is found to be lutein (peak 7) and its stereoisomers (peaks 8-10). Similar results were obtained with the extract from cooked kale. A comparison between the total xanthophyll content of raw and cooked Brussels sprouts shows that about 60% of the xanthophylls are destroyed as a result of cooking. The loss of the total xanthophylls for raw and cooked kale is about 68%. The application of heat affects violaxanthin most, and in comparison to the raw forms, only 10 and 12% of this component survives in cooked Brussels sprouts and kale, respectively. No significant stereochemical changes in the ratio of the *cis*- to *trans*-isomers of neoxanthin, lutein epoxide, and lutein is indicated. However, since the degradation of the xanthophylls is a competing process, which would also contribute to the changes in the ratio of *cis*- to *trans*-isomers, more carefully designed experiments must be conducted to investigate the thermally induced stereomutation of the various xanthophylls in the cooked vegetables. The destruction of xanthophylls in the cooked vegetables is not surprising. These compounds are epoxycarotenoids that are very sensitive to treatment with heat, light, and trace amounts of acids, and they are subjected to rearrangement, stereoisomerization, and degradation.

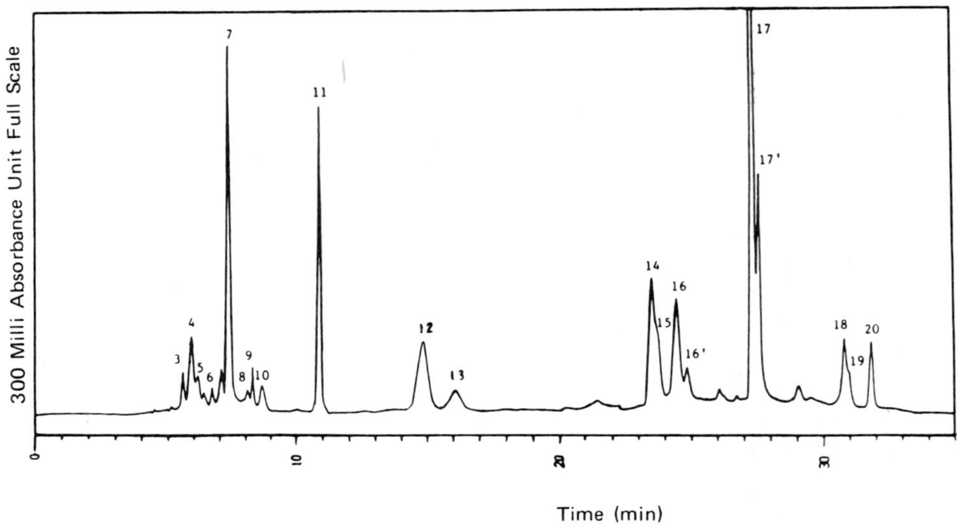

Fig. 14 Chromatographic profile of an extract from cooked Brussels sprouts. HPLC conditions (eluent A, Table 1) and peak identification are described in the tables. (Used with permission from Khachik et al., 1986.)

The cooking process also effects the conversion of chlorophyll *b* (peak 12) and chlorophyll *a* (peak 14) into pheophytin *b* (peak 16) and pheophytin *a* (peak 17), respectively (Fig. 14). On the other hand, the hydrocarbon carotenoids, all-*trans*-β-carotene (peak 18) and its 15,15′ *cis-isomer* (peak 19), are not greatly affected, and no significant stereoisomerization is observed with the application of heat. The losses of all-*trans*-β-carotene and its 15,15′ *cis*-isomer in cooked Brussels sprouts and kale were 15 and 14%, respectively. It must be stressed that the degradation, rearrangement, and stereoisomerization of carotenoids and chlorophylls are expected to be greatly influenced by the severity and the length of cooking as well as the means by which the vegetables were cooked (i.e., frying, steaming, boiling, microwave cooking, etc.). Therefore, these factors would be expected to effect the proportion of the various components in the cooked vegetables. At present, there are no available experimental data focused on the evaluation of individual carotenoids in cooked foods in such detail. For a review of the influence of food processing and cooking on carotenoid content of foods, the reader is referred to the publication by Klaui and Bauernfeind (1981). The effect of cooking and processing on the content of carotenoid isomers in several green and yellow-orange vegetables has been reported (Panalaks and Murray, 1970).

Recently observations on the effects of cooking and processing on the qualitative and quantitative distribution of carotenoids from extracts of several varieties of squash have revealed some interesting aspects of the stability of other classes of carotenoids. These are carotenol mono- and di-fatty acid esters, which are found to be among the abundant constituents in this vegetable. A comparison between the chromatographic profiles of the extract from raw and cooked acorn squash, shown in Fig. 6a and b, respectively, indicates that while mono-fatty acid esters of violaxanthin and violeoxanthin (9-*cis*-violaxanthin) are completely destroyed in the cooking process, the di-fatty acid esters of violaxanthin and violeoxanthin survived to some extent. No significant change in the ratio of *cis* to *trans*-isomers of violaxanthin di-fatty acid esters as a result of cooking is indicated. The conversion of violaxanthin and violeoxanthin di-fatty acid esters to their corresponding luteoxanthin and auroxanthin di-fatty acid esters is not affected as a result of heat treatment and no detectable amounts of these compounds are shown to be present in the cooked squash extract. From this study it is evident that the epoxycarotenoids that contain unsubstituted hydroxyl groups are extremely sensitive to heat treatment, whereas substitution of the hydroxyl groups with long chain fatty acids increases the thermal stability of these compounds. The presence of lutein mono- and di-fatty acid esters in the varieties of cooked and processed squash also indicates that these compounds (similar to their parent compound, lutein) survived the heat treatment to a great extent.

Recommendations for Presentation of Carotenoid Composition Data in Food Tables

Vitamin A and carotene values published in food tables during the past quarter century have generally been derived by use of methods similar to the official methods of the AOAC (Horwitz, 1980). For an outline of the analytic methods, calculations, and presentation of data according to these procedures see the publication by Beecher and Khachik (1984). Generally, in these methods, samples are subjected to alkaline hydrolysis followed by partitioning of the retinoids and carotenoids into a nonpolar solvent, such as n-hexane or petroleum ether. The resulting extracts are reduced in volume and the components are quantified directly or subjected to chromatography. Extracts that contain both retinoids (vitamin A) and carotenoids are chromatographed on aluminum oxide adsorption columns resulting in the separation of these two major classes of compounds. The retinoid fraction is quantified with colorimetric procedures, and the carotenoid fraction is either quantified with spectrophotometric procedures or separated into additional components on other adsorption columns and ultimately quantified. These procedures, which are long and laborious, separate the retinoids and carotenoids in foods only into major classes of compounds, i.e., retinoids, carotenes, and xanthophylls, rather than into individual retinoids and carotenoids. This constitutes one of the major sources of analytic errors in these procedures (Egberg, 1982). Other potential sources of error include incomplete solvent extraction, destruction and stereochemical changes during extraction and chromatography, and incomplete separation and recovery during chromatography. Despite all the pitfalls, these procedures have been widely used and at least provide an estimate of the total retinoid and carotenoid contents of foods. In food composition tables from several countries, i.e., United States (Haytowitz and Matthews 1984), United Kingdom (Paul and Southgate, 1978), West Germany (Souci et al., 1982), China (Institute of Occupational Health, 1980), and East Asia (Wu Leung et al., 1972), carotenoid data for several food groups have been presented in terms of vitamin A activity and/or total carotene content. Since these data have been generated by AOAC procedures, they do not reflect accurate quantitative and qualitative data on individual carotenoids. With advances in HPLC instrumentation and recent developments in carotenoid analytic techniques, food tables should be constructed to provide detailed information on both qualitative and quantitative data on individual naturally occurring carotenoids and retinoids in foods. One approach for construction of such food tables may be to list the abundant carotenoids and retinoids in various foods according to their chemical class. For example, the abundant caretnoids in fruits and vegetables, whose high consumption has been associated with a reduction in several types of cancers, may be divided into epoxycarotenoids, hydroxycarotenoids, hydrocarbons, and mono- and di-fatty acid esters. The various fruits and vegetables can be classified by traditional methods in food tables and data bases. Unfortunately, with the exception of the green leafy vegetables that basically contain the same carotenoids but at varying concentrations, there are no distinct patterns in distribution of carotenoids among various fruits and vegetables. It is this unpredictable pattern of the naturally occurring carotenoids in foods that contributes to difficulties in presentation of data in such food tables. It is essential for the food composition tables to contain information about the source of food samples and the methods of preparation and analysis. With regard to cooked foods, the length and means of cooking, as well as a comparison of carotenoid profile and levels with those of the raw food, can provide useful information about the effect of cooking and processing on the destruction and structural transformation of carotenoids in these foods. The data presented in such food tables will provide a better understanding of the correlation between carotenoids in various foods and their role, if any, in cancer prevention.

RETINOIDS

Naturally occurring vitamin A derivatives and retinoids are found in animal tissues and result from oxidative modification and cleavage of C-40-carotenoids, usually β-carotene. The major naturally occurring retinoid in the diet is retinol, often in the form of retinyl esters and supplied by foods of animal origin. all-*trans*-Retinol is the most active form of vitamin A, as evidenced by its ability to sustain a variety of biologic functions in higher animals, i.e., growth, vision, reproduction, mucus secretion, maintenance of differentiated epithelia, and gene expression of cells. As a result, all-*trans*-retinol has become the "reference compound" for the assessment of vitamin A activity and for the presentation of data in many food tables. Stereoisomerization of all-*trans*-retinol, induced by light, heat, or an appropriate catalyst, can result in several "unhindered" (i.e., 9-*cis*, 13-*cis*, 9,13-di-*cis*) and "hindered" (i.e., 11-*cis*, 11,13-di-*cis*) isomeric forms of this compound, which are known to possess lower vitamin A activity than their all-*trans*-compounds. Drastic structural changes in all-*trans*-retinol, e.g., oxidation to retinoic acid, can cause the molecule to display some, but not necessarily all, of the biologic activities of vitamin A represented by retinol (Sporn et al., 1976; DeLuca, 1979). Currently, a large number of synthetic retinoids are being tested as potential cancer chemotherapeutic and prophylactic agents (Mayer et al., 1978; Sporn and Newton, 1981). A few studies have been conducted with naturally occurring retinoids fed to animals. Results from these studies suggest that under certain circumstances natural retinoids (retinyl esters and retinoic acid) can prevent the development of epithelial cancer, but they have limited usefulness as agents for chemoprevention of cancer (Shekelle et al., 1981). A few, but not all, epidemiologic studies suggest an association between low serum retinol levels with an increased risk of cancer (Goodman, 1984; Willett, 1984). This possible association has encouraged the development of modern analytic techniques that can generate accurate food composition data on synthetic and naturally occurring retinoids. Several comprehensive reviews dealing with analytical methods for determination of synthetic and naturally occurring retinoids and related compounds have recently appeared in the literature (Taylor, 1983; Egberg et al., 1985; Lambert et al., 1985; Parrish et al., 1985; Simpson et al., 1985; Thompson, 1986). Since in these reviews various aspects of retinoids analyses have been described in detail, the present article will only deal briefly with some of the reported procedures for isolation and detection of these compounds.

Similar to carotenoids, analysis of retinoids involves isolation and extraction of these pigments from foods and animal sources followed by detection and separation by various chromatographic techniques. Some of the most important aspects of isolation and chromatographic procedures of retinoids and related compounds are discussed here.

Isolation

The extraction and isolation procedures for retinoids are very similar to those for carotenoids. Owing to the instability of retinoids in the presence of light, heat, and air, these pigments should be handled with great care. To prevent oxidative degradation and isomerization, the extraction of retinoids should be conducted under a nitrogen or argon atmosphere and subdued light. Heating solutions of retinoids above 40°C during solvent evaporation must be avoided and, when not in use, these solutions must be stored at −70°C. The general extraction procedures for retinoids from biologic or commercial sources follow the same pathways as carotenoids; these procedures have been adequately described by Davies (1976) and Liaaen-Jensen and Jensen (1966). Alkaline hydrolysis of retinoid extracts is often a necessary purification step in removal of lipids, however, in cases where retinoids may contain labile groups such as esters, other purification procedures have been employed (Taylor, 1983). In extraction of vitamin A from protected preparations, prior to organic solvent extraction, the coating must be penetrated by treatment with water and alkaline. There has been no evidence to suggest that saponification of retinoids may result in degradation and destruction of these pigments, however, in some saponification and extraction procedures that involve refluxing in alcoholic potassium hydroxide, stereoisomerization and structural transformation of these compounds may be inevitable. In recent laboratory studies, vitamin A has been shown to be stable for one week when kept in ethanolic KOH in pyrogallol (Thompson, 1986). Diethyl ether, hexane, or petroleum ether are among the most common extracting solvents for retinoids and vitamin A compounds. The incomplete removal of retinoids from biologic and commercial sources is often one of the major difficulties associated with the extraction of these pigments. Unlike carotenoids, whose incomplete extraction can be visually detected, the evaluation of the endpoint of extraction for retinoids that absorb light in the near UV region may be accomplished by monitoring the extract by HPLC. This requires establishing chromatographic conditions that have been optimized to separate the various naturally occurring retinoids. The efficiency of several extraction procedures for vitamin A has been reviewed by Thompson (1986).

Chromatography

Chromatographic techniques employed for the separation and purification of retinoids include open-column, thin layer, paper, gas liquid, and high performance liquid chromatography. Excellent reviews on various aspects of these procedures have been repoted by Taylor (1983) and Lambert et al. (1985). Among the various chromatographic methods, the separation of retinoids by HPLC is the most successful and widely used technique, which has gradually replaced other conventional methods. Normal phase and reversed phase adsorbents have both been used in separation of retinoids and related compounds by HPLC.

Retinol

all-*trans*-Retinol and several of its stereoisomers (i.e., 9-*cis*, 11-*cis*, 13-*cis*) have been separated by HPLC on a Zorbax SIL column employing various combinations of eluents, such as hexane, ethyl acetate, diethyl ether, and methylene chloride (Tsukida et al., 1977a). HPLC separation of standards of all-*trans*-retinol and its geometrical isomers has also been reported by Paanakker and Groenendijk (1979), who employed n-hexane-dioxane (95:5) as eluent and n-Silica 60 as adsorbent. In determination of retinol by HPLC in food substances in which retinol is present in the esterified form, saponification of the extracts has been carried out in the presence of antioxidants, such as hydroquinone (Fankel and Schmid, 1976) and ascorbic acids (Egberg et al., 1977). The retinol in the saponified extract has then been determined by HPLC employing Lichrosorb Si 60 as adsorbent and n-hexane-ethanol (97:3) as eluent (Fankel and Schmid, 1976). Similarly, retinol in saponified oil extract has been separated by HPLC on a Zorbax SIL column employing n-hexane-methylene chloride-isopropanol (300:200:1.5) as eluent (Egberg et al., 1977). The separation of all-*trans*-retinol from its 13-*cis* isomer in a saponified oil extract has also been accomplished on a Vydac ODS reversed phase column employing acetonitrile-water (65:35) as mobile phase (Egberg et al., 1977). In nonaqueous reversed phase chromatography of vitamins, Landen (1981) has employed ternary mixture of acetonitrile, methylene chloride, and methanol to separate a mixture of retinyl acetate, retinol, α-tocopheryl acetate, vitamin D_2, vitamin D_3, β-carotene, and retinyl palmitate.

Retinal

A mixture of standards of all-*trans*-retinol and several of its stereoisomers (13-*cis*, 11-*cis*, 9-*cis*, 7-*cis*) have been separated by HPLC employing Zorbax SIL (Tsukida et al., 1977b, 1978a) and shimadzu silica (Tsukida et al., 1978b) as adsorbents and hexane diethyl ether as eluent. Other workers have separated these isomeric retinals by HPLC on μ Porasil column (Rotman and Kropf, 1975; Waddell et al., 1976, 1979; Denny and Liu, 1977). Frolik et al. (1978a) have separated several naturally occurring retinoids (retinoic acid, retinol, retinal, retinyl acetate, retinyl palmitate) by HPLC on an Spherisorb ODS reversed phase column employing acetonitrile–1% ammonium acetate (60:40).

Retinyl Esters

Several chromatographic procedures have been reported that have separated all-*trans*-retinyl acetate and all-*trans*-retinyl palmitate and their stereoisomers on normal phase HPLC columns. Paanakker and Groenendijk (1979) have employed eluents consisting of hexane and dioxane to separate all-*trans*- and several *cis*-retinyl palmitates (13-*cis*, 11-*cis*, 9-*cis*) on a SI 60 HPLC column. Separations of all-*trans*-retinyl palmitate its mono- and di-*cis*-isomers (11,13-di-*cis* and 9,13-di-*cis*) on a Lichrosorb (AloxT) column with isooctane-diisopropyl ether as mobile phase have been reported by Steuerle (1981). Under these conditions several stereoisomers of all-*trans*-retinyl acetate as well as retinyl palmitate and retinyl oleate were also separated. A number of retinyl esters have been separated by reversed phase chromatography on a Spherisorb ODS column employing a mixture of acetonitrile and water (98:2) as mobile phase (Roberts et al., 1978).

Retinoic Acid

De Ruyter et al. (1979) have separated all-*trans*-retinoic acid as well as its 13-*cis* and 9-*cis* isomers in a serum extract by HPLC on a RSIL column employing petroleum ether, acetic acid, and acetonitrile as mobile phase. In these studies, all-*trans*-demethylretinoic acid (closely related to retinoic acid), was used as an internal standard for quantitative measurements of retinoic acid and its *cis*-isomers in a serum extract (De Leenheer and Lambert, 1981; De Leenheer et al., 1982). all-*trans*-Retinoic acid and its 13-*cis* isomer have also been separated by reversed phase HPLC on a Partisil (ODS-2) column with an eluent consisting of acetonitrile-1% ammonium acetate (60:40) (Frolik et al., 1978a). For other examples of the separation of retinoic acid and related compounds by reversed phase chromatography, the reader is referred to the publications by McCormick et al. (1979), Frolik et al. (1978b), and McKenzie et al. (1978).

PHENOLS, INDOLES, ISOTHIOCYANATES, AND FLAVONES

The development of analytical procedures for phenols, indoles, isothiocyanates, and flavones that are known to be present in some fruits and vegetables have received little attention. There are few literature reports on the detection of phenols (hydroxycinnamic and hydroxybenzoic acid derivatives) in green vegetables (Schmidtlein and Herrmann, 1975a,b). These methods employ open-column chromatography for separation and quantification of the phenolic compounds found in green vegetables of the *Brassica* family. The advances in separation and detection techniques and the application of HPLC in generating accurate and reproducible analytical data have replaced the need for conventional open-column chromatography. Although several reports on the HPLC separation of reference samples of phenols, indoles, and flavonoids have appeared in the literature (Brandl and Herrmann, 1983; Vande Casteele et al., 1983; Banwart et al., 1985), the application of these methods to the chromatographic separation of complex mixtures of these compounds in fruits and vegetables has not been investigated. One of the rare examples of the analysis of the UV-absorbing compounds in vegetables by HPLC has been recently reported by Bradfield and Bjeldanes (1987), who employed this technique for separation of anticarcinogenic indoles in vegetables of *Brassica oleracea*. Recent preliminary studies on an extract from raw broccoli have shown that the carotenoid and chlorophyll constituents of this vegetable can be removed by washing the meth-

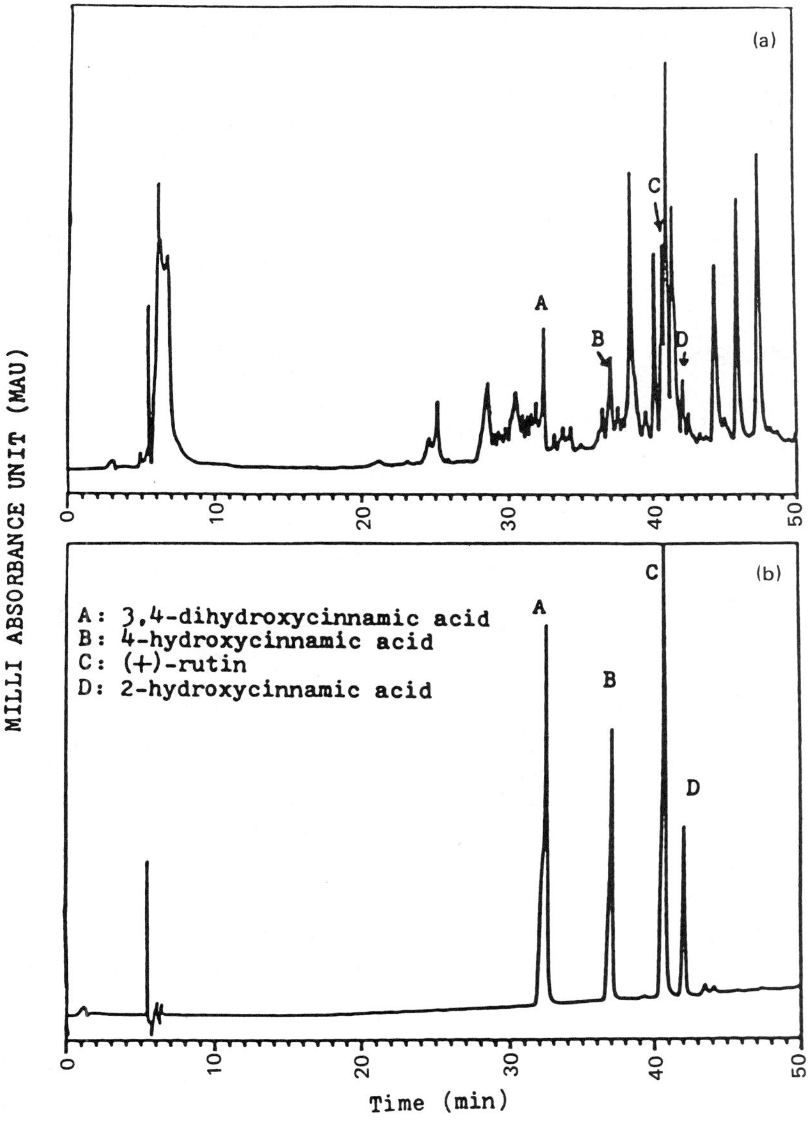

Fig. 15 (a) Upper trace, HPLC profile of the UV-absorbing compounds in the extract from raw broccoli monitored at 320 nm; (b) lower trace, HPLC profile of (+)-rutin and the reference samples of several phenolic compounds monitored under identical HPLC conditions. Chromatographic conditions (eluent G) are described in Table 1.

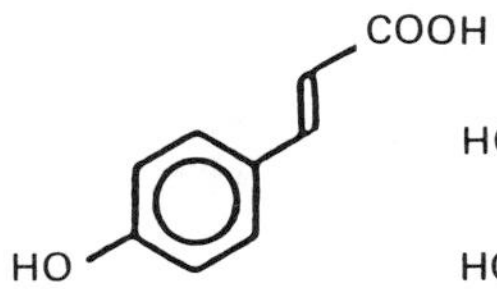

p-Coumaric Acid

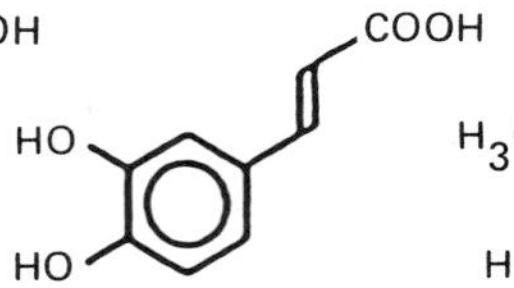

Caffeic Acid

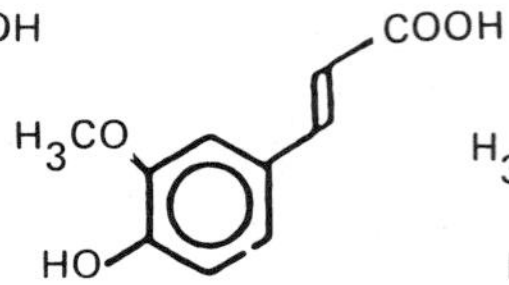

Ferulic Acid

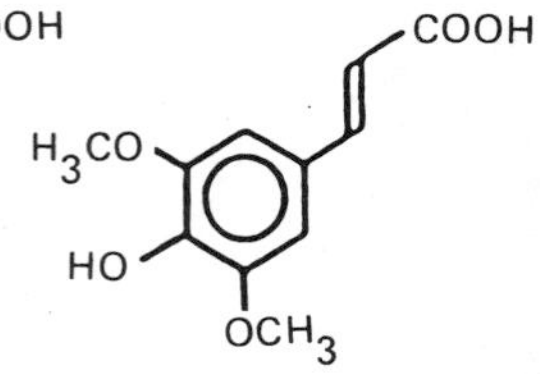

Sinapinic Acid

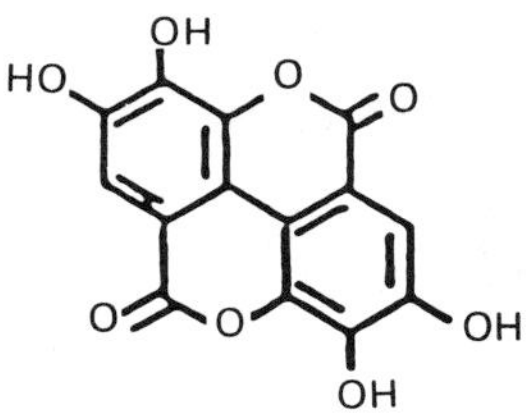

Ellagic Acid

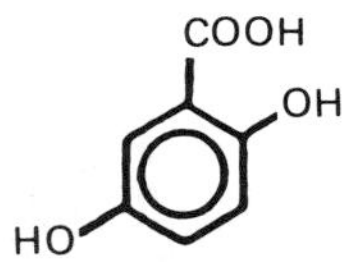

Gentisic Acid

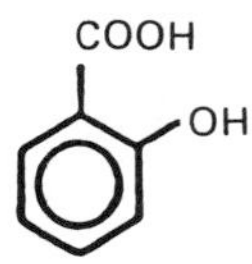

Salicylic Acid

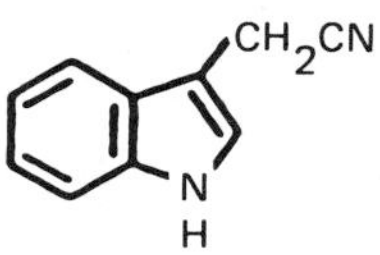

3-Indolylacetonitrile

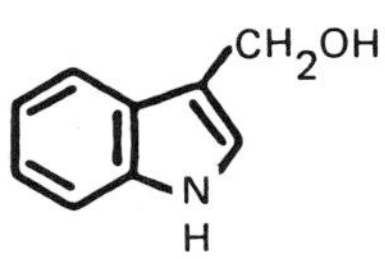

Indole-3-carbino

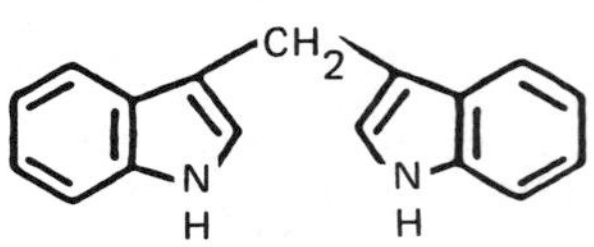

3.3′-Diindolylmethane

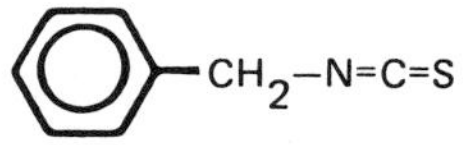

Benzyl Isothiocyanate

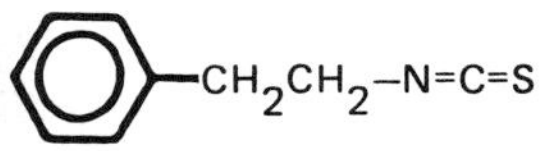

Phenethyl Isothiocyanate

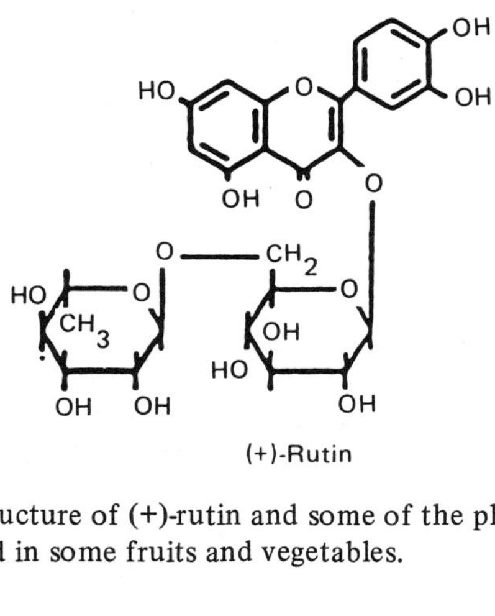

(+)-Rutin

Fig. 16 Chemical structure of (+)-rutin and some of the phenols, indoles, and isothiocyanates found in some fruits and vegetables.

anolic extract with light petroleum ether (Khachik and Beecher, unpublished results). The carotenoid and the chlorophyll-free methanolic solution of broccoli extract, which were shown to contain a number of UV-absorbing compounds, were monitored between 300-330 nm by HPLC on a C-18 reversed phase column. Employing gradient elution chromatography and a mobile phase consisting of water, formic acid, and methanol (eluent G), as many as 20 components were separated in the preliminary HPLC runs of the raw broccoli extract. The chromatographic profiles of the UV-absorbing compounds in raw broccoli extract and several reference samples of phenoliç compound obtained under identical HPLC conditions are shown in Fig. 15. Comparison of the retention times and absorption spectra of the various components in raw broccoli extract with those of the reference samples tentatively indicates that the major constituents of this vegetable are derivatives of hydroxycinnamic acid. The presence of 3,4-dihydroxycinnamic acid, 4-hydroxycinnamic acid, 2-hydroxycinnamic acid as well as (+)-rutin in the extract from raw broccoli is particularly noticeable. The chemical structure of (+)-rutin and some of the phenols, indoles, and isothiocyanates found in some fruits and vegetables are shown in Fig. 16. From this preliminary study, it is apparent that the existing analytical methods and HPLC separation of these components present in some fruits and vegetables requires a great deal of development. In addition, the development of improved analytical methods must also be accompanied by a more definite structural elucidation of the individually isolated, UV-absorbing components by various spectroscopic and chemical methods in these foods.

VITAMIN E

Structure, Nomenclature, and Activities of Tocopherols and Tocotrienols

Several closely related and naturally occurring organic compounds contribute to the "vitamin E activity" of foods. These compounds are members of two homologous series: (a) the tocopherols, with a saturated side chain, and (b) the tocotrienols, with a side chain unsaturated between carbons 3′ and 4′, 7′ and 8′, and 11′ and 12′. The structure and numbering of the basic compound of these series, tocol, are shown in Fig. 17. The various ring substitutions of tocol or tocotrienol and the resulting naturally occurring compounds possessing vitamin E activity are tabulated in Table 5. α-Tocopherol has the highest vitamin E activity and is the best known member of this group of eight compounds.

There are three asymmetric carbons in the tocol or tocotrienol molecule, at positions 2, 4′, and 8′, resulting in a possibility of eight diastereoisomers. Fortunately, the only naturally occurring stereoisomer of α-tocopherol hitherto discussed has a configuration of 2R, 4′R, 8′R and is designated RRR-α-tocopherol. This compound was formerly known as **d**-α-tocopherol. The double

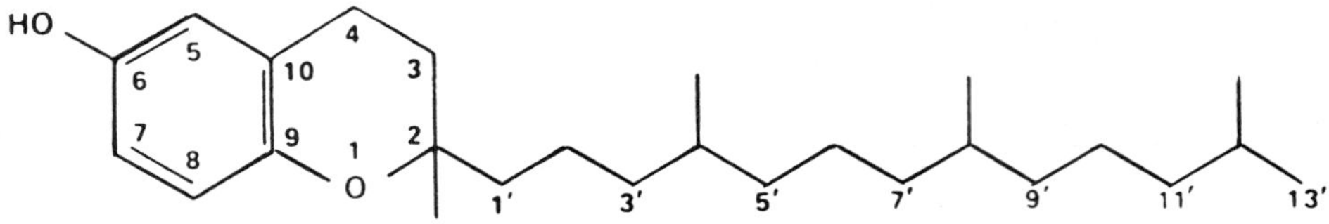

Fig. 17 Tocol—basic structure of tocopherol group.

bonds in the side chain of tocotrienols also introduce the possibility of *cis-trans* isomerism in these molecules. As far as is known, the naturally occurring tocotrienols in foods have an all-*trans* configuration (AIN Committee on Nomenclature, 1979).

Historically, vitamin E has been associated with sterility and reproduction, particularly in laboratory and farm animals (Dam, 1962). In human beings, inadequacy of dietary vitamin E does not result in specific clinical symptoms. Laboratory studies, however, suggest enhanced fragility of red blood cells in vitro when dietary and blood levels of vitamin E are low. Based upon these observations as well as levels of vitamin E in the blood and diets of normal healthy human beings, recommended dietary allowances for this vitamin have been established (Food and Nutrition Board, 1980). These guidelines have the units of α-tocopherol equivalents (α-TE), which relate to the summation of "vitamin E activity" of each tocopherol and tocotrienol in a food or mixed diet. Table 6 relates the weight of several common forms of vitamin E to their corresponding vitamin E activity.

Table 5 Nomenclature of Naturally Occurring Vitamin E Active Compounds

Ring substitution	Tocopherols[a]	Tocotrienols[a]
5,7,8-Trimethyl	α-Tocopherol (α-T)	α-Tocotrienol (α-T_3)
5,8-Dimethyl	β-Tocopherol (β-T)	β-Tocotrienol (β-T_3)
7,8-Dimethyl	γ-Tocopherol (γ-T)	γ-Tocotrienol (γ-T_3)
8-Monomethyl	δ-Tocopherol (δ-T)	δ-Tocotrienol (δ-T_3)

[a]Suggested abbreviations shown in parentheses (Brubacher et al., 1985).
Source: AIN Committee on Nomenclature, 1979.

Table 6 Vitamin E Activity of Various Tocopherols and Tocotrienols

Tocopherol or tocotrienol	Vitamin E activities		
Conventional IUPAC trivial name	Name	α-TE/mg[a]	IU/mg[b]
dl-α-tocopherol acetate (international std)	α-ambo-α-tocopherol acetate	–	1.0
dl-α-tocopherol acetate (totally synthetic)	all-rac-α-tocopherol acetate	–	1.0
dl-α-tocopherol (totally synthetic)	all-rac-α-tocopherol	–	1.1
d-α-tocopherol (naturally occurring)	RRR-α-tocopherol	1.0	1.49
d-α-tocopherol acetate	RRR-α-tocopherol acetate		1.36
β-tocopherol	β-tocopherol	0.5	–
γ-tocopherol	γ-tocopherol	0.1	–
δ-tocopherol	δ-tocopherol	0.01	–
α-tocotrienol	α-tocotrienol	0.3	–
β-tocotrienol	β-tocotrienol	0.05	–
γ-tocotrienol	γ-tocotrienol	0.01	–

[a]α-Tocopherol equivalent (RRR-α-tocopherol equivalents) per mg specific tocopherol or tocotrienol.
[b]International units per mg specific tocopherol.
Source: Data collated from McLaughlin and Weihrauch, 1979; Parrish, 1980; Food and Nutrition Board, 1980.

Another type of activity of tocopherols is as antioxidants (Parrish, 1980). The antioxidant capability of tocopherols in food preparations has been recognized for some time. They also may act as protective antioxidants in the gastrointestinal tract and in tissues of human beings and thus provide a "cancer protective" effect. The antioxidant activity of the naturally occurring tocopherols has the following order: $\delta = \gamma > \beta > \alpha$. Tocopherol esters, however, are devoid of antioxidant activity. A suggested mechanism of antioxidant action is the conversion of the 6-chromanol ring into a quinone, which increases the ability of the molecule to scavenge free radicals (Bauernfeind and Cort, 1974). Thus, the naturally occurring tocotrienols would be expected to have about the same antioxidant activity as the tocopherols.

It is important to note that the rank order for vitamin E activity of the various tocopherols and tocotrienols in foods (Table 6) is nearly the opposite of their antioxidant activity. Whereas α-tocopherol provides most of the vitamin E activity in mixed diets, δ- and γ-tocopherol also contribute significant antioxidant activity. As a result food tables are tabulated in units of α-TE; these data provide only a crude estimate of the antioxidant activity of the diet, which may be more appropriate in cancer prevention studies. These studies require food composition data bases which tabulate levels of all forms of added and naturally occurring tocopherols and tocotrienols in foods. Only after these data bases are in place will investigators and nutritionists be able to calculate the contribution of antioxidant activity to the diet from the various forms of vitamin E.

Colorimetric and Chromatographic Methods of Analyses

A number of analytic procedures have been used to quantify the vitamin E activity of foods (see reviews by Bunnell, 1967; Parrish, 1980). By far the most widely used procedure has been the colorimetric method developed by Emmerie and Engel (1938). This method relies on the ability of tocopherols to reduce ferric ions to ferrous and subsequently react with α-α′-dipyridyl to form a red complex. The intensity of the color is quantified at 520 nm and is proportional to the reducing material present. Because of the chemistry of the 6-chromanol ring, tocopheryl esters per se do not react, whereas tocotrienols would be expected to react positively and with similar intensity as tocopherols. Other reducing materials in foods may also react in a similar manner and a number of substances, including vitamin A, carotenoids, and fats, interfere in the color development. Nevertheless, this method has been used extensively to measure total tocopherols in foods, and much of the data currently tabulated in food tables and data bases has been generated using this method (J. Weihrauch, personal communication).

Accurate determination of the vitamin E or antioxidant activity of foods requires separation and quantification of each tocopherol and tocotrienol species that is present. Gas liquid chromatography (GLC) has been successfully employed for the separation and quantification of tocopherols and, to a limited extent, tocotrienols in foods. Parrish (1980) and Nelis et al. (1985) have reviewed analytical GLC procedures developed prior to 1982. A recent major techological advance in GLC has been the introduction of rugged wall-coated open tabular (WCOT) capillary columns. These columns have superior separation efficiency and in general provide increased sensitivity over conventional packed GLC columns. A typical procedure for separating and quantifying tocopherols and tocotrienols in foods using WCOT columns has been detailed by Slover et al. (1983). Excellent resolution of all of the tocopherols and sterols in a series of vegetable oils was attained with this procedure. In addition, this method also includes an internal standard, 5,7-dimethyltocol, and has the capacity to separate tocotrienols that may be present in foods.

Recent advances in high performance liquid chromatography (HPLC) instrumentation have moved it to the forefront as a technique for the separation and quantification of tocopherols and tocotrienols in foods. The great appeal of HPLC procedures over GLC methods are the relatively low operating temperatures of HPLC columns and the ability to chromatograph extracts of foods directly, without derivatization. Parrish (1980), Van Niekerk (1982), and Nelis et al. (1985) have reviewed HPLC procedures for quantifying vitamin E vitamers in foods. Table 7 is a tabulation of these procedures reported after 1980; see reports by Van Niekerk (1982) and Nelis et al. (1985) for earlier procedures. In general, HPLC systems equipped with normal phase columns, e.g., LiChromosorb, μ-Porasil, Spherisorb, have been employed to separate tocopherols and tocotrienols in foods. Mobile phases for these systems have been principally hexane or n-heptane with appropriate modifiers. Both free tocopherols and tocotrienols exhibit strong fluorescence and, because of the selectivity and sensitivity of this technique, it has been the HPLC detector of choice for these vitamers. Inclusion of dioxane or diethyl ether in the mobile phase increases fluorescence efficiency and reduces the limits of detection even more (Thompson and Hatina, 1979). A typical HPLC chromatogram of the vitamin E vitamers of palm oil is shown in Fig. 18.

Several foods are fortified with vitamin E in the form of tocopheryl acetate. Quantification of this vitamer requires either saponification followed by separation of α-tocopherol on normal phase HPLC columns or development of HPLC protocols which separate and quantify α-tocopheryl acetate directly. Both normal phase (Widicus and Kirk, 1979) and reversed phase (Barnett et al., 1980; Landen, 1981, 1982) HPLC systems have been developed to quantify this form of vitamin E (Table 7). Tocopheryl esters however, do not fluoresce and as a result ultraviolet absorption detectors have been used with these systems. Extracts of foods and vegetable oils have been shown to contain compounds which may interfere with tocopherol peaks and also give a positive response when an absorbance detector is used (Thompson and Hatina, 1979).

Sampling and sample preparation as well as analytical quality control are additional areas that require focused attention as part of vitamin E analysis of foods in order to assure high quality analytical data. Food samples must be transported, comminuted, and subsampled in a manner to minimize losses of tocopherols and tocotrienols yet ensure confidence that the subsample is representative of the food. Sample preparation procedures depend upon the nature of the food and the specific vitamin E vitamers present in the food (Parrish, 1980, Van Niekerk, 1982). Vegetable oils, which contain tocopherols in the unesterified form, may be diluted with HPLC mobile phase and injected onto the column directly. Solid food samples require either direct extraction

Table 7 HPLC Systems Used for Vitamin E Determinations in Foods, 1981-1986[a]

Compounds determined	Type of food	Sample preparation	Stationary phase[b]	Mobile phase[c]	Detector[d]	Reference
α-Tocopheryl acetate	Infant formulas	Extracted with isopropanol-methylene dichloride; removed lipids by gel permeation chromatography	Zorbax ODS 4.6 X 250	Methylene dichloride-acetonitrile-methanol (30:70:0.2)	UV 280 nm	Landen, 1981, 1982
α-, β-, γ-, δ-Tocopherols	Vegetable oils and shortening	Diluted with ethanol, saponified, analytes partitioned into hexane	Corasil II 4.6 X 250 Partisil PXS5 4.6 X 100	Hexane-isapropanol (98.6:1.4)	Fluorescence 200 nm/335 nm	Tangney et al., 1981
α-, γ-Tocopherols	Various	Extracted with methanol; partitioned analytes into chloroform	Zorbax ODS 4.6 X 250	Methanol	Fluorescence 292 nm/335 nm	Lehmann et al., 1986
α-, γ-, δ-Tocopherols	Soybeans and tofu	Extracted with ethanol; solubilized analytes into hexane followed by isooctane	Ultrasil NH 4.6 X 250 4.6 X 30	Hexane-2-propanol (99:1)	UV 280 nm	Guzman and Murphy, 1986
α-, β-, γ-, δ-Tocopherols	Mixed tocopherol concentrates	Diluted with mobile phase	Lichrosorb (SI-100) 4.6 X 250 μ Porasil 3.9 X 300	Hexane-2-propanol (0.2-0.5% 2-propanol,	UV 295 nm	Shen and Sheppard, 1986

			Spherisorb 4.6 X 100 Spherisorb 4.6 X 250	column dependent)		
α-, β-, γ-, δ-Tocopherols and α-, β-, γ-, δ-Tocotrienols	Several foodstuffs common with foods	Extracted with ethanol, saponified, partitioned analytes into petroleum ether	Chromegasphere (SI60) 4.6 X 150	Isooctane-tetrahydro furan (97.5:2.5)	Fluorescence 294 nm/326 nm	Cort et al., 1983
α-, γ-Tocopherols and α-, γ-tocotrienols	Corn	Suspended in ethanol, saponified, partitioned analytes into hexane	Ultrasphere-Si 4.6 X 250	Hexane-isopropanol (98.7:1.3)	Fluorescence 205 nm/330 nm	Weber, 1984
α-, β-, γ-, δ-tocopherols and α-, β-, γ-, δ-tocotrienols	Foods and oils	Foods suspended in methanol, saponified, analytes partitioned into diethyl ether; oils extracted with acetone	LiChromsorb (SI60) 4.0 X 125	n-Heptane-1,4-dioxane (96:4)	Fluorescence 296 nm/326 nm	Brubacher et al., 1985
	Oils, fats fish and fish products	Fish and fish products suspended in ethanol, saponified, partitioned analytes into hexane; oils and fats extracted with hexane	LiChromsorb (SI60) 4.0 X 250	Di-isopropyl ether gradient in hexane	Fluorescence 290 nm/325 nm	Syväoja et al., 1985c, 1986

[a] Van Niekerk (1982) and Nelis et al. (1985) have tabulated procedures published prior to 1981.
[b] Column size (mm) is tabluated below commercial name of stationary phase; where two sizes are listed, shorter column represents a guard column.
[c] Ratios of mobile phase constituents tabulated as proportions by volume.
[d] Wavelengths tabulated for fluorescence detectors represent excitation/emission.

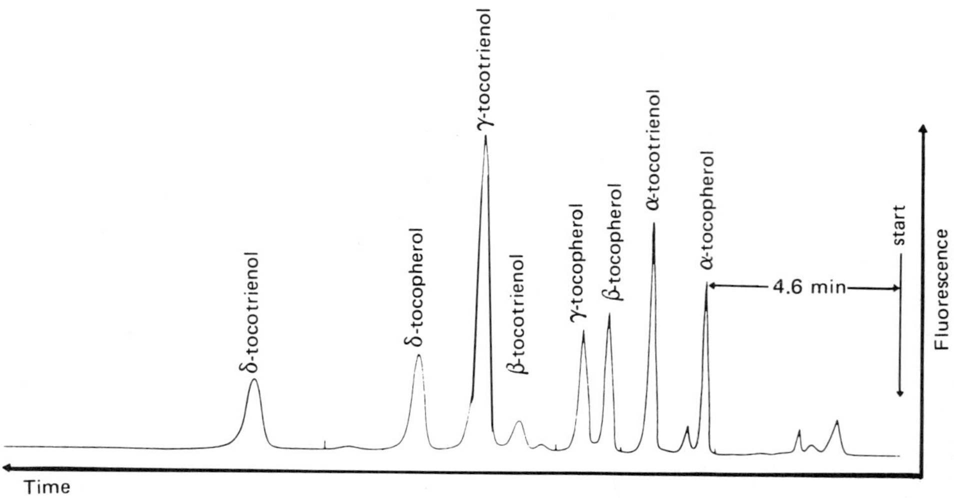

Fig. 18 Chromatogram of palm oil. Conditions: Column: LiChrosorb Si60 5 μm (Merck); Mobile phase: 1,4-Dioxane in *n*-heptane (40 ml/liter); Flow rate: 2 ml/min isocratically at room temperature; Pump: Latek Constametric III; Detector: Fluorimetric detector LS 5, Perkin-Elmer; Feed: 1 cm/min; Excitation: 296 nm; Emission: 326 nm. (Used with permission from Brubacher et al., 1985.)

with an appropriate organic solvent or saponification, to free the vitamers of glycerides and other materials, followed by organic solvent extraction. Landen (1982) has developed a chromatography procedure, in lieu of saponification, to separate fat-soluble vitamers from lipid material in extracts of infant flormulae. Sample manipulation during preparation, particularly saponification, may result in losses of tocopherols and tocotrienols by oxidation. Therefore, most procedures call for use of an antioxidant, i.e., pyrogallol, BHA, BHT, and liberal use of an inert gas such as nitrogen or argon. In an attempt to minimize losses as part of sample transfer, Slover et al. (1983) have developed procedures for saponification, extraction, and derivitization that are conducted in a single screw-capped test tube.

Analytic quality control refers both to peak identification and purity as well as analytic accuracy. Heretofore, GLC and HPLC peak identification have been based almost solely on retention time. Only rarely have tocopherol peaks from samples been identified by ancillary techniques (Tangney et al., 1981). The development and implementation of such instruments as HPLC photodiode array detectors, GC-MS, and HPLC-MS will provide analysts with substantial additional information to evaluate peak identification and purity. A few procedures and materials have been developed to improve the accuracy of measuring tocopherols in foods. Slover et al. (1983) used 5,7-dimethyltocol, Lehmann and Martin (1983) incorporated tocol, and Weber (1984) employed δ-tocopherol as an internal standard during their respective chromatographic separations of tocopherols and tocotrienols in extracts of foods. In addition, Slover and Thompson (1985) demonstrated that tocopherols were stable in margarine stored at –40 to –60°C for up to three years and have suggested that it may be used as an analytic quality control material during routine analyses of foods. Unfortunately, there are no standard reference materials with certified values for any of the tocopherols or tocotrienols (Wolf, 1987).

Tocopherol and Tocotrienol Contents of Foods

Food composition tables and data bases have a dearth of information relative to the individual vitamin E vitamer content of foods. The USDA handbook on the composition of fats and oils contains values for total tocopherol as well as α-tocopherol (Reeves and Weihrauch, 1979). Handbooks for foods of other countries contain total vitamin E values but for selected foods only (Paul and Southgate, 1978; Souci et al., 1982). The data base recently developed for the 1985 Continuing Survey of Food Intake by Individuals (Nationwide Food Consumption Survey) and the Hispanic Health and Nutrition Examination Survey (HHANES) contains total vitamin E values for all foods expressed as α-tocopherol equivalents (Nutrition Monitoring Division, 1986). Due to the lack of analytic values for many foods, a substantial number of those values were imputed (J. Weihrauch, personal communication). Perusal of the most recent index of food composition data bases for computer systems (Hoover, 1987) indicates that only a few contain data on the vitamin E content of foods.

Data on tocopherol and tocotrienol content of foods have been published as part of ongoing research and monitoring programs. McLaughlin and Weihrauch (1979) tabulated the then-available vitamer content of a large number of foods. Recently, Lehmann et al. (1986) reported the α- and γ-tocopherol contents of prepared foods used to formulate several menus as part of a large human diet study. The tocopherol and tocotrienol content of a many feed stuffs was quantified by Cort et al. (1983); Guzman and Murphy (1986) measured the tocopherols in soy beans and tofu; and Landen (1982) reported the level of α-tocopherol acetate in 32 commercial infant formulas.

A large study is currently ongoing to survey the vitamin E vitamer content of Finnish foods. Several reports have been published including data for complete diets (Piironen et al., 1984a, b), human milk and baby foods (Syväoja et al., 1985a), milk product and eggs (Syväoja et al., 1985b), fish and fish products (Syväoja et al., 1985c), meat (Piironen et al., 1985), cereals (Piironen et al., 1986), and oils and fats (Syväoja et al., 1986). These efforts will result in a complete data base on the vitamer content of foods and will be available to several professional groups in Finland.

REFERENCES

AIN Committee on Nomenclature (1979). *J. Nutr. 109*: 8.

Andrews, A. G., Liaaen-Jensen, S., Borch, G. (1974). *Acta Chem. Scand. B28*: 737.

Banwart, W. L., Porter, P. M., Granato, T. C., Hassett, J. J. (1985). *J. Chem. Ecol. 11(3)*: 383–395.

Barnett, S. A., Frick, L. W., Baine, H. M. (1980). *Anal. Chem. 52*: 610.

Bauernfeind, J. C., Cort, W. M. (1974). In *Encyclopedia of Food Technology*, Vol. 2, Johnson, A. H., Peterson, M. S. (Eds.). AVI: Westport, pp. 891-898.

Beecher, G. R., Khachik, F. (1984). *J. Natl. Cancer Inst. 73*: 1397.

Bradfield, C. A., Bjeldanes, L. F. (1987). *J. Agric. Food Chem. 35*: 46.

Brandl, W., Herrman, K. (1983). *J. Chromatog. 260*: 447-455.

Brubacher, G., Müller-Mulot, W., Southgate, D. A. T. (1985). In *Methods for the Determination of Vitamins in Food*. Elsevier, New York, pp. 97 and 107.

Budzikiewicz, H., Brzezinka, H., Johannes, B. (1970). *Monatsch. Chemie 101*: 579-609.

Bunnell, R. H. (1967). In *The Vitamins*, Gyorgy, P., Pearson, W. N. (Eds.). Academic Press, New York, p. 261.

Burton, G. W., Ingold, K. U. (1984). *Science 224*: 569-573.

Cort, W. M., Vicente, T. S. Waysek, E. N., Williams, B. D. (1983). *J. Agric. Food Chem. 31*: 1330.

Dam, H. (1962). *Vit. Horm. 20*: 527.

Davies, B. H. (1976). In *Chemistry and Biochemistry of Plant Pigments*, Vol. 2, Goodwin, T. W. (Ed.). Academic Press, New York, p. 38.

Davis, W. B. (1949). *Anal. Chem. 21*: 1500.

De Leenheer, A. P., Lambert, W. E. (1981). *Int. J. Vitamin Nutr. Res. 51*: 180.

De Leenheer, A. P., Lambert, W. E., Claeys, I. (1982). *J. Lipid Res. 23*: 1362.

DeLuca, H. F. (1979). *Fed. Proc. 38*: 2519.

Denny, M., Liu, R.S. H. (1977). *J. Am. Chem. Soc. 99*: 4865.

De Ruyter, M. G., Lambert, W. E., De Leenheer, A. P. (1979). *Anal. Biochem. 98*: 402.

Driskell, W. J., Bashor, M. M., Neese, J. W. (1983). *Clin. Chem. 29*: 1042.

Egberg, D. C. (1982). An assessment of the accuracy and precision of the methods used for the measurement of organic nutrients in cereal and grain products. In *Reference Materials for Organic Nutrients Measurement*, Margolis, S. A. (Ed.). NBS Special Publication No. 635, U. S. Government Printing Office, Washington, D.C., pp. 8-12.

Egberg, D. C., Heroff, J. C., Potter, R. H. (1977). *J. Agric. Food chem. 25*: 1127.

Egberg, D. C., Pelletier, O., Johnson, A. J., Thompson, J. N. (1985). In *Methods of Vitamin Assay*, Augustin, J., Klein, B. P., Becker, D., Venugopal (Eds.). John Wiley & Sons, New York, pp. 95–133.

Emmerie, A., Engel, C. (1938). *Rec. Trav. Chim. 57*: 1351.
Englert, G. (1982). In *Carotenoids Chemistry and Biochemistry*, Britton, G., Goodwin, T. W. (Eds.). Pergamon, Oxford, pp. 107-153.
Entschel, R., Karrer, P. (1958). *Helv. Chim. Acta 41*: 402.
Enzell, C. R., Francis, G. W., Liaaen-Jensen, S. (1969). *Acta Chem. Scand. 23*: 727-750.
Enzell, C. R., Wahlberg, I. (1980). In *Biochemical Application of Mass Spectrometry*, Waller, G. R., Dermer, O. C. (Eds.). Wiley-Interscience, New York, pp. 407-438.
Eugster, C. H., Trivedi, A. H., Karrer, P. (1955). *Helv. Chim. Acta 38*: 1359.
Eugster, C. H. (1982). In *Carotenoids Chemistry and Biochemistry*, Britton, G., Goodwin, T. W. (Eds.). Pergamon, Oxford, pp. 1-26.
Fankel, R., Schmid, K. (1976). *Landwirtsch. Forsch. 33(2)*: 283.
Food and Nutrition Board (1980). In *Recommended Dietary Allowances*, National Academy of Sciences, Washington, D.C., pp. 63-69.
Frolik, C. A., Tavela, T. E., Sporn, M. B. (1978a). *J. Lipid Res. 19*: 32.
Frolik, C. A., Tavela, T. E., Peck, G. L., Sporn, M. B. (1978b). *Anal. Biochem. 86*: 743.
Goodman, D. S. (1984). *N. Engl. J. Med. 310*: 1023.
Goodwin, T. W. (1980a). In *Biochemistry of the Carotenoids*, Vol. 1, Chapman and Hall, New York, p. 62.
Goodwin, T. W. (1980b). In *Biochemistry of the Carotenoids*, Vol. 1, Chapman and Hall, New York, p. 107.
Gregory, G. K., Chen, T. S., Philip, T. (1986). *J. Food Sci. 51(4)*: 1093.
Guzman, G. J., Murphy, P. A. (1986). *J. Agric. Food Chem. 34*: 791.
Haytowitz, D. B., Matthews, R. H. (1984). In *Composition of Foods: Vegetables and Vegetables Product-Raw, Processed, Prepared*. USDA Agriculture Handbook No. 8-11, USDA, Washington, D.C..
Hoover, L. W. (1987). *Nutrient Data Bank Directory*, 6th ed. University of Missouri, Columbia.
Horwitz, W. (Ed.) (1980). *Official Methods of Analysis of the Association of Analytical Chemists*. AOAC, Washington, D.C., pp. 230-231, 734-740.
Institute of Occupational Health, Environmental Health and Nutrition, Department of Nutrition (1980). *Table of Food Composition*. Chinese Acad. Med. Sci., Beijing.
Jamieson, G. R. (1970). In *Topics in Lipid Chemistry*, Gunstone, F. D. (Ed.). Pergamon Press, New York, p. 107.
Khachik, F., Beecher, G. R. (1985). *J. Chromatog. 346*: 237.
Khachik, F., Beecher, G. R., Whittaker, N. F. (1986). *J. Agric. Food Chem. 34*: 603.
Khachik, F., Beecher, G. R. (1986). *J. Ind. Eng. Chem. Prod. Res. Dev. 25*: 671.
Khachik, F., Beecher, G. R. (1987). *J. Agric. Food Chem., 35*: 732.
Khachik, F. and Beecher, G. R. (1988). *J. Agric. Food Chem.*, in press.
Khachik, F., Beecher, G. R., and Lusby, W. R. (1988a). *J. Agric. Food Chem.*, in press.

Khachik, F., Beecher, G. R., Vanderslice, J., and Furrow, G. (1988b). *Anal. Chem. 60*: 807.
Khachik, F., Beecher, G. R., (1988c). *J. Chromatog.*, in press.
Klaui, H., Bauernfeind, J. C. (1981). In *Carotenoids as Colorants and Vitamin A Precursors*, Bauernfeind, J. C. (Ed.). Academic, New York, p. 156.
Lambert, W. E., Nelis, H. J., De Ruyter, M. G. M., De Leenheer, A. P. (1985). In *Modern Chromatographic Analysis of the Vitamins*, Vol. 30, De Leenheer, A. P., Lambert, W. E., De Ruyter, M. G. M. (Eds.). Marcel Dekker, New York, pp. 1-72.
Landen, W. O., Jr., (1982). *J. Assoc. Off. Anal. Chem. 65*: 810.
Landen, W. O., Jr., (1981). *J. Chromatog. 211*: 155.
Lehmann, J., Martin, H. L. (1983). *Clin. Chem. 29*: 1840.
Lehmann, J., Martin, H. L., Lashley, E. L., Marshall, M. W., Judd, J. T. (1986). *J. Am. Diet. Assoc. 86*: 1208.
Liaaen-Jensen, S. (1971). In *Carotenoids*, Isler, O. (Ed.). Birkhauser Verlag, Basel, pp. 61-188.
Liaaen-Jensen, S., Jensen, A. (1966). *Prog. Chem. Fats 8*: 129.
Lime, B. J., Stephens, T. S., Griffiths, F. P. (1954). *Food Technol. 8*: 566.
MacGillivray, J. H. (1935). *Cancer 81*: 7.
Macrae, R. (1982). In *HPLC in Food Analysis*, Macrae, R. (Ed.). Academic Press, New York, p. 1.
Mayer, H., Bollag, W., Hanni, R., Ruegg, R. (1978). *Experimentia 34*: 1105.
Mayer, H., Isler, O. (1971). In *Carotenoids*, Isler, O. (Ed.). Birkhauser Verlag, Basel, pp. 325-575.
McCormick, A. M., Napoli, J. L., DeLuca, H. F. (1979). *Anal. Biochem. 86*: 25.
McKenzie, R. M., Hellwege, D M., McGregor, M. L., Rockley, N. L., Riquetti, Nelson, E. C. (1978). *J. Chromatog. 155*: 379.
McLaughlin, P. J., Weihrauch, J. L. (1979). *J. Am. Diet. Assoc. 75*: 647.
Nelis, H. J., De Bevere, V. O. R. C., De Leenheer, A. P. (1985). In *Modern Chromatographic Analysis of the Vitamins*, De Leenheer, A. P., Lambert, W. E., De Ruyter, M. G. M. (Eds.). Marcel Dekker, New York, pp. 129-200.
Noga, G., Lenz, F. (1983). *Chromatographia 17*: 139.
Nutrition Monitoring Division (1986). In *Machine-Readable Data Sets on Composition of Foods and Results from Food Consumption Surveys*. U.S. Department of Agriculture, Washington, D.C., HNIS Admin. Report No. 378, pp. 12-15, 20-21.
Paanakker, J. E., Groenendijk, G. W. T. (1979). *J. Chromatog. 168*: 125.
Panalaks, T., Murray, T. K. (1970). *Can. Inst. Food Technol. J. 3*: 145.
Parrish, D. B. (1980). *CRC Crit. Rev. Food Sci. Nutr. 13*: 161.
Parrish, D. B., Moffitt, R. A., Noel, R. J., Thompson, J. N. (1985). In *Methods of Vitamin Assay*, Augustin, J., Klein, B. P., Becker, D. Venugopal, P. B. (Eds.). John Wiley & Sons, New York, pp. 153-184.
Paul, A. A., Southgate, D.A. T. (1978). *The Composition of Foods*, Elsevier, Amsterdam, North-Holland.
Petracek, F. J. Zechmeister, L. (1956). *J. Am. Chem. Soc. 78*: 1427.

Piironen, V., Varo, P. Syväoja, E. L., Salminen, K., Koivistoinen, P. (1984a). *Int. J. Vit. Nutr. Res. 54*: 35.
Piironen, V., Varo, P., Syväoja, E. L., Salminen, K., Koivistoinen, P., Arvilommi, H. (1984b). *Int. J. Vit. Nutr. Res. 54*: 41.
Piironen, V., Syväoja, E. L., Varo, P., Salminen, K., Koivistoinen, P. J. (1985). *Agric. Food Chem. 33*: 1215.
Piironen, V., Syväoja, E. L., Varo, P., Salminen, K., Koivistoinen, P. (1986). *Cereal Chem. 63*: 78.
Reeves, J. B., III, Weihrauch, J. L. (1979). *Composition of Foods: Raw, Processed, Prepared: Fats and Oils*. Agriculture Handbook No. 8-4, United States Department of Agriculture, Washington, D.C.
Ritter, E. D., Purcell, A. E. (1981). In *Carotenoids as Colorants and Vitamin A Precursors*, Bauernfeind, J. C. (Ed.). Academic, New York, p. 883.
Roberts, A. B., Nichols, M. D., Frolik, C. A., Newton, D. L., Sporn, M. B. (1978). *Cancer Res. 38*; 3327.
Rotman, J. P., Kropf, A. (1975). *Vision Res. 15*: 1301.
Schmidtlein, H., Herrmann, K. Z. (1975a). *Lebensm. Unters. Forsch. 159*: 139.
Schmidtlein, H., Herrmann, K. Z. (1975b). *Lebensm. Unters. Forsch. 159*: 225.
Schwartz, S. J., Woo, S. L., Elbe, J. H. (1981). *J. Agric. Food Chem. 29*; 533.
Shekelle, R. B., Lepper, M., Liu, S., Oglesby, P., Shryock, A. M., Stamler, J. (1981). *Lancet 2*: 1185.
Shen, C-S. J., Sheppard, A. J. (1986). *J. Micronutr. Anal. 2*: 43.
Simpson, K. L., Tsou, S. C. S., Chichester, C. O. (1985). In *Methods of Vitamin Assay*, Augustin, J., Klein, P. B., Becker, D., Venugopal, P. B. (Eds.). John Wiley & Sons, New York, pp. 185-220.
Slover, H. T., Thompson, R. H., Jr., Merola, G. V. (1983). *J. Am. Oil Chem. Soc. 60*: 1524.
Slover, H. T., Thompson, R. H., Jr., (1985). In *Biological Reference Materials*, Wolf, W. R. (Ed.). John Wiley, New York, p. 239.
Snyder, L. R., Kirkland, J. J. (1979). In *Introduction to Modern Liquid Chromatography*. John Wiley, New York, p. 791.
Souci, S. W., Fachmann, W., Kraut, H. (1982). *Food Composition and Nutrition Tables 1981/82*. Wisenschaftliche Verlagsgesellschaft, Stuttgart.
Sporn, M. B., Dunlop, N. M., Newton, D. L., et al. (1976). *Fed. Proc. 35*: 1332.
Spron, M. B., Newton, D. L. (1981). In *Inhibition of Tumor Induction and Development*, Zedeck, M. S., Lipkin, M. (Eds.). Plenum Press, New York, p. 71.
Stancher, B., Zonta, F. (1982). *J. Chromatog. 238*: 217.
Steuerle, H. (1981). *J. Chromatog. 206*: 319.
Straub, O. (1987). In *Key to Carotenoids*, Pfander, H. (Ed.) in collaboration with Gerspacher, M., Rychener, M., and Schwabe, R. 2nd enlarged and revised edition, Birkhauser Verlag, Basel.
Surmatis, J. D., Ofner, A. (1961). *J. Org. Chem. 26*: 1171.
Syväoja, E. L., Piironen, V., Varo, P., Koivistoinen, P., Salminen, K. (1986). *J. Am. Oil Chem. Soc.* 63, 328.

Syväoja, E. L., Salminen, K., Püronen, V., Varo, P., Kerojoki, O., Koivistoinen, P. (1985c). *J. Am. Oil Chem. Soc. 62*: 1245.
Syväoja, E. L., Püronen, V., Varo, P., Koivistoinen, P., Salminen, K. (1985a). *Int. J. Vit. Nutr. Res. 55*: 159.
Syväoja, E. L., Püronen, V., Varo, P., Koivistoinen, P., Salminen, K. (1985b). *Milchwissenschaft 40*: 467.
Sweeney, J. P., Marsh, A. C. (1971). *J. Am. Dietet. Assoc. 59*: 238.
Tangney, C. C., McNair, H. M., Driskell, J. A. (1981). *J. Chromatog. 224*: 389.
Taylor, R. F. (1983). In *Advances in Chromatography*, Giddings, J. C., Grushka, E., Cazes, J., Brown, P. R. (Eds.). Marcel Dekker, Inc., New York, pp. 157-213.
Thompson, J. N. (1986). *J. Assoc. Off. Anal. Chem. 5*: 727.
Thompson, J. N., Hatina, G. J. (1979). *Liquid Chromatog. 2*: 327.
Ting, S. V., Deszyck, E. J. (1958). *Proc. Am. Soc. Hortic. Sci. 71*: 271.
Tsimidou, M., Macrae, R. (1985). *J. Chromatog. 23*: 155
Tsukida, K., Kodama, A., Ito, M. Kawamoto, M., Takahashi, K. (1977a). *J. Nutr. Sci. Vitaminol. 23*: 263.
Tsukida, K., Kodama, A., Ito, M. (1977b). *J. Chromatog. 134*: 331.
Tsukida, K., Ito, M. Kodama, A. (1978a). *J. Nutr. Sci. Vitaminol. 24*: 143.
Tsukida, K., Kodama, A., Ito, M. (1978b). *J. Nutr. Sci. Vitaminol. 24*: 593.
Tsukida, K., Saiki, K., Takii, T., Koyama, Y. (1982). *J. Chromatog. 245*: 359.
Tsukida, K., Saiki, K. (1983). *J. Nutr. Vitaminol. 29*: 111.
Vande Casteele, K., Geiger, H., Van Sumere, C. F. J. (1983). *Chromatog. 258*: 111-124.
Van Niekerk, P. J. (1982). In *HPLC in Food Analysis*, Macrae, R. (Ed.). Academic Press, New York, p. 187.
Vetter, W., Englert, G., Riggassi, N., Schwieter, U. (1971). In *Carotenoids*, Isler, O. (Ed.). Birkhauser Verlag, Basel, pp. 189-266.
Vogele, A. C. (1937). *Plant Physiol. 12*: 929.
Waddell, W. H., Crouch, R., Nakanishi, K., Turro, N. J. (1976). *J. Am. Chem. Soc. 98*: 4189.
Waddell, W. H., Dawson, P. M., Hopkins, D. L., Rach, K. L., Uemura, M., West, J. L. (1979). *J. Liquid Chromatog. 2*: 1205.
Weber, E. J. (1984). *J. Am. Oil Chem. Soc. 61*: 1231.
Weedon, B. C. L. (1971). In *Carotenoids*, Isler, O. (Ed.). Birkhauser Verlag, Basel, pp. 267-323.
Widicus, W. A., Kirk, J. R. (1979). *J. Assoc. Off. Anal. Chem. 62*: 637.
Willett, W. C. (1984). *N. Engl. J. Med. 310*: 633-638, 697-701.
Wolf, W. R. (1987). *Fresenius Z Anal. Chem. 326*: 597.
Wright, S. W., Shearer, J. D. (1984). *J. Chromatog. 294*: 281.
Wu Leung, W. T., Butrum, R. R., Chang, F. H. et al. (1972). Food composition table for use in East Asia. Rome: FAO, 1-189.

6
Dietary Assessment Methods

GLADYS BLOCK and ANNE M. HARTMAN
National Cancer Institute, National Institutes of Health, Bethesda, Maryland

The ability to uncover relationships between diet and disease, the ability to monitor diet change in intervention studies, and the ability to control for dietary factors in studies of other risk factors all depend profoundly on the appropriateness and adequacy of the dietary assessment methods chosen. This chapter will discuss the dietary methods available, the evidence for their validity, and the limitations and appropriate uses of the types of data they produce. Before turning to the specific methods, however, it may be useful to consider two overriding issues—the nutrients to be assessed, and the need for data representative of the usual diets of individuals.

SPECIFIC DIETARY CONSTITUTENTS OR THE WHOLE DIET?

There are some situations in which collecting information on one or a few nutrients may be justified. However, for etiologic research or for research in which baseline data are collected for future outcome analysis, control of confounding or examination of effect modification, it is usually unwise and poor economy to restrict data collection to a limited list of a few nutrients. Current laboratory or epidemiologic data (Committee on Diet, Nutrition, and Cancer, 1982) suggest relationships between cancer and a number of micronutrients, including vitamins A, C, E, carotenoids, folacin, and trace minerals including selenium and zinc. Other dietary components of potential significance include total calories, total fat, percent of calories derived from fat, specific fat fractions such as polyunsaturated fatty acids, cholesterol, dietary fiber and fiber fractions, alcohol, and others. It is important to recognize that a few years ago the list would have been different; a few years in the future the list will again be different. If we ask only about one or two nutrients, we forego all ability to reanalyze data later for nutrients which may become of interest—or even be discovered—in the future.

Studies that do not attempt to assess the whole diet may, at the worst, result in erroneous conclusions. Foods contain many nutrients simultaneously. If we only ask about vitamin x we may conclude that a protective effect is due to vitamin x, when instead it may simply be that vitamin x is positively (or negatively) associated with the true etiologic factor. A great deal of effort, expense, and public credibility may then be wasted conducting interventions on the wrong dietary factor.

At best, studies collecting data on only a few elements of the diet leave a great many questions unanswered and produce small and ambiguous, rather than large and complex, advances in our understanding. Vitamin C and carotenoids are both antioxidants; is a low intake of carotenoids only deleterious if vitamin C is simultaneously low, or can they substitute for each other? Or conversely, must both be present in adequate amounts because they act preferentially on different oxidants or radicals in a cascade? The answer is important to public health and can only be answered if data on both vitamin C and carotenoids have been collected.

The above example is a simple one, because we often do collect data on both vitamin C and carotenoid sources; but the same principle applies to *all* of the dietary factors we wish to study. Is a high polyunsaturated fat intake only harmful in the presence of a low intake of vitamin E, a lipid antioxidant? Is it fiber or something else contributed by the vegetable kingdom which is protective against colon cancer? Is the effect of selenium dependent on levels of vitamin E (Willett et al., 1983; Menkes et al., 1986) or retinol (Willett et al., 1983)? Only by capturing the whole diet can new hypotheses be generated and tested, and existing hypotheses tested adequately. And only by capturing the whole diet can we begin to examine dietary interactions such as those noted above, an area where our understanding is minimal at best. "Perhaps the most striking impression received from an evaluation of the literature is that hardly any study undertaken with any pair of nutrients has failed to show a significant interaction in terms of some nutritional or biochemical criterion" (Harte and Chow, 1964).

"An Individual's Usual Diet"

Individual vs. Group Data

For some, primarily nonetiologic, purposes data on the mean intake of groups may be needed. Group means may be used to compare the progress of two randomized diet groups, for example, or to examine the balance on baseline dietary characteristics. Or they may be used to assess whether the mean intake of a population subgroup meets the RDA for a given nutrient, in which case the nutrient estimate is needed with accuracy and precision, but at the group mean level. Even in those cases, however, more useful information would be obtained by describing the *distribution* of intakes, what proportion is below the RDA, something for which the mean alone is useless (Subcommittee on Criteria for Dietary Evaluation, 1986). The United States Department of Agriculture, charged with the description of the population's intake, has recognized the need to go beyond simple means; the Nationwide Food Consumption Survey (USDA, 1984) thus collects three days of diet data, so as to be able to describe the population's *distribution* of intake, e.g., what proportion is habitually consuming less than 100% of the RDA, less than 75%, less than 50%. Surveys charged with going beyond description of group means to analysis and explanation need data representative of individuals.

To study the relationship between diet and disease or other physiologic characteristics with adequate statisitical power, data are needed at the level of the individual. As Lilienfeld has said, "In studying *group* characteristics, . . . the results of such studies provide *clues* to etiologic hypotheses" (emphasis in the original) but "may suffer from an 'ecologic fallacy'. . . . Associations established by studying characteristics of population groups have a greater chance of being indirect than those established by studying characteristics in individuals. In other words, it is preferable to have an association based on data obtained at the level of the individual and not at . . . the level of a population or group" (Lilienfeld and Lilienfeld, 1980).

It may be thought that epidemiologists and other medical researchers study groups—cases and controls, for example—and consequently group data may be appropriate. It is important to note, however, that analytic epidemiologic studies, including *case-control studies* and *prospective studies*, involve not the examination of group means but the *categorization* of *individuals* into exposed or nonexposed. Dietary methods that cannot at least place individuals into the correct quartile or so of the distribution of intake of a nutrient will not permit studies of this sort with any statistical power.

The same argument applies to the *cross-sectional study* of the relationship between diet and serum values or behavioral characteristics. For example, little progress has been made in understanding the degree to which dietary fat is related to serum cholesterol in datasets using 24-hour recalls (Nichols et al., 1976; National Center for Health Statistics, 1983). Although little or no relationship was observed, the diet data on which they are based support only group data, affording neither support for a relationship nor support for lack of a relationship. Only the unresolved question remains.

Intervention studies or clinical trials may use group-level data for the purpose of monitoring if study groups are adhering to a prescribed diet or evaluating balance between the groups. However, to identify individuals needing counseling or to investigate whether the effect of the intervention may be different in subsets with high or low dietary intake (effect modification), individually valid data are needed.

It is necessary to consider this issue of group vs. individual, because the various dietary assessment methods vary in their ability to measure validly the usual intake of an individual. As will be seen, one-day methods clearly provide the weakest data on an individual's diet. For multiple-day methods, the strength of the data for an individual depends on the number of days and the day-to-day variability of intake of the particular nutrient (Liu et al., 1978; Beaton et al., 1979, 1983; Sempos et al., 1985).

"Usual" Diet

Very recent diet may be relevant to certain labile serum or urine values. Chronic disease states, however, if they are related to diet at all, are almost certain to be related not to a particular point on a fluctuating pattern of intake, but to some sort of long-term averaged usual intake. It is always important, therefore, to weigh carefully the precision that can be obtained for short-term intake against its relevance or irrelevance for chronic disease or physiologic characteristics.

DIETARY ASSESSMENT METHODS: DESCRIPTION AND VALIDITY

This has been reviewed extensively elsewhere (Burk and Pao, 1976; James, Bingham, and Cole, 1981; Block, 1982).

24-Hour Recalls

In this method, the respondent is asked to report his complete dietary intake of all foods and beverages consumed over the past 24 hours. Its strength lies in the fact that, if properly performed, it can provide information detailed enough to permit extremely precise coding of the foods consumed, and thus of the nutrients consumed. This accuracy is, however, dependent on a number of factors. First, portion size must be obtained accurately, ideally with three-dimensional models or picture booklets, since research indicates that individuals of all ages are poor estimators of their portion sizes (Guthrie, 1984). Second, precision in coding requires interviewers with nutrition experience and careful probing for exact food type and preparation method to minimize use of "Not Further Specified" codes, an important source of imprecision in group estimates. Third, the data base must be detailed enough to permit coding of the great variety of foods, cuts of meat, preparation methods, etc. Values for "Not Further Specified" codes should be assigned based on foods that are most commonly eaten rather than by the so-called "conservative" approach, which uses the most extreme value in the data base (the fattiest cuts of meat, for example) regardless of its frequency of consumption.

The 24-hour-recall method thus requires a highly trained interviewer and usually takes 20-30 minutes to perform. The coding of the completed interview also requires considerable time and well-trained coders. Some investigators have used it with telephone interviews, and Posner et al. (1982) have developed two-dimensional models and pictures, which are sent to the respondent ahead of time to enhance portion size accuracy.

The method has been validated by comparing the nutrient extimates with those produced by collecting and weighing duplicate meals (Madden, Goodman, and Guthrie, 1976; Gersovitz, Madden, and Smiciklas-Wright, 1978), or by detailed food diaries (Young et al., 1952). It generally produces estimates of the mean nutrient intake of a group that are similar to those of a reference method. However, there is also evidence (Madden, Goodman, and Guthrie, 1976; James, Bingham, and Cole, 1981) that forgetting may produce underestimation of nutrient intake.

The chief drawback of the 24-hour recall for research on the relationship between diet and disease or diet and serum levels is that it does not provide valid esimates of the *usual* diet of *individuals* (Beaton et al., 1979, 1983; Todd, Hudes, and Calloway, 1983). This is a result of the day-to-day variability in ordinary diets, an issue which will be discussed extensively below under "Precision and Misclassification Issues." Thus, the 24-hour recall is primarily useful only to measure the *mean* intake of groups. Under some circumstances it might be useful as a monitoring tool, in a dietary intervention study, for example, to assess whether the two *groups* were maintaining their group assignments. For etiologic studies of diet and disease, however, or for cross-sectional studies that seek to elucidate the relationship between diet and some serum or other physiologic factor, 24-hour recalls provide the weakest basis for valid inference.

Diet Records

In this method respondents are asked to record their diet as they are consuming it, thus minimizing errors of memory. Records of longer than a single day provide diet data more representative of the individual's usual intake than one-day records or recalls. When a diet record is performed carefully, it can capture components of diet which might be overlooked by a recall, and affords the opportunity to obtain more accurate portion size estimation through measuring or weighing. It requires that respondents be reasonably literate and comfortable with the idea of careful record keeping and be sufficiently committed to the goals of the study to perform the record keeping conscientiously.

Gersovitz et al. (1978) examined the validity of diet records by instructing 44 elderly persons to record their diets for seven days and then comparing the recorded lunches with the lunches they had actually consumed during that period at a congregate meal site. For 8 of 10 nutrients, the group means were not significantly different. However, the investigators also found evidence that the accuracy of the recorded values declined after the first two days. Because of this, and because consecutive days probably provide less information about usual diet than the same number of nonconsecutive days, multiple-day food records should be in the form of 1-2-day units scattered over a longer period of time.

Multiple-day records demand the time and cooperation of the respondents. Thus, they are of limited use in large-scale population studies, in which the sample that could be induced to participate would be small and unrepresentative. They also require careful instruction beforehand by a nutritionist, careful review afterwards, and are extremely demanding of expert time in the coding process. For studies that can afford them, multiple-day records, like 24-hour recalls, can provide reasonably valid data on the mean intake of groups. If data on the usual intake of individuals is required—to identify those in need of extra counseling, to use as exposure data for subsequent outcome analysis, or to use in control of confounding—their validity depends on the length of the record, discussed under "Precision and Misclassification Issues" below.

Frequency Questionnaires

In this method the respondent is asked to indicate his usual frequency of consumption of each of a list of foods or, sometimes, food groups. If quantified (so that nutrients are estimated, in addition to simple frequencies), a weighting factor such as nutrient quantity in a "standard portion" is multiplied by the frequency of consumption to obtain a nutrient score or estimate of the quantitative nutrient content of the diet.

The food list has, in the past, often been targeted toward the assessment of a single nutrient or a few nutrients, such as vitamin A, and then would include only foods designed to capture that nutrient. That is not a necessary feature of frequency questionnaires, however, and food lists can be designed to capture all of the important nutrients in an individual's diet. To do so, the food list must reflect the population's major sources of those nutrients, and the food items must be kept reasonably distinct (Block et al., 1986).

Food frequency questionnaires can be administered by nonnutritionist interviewers or can be self-administered (Willett et al., 1985). It is thus possible to use them in large population studies in which the purpose is to categorize individuals broadly with respect to usual intake. Coding of such questionnaires is usually relatively fast and does not require nutritional expertise, and can even be made machine-readable (Willett et al., 1985).

While several investigators have evaluated the validity and reliability of frequency questionnaires at measuring purely the *frequency* of consuming foods (Hankin, Rhoads, and Glober, 1975; Axelson and Csernus, 1983; Graham, Lilienfeld, and Tidings, 1967), the validity of these instruments at estimating usual *nutrient* intake is more difficult to assess, because the reference method itself must be a good estimator of usual intake. Consequently, very few investigators have actually validated pure frequency questionnaires using adequate reference methods. Two groups who have done so are Willett et al. (1985) and Pietinen et al. (1988). Willett et al. administered a 61-item questionnaire and compared nutrient estimates with those produced by four seven-day records obtained over the course of a year. The questionnaire nutrient estimate was obtained by multiplying the reported frequency by the nutrient amount in a portion stated on the questionnaire (e.g., "cream cheese, 1 oz.").

Correlations between this food frequency questionnaire, collected at the end of the one-year period, and the four seven-day records collected over the same time period were approximately 0.45 without adjustment for reported caloric intake, and about 0.53 after adjustment for calories. These figures are for estimates excluding vitamin supplements; since populations vary in the extent to which they use vitamin supplements, it is important to evaluate the performance of diet instruments for the assessment of diet alone.

Pietinen et al. (1988) evaluated the validity of a 44-item frequency questionnaire targeted at eight macro- and micronutrients in a study in Finland. They used as the reference data 12 two-day food records collected over a period of six months. The average of the correlation coefficients for the eight nutrients was 0.51, and was 0.58 after adjustment for calories.

Thus it is possible to obtain, from pure frequency questionnaires, nutrient estimates which indicate a fair ability to categorize individuals at the extremes. For example, 40-50% of individuals who were in the lowest quintile of intake by diet record were also in the lowest quintile by the Willett frequency questionnaire. For most nutrients, however, levels of validity for pure frequency questionnaires appear to be in a range which entails such a degree of misclassification as to seriously weaken the power of a study. The effect of such misclassification will be discussed further below.

If data are needed simply on the actual frequency of consumption of certain foods—to evaluate the success of an educational project, for example—then pure frequency questionnaires offer a fairly inexpensive method, easily usable in the general population. If data are needed on individual nutrient intakes for etiologic purposes, however, the addition of some form of portion size assessment will usually produce more accurate nutrient estimates and more accurate ranking. The instrument, if designed to assess the whole diet of an individual, then becomes a diet history questionnaire.

Diet History Questionnaires

This term has been applied to a wide variety of approaches. The characteristics which define a method as a diet history are that it is designed to elicit quantitative information about the individual respondent's usual dietary intake over an extended period of time, with an attempt at quantitation of the individual's usual portion sizes of the foods in his diet. The quantitation may require the respondent to report his usual portion size of each food in household measures, or he may select a three-dimensional model or a photograph that most closely resembles his usual portion.

The use of the word "history" does not indicate that diet information is sought for some time in the past. Such past-diet assessments are more usually termed "retrospective diet assessment," and are discussed below. Rather, as "diet history" is usually used, the method attempts to elicit information about the respondents' customary dietary intake at this general period in their lives. The time frame often specified is the past year, a period long enough to encompass normal seasonal variation and to smooth out shorter-term aberrations. Sometimes diet histories focus the respondent on a shorter time period, such as the past month, in the belief that recall over a shorter, more recent time may be more accurate. While this has not been definitively studied, a shorter time frame runs the danger of reflecting an unrepresentative seasonal peak or trough, or a time when a certain food was eaten with atypical frequency. Furthermore, restricting the reported period to a shorter time may lead the respondent to attempt to *remember* rather than report a usual pattern of frequency.

One often hears the objection, "I can't remember what I ate yesterday; how could anyone remember what they ate in the past year?" However, this reflects a misunderstanding of the cognitive process involved. Unlike the 24-hour recall, responses to frequency questionnaires or diet histories do not invoke *memory* and do not involve the remembering of instances or events. Rather, they involve the recognition and reporting of a *pattern* of behavior. When asked, "How often do you eat eggs?," the respondent does not attempt to remember each instance of egg-eating over the past year. Rather, he reports a pattern, "I eat eggs about twice a week."

Burke's original method (Burke and Stuart, 1938) was primarily menu-based, with lists and recalls used for cross-checking. Menu-based approaches require a high degree of interviewer time and expertise to ensure that all of the constituents of the respondent's diet are incorporated, and usually take 1 to 1½ hours. They may also be heavily influenced by the individual's diet of the past few days (Balogh et al., 1968). Furthermore, menu-based approaches may produce some optimization of the reported diet, since the emphasis on meals may disguise the fact that modern diets are less orderly and often fail to include three square meals a day. This may be the source of the overestimates reported by some investigators of the method.

Many current approaches to diet history interviews are primarily list-based and structured, requiring a shorter time and nonnutritionist interviewers. That is, the individual is prompted with a list of specific foods, and then his frequency of consumption and portion size is obtained for those he reports consuming. List-based approaches, while requiring less time and sophistication on the part of the interviewer, are dependent on the adequacy of the list of foods and their quantitation.

The key distinction between this form of diet history and a frequency questionnaire with an extensive food list designed to capture a broad range of nutrients is that the list-based diet history attempts to get some measure of the respondent's usual portion size of each food, and the frequency questionnaire does not. Most of the instruments usually cited in this connection as "frequency questionnaires"–e.g., those of Balogh (1968), Jain (1982), Browe (1966) and Epstein (1970)–actually contained some individualized quantitation of the respondent's usual portion sizes, and thus will be discussed here under "Diet Histories."

Validity

As with food frequency questionnaires, it is actually meaningless to speak of the validity of *the* diet history or *the* food frequency questionnaire. In both cases, validity is profoundly dependent on the particular food list and the particular quantitation method of each instrument. Observed correlations may be as much a function of imperfect portion size assumptions made by the investigators, for example, as a function of the respondent's ability to report his usual diet. Further, as mentioned above, the appropriateness of the reference method must be carefully examined. Because of day-to-day variability, it is likely that even a seven-day record, for example, may not be an appropriate "truth" measure for long-term usual diet for many nutrients, against which a test instrument is to be judged. Low correlations found in some validation studies may be in part a reflection of unrepresentative reference periods rather than unreliable questionnaires. (In Beaton's data (1979), for example, only percent of calories from carbohydrate and fat could be obtained from both men and women in seven days to an accuracy of ±20% of the individual's true long-term intake.)

Several investigators have developed brief diet history questionnaires including some quantitation of the individual's usual portion sizes. Jain et al. (1982) and Balogh et al. (1968), for example, used pictures of different portion sizes. Browe et al. (1966) had the subject "compare his usual portion with (a stated standard portion) and make appropriate changes on the questionnaire." Epstein et al. (1970) also state that they collected "the size of the usual portion." Such approaches–structured, list-based, and with variable portion-size assessments–can provide reasonably accurate quantitation of an individual's usual

Table 1 Validation Studies of List-Based Diet Histories (LBDH)

Validation Study	Pearson correlation
Balogh[a]	
LBDH vs. 7-day weighed records	.7-.9
Macronutrients	
Balogh[a]	
LBDH vs. 8+ days records	.6-.8
Macronutrients	
Jain[b]	
69-item LBDH vs. interview	.6-.7
Macro, micronutrients	
Hankin[c]	
LBDH vs. interview	.6-.7
Fats	
Block	
LBDH vs. 7-day records, calcium[d]	.75
Pietinen	
LBDH vs. 24 days of records	.5-.7
Macro, micronutrients	

[a]Balogh et al., 1968, 1971.
[b]Jain et al., 1982.
[c]Hankin et al., 1975.
[d]Cummings et al., 1987.
[e]Pietinen et al., 1988.
Values are higher when corrected for attenuation, but are presented here uncorrected for comparison with other studies.

diet in a shorter interview time than required for a traditional diet history interview and without the need for a nutritionist interviewer.

Burke herself (generally considered to be the originator of the traditional diet history interview) (1943) and Reed and Burke (1954) evaluated the method against clinical criteria and found excellent agreement. When compared with seven-day records, some but not all investigators have found that the history method gives higher mean values, while correlations have generally ranged from 0.4 to 0.8. Some validation studies are summarized in Table 1.

Balogh et al. (1971) found correlations ranging from 0.6 (for total carbohydrate) to 0.8 (for fats) between the mean of eight or more days over a year and a diet history based on 69 food items. Jain et al. (1982) validated a different 69-item self-administered questionnaire, quantified by the respondent's choice among sets of photographs of different portion sizes, against a more extensive one-hour interview. They reported correlations of 0.6 to 0.7 for nine macronutrients, vitamin C, and fiber. When compared with a detailed diet interview, Hankin (1967) also found correlations in this range for a short diet history questionnaire targeted toward dietary fat, in which respondents selected photographs of small, medium, and large portions. (See Block, 1982, for a more extensive review of these studies.)

Pietinen et al, (1988) have developed an extensive self-administered questionnaire and food picture book, taking approximately 2½ hours to self-administer, for assessment of the Finnish diet. The average correlations with multiple-day food records for 13 nutrients often assessed by other investigators were 0.59 before adjustment for calories and 0.61 after adjustment.

Other list-based diet histories have been developed by other investigators. Byers et al. (1985), for example, describe a 128-item questionnaire. Although they usually administer it as an extensive interview, they have developed shorter versions targeted toward specific nutrients. Similar extensive instruments have been used by others (Van Horn, 1986).

Block et al. (1986) developed a list-based diet history, which can be self- or interviewer-administered. By using a data-based approach, selecting foods on the basis of their population contribution to calories and 17 other major nutrients, and keeping the food items reasonably distinct, the instrument is designed to capture all of the major nutrients in the diet with the most parsimonious food list. In addition, portion sizes were developed for it on the basis of age- and sex-specific data from NHANES II, thus making use of large-population data based on three-dimensional models. The questionnaire can produce group mean estimates which closely reflect the age and sex differences in intake seen in the NHANES II data (Block et al., 1986). In addition, the ability to rank individuals correctly is supported by good correlations with reference data (Cummings et al., 1987; Sobell et al., 1989).

Individuals are asked to quantify their usual portion of each food by indicating whether it is small, medium, or large with respect to a stated medium portion. An open-ended section in which foods not on the main list can be reported enhances its usefulness for individuals with ethnic or idiosyncratic diets. The questionnaire is administered in an average of 25-35 minutes, can be self-administered, and does not require a person with nutrition expertise for either interviewing or coding. Thus, the work of Hankin, Jain, Balogh and others, as well as our work at NCI, all suggests that correlations in the range of 0.6 to 0.8 can be achieved with list-based diet histories, quantified either with photographs or with a "small-medium-large" approach.

RETROSPECTIVE DIET ASSESSMENT

There is evidence that some dietary factors may play a role in the delay or prevention of the late stages of carcinogenesis, the promotion/progression stages, in which case recent diet may indeed be relevant. Vitamin A, provitamin A, and their analogues appear to be examples of nutritents that exert their anticancer effect at the promotion stage (Peto et al., 1981).

However, for many chronic diseases, one suspects that the relevant dietary patterns took place not in the present but perhaps in the distant past. Among Americans, at least, atherosclerosis begins in adolescence (Blumenthal, 1973), and it is likely that if diet is a factor, its influence begins then as well. Many cancers have long latent periods, 20 years or more, between cancer initiation and the manifestation of frank disease (Higginson, 1975). If diet plays a role in cancer initiation, it is the diet in the past which is important. Vitamin C, for example, in its role as a preventor of nitrosation, presumably acts at the initiation stage (Weisburger et al., 1980).

Several studies of the validity of retrospective dietary assessment have been reported (Byers et al., 1983; Van Leeuwen et al., 1983; Jensen et al., 1984; Rohan and Potter, 1984; McKeown-Eyssen, Yeung, and Bright-See, 1986), with most producing low to moderate correlations (0.3-0.6) with the reference data from the past. Studies in which the reference data were obtained in the same manner as the new data (both were frequency questionnaires, for example) can be expected to produce higher correlations than those in which the reference data were from diet records and the new data are from a diet history or frequency questionnaire.

Sobell and Block (1989) have studied the agreement between 14 days of diet records collected 10-15 years in the past and a list-based diet history developed as reported above (Block et al., 1986). Interviewer-administered correlations in the range of 0.5 to 0.65 were obtained. Correlations in this range support the possibility of obtaining diet from the distant past, but have significant sample-size implications as discussed under "Precision and Misclassification" below.

PRECISION AND MISCLASSIFICATION ISSUES

All dietary assessment methods entail imprecision in the estimate of an individual's usual dietary intake and entail misclassification of individuals with respect to their place along the distribution of long-term dietary intake. In this context *imprecision* means that the absolute value of the nutrient estimate (of calories, for example) differs from the true nutrient intake of the individual to some degree. A questionnaire or a few-day record, for example, may produce a caloric estimate which differs from the individual's true long-term intake by several hundred calories. Imprecision is undesirable if one wishes to counsel individuals regarding their dietary intake, for instance, or identify persons at risk because of nutrient deficiency or excess; it may be less serious in a study of diet-disease relationships (unless combined with misclassification).

Misclassification means that individuals are not categorized correctly along the distribution of intake. That is, persons with high intake in relation to others in the population may be miscategorized as having lower intake. A dietary assessment method may be imprecise in terms of the level of the estimates it produces but still be perfectly satisfactory at classifying or categorizing individuals correctly. For example, all of the estimates may be several hundred calories too low, but the ranking of individuals may be undisturbed. Conversely, two methods may produce similar group means, but nevertheless have very poor ability to classify individuals similarly.

Misclassification has a profound impact on the power of a study, the sample size needed, and the ability to detect true relationships if they exist. It is an aspect of dietary research which cannot be overlooked and which must be included in all considerations of study design and selection of dietary assessment methods.

All methods entail imprecision and misclassification, but the sources of the misclassification are different for the various methods, and the available remedies are different. For one-day or multiple-day methods, the source of misclassification is intraindividual variability—that is, the fact that individuals vary from day to day in their dietary intake. Intraindividual variability makes it difficult to detect differences between groups or individuals and to categorize persons accurately, because it introduces noise into the system. For any given nutrient, the greater the day-to-day variability in intake, the more days are required to adequately represent the long-term diet. In this case the remedy is increasing the number of days. For food-frequency questionnaires or list-based diet histories, the source of imprecision and misclassification is inadequate or inappropriate food lists and the quantitation of them, and the imperfect ability of respondents to report their frequency of consumption. Thus, while there are different sources of error arising from different methods, the adverse effects on the ability to estimate absolute levels or classify individuals are the same.

Since one day provides inadequate characterization of an individual's usual intake, numerous investigators have used three or more consecutive days of diet, either by record or a combination of record and recall, in an attempt to achieve both quantitative precision and greater representativeness of usual diet. How many days, then, are required to obtain adequate representativeness of an individual's usual diet?

Precision

This issue will first be discussed with respect to precision—how many days are required to provide an estimate which is "close to" the actual level of the in-

Table 2 Precision of Multiple-day Nutrient Estimates[a]

Nutrient	Beaton[b] Male	Beaton[b] Female	Balogh[c] Male	Todd[d] Male	Chalmers[e] Male	Chalmers[e] Female
Calories	7	10	9	7	14	11
Protein	13	10	27	11		
Fat	10	16	23			
Fat (% of cals.)	3.1	5				
Cholesterol	27	30	45			
Calcium	17	19				
Thiamin	19	28				
Vitamin C	45	42				

[a]Number of days required to produce a nutrient estimate for an individual which is ±20% of his true long-term usual intake.
[b]Data based on six nonconsecutive days, among 30 males and 30 females, aged 25-44 years. Beaton et al., 1979, 1983.
[c]Data based on 2-11 random days over one year, among 100 Israeli males. Balogh et al., 1971.
[d]Data based on three-day records, among 18 males aged 22-31 years. Todd et al., 1983.
[e]Data based on seven-day records, among "youth." Chalmers et al., 1952.

dividual's usual intake. Although first studied by Chalmers in 1952, this question has been studied intensively in the last decade (Hunt et al., 1983; Liu et al., 1978; Sempos et al., 1985; James et al., 1981). Some results are summarized in Table 2. The data all indicate that a small number of days of diet information does not represent an individual's longer-term usual intake with any precision. The results are extremely consistent across all of these investigators and their different study populations.

Beaton et al. (1979, 1983) found that to be 95% confident of producing an estimate within ±20% of the true usual intake (a rather generous criterion representing, e.g., being between 1600 and 2400 for a true usual intake of 2000 calories), it would require 7 days for males and 10 days for females. For protein, it would be 13 days for males and 10 days for females. For percent of calories from fat, it would require three days in males but five in females. For most micronutrients the situation is even worse: for cholesterol, 27 days for men, 30 for women; for vitamin C, 45 days for men, 42 for women. And if one wanted precision to within ±10%, a great many more days would be required.

Other investigators have found similar results. Balogh, Kahn, and Medalie (1971) found that in order to be within ±20% for 90% of the population it would take 9 days for calories, 45 for cholesterol. And Chalmers et al. (1952), in 1952, calculated that to have a 95% confidence interval equal to ±15% of the then-RDA for calories, one would need 14 days for men, 11 for women. That is to say, to assess with precision the actual level of intake of an individual, *many* days are required.

This inability of a single day's intake to represent usual diet is only somewhat relieved by restricting analysis to nutrients as a percent of calories. Beaton et al. (1979) indicated that "the elimination of the effect of energy intake by calculation of the ratio of nutrient:energy could be expected to reduce variability. Nevertheless, the relatively high intraindividual variability (of nutrients expressed per 1000 kilocalories) suggests wide variation, day by day, in the *composition* (emphasis added) of self-selected diet." James et al. (1981) also concluded that "an individual's variable intake of protein and energy is sufficient from day to day to limit the possibility of using nutrient density rather than absolute intakes as discriminators between individuals" (on usual intake).

Classification

With regard to the ability of a given number of days to classify correctly, some results are summarized in Table 3. Liu et al. (1978) examined the ability to classify individuals into quintiles of the distribution of cholesterol intake. In order to have less than a 5% chance of grossly misclassifying someone from the first to the fifth quintile, again a rather generous criterion, it would require seven days of diet information. In order to avoid misclassifying someone from the first to the third quintile or vice versa, it would require 11 days.

Sempos et al. (1985) used a somewhat different criterion. Suppose one wanted to ensure that an observed correlation between a dietary factor and a physiologic factor such as serum cholesterol was at least as much as 90% of the real correlation. Then it would take seven days for calories, nine for protein, six for calcium, and at least 15 days for micronutrients, such as the B vitamins.

James et al. (1981) in England found that to correctly classify 80% of men into the correct *third* of the distribution would require five days for calories, nine for fat, and 18 days for percent of calories from fat.

It would appear that in terms of both precision and classification, a substantial number of days of diet records would be needed in order to have a high probability of accurately reflecting an individual's true long-term intake. Furthermore, most of the data quoted above give the best cases, the macronutrients that one would suppose were reasonably stable from day to day or over a few days. For most of the micronutrients, investigators have found 10, 15, 20, or more days to be needed. For vitamin A, the situation is totally hopeless.

It is not possible to make similar calculations for food frequencies and diet histories in general, because different instruments vary both in the level of the

Table 3 Classification with Multiple-day Nutrient Estimates[a]

Nutrient	Avoid misclass. from first to fifth quintile	Correct tertile		Estimate of diet-serum relationship at least 90% of true correlation	
		James[c]			
	Liu[b] Male	Male	Female	Liu[b] Male	Sempos[d] Female
Calories		5	4		7
Protein		5	5		9
Fat		9	6		
Fat (% cals.)		18	7		
Cholesterol	7			9	
Calcium		4	4		6
Thiamin		6	9		17
Vitamin C		6	6		11

[a]Number of days required to achieve stated ability to classify individuals or estimate correct diet-serum correlations.
[b]Data based on seven-day records, among 448 Chicago males. Liu et al., 1978
[c]To classify 80% of subjects into correct tertile. Data based on seven-day weighed records, among 31 males, 30 females, England. James et al., 1981.
[d]Data based on 24 random days in each of two years, among 151 women. Sempos et al., 1985.

estimates they produce and in their ability to classify individuals correctly. It is possible, however, to compare correlations with usual intake which a given method produces, and such work is in progress. In general, it appears that good list-based diet histories can classify individuals approximately as well as a few days of diet records for the most stable nutrients, and approximately as well as several days of records, for the less stable nutrients.

Effect of Misclassification on Statistical Power

As indicated above, misclassification can have a profoundly deleterious impact on the power of a study and consequently on the sample size needed to detect a true relationship. To assess the degree of this impact, it is necessary to consider the degree of misclassification which results when individuals are classified into quantiles of the nutrient distributions. This can be accomplished by cross-classifying or correlating the intakes derived from the proposed dietary assessment instrument with those from a reference measure of "true" usual diet (Walker and Blettner, 1985). While "true" usual intake is not known, it can be estimated from the mean of several days of dietary records (which are themselves imperfect), combined with knowledge about the intra- and interindividual variability in daily intake from these records or recalls (Liu et al., 1978; Beaton et al., 1979). If the estimate of intraindividual variability is itself based on a large enough number of days (Balogh, Kahn, and Medalie, 1971), it is possible to estimate the number of days required to measure usual intake with good precision, which can then be used as the reference method.

Walker and Blettner (1985) have illustrated how misclassification (as reflected in correlations between a diet instrument and standard or "true" measures of intake) influences the resulting estimate of relative risk (RR). For illustration, they assume a true RR of 3.0 and a linear trend in risk across quintiles. For a diet instrument in a cohort study which correlated at 0.7 with truth, the corresponding patterns of misclassification would be such that in the extreme quintiles of the distribution only 57% would be correctly classified. The true relative risk of 3.0 would be attenuated by 35%, resulting in an observed RR = 2.0. For a diet instrument which correlated at only 0.4 with the truth, only 38% of those in the extreme quintiles would be correctly classified, and the RR would be attenuated by 51%, to an observed RR = 1.5.

These attenuations also affect the sample size needed to detect as statistically significant a true dose-response trend in relative risk across the exposure categories. If there were a linear trend in risk and RR = 3 from top to bottom quintile, a diet instrument which correlated at 0.7 with the truth would require a 2.4-fold increase in sample size, above the sample size estimated in the standard calculations which assume no error in the measurement of the exposure variable. For an instrument which correlated at 0.4 with true long-term diet, one would need almost an 8-fold increase in sample size (Walker and Blettner, 1985). Changing the assumptions about the true relative risk further changes the attenuation. If the true RR were 9.0, the observed RR would be attenuated by 63% and by 79% with the diet instrument which correlated at 0.7 or 0.4, respectively, with the truth.

Regardless of whether a diet measure is the average of multiple days of records or daily consumption calculated from a frequency questionnaire or diet history, the correlation between that measure and "true" usual intake reflects both the method's validity (ability to measure "true" usual intake) and its reliability (reproducibility on subsequent occasions assuming no change in intake has taken place). The attenuation associated with imperfect reliability can be calculated from the ratio of intra- to interindividual variability (Liu et al., 1978). Wu et al. (1986) have also shown the relationship between an instrument's reliability and attenuation in the true odds ratio estimate.

It is clear, therefore, that all dietary assessment methods involve imprecision and misclassification. Numerous days of recalls or records are required to estimate an individual's correct long-term intake. Diet histories or frequency questionnaires also entail imprecision and misclassification, although the extent varies with the particular instrument, and further work remains to be done to establish the dimensions of error for these instruments and to improve their ability to classify individuals. In planning research involving dietary assessment, investigators now have better information on which to base their decisions regarding methods. Every proposed method entails a given correlation with the "truth". For *n* multiple days, that correlation can be estimated using data from Beaton et al. (1979) and Liu et al. (1978). For diet histories and frequency questionnaires, that correlation can be estimated from published validation studies, combined with adjustment for imperfect reference methods (Liu et al., 1978). Finally, Walker and Blettner (1985) provide formulae with which to calculate the sample size needed to detect an effect, given that the dietary intake is measured with some degree of error, as reflected in those correlations with the truth. Such sample size estimates are invariably several times the sample size calculated under the assumption of perfect measurement. Investigators can then balance requirements, in terms of research goals and desired precision, against the cost in dollars and human resources.

In addition to the use of these data at the planning stage, investigators can also make use of recent work, particularly that of Walker and Blettner (1985), at the analysis stage. Standard calculations of confidence intervals are, again, always based on the assumption of measurement without error, clearly an incorrect assumption in the case of dietary assessment. Not only are estimates of relative risk biased towards 1.0, but the confidence limits which should be placed around those estimates are in fact much wider than the standard calculations would produce. Progress in our understanding of the relationship between diet and disease requires that we have an accurate reflection of the strength of our conclusions.

CONCLUSION

A great deal has been said here about the errors inherent in dietary assessment; when investigators take these errors into account in estimating confidence limits, the obvious uncertainty in dietary research may be discouraging. When viewed as a challenge rather than a barrier, however, a clear understanding of the limitations is a necessary first step in overcoming them. With that understanding, methods can and will be found to reduce the expense and improve the validity of dietary assessment. In the meantime, a great deal of useful research has been and will continue to be done.

REFERENCES

Axelson, J. M., Csernus, M. M. (1983). Reliability and validity of a food frequency checklist. *J. Am. Diet. Assoc. 83*: 152.

Balogh, M., Medalie, J. H., Smith, H., Groen, J. J. (1968). The development of a dietary questionnaire for an ischemic heart disease survey. *Israel J. Med. Sci. 4*: 195.

Balogh, M., Kahn, H., Medalie, J. H. (1971). Random repeat 24-hour dietary recalls. *Am. J. Clin. Nutr. 24*: 304.

Beaton, G. H., Milner, J., Corey, P., McGuire, V., Cousins, M., Stewart, E., deRamos, M., Hewitt, D., Grambsch, P. V., Kassim, N., Little, J. A. (1979). Sources of variance in 24-hour dietary recall data: implications for nutrition study design and interpretation. *Am. J. Clin. Nutr. 32*: 2456.

Beaton, G. H., Milner, J., McGuire, V., Feather, T. E., Little, J. A. (1983). Sources of variance in 24-hour dietary recall data: implications for nutrition study design and interpretation. Carbohydrate sources, vitamins, and minerals. *Am. J. Clin. Nutr. 37*: 986.

Block, G. (1982). A review of validations of dietary assessment methods. *Am. J. Epidemiol. 115*: 492.

Block, G., Hartman, A. M., Dresser, C. M., Carroll, M. D., Gannon, J., Gardner, L. (1986). A data-based approach to diet questionnaire design and testing. *Am. J. Epidemiol. 124*: 453.

Blumenthal, S., (1973). Prevention of atherosclerosis. *Am. J. Cardiol. 31*: 591.

Browe, J. H., Gofstein, R. M., Morlley, D. M., McCarthy, M. C. (1966). Diet and heart disease study in the cardiovascular health center. *J. Am. Diet. Assoc. 48*: 95.

Burk, M. C., Pao, E. M. (1976). Mehhodology for Large-scale Surveys of Household and Individual Diets. Home Economics Research Report No. 40. Consumer and Food Economics Institute, Agriculture Research Service, U.S. Department of Agriculture, Washington, D.C. GPO No. 001-000-03620-3.

Burke, B. S., Stuart, H. C. (1938). A method of diet analysis. *J. Pediatr. 12*: 493.

Burke, B. S., Beal, V. A., Kirkwood, S. B., Stuart, H. C. (1943). Nutrition stud-493.

Burke, B. S., Beal, M. A., Kirkwood, S. B., Stuart, H. C. (1943). Nutrition studies during pregnancy. *Am. J. Obstet. Gynecol. 46*: 38.

Byers, T. E., Rosenthal, R. I., Marshall, J. R., Rzepka, T. F., Cummings, K. M., Graham, S. (1983). Dietary history from the distant past: A methodologic study. *Nutr. Cancer 5*: 69.

Byers, T., Marshall, J., Fiedler, R., Zielezny, M., Graham, S. (1985). Assessing nutrient intake with an abbreviated dietary interview. *Am. J. Epidemiol. 122*: 41.

Chalmers, F. W., Clayton, M. M., Gates, L. O., Tucker, R. E., Werts, A. W., Young, C. M., Foster, W. D. (1952). The Dietary Record—How many and which days? *J. Am. Dietetic Assoc. 28*: 711.

Committee on Diet, Nutrition, and Cancer (1982). National Research Council. *Diet, Nutrition, and Cancer.* National Academy Press, Washington, D.C.
Cummings, S., Block, G., McHenry, K., Baron, R. B. (1900). Evaluation of two food frequency methods of measuring dietary calcium intake. *Am. J. Epidemiol. 126*: 796.
Epstein, L. M., Reshef, A., Abramson, J. H., Bialik, O. (1970). Validity of a short dietary questionnaire. *Israel J. Med. Sci. 6*: 589.
Gersovitz, M., Madden, J. P., Smiciklas-Wright, H. (1978). Validity of the 24-hour dietary recall and seven-day record for group comparisons. *J. Am. Diet. Assoc. 73*: 48.
Graham, S., Lilienfeld, A. M., Tidings, J. E. (1967). Diet and purgation factors in the epidemiology of gastric cancer. *Cancer 20*: 2224.
Guthrie, H. A. (1984). Selection and quantification of typical food portions by young adults. *J. Am. Diet. Assoc. 84*: 1140.
Hankin, J. H., Reynolds, W. E., Margen, S. (1967). A short dietary method for epidemiologic studies. II. Variability of measured nutrient intakes. *Am. J. Clin. Nutr. 20*: 935.
Hankin, J. H., Rhoads, G. G., Glober, G. A. (1975). A dietary method for an epidemiological study of gastrointestinal cancer. *Am. J. Clin. Nutr. 28*: 1055.
Harte, R. A., Chow, B. Dietary interrelationships. In *Modern Nutrition in Health and Disease*, third edition, Wohl, M. G., and Goodhart, R. S. (Eds.). Philadelphia, Lea and Febiger, pp. 534-544.
Higginson, J. (1975). Cancer etiology and prevention. In *Persons at High Risk of Cancer*, Fraumeni, J. F. (Ed.). Academic Press, New York.
Hunt, W. C., Leonard, A. G., Garry, P. J., Goodwin, J. S. (1983). Components of variance in dietary data for an elderly population. *Nutr. Res. 3*: 433.
Jain, M., Howe, G. R., Johnson, K. C., Miller, A. B. (1980). Evaluation of a diet history questionnaire for epidemiologic studies. *Am. J. Epidemiol. 111*:212.
Jain, M. G., Harrison, L., Howe, G. R., Miller, A. B. (1982). Evaluation of a self-administered dietary questionnaire for use in a cohort study. *Am. J. Clin. Nutr. 36*: 931.
James, W. P. T., Bingham, S. A., Cole, T. J. (1981). Epidemiological assessment of dietary intake. *Nutr. Cancer 2*: 203.
Jensen, O. M., Wahrendorf, J., Rosenqvist, A., Geser, A. (1984). The reliability of questionnaire-derived historical dietary information and temporal stability of food habits in individuals. *Am. J. Epidemiol. 120*: 281.
Lilienfeld, A. M., Lilienfeld, D. E. (1980). *Foundations of Epidemiology*. Oxford University Press, Inc., New York, p. 14, 291.
Liu, K., Stamler, J., Dyer, A., McKeever, J. , McKeever, P. (1978). Statistical methods to assess and minimize the role of intra-individual variability in obscuring the relationship between dietary lipids and serum cholesterol. *J. Chron. Dis. 31*: 399.
Madden, J. P., Goodman, S. J., Guthrie, H. A. (1976). Validity of the 24-hour recall. Analysis of data obtained from elderly subjects. *J. Am. Diet. Assoc. 68*: 143.

McKeown-Eyssen, G. E., Yeung, K. S., Bright-See, E. Assessment of past diet in epidemiologic studies. *Am. J. Epidemiol. 124*: 94.

Menkes, M. S., Comstock, G. W., Vuilleumier, J. P., Helsing, K. J., Rider, A. A., Brookmeyer, R. (1986). Serum beta-carotene, vitamins A and E, selenium, and the risk of lung cancer. *N. Engl. J. Med. 315*: 1250.

National Center for Health Statistics: Harlan, W. R., Hill, A. L., Schmouder, R. P., et al. (1983). Dietary intake and cardiovascular risk factors, part II. Serum urate, serum cholesterol and correlates: United States, 1971-75. Vital and Health Statistics, Series 11, No. 227. DHHS Pub. No. (PHS) 83-1677. Public Health Service, Washington, U.S. Government Printing Office.

Nichols, A. B., Ravenscroft, C., Lamphiear, D. E., et al. (1976). Independence of serum lipid levels and dietary habits: The Tecumseh Study. *J.A.M.A. 236*: 1948.

Peto, R., Doll, R., Buckley, J. D., Sporn, M. (1981). Can dietary beta-carotene materially reduce human cancer rates? *Nature 290*: 201.

Pietinen, P., Hartman, A. M., Haapa, E., Räsänen, L., Haapakoski, J., Palmgren, J., Albanes, D., Virtamo, J. (1988). Validity and reproducibility of dietary assessment instruments: II. A qualitative food frequency questionnaire. *Am. J. Epidemiol.* (In press).

Pietinen, P., Hartman, A. M., Haapa, E., Räsänen, L., Haapakoski, J., Palmgren, J., Albanes, D., Virtamo, J. Huttunen, J. K. (1988). Validity and reproducibility of dietary assessment instruments: I. A self-administered food use questionnaire with a portion size picture booklet. *Am. J. Epidemiol.* (In press).

Posner, B. M., Borman, C. L., Morgan, J. L., Borden, W. S., Ohls, J. C. (1982). The validity of a telephone-administered 24-hour dietary recall methodology. *Am. J. Clin. Nutr. 36*: 546.

Reed, R. B., Burke, B. S. (1954). Collection and analysis of dietary intake data. *Am. J. Public Health 44*: 1015.

Rohan, T. E., Potter, J. D. (1984). Retrospective assessment of dietary intake. *Am. J. Epidemiol. 120*: 876.

Sempos, C. T., Johnson, N. E., Smith, E. L., Gilligan, C. (1985). Effects of intraindividual and interindividual variation in repeated dietary records. *Am. J. Epidemiol. 121*: 120.

Sobell, J., Block, G., Koslowe, P., et al. (1989). Retrospective assessment of diet 15 years in the past. *Am. J. Epidemiol.* (In press).

Subcommittee on Criteria for Dietary Evaluation, Food and Nutrition Board, National Research Council (1986). *Nutrient Adequacy-Assessment Using Food Consumption Surveys.* National Academy Press, Washington, D.C.

Todd, K. S., Hudes, M., Calloway, D. H. (1983). Food intake measurement: problems and approaches. *Am. J. Clin. Nutr. 37*: 139.

U.S. Department of Agriculture, Consumer Nutrition Center (1984). Nutrient intakes: Individuals in 48 states, year 1977-78. Nationwide Food Consumption Survey 1977-75, NFCS Report I-2. Hyattsville, Md.

Van Horn, L. (1986). Personal communication.

Van Leeuwen, F. E., DeVet, H. C. W., Hayes, R. B., Van Staveren, W. A., West, C. E., Hautvast, J. G. A. J. (1983). An assessment of the relative validity of retrospective interviewing for measuring dietary intake. *Am. J. Epidemiol. 118*: 752.

Van Staveren, W. A., West, C. E., Hoffman, M. D. A. F., Bos, P., Kardinaal, A. F. M., Van Poppel, G.A. F. C., Schipper, H. J. A., Hautvast, J. G. A. J., Hayes, R. B. (1986). Comparison of contemporaneous and retrospective estimates of food consumption made by a dietary history method. *Am. J. Epidemiol. 123*: 884.

Walker, A. M., Blettner, M. (1985). Comparing imperfect measures of exposure. *Am. J. Epidemiol. 121*: 783.

Weisburger, J. H., Marquardt, H., Mower, H. F., Hirota, N., Mori, H., Williams, G. (1980). Inhibition of carcinogenesis: Vitamin C and the prevention of gastric cancer. *Prev. Med. 9*: 352.

Willett, W. C., Polk, B. F., Morris, J. S., Stampfer, M. J., Pressel, S., Rosner, B., Taylor, J. O., Schneider, K., Hames, C. G. (1983). Prediagnostic serum selenium and risk of cancer. *Lancet 2*: 130.

Willett, W. C., Sampson, L., Stampfer, M. J., Rosner, B., Bain, C., Witschi, J., Hennekens, C. W., Speizer, F. E. (1985). Reproducibility and validity of a semiquantitative food frequency questionnaire. *Am. J. Epidemiol. 122*: 51.

Wu, M. L., Whittemore, A. S., Jung, D. L. (1986). Errors in reported dietary intakes. I. Short-term recall. *Am. J. Epidemiol. 124*: 826.

Young, C. M., Hagan, G. C., Tucker, R. E., Foster, W. D. (1952). A comparison of dietary study methods. II. Dietary history vs. seven-day record vs. 24-hour recall. *J. Am. Diet. Assoc. 28*: 218.

7

Methods for Determination of Retinoids, α-Tocopherols, and Carotenoids in Human Serum, Plasma, and Other Tissues

DAVID W. NIERENBERG
Dartmouth Medical School, Hanover, New Hampshire

YEI-MEI PENG AND DAVID S. ALBERTS
The University of Arizona College of Medicine, Tucson, Arizona

INTRODUCTION

The evidence that retinol (R), β-carotene (CAR), α-tocopherol (E), and selenium may prevent certain types of cancer has been presented in other chapters of this book. Some of the evidence obtained thus far in humans involves the determination of serum or plasma concentrations of these analytes in specific populations, and demonstrating that there exists an inverse correlation between the analyte of interest and the risk of developing cancer. In a recent publication concerning the relationship between serum levels of these analytes and the risk of lung cancer (Menkes et al., 1986), reference was made to nine prior studies concerning retinol levels, three prior studies of β-carotene levels, and five prior studies of α-tocopherol levels.

The National Cancer Institute is currently funding over 22 clinical trials (Greenwald et al., 1984) in which these and other substances are being administered to subjects in an effort to demonstrate cancer preventive effects. In many of these studies, serum or plasma levels are being drawn at baseline and again at intervals during the study. Such analysis may well assist in the assessment of patient compliance, the establishment of a preventive range, and the establishment of a toxic range of the substance being tested.

It is possible that actual tissue levels of a potential cancer preventive agent may be more important than serum or plasma levels. For examples, levels of R and CAR in human skin have been studied (Vahlquist et al., 1982) and may be important in determining the preventive effects of those substances. When α-tocopherol acetate has been given in an effort to prevent colonic polyps or colonic cancer, it is possible that colonic or fecal levels of free α-tocopherol may be more important than serum levels in determining the subsequent risk of polyps or cancer (Nierenberg, Lester, and Colacchio, 1987).

For all of the reasons outlined above, there has been increasing interest in measuring concentrations of R, E, and CAR in human serum, plasma, and other tissues. This interest has carried over into the measurement of other retinoids and carotenoids. It is clear that high pressure liquid chromatography (HPLC) has become the method of choice for separating these analytes of interest from other substances, and UV detection has emerged as the most widely used method for quantifying the analytes separated by the chromotographic procedure. HPLC has allowed increased sensitivity and specificity relative to older spectrophotometric or fluorometric techniques. UV detection can be utilized because most of these compounds of interest have relatively high extinction coefficients in the UV range.

Nevertheless, there is still a lack of consensus concerning the "best" method for determining any of these analytes. In fact, it is unlikely that any "best" method will be determined. Each method represents a compromise between technical difficulty, time required, expense of equipment, volume of sample required or available, number of analytes measured simultaneously, sensitivity, specificity, same-day precision, between-day precision, and accuracy. Thus, the method of choice for a general survey of the nutritional status of a large population may not be the method of choice for very accurate determination of only one analyte in several hundred subjects.

Finally, there are many technical questions for which answers are still evolving. Are there differences between analyte levels in serum and plasma? How labile are these samples during sample preparation, chromatography, and freezer storage over long periods of time? Do certain types of solvents actually hasten destruction of the analyte of interest? Is there agreement on the best UV extinction coefficients for these analytes, and can they be obtained commercially in pure form?

While the answers to many of these questions are still evolving, we hope to summarize the current state-of-the-art methods in the analysis of retinol, α-tocopherol, and β-carotene. Some methodologic issues in the analysis of selenium in biological tissues are discussed in Chapters 14 and 19.

DETERMINATION OF RETINOL AND RETINOIDS

Background

The application of HPLC to the separation and detection of retinoids in biological samples has proven to be a powerful and valuable tool for pharmacologic studies. The use of HPLC offers several advantages over conventional methods such as colorimetry, thin layer chromatography (TLC), gas chromatography (GC), or GC/mass spectromotry (GC/MS). Rapid separation, excellent resolution, quantitative recovery, and the capability of separating a wide range of retinoids and metabolites with only minor manipulation of the chromatographic conditions are a few of these advantages.

A number of HPLC methods for the measurement of retinoids have been published (Frolik, Tavela, and Sporn, 1978; McCormick, Napoli, and Deluca, 1978; Besner, LeClaire, and Band, 1980; Chian, 1980; Davis et al., 1982; Driskell et al., 1982; McClean et al., 1982; Yane, Stoltenborg, and Bugge, 1982; Biesalski et al., 1983; Catignani and Bieri, 1983; Vuilleumier et al., 1983; Collins and Chow, 1984; Frolik and Olson, 1984; Furr, Amedee-Manesme, and Olson, 1984; Nierenberg, 1984; Miller and Yang, 1985; Peng, Xu, and Alberts, 1987). In this section, several aspects of these methods for separating and measuring retinoids will be examined. To keep the reference list within bounds, some older citations have been omitted.

Because retinoids are extremely sensitive to photosiomerization and oxidation, we emphasize the importance of the proper collection, handling, and storage of biological samples in avoiding artifacts. Precautions must likewise be taken when working with reference standards.

Sample Clarification

Methods for extraction of retinoids from biological samples can be broadly classified into two categories: saponification and direct extraction.

Saponification

The general procedure for saponification (Frolik and Olson, 1984) consists of adding to the sample (serum, plasma, lyophilized or homogenized tissues) 1-4 parts of an aqueous or ethanolic potassium hydroxide solution. Ascorbic acid (1-10 mg/ml) may be added as an antioxidant and the mixture flushed with nitrogen prior to heating at 60-100°C for 15-45 minutes. After cooling the digest, retinoids are extracted by the addition of 1 part of water and 3-5 parts of hexane or ether. After mixing and centrifugation, the organic layer is removed and saved (the aqueous layer may be re-extracted). The combined organic phase is evaporated under a stream of an inert gas, and the residue is resuspended in an appropriate solvent. A set of standards should be carried through the procedure each time it is performed. In addition, extreme caution must be taken to exclude light and oxygen during the digestion process to prevent degradation of the retinoids.

Saponification is recommended only when the level of total retinol is sought without regard to whether it is present in its free or esterified form. When determining the concentration or retinyl esters or the more polar retinoids, the less destructive direct extraction methods described below are preferred.

Direct Extraction

The variations on procedures described in the literature for the direct extraction of retinoids from biological samples are almost limitless. Although there are many different modifications of the extraction procedure, they are all based upon the precipitation of the protein material present in the biological sample, followed by the removal of the lipid-soluble material by extraction into an organic solvent phase. The choice of solvent depends on the polarity of the retinoids of interest. However, it is important to remember that retinoids vary widely in terms of their solubility and stability in various organic solvents.

A common direct extraction procedure involves taking the plasma sample (0.1-0.5 ml) and mixing it with an equal volume of ethanol (methanol or acetonitrile have also been used) to precipitate plasma proteins. After thorough mixing, 1-4 parts of hexane are added to the mixture. After mixing and centrifugation, the upper organic phase is carefully removed and either injected directly onto the HPLC apparatus or evaporated to dryness under a stream of nitrogen. The dried residue is reconstituted with a small volume of HPLC mobile phase solvent prior to analysis.

The evaporation and resuspension step is required only when the extraction organic solvent is not compatible with the HPLC system or when the sensitivity of the assay must be increased. Other organic solvents used to extract retinoids from plasma samples have included ethyl acetate, ethyl acetate/butanol, butanol/acetonitrile, butanol/methanol, chloroform/methanol, and hexane/methylene chloride/isopropanol mixtures. Using these extraction matrices, recoveries of retinol and its fatty acid esters from plasma have been greater than 90% (McLean et al., 1982; Biesalski et al., 1983; Collins and Chow, 1984; Nierenberg, 1984).

The extraction of polar retinoids such as 13-*cis* retinoic acid (13-CRA) and its major metabolite 4-oxo-13-*cis* retinoic acid (4-oxo-CRA) is pH-dependent. At basic pH, the retinoid remains in the aqueous layer while acidification of the mixture allows the retinoid to be extracted into the organic phase more readily (Chiang, 1980; Frolik and Olson, 1984). For this reason, we have used perchloric acid in one of our laboratories to acidify the serum or plasma sample and to precipitate protein during the extraction procedure (Peng, Xu, and Alberts, 1987). Briefly, the addition of 50 μl of a 5% perchloric acid solution to

500 μl of serum or tissue sample precipitates protein; retinoids are then extracted into an ethyl acetate organic phase, which can be injected directly onto the HPLC apparatus.

Chromatographic Analysis and Detection

Both normal-phase and reverse-phase chromatographic systems have been employed for the separation and measurement of retinoids. Normal-phase HPLC has generally been used to separate closely related retinoids that are not highly polar such as retinol, retinyl esters, and their analogues. With this mode, retinoids that differ only by the isomeric configuration of their side chain can be easily separated even with an isocratic mobile phase. Hexane, with minor amounts of a more polar organic modifier such as isopropanol, has been chosen most frequently for the mobile phase (McCormick, Napoli, and Deluca, 1978; Biesalski et al., 1983; Vuilleumier, Keller, Gysel and Hunziker, 1983).

When dealing with mixtures of retinoids that contain both polar and nonpolar compounds, a solvent gradient is usually needed to obtain adequate separation of the nonpolar retinoids, while still permitting elution of the more polar compounds (Bridges, Fong, and Alvarez, 1980). The use of solvent gradients with normal-phase silica columns, however, may sometimes create irreproducible retention times (Frolik, Tavela, and Sporn, 1978). This apparently is due to the removal of the water from the silica by the more polar solvent, thereby continually changing the adsorption characteristics of the column (Snyder and Kirkland, 1974).

Reverse-phase HPLC is not sensitive to the presence of water either in the sample or in the mobile phase. Thus, mobile phase gradients can be used with reproducible retention times. For this reason, reverse-phase HPLC would be the preferred choice for the separation of a mixture of retinoids with a wide range of polarity and for the analysis of biological extracts which contain high water content.

A wide range of columns is available for reverse-phase separation of retinoids. Methods using a variety of isocratic, discontinuous step, and continuous gradient elution methods have been described. The choice of column and solvent system depends mainly on the particular needs of the investigator. The solvent systems most often used in reverse-phase HPLC are mixtures of either acetonitrile or methanol and water. Addition of a salt (usually 0.1-1.0% ammonium acetate) may be required to reduce tailing of retinoid peaks.

Retinoid detection is usually accomplished by measuring UV absorption between 310 and 365 nm. Fluorescence using a 470 nm emission filter with excitation at 348 nm can also be used to detect retinol and its esters (Collins and Chow, 1984). Retinoic acids, however, show only very weak fluorescence at these wavelengths. Detection with UV absorption also has the advantage of permitting measurement simultaneously at two wavelengths, thus permitting the calculation of an absorption ratio. The plotting of dual wavelength absorbance ratios allows the confirmation of peak identity and the detection of any possible co-eluting peaks with different absorpbance spectra.

Other Issues

Availability of Pure Substances

Reference standards should be of the highest purity available. Concentrations of standard solutions should be determined spectrophotometrically using a gnerally accepted extinction coefficient. The extinction coefficient (E 1%, 1 cm in ethanol) recommended by the National Bureau of Standards is 1850. Several sources of all-*trans* retinol are available; we have found that supplied by Sigma Chemical (St. Louis, MO) to be generally satisfactory.

Recovery

Using the type of extraction procedure described above, we have observed 90–95% recovery of retinoids, including 13-CRA and 4-oxo-CRA, retinol, and its fatty acid ester retinyl palmitate (Davis et al., 1982; Goodman et al., 1982; Peng, Xu, and Alberts, 1987). Similar retinoid recoveries have been observed with other methods as well (Nierenberg, 1984).

Use of Internal Standards

As with the analysis of other endogenous substances in serum or plasma, the addition of an internal standard to the sample prior to the extraction procedure is desirable. Retinol (retinyl) acetate has most often been chosen as an appropriate internal standard because it is not present in human serum or plasma; it has retention properties similar to that of retinol; and it has UV absorption properties similar to that of retinol.

Precision and Accuracy

Various methods reported different values of coefficients of variation. Most of the methods cited above have achieved same-day (within-run) precision near 3% and between-day precision near 5%.

As yet, there has not been a gold stand for determining the absolute accuracy of these different methods. The preliminary data from the quality control program administered by the National Bureau of Standards suggest that most of the methods for the measurement of retinol outlined above produce results that are generally in good agreement with mean values derived from results obtained from all participating laboratories.

Sensitivity and Specificity

The degree of sensitivity of methods for the measurement of retinol in plasma outlined above is usually satisfactory since typical values for retinol in human plasma are 400-800 ng/ml. Methods that are unable to achieve sensitivities of 5-25 ng/ml may have difficulty measuring other retinoids such as retinyl palmitate in normal healthy individuals.

The peaks in the chromatogram identified as retinol or other retinoids have been confirmed as those substances, based upon their retention times, co-elution with known standard compounds, determination of peak absorbance ratios at two wavelengths (Nierenberg and Lester, 1986), and mass spectrometry identification (Davis et al., 1982).

Use of Stabilizers During Clarification

For added protection of retinoids against oxidation during extraction and clarification procedures, a number of soluble antioxidants such as butylated hydroxytoluene (BHT) or ascorbic acid (AA) have been used. The inclusion of these compounds seems to be necessary in some extraction procedures (Driskell, Bashor, and Neese, 1985) but not in others (Nierenberg, 1984; Nierenberg and Lester, 1986).

Sample Stability

Several groups have demonstrated that retinol in serum or plasma is stable whether the blood samples are centrifuged immediately, stored on ice, or kept at room temperature in the dark for up to 24 hours (Mejia and Arrouave, 1983; Nierenberg, 1984; Rider, Foard and Sommer, 1984; Peng, Xu, and Alberts, 1987). While it remains good general laboratory practice to protect blood samples from extreme heat and light prior to serum or plasma separation, and to conduct such separation within a few hours of blood collection, in fact it appears to be acceptable to leave blood samples on ice or at room temperature in the dark for up to 24 hours prior to plasma separation. However, care should be taken to prevent hemolysis. Also, other retinoids or carotenoids may not be as stable as retinol appears to be.

Most workers have recommended that serum or plasma samples be stored in polypropylene freezer tubes (tightly capped) at or below -20°C prior to measurement of retinol. Since photoisomerization of retinol can occur rapidly under normal laboratory lighting conditions, it appears to be important to carry out sample collection, handling, storage, and analysis in the absence of light (Goodman et al., 1982). Most workers have recommended the use of a low intensity yellow or gold incandescent bulb for illumination.

The stability of retinol in plasma or serum samples stored over years has been a potential problem acknowledged in at least two clinical studies (Wald et al.,

1980; Kark et al., 1981). Retinol and retinyl palmitate appear to be stable if stored below -20°C for one year (Peng, Xu, and Alberts, 1987). However, levels of 13-CRA fell by 20-30% in plasma samples stored at -17°C for 5 months (Vane, Stoltenborg, and Bugge, 1982). This loss in 13-CRA was progressive with time, and was due only in part to its conversion to the all-*trans* isomer (TRA).

General recommendations for the storage of serum samples include: (1) documenting the history of freezing/thawing for samples; (2) proper indelible labeling of specimens; (3) including an assayed reference sample of serum or plasma with endogenous retinoids, and (4) storing samples at the lowest temperatures possible.

Choice of Serum or Plasma

Several investigators (McClean et al., 1982; Nierenberg, 1984) have reported that plasma anticoagulated with heparin and serum yield equivalent values of retinol and retinoids. However, it has been documented that recovery of retinol is slightly less when EDTA is used as the anticoagulant and is much less when oxalate or citrate are used as anticoagulants (Nierenberg, 1984; Peng, Xu, and Alberts, 1987).

Retinoid Levels in Tissues

Under usual conditions, > 90% of the total body reserve of vitamin A is stored in the liver in the form of retinyl esters. Therefore, measurement of liver concentrations of retinol and retinyl plamitate gives a good indication of total body vitamin A reserves (Olson, 1982). Similar determinations in skin or cutaneous fat, if obtainable in clinical studies, might also give a good indication of body reserves.

All tissue samples, unless processed and analyzed immediately, should be frozen in liquid nitrogen and stored in foil-wrapped sealed containers at -20°C or lower. Retinoids are very stable in frozen tissues. During 6-month periods of storage, no differences in retinol or retinyl palmitate concentrations were noted in liver (Parkinson and Gal, 1972) or skin (Peng and Alberts, unpublished data). However, one must remain concerned about tissue dehydration during prolonged storage. In addition, any blood, fat, or other adhering material should be carefully removed from the frozen samples before an aliquot is taken for analysis.

All tissues must be homogenized and/or lyophilized prior to the extraction of retinoids. For homogenization, we have adopted the procedure of Kalin (Kalin, Starling, and Hill, 1981) with slight modification (Peng et al., 1986). Briefly, tissue samples are suspended in an aqueous solution containing EDTA and ascorbic acid (0.5-0.1 mg/ml of each). Tissue suspensions are homogenized on ice in a polytron tissue homogenizer. The ratio of tissue (g wet weight) to EDTA-

Table 1 Concentration of Retinol and Retinyl Palmitate in Skin and Subcutaneous Fat Biopsies from Normal, Healthy Females with No Vitamin A Supplementation Prior to Facial (Cosmetic) Surgery

Subject (no.)	Age (years)	Retinol (ng/g)				Retinyl palmitate (ng/g)			
		Epi	Derm	Whole skin	Subcut. fat	Epi	Derm	Whole skin	Subcut. fat
1	60	73	70	38	357	16	16	16	446
2	60	260	87	94	1136	74	32	0	1761
3	60	108	126	131	177	16	16	16	96
4	57	111	150	125	408	45	64	40	307
5	61	93	29	95	1352	0	0	0	1388
6	63	84	165	100	498	68	200	58	437
7	64	133	214	158	361	31	0	0	153
8	53	90	117	165	590	32	78	48	680
9	64	86	67	165	999	16	65	16	146
10	62	29	35	48	380	0	0	0	160
Mean				112	626			19	557

Epi = epidermis; Derm = dermis; Whole skin = epidermis + dermis unseparated; Subcut. fat = Subcutaneous fat.

ascorbate solution (ml) were 1:10 for liver, and 1:2 for skin, fat, or other tissues. The resulting homogenate can be used directly for the extraction of retinoids, or can be lyophilized to remove tissue water and extracted later.

While several studies describe epidermal levels of retinol in patients with various dermatologic disorders (Rollman and Vahlquist, 1983; Rollman and Vahlquist, 1986), little data exist concerning the concentrations of retinol and retinyl palmitate in skin and subcutaneous fat of normal subjects. One of our laboratories (Peng and Alberts, unpublished data) has determined retinol and retinyl palmitate concentrations in skin and subcutaneous fat biopsies from healthy females ages 53-64 who were undergoing facial cosmetic surgery; none of these normal subjects had been taking vitamin A supplements prior to skin removal.

In Table 1 are shown the retinol and retinyl palmitate concentrations in various tissues in this study. Note that retinol concentrations in whole skin were almost tenfold greater than those of retinyl palmitate. In contrast the levels of the two vitamin A compounds were similar, though much higher, in subcutaneous fat. Retinol and retinyl palmitate concentrations average 112 and 19 ng/g whole skin and 626 and 557 ng/g subcutaneous fat, respectively. These data can serve as baseline values of retinoid concentrations in normal integument. It will be interesting to compare such values with retinoid levels achieved in the skin from patients entered into various skin cancer prevention trials using supplemental vitamin A compounds.

DETERMINATION OF α-TOCOPHEROL

Background

α-Tocopherol (E) is the most abundant of the tocopherol isomers present in human serum and plasma (Mandel and Cohn, 1985). Most recent developments in its analysis have exploited the excellent ability to separate E from other serum components using HPLC, and tocopherol's combination of high serum levels and adequate UV absorption near 292 nm. In addition, since E and R have similar retention times on reverse-phase columns and similar absorption maxima (292 nm and 325 nm, respectively), many methods for determining E levels also measure R levels at the same time.

Almost all methods reported thus far dealing with human material concentrate on measuring E (and R) levels in serum or plasma, probably because of the difficulty in obtaining solid tissues. Methods have been reported for determining E levels in platelets (Lehmann and Martin, 1982) and red blood cells (Lehmann and Martin, 1983). One paper reported a method for determining tocopherol and tocopherol acetate (EA) in human feces (Nierenberg, Lester, and Colacchio, 1986). Several recent papers discussed techniques for extracting E from solid animal tissues, using either solvent extraction of dried or frozen tissue (Zaspel and Csallany, 1983; Mostow et al., 1985; Omaye and Chow, 1986), or direct alkaline digestion of the tissue (Buttriss and Diplock, 1984; Desai, 1984). Since most recent work using human samples has focused on determining E levels in serum or plasma, we will pay particular attention to that application.

Sample Clarification

Since 1979, most investigators have used a standard technique for clarifying serum or plasma prior to the actual chromatographic step (Bieri, Tolliver, and Catignani, 1979; De Leenheer et al., 1979; Cantignani and Bieri, 1983; Driskell et al., 1982; Howell and Wang, 1982; Chow and Omaye, 1983). This method involves the addition of 100 μl ethanol to 100 μl of the sample of serum or plasma to precipitate protein. The analytes of interest are then extracted into 100–1000 μl of hexane (or heptane); most of the hexane layer is recovered after separation by centrifugation, and evaporated to dryness using either a centrifugal vacuum evaporator system, or a water bath under a stream of nitrogen. The resultant residue is then resuspended in an organic solvent, usually ethanol or the mobile phase for the HPLC system.

Two methods of sample clarification have been reported which were designed to avoid the solvent evaporation step. Lehmann and Martin (1982) mixed 50 μl of plasma with 3 ml of methanol. After centrifugation, a small amount of the resultant supernatant could be injected directly onto the HPLC system. Nierenberg and Lester (1985) took 500 μl of serum or plasma and precipitated protein with 100 μl of acetonitrile. After vortexing, 250 μl of an organic matrix consisting of butanol-ethyl acetate (1:1) was added, with further vortexing. Finally, 150 μl of an aqueous solution of dipotassium monohydrogen phosphate (1.2 g/ml) was added, the solution mixed and centrifuged once again, and a portion of the upper organic matrix was then injected directly onto the HPLC apparatus.

The methods which avoid the solvent evaporation step are simpler and quicker, important considerations for laboratories which process thousands of samples each year. The hexane evaporation methods have been in use longer—for more than seven years. Informal comparisons of one method with another suggest that results obtained are quite similar. The quality control program administered by the National Bureau of Standards will ultimately be able to determine which laboratories (and which methods) produce the greatest accuracy and precision.

Chromatographic Analysis and Detection

Essentially every method utilizes a C18 reverse-phase column for the solid phase of the HPLC system. More recent methods employed 5 μm spherical packing material, while older methods used 10 μm particulate material. Several different column sources (e.g., Waters, Altex/Beckman, DuPont, Whatman, and others) were used, and results appeared comparable though not identical. Almost all investigators employed a binary isocratic mobile phase consisting of methanol (87–99%) and water (13–1%). By adjusting the composition of the mobile phase and the flow rate, most chromatographic runs were completed within 12 minutes.

Detection was usually accomplished by measuring UV absorption of the column eluate. Variable wavelength detectors were usually set to 292 nm, the $lambda_{max}$ for E; fixed-wavelength detectors were usually equipped with a 280 nm filter. A few authors (Lehmann and Martin, 1982; Lehmann and Martin, 1983; Zaspel and Csallany, 1983) utilized fluorometric detection. However, while UV detection may be confounded by non-E UV-absorbing material with similar column retention times, this was not a problem in most of these studies.

Other Issues

Availability of Pure Substances

Most investigators were able to purchase relatively pure R and E from commercial suppliers. Crystalline all-*trans* retinol was often purchased from Sigma (St. Louis, MO), while d-α-tocopherol was often purchased from Kodak (Rochester, NY). Extinction coefficients for these substances in ethanol (E1%, 1 cm) were generally accepted to be 1850 at 325 nm for R and 75.8 at 292 nm for E. These values have been tentatively accepted for use by the National Bureau of Standards as well.

Recovery

Recoveries of E (and R) achieved by these methods were determined in different ways. Most authors reported greater than 80% recovery of both analytes when exogenous material was added to plasma or serum samples. Nierenberg and Lester (1985) found that recoveries of exogenous R, E, and EA from serum samples (compared to recoveries from aqueous samples) averaged 102.6%, 96.9%, and 96.5%, respectively.

Use of Internal Standards

Most investigators added one or more compounds as internal standards at the beginning of the sample clarification process. Tocol was used by several investigators, but was not widely used because it was not commercially available. Retinol acetate (RA) was available in pure form (Sigma, St. Louis, MO). However, Nierenberg and Lester (1985) noted that the RA peak was coincident with another peak on the chromatogram which probably represented a phthalate plasticizer present in blood samples (Pollack et al., 1984). Therefore, they used d-α-tocopherol acetate (Sigma) as an internal standard, since there were no such interfering peaks. While some groups used both RA and EA as internal standards, there seemed to be no advantage in using two standards.

Precision and Accuracy

Various methods reported different values of coefficients of variation for same-day and between-day precision. Most groups were able to achieve same-day precision near 3% and between-day precision near 5%.

As yet, there has not been a gold standard for determining the absolute accuracy of these different methods for measuring E (and R) in serum and plasma. At this point, we have only preliminary data from the quality control program administered by the National Bureau of Standards. This preliminary evidence suggests that most of the methods outlined above produce results which are generally in good agreement with mean values derived from results obtained from all participating laboratories.

Sensitivity and Specificity

Most of the methods described were able to achieve sensitivities of at least 0.6 μg/ml for E, and 60 ng/ml for R. This degree of sensitivity is usually satisfactory since typical values for E and R in human plasma are 5–25 μg/ml and 400–800 ng/ml, respectively. The peaks in the chromatogram identified as R and E have been confirmed as those substances, based upon their retention times, co-elution with known standard compounds, and determination of peak absorbance ratios at two wavelengths (Nierenberg and Lester, 1986). While diode-array UV detectors are considerably more expensive than conventional detectors, their use has confirmed that when vegetable oils are analyzed, peaks identified as E have UV spectra identical to known E standard solutions (Mulholland, 1986).

Use of Stabilizers During Clarification

Several groups which used hexane evaporation methods found it advantageous to add antioxidants to the serum sample prior to clarification. Substances evaluated included pyrogallol (Bieri, Tolliver, and Catignani, 1979; Chow and Omaye, 1983; Lehman and Martin, 1983), butylated hydroxytoluene (BHT), or ascorbic acid (Chow and Omaye, 1983). When an evaporation step was not used, the addition of BHT did not improve recovery of R, E, or EA (Nierenberg and Lester, 1985). Also, perhaps the most widely used hexane evaporation method (Catignani and Bieri, 1983) did not mention use of an antioxidant. However, recent work (Driskell, Bashor and Neese,1985) has demonstrated that in serum samples stored at -20°C for 2-6 years, E and R began to degrade during the extraction step immediately after ethanol was added to the serum, possibly due to free radical oxidation of the polyunsaturated vitamins. Such losses of E and R could be prevented by adding ascorbic acid (0.1% w/v) to the ethanol before it was used in the preassay extraction. Catignani (1986) has recently agreed with that recommendation.

Sample Stability

Nierenberg and Lester (1985) found that both R and E were stable in fresh heparinized plasma stored under subdued incandescent light for up to 48 hours at room temperature. Both E and R in serum were stable during 17 repeated freezing (-20°C) and thawing cycles over 5 weeks (Catignani, 1986). Catignani also reported that both R and E were stable in serum for 4 weeks at 4°C, and for up to one year at -20°C or colder. There is at least indirect data that R and E are stable in human serum for as long as 10 years, although β-carotene levels may not be as stable (Menkes et al., 1986).

Choice of Serum or Plasma

Nierenberg and Lester (1985) specifically evaluated the recoveries of R and E from two types of serum collection tubes, and tubes anticoagulated with heparin, EDTA, citrate, or oxalate. Results were very similar to those previously reported for R alone (Nierenberg, 1984). Concentrations of R and E were approximately 2% higher in serum than in heparinized plasma. When any other type of anticoagulant was used, concentrations of R and E fell by 9-24%, compared to concentrations in serum.

DETERMINATION OF β-CAROTENE AND CAROTENOIDS

Background

The determination of the content of β-carotene and other carotenoids in vegetables led to some of the original applications of HPLC to carotenoid analysis (Zakaria et al., 1979). While the application of these techniques to plant analysis is discussed in a prior chapter, it is important to stress that recent work in this area (Krinsky and Welankiwar, 1984; Bushway, 1986) continues to be useful and relevant to the determination of these compounds in human samples as well. Several methods have been reported (Lee et al., 1975; Vahlquist et al., 1982; Chew, Holpuch, and O'Fallon, 1984; Stich, Hornby, and Dunn, 1986) which describe techniques for measuring carotenoids in solid human or animal tissues. However, since most recent work has focused on the determination of CAR in human serum or plasma, we will concentrate our discussion on that area as well.

Traditionally, the serological tests of serum "carotene" or "β-carotene" have really been assays of total carotenoids. Serum is deproteinized by the addition of ethanol, and the complex mixture of carotenoids is extracted into hexane. The UV absorbance of the hexane supernatant is measured spectrophotometrically (usually at 450-452 nm), and total carotenoid concentration determined using a representative extinction coefficient for β-carotene.

In a description of one of the earlier HPLC methods (Driskell, Bashor and Neese, 1983), it was demonstrated that β-carotene levels measured by HPLC were always less than total carotenoid levels determined by spectrophotometry and made up a variable fraction of the total carotenoids present. Katrangi and coworkers (1984) confirmed that β-carotene results obtained by HPLC averaged 23.4% ± 7.9% as great as the results obtained by a colorimetric assay. In addition, they found that only 20.5% (on average) of the total area of all peaks of the chromatogram was due to β-carotene. Another group (Bieri, Brown, and Smith, 1985) determined that when six discrete carotenoid peaks were measured, more than 90% of the total extractable carotenoids in plasma were accounted for. Again, β-carotene composed a small and variable fraction or total carotenoid content.

Most currently used methods separate and quantitate β-carotene concentration in human serum or plasma samples. Some methods also quantitate lycopene and α-carotene (Broich, Gerber, and Erdman, 1983; Katrangi, Kaplan, and Stein, 1984; Tangney, 1984), and a few methods allow the measurement of up to six or more discrete carotenoid peaks (Nelis and De Leenheer, 1983; Bieri, Brown, and Smith, 1985). While attention in epidemiological and chemoprevention studies has focused on β-carotene, it appears that greater efforts will be made to examine possible relationships between other carotenoids and cancer risk.

Sample Clarification

Recently reported methods for determinating β-carotene levels in serum or plasma have clarified the sample in one of two ways. Most methods reported (Drisekll, Bashor, and Neese, 1983; Nelis and De Leenheer, 1983; Katrangi, Kaplan, and Stein, 1984; Tangney, 1984; Bieri, Brown, and Smith, 1985) use an extraction protocol similar to that described in the sections dealing with retinol and α-tocopherol. Serum or plasma (usually 100 μl) is deproteinated with an equal volume of ethanol. β-Carotene and other carotenoids are then extracted into hexane (120–600 μl). After the hexane is evaporated, the residue is resuspended in ethanol or mobile phase, and injected onto the HPLC system.

Four methods have been described which were designed to avoid the solvent evaporation system. The method reported by Meyer's group (Meyer et al., 1985) is identical to that described above, but the hexane can be injected directly onto their HPLC system since hexane is used in the mobile phase of a normal-phase chromatography system. The method described by Peng's group (Peng et al., 1983) and subsequently modified (Nierenberg, 1985) deproteinizes 500 μl of serum or plasma with the addition of 100 μl of a 5% solution of perchloric acid. Carotenoids are then extracted into 500 μl of an organic phase of preserved tetrahydrofuran:ethyl acetate (1:1) and injected directly onto the HPLC system. The method reported by Broich's group (Broich, Gerber, and Erdman, 1983) deproteinates 100 μl of serum by the addition of 100 μl methanol, and extracts carotenoids into 200 μl of chloroform, which is then injected directly onto the HPLC system.

As was true with R and E assays, the CAR assays involving extraction into hexane with evaporation and resuspension are apparently used by many groups. The methods which avoid solvent evaporation are used by fewer groups, but have the advantage of simpler and quicker sample preparation, especially important in laboratories handling several thousand assays each year. Again, there is as yet no gold standard for the measurement of β-carotene. However, preliminary and informal results of comparison with several different laboratories using different assay methods suggest that β-carotene determinations of aliquots of identical serum or plasma samples yield comparable results.

Chromatographic Analysis and Detection

With two exceptions (Toth, 1984; Meyer et al., 1985), all methods described utilized reverse-phase HPLC. It appears that reverse-phase systems usually offer better separation of individual carotenoids, longer column life, and the use of mobile phases which are safer and easier to handle in the laboratory (benzene, hexane, or methylethylketone were required in the mobile phases of the two methods cited above).

The methods reported which employed reverse-phase chromatography generally used columns 25 cm in length, filled with 5 μm diameter packing material of the C18 variety. A variety of column manufacturers was cited in the various papers. The isocratic mobile phase was usually acetonitrile, modified with other solvents. Binary systems included acetonitrile modified with dichloromethane (Driskell, Bashor, and Neese, 1983) or chloroform (Katrangi, Kaplan, and Stein, 1984). Ternary systems included acetonitrile and methanol modified with dichloromethane (Nelis and De Leenheer, 1983; Bieri, Brown, and Smith, 1985), chloroform (Broich, Gerber, and Erdman, 1983), or tetrahydrofuran (Tangney, 1984). The few quaternary systems reported included acetonitrile modified with methanol, tetrahydrofuran, and an aqueous solution of ammonium acetate (Peng et al., 1983; Nierenberg, 1985).

Detection was accomplished by monitoring UV absorption at either 436 nm (with fixed wavelength detectors) or 450–452 nm (for variable wavelength detectors). Results were recorded as peak heights using strip-chart recorders, or peak areas using recorder-integrators. There is data suggesting that peak area measurements are preferable to peak height measurements (Nierenberg and Lester, 1986; Pauls et al., 1986).

Other Tissues

While the techniques for measuring β-carotene in serum and plasma appear straightforward, in fact many methodological problems have been reported or suspected with most if not all of the assays. Most laboratories measuring R, E, and β-carotene experience more difficulties with the carotene assay than with the other two. Some of the methodological issues are mentioned below.

Availability of Pure Substances

Reasonably pure all-*trans* β-carotene (greater than 99% UV absorption present under one peak upon HPLC analysis) may be purchased from Sigma Chemical (Type IV), although some groups have recommended purification of the β-carotene prior to use. The β-carotene may be easily dissolved in benzene or toluene, and further diluted into hexane or ethanol. Such solutions can be easily filtered to remove insoluble particulate matter and are stable with or without the presence of BHT (Nierenberg, 1985). Chloroform solutions of β-carotene are not stable and are not recommended (personal communication, Robert Schaffer Ph D, National Bureau of Standards). While many different values for the extinction coefficient of β-carotene have been reported, the National Bureau of Standards is currently suggesting extinction coefficients (E 1%, 1 cm) of 2592 at 450 nm in hexane, and 2560 at 452 nm in ethanol.

Recovery

Absolute recoveries of β-carotene during extraction procedures are difficult to measure. Recoveries of β-carotene added to serum or plasma are usually greater than 90%, and re-extraction of serum or plasma has usually yielded less than 3% more β-carotene. Exogenous β-carotene added to serum or plasma does not adsorb to the walls of polypropylene tubes, and recoveries do not decrease with increasing incubation time (Nierenberg and Lester, 1986).

Use of Internal Standards

Use of internal standards is helpful in assays which do not involve a solvent evaporation step, although external standards can also be used. In one such assay, torulene was used for quality control purposes (Nierenberg and Lester, 1986). In assays which involve a solvent evaporation step, the use of an internal standard is more important. Compounds which have been recommended include dimethyl β-carotene (Driskell, Bashor, and Neese, 1983), echininone (Nelis and De Leenheer, 1983; Bieri, Brown, and Smith, 1985), retinyl acetate (Broich, Gerber, and Erdman, 1983), β-apo-8-carotenoic ethyl ester (Tangney, 1984), and decapreno β-carotene (Khachik and Beecher, 1985). Of the above alternatives, only retinyl acetate is commercially available, but it must be monitored at a different wavelength. It has been difficult to demonstrate similar recoveries of exogenous in-

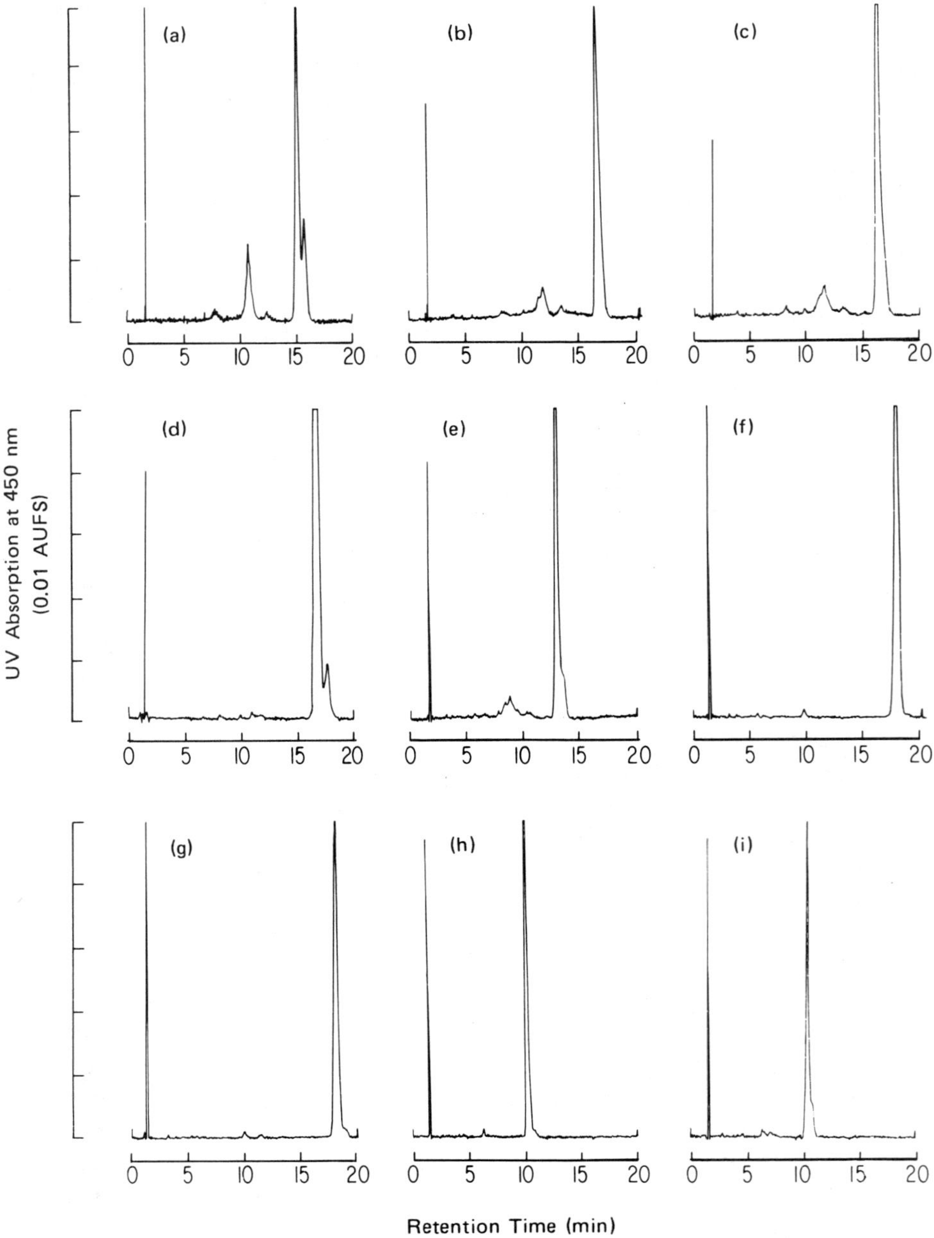

UV Absorption at 450 nm
(0.01 AUFS)
(a)
(b)
(c)
(d)
(e)
(f)
(g)
(h)
(i)
0 5 10 15 20
Retention Time (min)

Fig. 1

ternal standard and endogenous carotenoids. While use of an internal standard is theoretically beneficial, many groups continue to use external standards for quantitating peak areas.

Precision and Accuracy

Almost all of the methods cited above have achieved same-day (within-run) precision near 3%, and between-day precision near 5%. Such precision is adequate for the types of studies being carried out by most groups.

As yet there is no gold standard method for measuring β-carotene. The National Bureau of Standards has been very helpful in this area, sponsoring yearly quality control workshops. It appears that many of the methods cited above can be used to determine CAR concentrations in aliquots of plasma with comparable results (within 10% of the group mean value), although some laboratories report results which differ by as much as 200%.

Sensitivity and Specificity

The above methods achieve detection limits of 5-25 ng/ml in serum or plasma. Since healthy individuals have CAR levels in the range of 50–750 ng/ml (mean values about 225 ng/ml), such sensitivity is usually adequate. Methods which are unable to determine β-carotene levels in the 5–50 ng/ml range may have difficulty with the occasional individual who has a very low CAR level.

These assays also appear to be quite specific for β-carotene. Most of the assays are able to resolve α-carotene from β-carotene, although they have more difficulty distinguishing all-*trans* β-carotene from its 15–15′ *cis* isomer. The identity of the peaks identified as β-carotene have been confirmed by determining absorption spectra (Katrangi, Kaplan, and Stein, 1984) or multichannel

---

Fig. 1 Representative chromatograms of β-carotene in ethanol injected onto an HPLC column under different solvent conditions, illustrating on-column isomerization and degradation. The different mobile phases consisted of: (a) Acetonitrole:unpreserved dichloromethane:methanol (70:20:10), flow rate 1.7 ml/min. (b) Acetonitrile:preserved dichloromethane: methanol (70:20:10) at 1.7 ml/min. (c) Acetonitrile:preserved dichloromethane:methanol (70:20:10) plus BHT 125 μg/ml at 1.7 ml/min. (d) Acetonitrile:preserved dichloromethane: methanol (70:20:10) plus hydroquinone 100 μg/ml at 1.7 ml/min. (e) Acetonitrile:preserved THF:methanol (70:20:10) at 1.7 ml/min. (f) Acetonitrile:preserved THF:methanol:1% ammonium acetate aqueous solution (65:25:6:4) at 2.0 ml/min. (g)Acetonitrile:preserved THF:methanol:water (65:25:6:4) at 2.0 ml/min. (h) Acetonitrile:preserved THF:methanol:1% ammonium acetate aqueous solution (65:25:9:1) at 1.7 ml/min. (i) Acetonitrile:preserved THF:methanol:water (65:25:9:1) at 1.7 ml/min.

Table 2 Stability of β-Carotene in Heparinized Plasma from One Subject Over 22 Months when Stored at Three Different Temperatures

Months	-7°C	-35°C	-75°C
0	168 (7)	168 (7)	168 (7)
1	150 (4)	172 (7)	172 (16)
6	155 (2)	175 (7)	174 (0)
12	85 (1)	154 (1)	156 (5)
22	63 (1)	176 (4)	170 (6)

Each aliquot was measured in duplicate. Results are expressed as mean (SD) in ng/ml.

wavelength analysis with determination of absorption ratios (Nierenberg and Lester, 1986).

Use of Stabilizers During Clarification

Because of the vulnerability of β-carotene to isomerization and oxidation, one group has recommended that an antioxidant such as BHT be used to preserve CAR during storage in organic solvents, during the sample clarification process, and during the HPLC assay itself (Nierenberg, 1985; Nierenberg and Lester, 1986). Another group (Driskell, Bashor, and Neese, 1983; Driskell, Bashor, and Neese, 1985) used ascorbic acid during the clarification step, and Tangney (1984) used both BHT and ascorbic acid.

β-Carotene may be destroyed during the sample clarification process or during the actual chromatography itself. This on-column destruction has been caused by either impure solvents such as THF (containing peroxides) or chloroform (containing HCl), or column frits made of stainless steel rather than a more inert alloy such as Hastelloy (Nierenberg and Lester, 1986). Other solvents can lead to formation of oxidation products or isomers of CAR as well. In one study, it was demonstrated that formation of *cis* isomers of retinol and retinyl palmitate by photoisomerization was increased in chlorinated solvents (methylene chloride and chloroform), THF, acetone, or methanol relative to hexane, and was increased after exposure to white light relative to exposure to gold light (Landers and Olson, 1986). Furthermore, addition of free-radical scavengers (α-tocopherol, hydroquinone, or BHT) did not protect retinyl plamitate in chloroform exposed to white light. The National Bureau of Standards (Robert Schaffer, personal communication) also recommends against dissolving β-carotene in chloroform, because of the rapid loss of the compound itself.

Finally, one of us (DWN) has attempted to repeat the analysis of multiple carotenoids previously reported (Nelis and De Leenheer, 1983; Bieri, Brown, and Smith, 1985). When their mobile phase of acetonitrile:methylene chloride: methanol (70:20:10) was used, many extra peaks appeared on the chromatogram, compared to the peaks seen when our standard mobile phase of acetonitrile:THF (with BHT):methanol:aqueous solution of ammonium acetate (65:25:6:4) was used (see Fig. 1). On-column photoisomerization or oxidation was minimally improved by using methylene chloride preserved with cyclohexane, BHT, hydroquinone, or THF. In fact, some of the degradation products formed on-column eluted from the precolumn, and occluded the inlet frit of the analytical column on several occasions. This on-column degradation could be eliminated by including water or an aqueous solution of ammonium acetate in the mobile phase (1% or 4%, as shown in Fig. 1). In addition, a mobile phase consisting of methanol:acetonitrile:THF (50:45:5) did not cause such on-column degradation of CAR. Thus, choice of mobile phase remains critical in the analysis of β-carotene and other carotenoids as well.

Sample Stability

Total carotenoids were stable in plasma for brief periods at room temperature, but were not stable at -20°C for 6 months or 10 years (Mathews-Roth and Stampfer, 1984). This instability has been noted by others as well (Willett et al., 1984). A more recent study using a specific HPLC assay demonstrated that serum stored for 10 years at -74°C exhibited substantial loss of β-carotene content (Menkes et al., 1986).

One of us has previously demonstrated that CAR is stable in serum or plasma for up to 4 hours at room temperature with exposure to light (Nierenberg, 1985). The same study demonstrated that CAR was stable in plasma during 7 freeze-thaw cycles, consistent with work previously reported (Broich, Gerber, and Erdman, 1983). We also found that β-carotene was stable in plasma for 6 months when stored at -35°C or -75°C, although storage at -7°C led to some loss (Nierenberg, 1985). We have now extended those observations to 22 months, and found that CAR in the plasma from one subject was stable at -75°C and -35°C, but not at -7°C (see Table 2).

Choice of Serum or Plasma

β-Carotene concentrations are 2-4% higher in serum than in heparinized plasma (Nierenberg, 1985; Nierenberg and Lester, 1986). Use of other anticoagulants such as EDTA, oxalate, or citrate is not recommended, since CAR concentrations are 8-21% less than those seen in either serum or heparinized plasma (Nierenberg, 1985).

SIMULTANEOUS DETERMINATION OF ANALYTES

Background

Because of the interest in measuring R, E, and CAR levels in serum from study participants, several methods have been reported which allow the simultaneous determination of all three analytes using one assay. While different structurally, all three analytes share properties of high lipid solubility and relatively high UV absorbance. However, they differ in their relative affinity for normal and reverse-phase HPLC solid phases, and in their wavelengths of peak UV absorption.

Recognizing these differences, one group extracted all three analytes from the same sample of serum into hexane, then split the extract and injected aliquots onto three separate HPLC systems, each optimized for the detection of one of the analytes (Vuilleumier et al., 1983). In essence, this method represented three separate assays which shared a common clarification step. Three other methods have been recently published which allow all three analytes to be measured using the same HPLC assay.

Sample Clarification

Three recently reported methods (Miller, Lorr, and Yang, 1984; Miller and Yang, 1985; Milne and Botnen, 1986) all deproteinized plasma with an equal volume of ethanol, and extracted compounds of interest into a volume of hexane or petroleum ether approximately twice the plasma volume. After evaporation under nitrogen, the residue was resuspended in a small volume of ethanol, and injected directly onto the HPLC apparatus.

Chromatographic Analysis and Detection

The earliest of these assays (Miller, Lorr and Yang, 1984) was able to separate R, E, lycopene, α-carotene, and β-carotene with the use of a step gradient. Elution was begun with 100% methanol at 1 ml/min for 8 minutes, and then switched to methanol:acetonitrile:chloroform (47:42:11) at 2 ml per minute. The column was a 5 mm × 10 cm RP-18 column with 10 μm packing. For the first 8 minutes (until E had eluted), UV absorption was measured at 280 nm, while for the last 7 minutes, absorption was measured at 436 nm. The method did not achieve baseline separation of α- and β-carotene, each run required 16 minutes, and 15 minutes equilibration time was required between runs.

The same group published an improved method the next year (Miller and Yang, 1985). Using an 8 mm × 10 cm RP-18 column with 5 μm packing, they were able to separate the same analytes as in their previous method. However, the mobile phase was now an isocratic one consisting of acetonitrile:methanol: chloroform (60:25:15) at 1.5 ml/min, and each run required 16 minutes. Detection was again accomplished with monitoring at 280 nm for the first portion of the run, and 436 nm for the second portion of the run (alternatively, a programmable photodiode-array HPLC detector was used).

In the final method (Milne and Botnen, 1986), the authors were able to simultaneously determine R, E, lycopene, α-carotene, and β-carotene using a 4.6 mm X 6 cm RP-18 column with 3 μm packing. The mobile phase was 100% methanol, flowing at 0.9 ml/min; each run required 9 minutes. Detection was accomplished at 305 nm, 290 nm, and 460 nm sequentially by a programmable diode array detector.

Other Issues

Recovery of exogenous analytes added to plasma were in general close to 100% except for R, which in one method achieved only 91% recovery (Miller, Lorr, and Yang, 1984). Internal standards used included retinyl acetate (Miller, Lorr, and Yang, 1984; Milne and Botnen, 1986), and α-tocopherol acetate (Miller and Yang, 1985). Same-day and between-day precision was 3–10% for all three methods. As with other methods discussed, absolute accuracy could not be determined.

The sensitivity of these assays was not specifically recorded. The specificity of two of the assays (Miller and Yang, 1985; Milne and Botnen, 1986) was confirmed by spectral analysis of peaks of interest. The need for preservatives during the extraction procedures was investigated by Milne and Botnen (1986), who found that the addition of BHT did not alter levels of E or the carotenoids, but did interfere with the determination of R. The same group also recommended the use of either serum or heparinized plasma, since the use of other anticoagulants variably reduced the recovery of several of the analytes.

CONCLUSION

Determination of serum or plasma levels of retinol, other retinoids, α-tocopherol, β-carotene, and other carotenoids is now essential for the conduct of both observational (e.g., case control) and experimental (e.g., intervention) studies. While determination of these analytes in tissue samples may ultimately offer more information, at present the best described methods utilize either serum or heparinized plasma.

The method of choice in each case is usually a sample clarification step followed by high pressure liquid chromatography with UV detection. Simplicity is maximized by the use of an isocratic mobile phase, reverse-phase chromatography, and UV detection at only one wavelength. However, gradient mobile phases have been used by some groups; normal-phase chromatography has occasionally been employed; and simultaneous monitoring at multiple wavelengths offers several advantages.

The methods described offer generally acceptable analyte recovery, precision, sensitivity, and specificity. Questions remain concerning absolute accuracy of each method; an ongoing quality control program with voluntary participation by research laboratories, sponsored by the National Bureau of Standards and the National Cancer Institute, continues to be a great help in this regard.

Remaining problems include finding acceptable commercial sources of pure analytes and internal standards. Destruction of compounds of interest by isomerization or oxidation, either during the clarification step or during the actual chromatography, is a constant concern. In some situations, the use of antioxidants or other stabilizers has proven to be useful. Most groups have found comparable results when serum or heparinized plasma has been used; the use of plasma anticoagulated with citrate, oxalate, or EDTA is not recommended.

The future will probably see further refinement in the measurement of these analytes in several ways. First, the methods which have been reported which can simultaneously measure R, E, and CAR will need to be confirmed in the hands of other investigators. Second, there will probably be further efforts made to analyze not only β-carotene, but other carotenoids as well. Third, relationships between tissue levels and drug effects may prove to be equally or more interesting than the relationship between serum levels and drug effects.

Which of the many methods described above should be used in a particular laboratory? It is still too early to know which methods will ultimately prove to have the greatest accuracy. However, preliminary data suggest that many of these methods are able to achieve comparable levels of accuracy. When methods yield grossly disparate results, it may well be the result of quality control problems within the laboratory rather than the method per se. Methods have been reported for the determination of R, R and E, or CAR which avoid a solvent evaporation step. On the other hand, all methods which determine multiple analytes seem to require a solvent evaporation step. Ultimately, each researcher will have to balance the cost (in time, equipment, and personnel) of each method with the number and accuracy of assays which must be conducted.

REFERENCES

Besner, J. G., LeClaire, R., Band, P. R. (1980). High performance liquid chromatography of 13-cis-retinoic acid and of endogenous retinol in human plasma. *J. Chromatog. 183*:346.

Bieri, J. G., Brown, E. D., Smith, J. C. (1985). Determination of individual carotenoids in human plasma by high performance liquid chromatography. *J. Liq. Chromatog. 8*:473.

Bieri, J. G., Tolliver, T. J., Catignani, G. L. (1979). Simultaneous determination of alpha-tocopherol and retinol in plasma or red cells by high pressure liquid chromatography. *Am. J. Clin. Nutr. 32*:2143.

Biesalski, H. K., Ehrenthat, W., Gross, M., Hafner, G., Harth, O. (1983). Rapid determination of retinol (vitamin A) in serum by high pressure liquid chromatography (HPLC). *Vit. Nutr. Res. 53*:130.

Bridges, C. D. B., Fong, S. L., Alvarez, R. A. (1980). Separation by programmed-gradient high pressure liquid chromatography of vitamin A isomers, their esters, aldehydes, oximes and vitamin A2: presence of retinyl ester in dark-adapted goldfish pigment epithelium. *Vision Res. 20*:355.

Broich, C. R., Gerber, L.E., Erdman, J. W. (1983). Determination of lycopene, alpha- and beta-carotene and retinyl esters in human serum by reversed-phase high performance liquid chromatography. *Lipids 18*:253.

Bushway, R. J. (1986). Determination of alpha- and beta-carotene in some raw fruits and vegetables by high-performance liquid chromatography. *J. Agric. Food Chem. 34*:409.

Buttriss, J. L. and Diplock, A. T. (1984). High-performance liquid chromatography methods for vitamin E in tissues. *Methods Enzymol. 105*:131.

Catignani, G. L. (1986). An HPLC method for the simultaneous determination of retinol and alpha-tocopherol in plasma or serum. *Methods Enzymology 123*:215.

Catignani, G. L. and Bieri, J. G. (1983). Simultaneous determination of retinol and alpha-tocopherol in serum of plasma by liquid chromatography. *Clin. Chem. 29*:708.

Chew, B. P., Holpuch, D. M., O'Fallon, J. V. (1984). Vitamin A and beta-carotene in bovine and procine plasma, liver, corpora lutes, and follicular fluid. *J. Dairy Sci. 67*:131.

Chiang, T. C. (1980). Gas chromatographic-mass spectrometric assay for low levels of retinoic acid in human blood. *J. Chromatog. 182*:335.

Chow, F. I. and Omaye, S. T. (1983). Use of antioxidants in the analysis of vitamins A and E in mammalian plasma by high performance liquid chromatography. *Lipids 18*:837.

Collins, C. A. and Chow, C. K. (1984). Determination of vitamin A and vitamin A acetate by high-performance liquid chromatography with fluorescence detection. *J. Chromatog. 317*:349.

Davis, T. P., Peng, Y. M., Goodman, G. E., Alberts, D. S. (1982). HPLC, MS, and pharmacokinetics of melphalan, bisantrene, and 13-cis-retinoic acid. *J. Chromatog. Sci. 20*:511.

De Leenheer, A. P., De Bevere, V. O. R. C., De Ruyter, M. G. M., Claeys, A. E. (1979). Simultaneous determination of retinol and alpha-tocopherol in human serum by high-performance liquid chromatography. *J. Chromatog. Biomed. Appl. 162*:408.

Desai, I. D. (1984). Vitamin E analysis methods for animal tissues. *Methods Enzymol. 105*:138.

Driskell, W. J., Bashor, M. M., Neese, J. W. (1983). Beta-carotene determined in serum by liquid chromatography with an internal standard. *Clin. Chem. 29*:1042.

Driskell, W. J., Bashor, M. M., Neese, J. W. (1985). Loss of vitamin A in long-term stored, frozen sera. *Clin. Chim. Acta 147*:25.

Driskell, W. J., Neese, J. W., Bryant, C. C., Bashor, M. M. (1982). Measurement of vitamin A and vitamin E in human serum by high-performance liquid chromatography. *J. Chromatog. Biomed. Appl. 231*:439.

Frolik, C. A., Olson, J. A. (1984). Extraction, separation, and chemical analysis of retinoids. In *The Retinoids*, Sporn, M. B., Roberts, A. B., Goodman, D. S. (Eds.). Academic Press, New York, pp. 181–233.

Frolik, C. A. Tavela, T. E., Sporn, M. B. (1978). Separation of the natural retinoids by high-pressure liquid chromatography. *J. Lipid Res. 19*:32.

Furr, H. C., Amedee-Manesme, O., Olson, J. A. (1984). Gradient reversed-phase high-performance liquid chromatographic separation of naturally occurring retinoids. *J. Chromatog. 309*:299.

Goodman, G. E., Einspahr, J. G., Alberts, D. S., Davis, T. P., Leigh, S. A., Chen, H. S., Meyskens, F. L. (1982). Pharmacokinetics of 13-cis-retinoic acid in patients with advance cancer. *Cancer Res. 42*:2078.

Greenwald, P., DeWys, W. D., Carrese, L. M., Murray, B. (1984). Chemoprevention programs of the National Cancer Institute. In *Vitamins, Nutrition, and Cancer*, K. N. Prasad (Ed.). A. G. Karper, Basel, Switzerland, p. 282.

Howell, S. K., Wang, Y. M. (1982). Quantitation of physiological alpha-tocopherol, metabolites, and related compounds by reversed-phase high-performance liquid chromatography. *J. Chromatog. Biomed. Appl. 227*:174.

Kalin, J. R., Starling, M. E., Hill, D. L. (1981). Disposition of all-trans-retinoic acid in mice following oral doses. *Drug, Metabolism and Disposition 9*:196.

Kark, J. D., Smith, A. H., Switzer, B. R., Hames, C. G. (1981). Serum vitamin A (retinol) and cancer incidence in Evans County, Georgia, *J. Nat. Cancer Inst. 66*:7.

Khachik, F. Beecher, G. R. (1985). Decapreno-beta-carotene as an internal standard for the quantification of the hydrocarbon carotenoids by high-performance liquid chromatography. *J. Chromatog. 346*:237.

Katrangi, N., Kaplan, L. A., Stein, E. A. (1984). Separation and quantitation of serum beta-carotene and other carotenoids by high performance liquid chromatography. *J. Lipid Res. 25*:400.

Krinsky, N. I. and Welankiwar, S. (1984). Assay of carotenoids. *Methods Enzymol. 105*:155.

Landers, G. M., Olson, J. A. (1986). Absence of isomerization of retinyl palmitate, retinol, and retinal in chlorinated and nonchlorinated solvents under gold light. *J. Assoc. Off. Anal. Chem. 69*:50.

Lee, R., Mathews-Roth, M. M., Pathak, M. A., Parrish, J. A. (1975). The detection of carotenoid pigments in human skin. *J. Invest. Dermatol. 64*:175.

Lehmann, J., Martin, H. L. (1982). Improved direct determination of alpha- and gamma-tocopherols in plasma and platelets by liquid chromatography, with fluorescence detection. *Clin. Chem. 28*:1784.

Lehmann, J., Martin, H. L. (1983). Liquid-chromatographic determination of alpha- and gamma-tocopherols in erythrocytes, with fluorescence detection. *Clin. Chem. 29*:1840.

Mandel, H. G., Cohn, V. H. (1985). Fat-soluble vitamins. In *The Pharmacological Basis of Therapeutics*, 7th Ed., A. G. Gilman, L. S. Goodman, T. W. Rall, F. Murad (Eds.). Macmillan, New York, pp. 1573–1591.

Mathews-Roth, M. M., Stampfer, M. J. (1984). Some factors affecting determination of carotenoids in serum. *Clin. Chem. 30*:459.

McClean, S. W., Ruddel, M. E., Gross, E. G., Degiovanna, J. J., Peck, G. L. (1982). Liquid-chromatographic assay for retinol (vitamin A) and retinol analogs in therapeutic trials. *Clin. Chem. 28*:693.

McCormick, A. M., Napoli, J. L., Deluca, H. F. (1978). High-pressure liquid chromatographic resolution of vitamin A compounds. *Anal. Biochem. 86*:25.

Mejia, L. A., Arroyave, G. (1983). Determination of vitamin A in blood. Some practical considerations on the time of collection of the specimens and the stability of the vitamin. *Amer. J. Clin. Nutr. 37*:147.

Menkes, M. S., Comstock, G. W., Vuilleumier, J. P., Helsing, K. J., Rider, A. A., Brookmeyer, R. (1986). Serum beta-carotene, vitamins A and E, and the risk of lung cancer. *New Engl. J. Med. 315*:1250.

Meyer, J. C., Grundmann, H. P., Seeger, B., Schnyder, U. W. (1985). Plasma concentrations of beta-carotene and canthaxanthin during and after stopping intake of a combined preparation. *Dermatologica 171*:76.

Miller, K. W., Lorr, N. A., Yang, C. S. (1984). Simultaneous determination of plasma retinol, alpha-tocopherol, lycopene, alpha-carotene, and beta-carotene by high-performance liquid chromatography. *Anal. Biochem. 138*:340.

Miller, K. W., Yang, C. S. (1985). An isocratic high-performance liquid chromatography method for the simultaneous analysis of plasma retinol, alpha-tocopherol, and various carotenoids. *Anal. Biochem. 145*:21.

Milne, D. B., Botnen, J. (1986). Retinol, alpha-tocopherol, lycopene, and alpha- and beta-carotene simultaneously determined in plasma by isocratic liquid chromatography. *Clin. Chem. 32*:874.

Mostow, N. D., O'Neill, R., Noon, D. L., Bacon, B. R. (1985). Determination of alpha-tocopherol in rat liver by high-performance liquid chromatography utilizing ultraviolet detection. *J. Chromatog. Biomed. Appl. 344*:137.

Mulholland, M. (1986). Linking low dispersion liquid chromatography with diode-array detection for the sensitive and selective determination of vitamins A, D, and E. *Analyst. 111*:601.

Nelis, H. J. C. F. De Leenheer, A. P. (1983). Isocratic nonaqueous reversed-phase liquid chromatography of carotenoids. *Analy. Chem. 55*:270.

Nierenberg, D. W. (1985). Serum and plasma beta-carotene levels measured with an improved method of high-performance liquid chromatography. *J. Chromatog. Biomed. Appl. 339*:273.

Nierenberg, D. W., Lester, D. C. (1985). Determination of vitamins A and E in serum and plasma using a simplified clarification method and high-performance liquid chromatography. *J. Chromatog. Biomed. Appl. 345*:275.

Nierenberg, D. W., Lester, D. C. (1986). High-pressure liquid chromatographic assays for retinol and beta-carotene: potential problems and solutions. *J. Nutr. Growth Cancer 3*:215.

Nierenberg, D. W., Lester, D. C., Colacchio, T. A. (1987). Determination of tocopherol and tocopherol acetate concentrations in human feces using high-performance liquid chromatography. *J. Chromatog. Biomed. Appl. 413*:79.

Olson, J. A. (1982). New approaches to methods for the assessment of nutritional status of the individuals. *Am. J. Clin. Nutr. 35*:1166.

Omaye, S. T., Chow, F. I. (1986). Distribution of vitamins A and E in blood and liver of rats depleted of vitamin A or vitamin E. *Lipids 21*:465.

Parkinson, C. E., Gal, I. (1972). Factors affecting the laboratory management of human serum and liver vitamin A analysis. *Clin. Chim. Acta 40*:83.

Pauls, R. E., McCoy, R. W., Ziegel, E. R., Wolf, T., Fritz, G. T., Marmion, D. M. (1986). Results of a cooperative study comparing the precision of peak height and area measurements in liquid chromatography. Part II. *J. Chromatog. Sci. 24*:273.

Peng, Y. M., Beaudry, J., Alberts, D. S., Davis, T. P. (1983). High-performance liquid chromatography of the provitamin A beta-carotene in plasma. *J. Chromatog. Biomed. Appl. 273*:410.

Peng, Y. M., Alberts, D. S., Xu, M. J., Watson, R. R., Gensler, H. L., Bowden, G. T. (1986). Effects of high dietary retinyl palmitate and selenium on tissue distribution of retinoids in mice exposed to tumor initiation and promotion. *J. Nutr. Growth Cancer 3*:33.

Peng, Y. M., Xu, M. J., Alberts, D. S. (1987). Analysis and stability of retinol in plasma. *J. Nat. Cancer Inst. 78(1)*:95.

Pollack, G. M., Slaughter, R. L., Buchanan, J. F., Shen, D. D. (1984). High-performance liquid chromatographic procedure for the determinatin of di-(2-ethylhexyl)phthalate in human blood specimens. *J. Chromatog. Biomed. Appl. 311*:101.

Rider, A. A., Foard, M. A., Sommer, A. (1984). Studies on the stability of vitamin A and related compounds in blood subjected to adverse conditions prior to serum separation. *Nutr. Rep. Internat. 29*:1307.

Rollman, O. and Vahlquist, A. (1985). Vitamin A in skin and serum-studies of acne vulgaris, a topic dermatitis ichthyosis vulgaris and lichen planus. *Br. J. Derm. 113*:405–413.

Rollman, O. and Vahlquist, A. (1986). Oral isotretinoin (13-cis-retinoic acid) therapy in severe acne. Drug and vitamin A concentrations in serum and skin. *Soc. Invest. Derm*: 384–389.

Snyder, L. R., Kirkland, J. J. (Eds.). (1974). *Introduction to Modern Liquid Chromatography*, Wiley, New York, pp. 239.

Stich, H. F., Hornby, P., Dunn, B. P. (1986). Beta-carotene levels in exfoliated mucosa cells of population groups at low and elevated risk for oral cancer. *Int. J. Cancer 37*:389.

Tangney, C. C. (1984). Individual carotenoid determination in human plasma by high-performance liquid chromatography. *J. Liq. Chromatog. 7*:2611.

Toth, G. (1984). Determination of vitamin A, vitamin A precursors and cytoprotective carotenoids in animal and human blood. *Acta Physiologica Hungarica 64*:319.

Vahlquist, A., Lee, J. B., Michaelsson, G., Rollman, O. (1982). Vitamin A in human skin: II. Concentrations of carotene, retinol and dehydroretinol in various components of normal skin. *J. Invest. Dermatol. 79*:94.

Vane, F. M., Soltenborg, J. K., Bugge, C. J. L. (1982). Determination of 13-cis-retinoic acid and its major metabolites, 4-oxo-13-cis-retinoic acid, in human blood by reverse-phase high performance liquid chromatography. *J. Chromatog. 227*:471.

Vuilleumier, J. P., Keller, H. E., Gysel, D., Hunziker, F. (1983). Clinical chemical methods for the routine assessment of the vitamin status in human populations. *Internat. J. Vit. Nutr. Res. 53*:263.

Wald, N., Idle, M., Boreham, J., Bailey, A. (1980). Low serum vitamin A and subsequent risk of cancer. *Lancet ii*:813.

Willett, W. C., Polk, B. F., Underwood, B. A., Hames, C. G. (1984). Hypertension detection and follow-up program study of serum retinol, retinol-binding protein, total carotenoids, and cancer risk: a summary. *J. Nat. Can. Inst. 73*: 1459.

Zakaria, M., Simpson, K., Brown, P. R., Krstulovic, A. (1979). Reversed-phase high-performance liquid chromatographic analysis for the determination of provitamin A carotenes in tomatoes. *J. Chromatog. 176*:109.

Zaspel, B. J., Csallany, A. S. (1983). Determination of alpha-tocopherol in tissues and plasma by high-performance liquid chromatography. *Anal. Biochem. 130*:146.

Part Three

EVIDENCE ON MICRONUTRIENTS AND CANCER PREVENTION

8
Foods, Micronutrients, and Reduction of Human Cancer

MARC S. MICOZZI
Armed Forces Institute of Pathology, Washington, D.C.

INTRODUCTION

Current clinical investigations focusing on micronutrients, such as β-carotene (provitamin A), as potential cancer-preventive agents, have been stimulated by laboratory findings on the possible cancer-modifying activity of these natural substances (Micozzi et al., 1985). For example, interest in the role of vitamin A as a possible cancer-preventive agent can be tracked back to the experiments of Wolbach and Howe in the 1920s (Wolbach and Howe, 1925). They observed that dietary deprivation of vitamin A, with consequent vitamin A deficiency, in rats caused squamous metaplasia (a "preneoplastic" lesion) in tracheobronchial mucosa and in other epithelial tissues. The growth activity of metaplastic epithelium was not diminished and, in fact, appeared to be enhanced, suggesting the acquisition of neoplastic properties in vitamin A-deprived tissues. Since the mid-1960s, numerous animal experiments have demonstrated that pharmacologic doses of retinol (vitamin A) and retinoids (synthetic derivatives and analogs of retinol) can prevent the development of tracheobronchial squamous metaplasia and squamous cell tumors (Saffiotti et al., 1967; Thompson et al., 1981). Vitamin A is currently suggested to participate in the regulation of cell differentiation (Sporn et al., 1976, 1981).

For a considerable period of time, epidemiologic studies on diet and cancer also investigated relations between the consumption of certain foods, or classes of foods (e.g., green vegetables) with the risk of various epithelial cancers in humans. All of the foods identified in theses studies were presumed to have high "vitamin A activity." Distinctions have been drawn in some investigations between intake of foods from animal sources, high in preformed vitamin A (retinol), versus intake of foods from plant sources, high in provitamin A activity (β-carotene). These investigations moved Peto et al. (1981) to pose the rhetorical question, "Can dietary β-carotene materially reduce human cancer rates?" More specifically, if individuals consuming diets high in β-carotene-containing foods have a lower risk of cancer, can β-carotene reduce the risk of cancer? Apparent assumptions about the carotenoid content of various foods found to be protective against cancer has led to further investigations, specifically focused upon β-carotene, made possible by new analytical techniques and by the commercial availability of this carotenoid.

In fact, the carotenoids consist of a broad class of chemical compounds with differing chemical structures and activities. Different foods contain differing amounts of various carotenoids, and carotenoid-containing foods may or may not contain significant levels of β-carotene. The construction of accurate dietary intake indices for "vitamin A," total carotenoids, and β-carotene had been difficult where the specific carotenoid content of various foods had not been established. Recent analysis of the carotenoid composition of various foods, using new methodologies and analytic techniques, (Khachik and Beecher, 1986) has helped to refine aspects of our understanding of nutrient composition relative to cancer risk in humans.

Analyzing *foods* found to be protective against cancer (rather than presumed dietary intake of a specific component) from review of the epidemiologic studies on diet and cancer is a new approach. People consume (and epidemiologic studies inquire about) foods, culturally processed in various ways, as opposed to nutrients. The cultural processing of foods includes agriculture (domestication, cultivation, harvesting, storage), cuisine (preparation, seasoning, cooking, and eating) and various intermediate processes. These cultural processes may introduce variability into nutrient composition and nutrient bioavailability of foods, in addition to the variability introduced by environmental factors (climate, soil, rainfall, seasonality, etc.).

Using new technologies, the levels of individual carotenoids and other micronutrients in these foods can be determined, and the results can be used to observe the patterns of occurrence of carotenoids and other micronutrients in those foods that may be protective against cancer. It is also important to recognize that carotenoid-containing foods may also contain a variety of noncarotenoid constituents such as fiber, indoles, flavones, isothiocyanates, phenols, and other chemicals which have also been suggested to be protective against cancer (Wattenberg, 1978).

The purpose of this chapter is to present analyses of the carotenoid content of foods widely found to be protective against various cancers in human epidemiologic studies and preliminary findings on the effects of food preparation on the carotenoid content of these foods as consumed by humans; and to move beyond the question of Peto et al. (1981) to evaluate the possibilities of various chemical constituents of foods being responsible for observed reduction in human cancer rates.

DIET AND CANCER PREVENTION

While U.S. rates of coronary heart disease and stroke decrease, rates for incidence of all cancer sites combined have increased significantly over the past decade to nearly one million new cases per year (Sondik et al., 1985). The majority of cancer deaths in the United States are due to a few relatively common cancer sites: prostate and bladder in men, breast in women, and colorectal and lung in both. Certain risk factors for cancer which have large relative risks in defined subsets of the population, such as smoking, genetic susceptibility, and various occupational exposures to industrial carcinogens, have been previously recognized in human epidemiologic studies. More recently, epidemiologic studies have begun to investigate other potential risk factors, such as human diet and nutrition, which have small relative risks, but may be common to the entire population, thus carrying significant population-attributable risks. Within the United States, it has been estimated that 80–90% of cancer incidence may be attributable to environmental risk factors, and that dietary and nutritional factors may account for approximately 35% of attributable risk for cancer (Doll and Peto, 1981). However, dietary factors are regarded as "effect modifiers," which modify cancer risk after exposure to primary carcinogens. Tests of diet-cancer hypotheses will lack specificity unless exposures to cancer risk factors can be controlled in the analysis. Hypotheses that lack specificity often lead to associations with small relative risks.

Therefore, epidemiologic analyses must be performed on a relatively large population sample in order to adequately test specific hypotheses and to control for exposures to primary carcinogens. Wynder and Bross (1961) pointed out in their early investigations into diet and cancer that studies on small samples would not be expected to show an effect of diet. Constraints on the degree of dietary variability observable within a population may also impose the requirement for large sample size to adequately detect small but significant differences in diet and cancer in the population. As emphasized by Wynder and Bross (1961) and Haenszel et al. (1972), studies of homogeneous populations within a single area cannot be expected to specifically identify the effects of risk factors to which there is relatively uniform exposure or a limited range of exposures. As heterogeneity in dietary habits and large sample sizes are sought and the detection limits of nutritional assessment technologies improve, smaller significant risks in the population may be observed for testing diet-cancer hypotheses.

These considerations have generally directed investigations of diet and cancer to the more common cancer sites listed above. A comprehensive review of epidemiologic studies on diet and these cancer sites performed over the last half-century has revealed a fairly consistent pattern of foods that appear to be protective against cancers in human populations. Studies on serum nutrient levels and cancer have also helped to answer questions about which nutrients may be protective against cancer.

SERUM STUDIES OF RETINOL, CAROTENOIDS, AND β-CAROTENE

Recent evidence has indicated that dietary intake of carotenoids in well-nourished populations is highly correlated to serum carotenoid levels (Brown et al., 1986). Studies on serum levels of micronutrients have shed light on the possible protective effects of retinol, total carotenoids, and β-carotene against cancer. Early serum studies were conducted in the context of case-control studies and focused upon vitamin A or retinol. Wahi et al. (1962) found significantly decreased retinol levels in 60 patients with oral cancer in India, where retinol deficiency is common. However, in a case-control study of 35 patients with cancer of various sites (gastrointestinal, lung, breast, and brain) in the United Kingdom, Basu et al. (1974) found low retinol and β-carotene levels only in patients with gastrointestinal cancer. They explained this observation on the basis of the effects of low dietary fat intake and low serum cholesterol levels on fat-soluble vitamin absorption and transport in these patients. In their subsequent study of 28 lung cancer patients (Basu et al., 1976), squamous cell carcinoma (but not other lung cancer histologic types) was associated with decreased retinol levels. Subsequently, this same group of investigators attributed low levels of serum vitamin A in 26 newly diagnosed lung cancer patients to decreased serum levels of zinc which may reduce mobilization of hepatic vitamin A stores (Atukorala et al., 1979).

A study by Cohen et al. (1977) on 67 newly diagnosed, unoperable lung cancer patients in the United States suggested that vitamin A deficiency was not implicated in pulmonary carcinogenesis. At the same time, a larger study on over 200 patients with oral cancer in Pakistan (Ibrahim et al., 1977) showed significantly decreased levels of both retinol and β-carotene in cancer patients. Any true protective effect of retinol may be most apparent in malnourished populations (Peto et al., 1981), due to the wide range of serum retinol levels in populations with vitamin A deficiency, as in India (Wahi et al., 1962) and Pakistan (Ibrahim et al., 1977). However, serum β-carotene levels can be assessed independently from retinol levels only in relatively well-nourished populations where variations in β-carotene intake have little effect on serum retinol levels.

Table 1 Summary of Studies on Serum Retinol, Carotenoids, and β-Carotene and Cancer Risk

Study	Cohort size	Year(s) collected	Storage temp. (°C)	Interval collection to: Cancer Dx (yrs)	Interval collection to: Analysis	Cancer protective effects: Retinol	Cancer protective effects: Tot. carot.	Cancer protective effects: β-Carotene
Wald et al. 1980, London	16,000	1975–78	–40	1–4	1–4[a]	+($p < 0.005$)	–	–
Kark et al. 1981, Georgia	3,102	1960–62	–18	12–14	14–16	+	–	–
Willett et al., 1984, HDFP	4,480	1973–74	–70	5	9	0	0	–
Stahelin et al., 1984, Basel	4,224	1971–74	?	3.7–4.9 (ave.)	0	0	–	+[b]($p < 0.05$)
Wald et al., 1984, Guernsey	5,004	1968–75	–20	7–14	8–15	0	–	ns
Menkes et al., 1984, Maryland	?	1974	?	8	9[a]	0	–	0
Nomura et al., 1985, Hawaii	6,860	1971–74	–75	10 (ave.)	10	0	–	+[b]($p < 0.005$)
Salonen et al., 1985, Finland	12,155	1977	–20	3	7	0	–	–
Menkes et al., 1986, Maryland	25,802	1974	–73	8	9[a]	+	–	+[b]
Friedman et al., 1986	143,574	1964–71	–23	2	12–19	0	–	–

+, protective effects; 0, not protective; –, not analyzed; ns, not significant.

[a]Did not indicate the year in which samples were analyzed; assumed analyzed one year prior to publication of results.

[b]Lung and gastric cancers only.

The interpretation of these case control studies generally is limited by a number of analytical considerations, including small sample size, the effects of disease on micronutrient status, and other limitations (Micozzi et al., 1985). The inconsistent results and analytic limitations of these case-control studies permit no firm conclusions to be drawn regarding serum retinol, β-carotene, and cancer risk.

A more specific approach to assessment of serum micronutrient levels and cancer risk was taken in 10 prospective studies on relatively well-nourished population samples, summarized in Table 1. All these studies reported serum retinol levels. In addition, five measured β-carotene, and one measured total carotenoid levels as well. These studies involved collection of serum samples on large cohorts of individuals who were free of disease. The samples were then stored frozen at varying temperatures (-18°C to -73°C) for variable lengths of time (one to fourteen years) and subsequently thawed to perform serum analyses for individuals who had developed cancer, as well as for a sample of controls who remained free of disease.

These studies considered cancers of one or more common sites, primarily lung, gastrointestinal, and breast cancer. Aside from the two initial studies, (Wald et al., 1980; Kark et al., 1981), increased serum retinol levels have consistently not been found to protect against the development of cancer in prospective studies. In addition, the initial study of Kark et al. (1981) used sera that had been repeatedly frozen and thawed and stored over a very long period of time at relatively high temperature. When this study was repeated by Peleg et al. (1984), serum retinol was not found to be protective against cancer.

The results on serum β-carotene levels are inconsistent. One study (Willett et al., 1984a,b) that measured total carotenoids found no protective effect. It was suggested by Peto et al. (1981) that total carotenoid levels might not be a good index of β-carotene levels specifically, and thus would not discriminate as to those at risk or not at risk by this hypothesis. We and others have subsequently found that serum total carotenoid levels provide a reliable index of serum β-carotene levels (Russell-Briefel et al., 1985; Brown et al., 1986). However, they are not highly correlated to levels of some other carotenoids (that may be important for cancer risk) and are independent of serum retinol in well-nourished populations (Brown et al., 1986). Therefore, the negative study on total carotenoids was probably testing the effects of β-carotene, but not all other carotenoids. These studies on serum retinol, total carotenoids, and β-carotene suggest that serum vitamin A activity, as reflected in retinol and β-carotene levels, may not be protective against cancer or may be protective only in specific populations under specific circumstances.

FOODS PROTECTIVE AGAINST CANCER

Initial studies of diet and cancer took a broad approach to dietary assessment. During 1929-1932, Stocks and Karn (Stocks, 1957) conducted a case-control study of diet and all-sites cancer on nearly 500 cancer patients in Wales, and found beetroot, bread (whole meal), cabbage, carrots, cauliflower, milk (unboiled), onions, turnips, and watercress to be protective against cancer. No associations were found for 25 other food items. They suggested that milk and green vegetables might contain a cancer protective factor. Stock's remarks provide a useful framework for considering subsequent studies:

> Little work has been done to investigate the possible influences of dietary habits on the incidence of cancer. . . . Such studies are difficult because it is to be expected that carcinogenic action of a particular kind of food would become manifest only after a long period of years, and histories have to be retrospective and must be compared with those of control groups of people without cancer. In such enquiries, error can arise from poor memory and careless answers, changes in habits which may be connected with onset of a pre-cancerous condition, manners of putting the question by the interviewer and differences of interpretation of it by patient and informant. . . .

Stocks (1957) repeated the study 15 years later in over 1750 cancer cases, ages 45-74, in North Wales and Liverpool. There were inverse associations between daily consumption of green vegetables and lung, gastric, intestinal, and other cancers. Eating green vegetables less often than once a day had a relative risk of 1.6 ($p < 0.01$) for gastrointestinal cancer. However, these negative associations were found only in areas where average green vegetable intake was highest. These results and the results of subsequent studies are summarized in Table 2.

In 1961, Wynder and Bross suggested that increased dietary intake of green and yellow vegetables was protective against cancer of the esophagus. Subsequently, Graham et al. (1972) made use of a heterogeneous dietary intake index, including a spectrum of red, orange, yellow, and green vegetables in studies of gastric cancer. Among these vegetables they found consumption of raw carrots, cole slaw, red cabbage, lettuce, and tomatoes to be protective.

Studies of diet and gastric cancer in Japan and Japanese Hawaiians (Haenszel et al., 1972) found increased fruit and vegetable intake to be protective. Low risks were suggested for several Western-style vegetables, many of which were eaten raw. The associations for uncooked vegetables appeared to be independent of those found for pickled vegetables, and persisted after controlling other aspects of vegetable consumption. Nine food items were analyzed in detail, and tomatoes and corn exhibited inverse dose-response relationships with gastric

Table 2 Summary of Epidemiologic Studies on Dietary Intake and Cancer Rates

Study	n	Cancer site	Protective foods or diet	Relative risk low/high consumption[a]
Stocks, 1957, Wales, U.K.	1750	all sites, GI	milk, green vegetables	1.6 ($p < 0.01$)
Wynder & Bross, 1961, United States	150	esophagus	green and yellow vegetables	1.4 ($p < 0.05$)
Graham et al., 1972, Buffalo, N.Y.	228	stomach	raw vegetables[b]	1.7 ($p < 0.01$)
Haenszel et al., 1972, Japanese-Americans, Hawaii	220	stomach	beans, green	1.6
			celery	1.7
			corn	1.4
			cucumber	1.5
			eggplant	1.4
			lettuce	1.6
			milk	1.4
			onion, green	1.5
			potatoes, sweet	1.7
			tomatoes	2.0
Modan et al., 1974, Israel	166	stomach	eggplant	
			squash	
Modan et al., 1975, Israel	198	colon	fruits and vegetables	
Bjelke, 1975[c],	53	lung	"vitamin A" index (carrots, eggs, milk) green vegetables	3.2 ($p < 0.01$)

Phillips, 1975[d], 7th Day Adventists, U.S.A.	41	colon (all sites)	green leafy vegetables	2.0 ($p < 0.05$)
			milk	3.3 ($p < 0.05$)
Haenszel et al., 1976, Japan	783	stomach	fruits and vegetables	1.3 ($p < 0.05$)
			lettuce	1.7 ($p < 0.05$)
			celery	3.3 ($p < 0.01$)
			Japanese pear	1.5 ($p < 0.06$)
			plum	1.2 ($p < 0.05$)
			pineapple	1.4 ($p < 0.01$)
Cohen et al., 1977, Washington, D.C.	67	lung	"vitamin A index" (milk, eggs)	1.0
Mac Lennan et al., 1977, Singapore Chinese	233	lung	eggplant	1.0
			kale	1.3
			mustard greens	2.3
			long beans	1.9
			vegetables index (all four above)	2.2
Tuyns et al., 1978, Brittany, France	200	esophagus	β-carotene retinol	1.0
Graham et al., 1978, Buffalo, New York	470	colon	raw vegetables[b]	1.7 ($p < 0.01$)
	512	rectum	broccoli, Brussels sprouts, cabbage, coleslaw, and sauerkraut	3.0 ($p < 0.01$)
Cook-Mozaffari et al., 1979, Iran	344	esophagus, all sites	fresh fruits and vegetables[e]	
			cucumbers	2.0 ($p < 0.001$)
			lemons, dried	2.0 ($p < 0.001$)
			oranges	2.2 ($p < 0.001$)
			tomatoes	1.6 ($p < 0.001$)
			vegetables, green, raw	1.8 ($p < 0.001$)

Table 2 (continued)

Study	n	Cancer site	Protective foods or diet		Relative risk low/high consumption
Mettlin et al., 1979, Buffalo, New York	292	lung	"vitamin A' index"[f] (green and yellow vegetables)		1.4 nonsmokers 4.0 smokers
			carrots		0.9 nonsmokers 2.0 smokers
			milk		1.5 nonsmokers
Hirayama, 1979,[i] Japan	807	lung stomach prostate	yellow/green vegetables		1.4 ($p < 0.01$)
Mettlin and Graham, 1979, Buffalo, N.Y.	569	bladder	carrots		3.2 ($p < 0.05$)
			cruciferous vegs.[g]		1.4 ($p < 0.01$)
			milk		2.1 ($p < 0.01$)
			"vitamin A index"		3.0 ($p < 0.01$)
Graham et al., 1981, Buffalo, N.Y.	374	larynx	green/yellow vegs.		2.1 ($p < 0.01$)
Mettlin et al., 1981, Buffalo, N.Y.	147	esophagus	fruits, vegetables		1.3 ($p < 0.05$)
Shekelle et al., 1981,[j] Chicago, Ill.	33	lung	"β-carotene" index[h]		1.3 ($p < 0.01$)
				hospital controls	community controls
Schuman et al., 1982, Minneapolis, Minn.	358	prostate	beans, green	1.0	1.3
			cabbage	1.2	1.4

			carrots	1.0	2.2 ($p < 0.05$)
			cauliflower	1.1	1.2
			peas	1.2	1.5
			rutabaga and kohlrabi	1.5	1.0
			tomatoes	1.1	1.4
Graham et al., 1982, Buffalo, N.Y.	2024	breast	"vitamin A index"		1.3 ($p < 0.05$)
			cruciferous vegetables		1.0 ($p < 0.05$)
Kvale et al., 1983	168	lung	"vitamin A index"[k]		1.6 ($p < 0.05$)
Graham et al., 1983, Buffalo, N.Y.	260	prostate	"vitamin A index"		ns (< 70 yrs)
			cruciferous vegetables		ns
Byers et al., 1984	427	lung	"vitamin A index"		
Winn et al., 1984, North Carolina	277	oral and pharyngeal	fruits and vegetables		2.0 ($p < 0.01$)
			fresh fruit		1.7 ($p < 0.01$)
			green leafy vegetables		1.4 ($p = 0.06$)
			other vegetables		1.4 ($p = 0.08$)
				total	smokers
Ziegler et al., 1984, New Jersey	763	lung	dairy products	1.3	0.9
			vegetables and fruit	1.3	1.8
			fruit (only)	–	1.2
			vegetables (only)	1.4	1.7
			dk green vegs.	1.5	1.8
			dk yellow/orange vegs.	1.5	2.2
			dk gr/yel/orange vegs.	–	3.1
Stehr et al., 1985, Pittsburgh, Pa.	111	stomach	"vitamin A"		1.7 ($p < 0.05$)

Table 2 (continued)

Study	*n*	Cancer site	Protective foods or diet		Relative risk low/high consumption
Colditz et al., 1985 Massachusetts	1271 (elderly)	all sites	broccoli		1.3
			carrots or squash		1.0
			dried fruits (apricots, prunes, raisins)		1.7
			salads		0.9
			strawberries		3.3
			tomatoes		2.0
				total	smokers
Ziegler et al., 1986 New Jersey	763	lung	retinol	0.8	1.0
			vitamin A (IU)	1.0	1.5
			vitamin A (retinol equiv.)	0.9	1.2
			carotenoids	1.3	1.7

[a]Some studies did not report relative risks and/or *p* values.
[b]Carrots, coleslaw, lettuce, red cabbage, tomatoes.
[c]Five-year follow-up on 8278 men with prospective dietary data.
[d]Two-year follow-up on 100,000 Seventh-Day Adventists with prospective dietary data.
[e]Apples (*rr* = 2.0), cherries (*rr* = 1.6), cooked green vegetables (*rr* = 1.2), grapes (*rr* = 1.5), melons (*rr* = 1.9), onions (*rr* = 1.4), peas and beans (*rr* = 1.5), plums (*rr* = 2.3), pumpkin (*rr* = 1.6), quince (*rr* = 1.5), wild fruits (*rr* = 2.0).
[f]Vitamin A index: beef, beets, broccoli, Brussels sprouts, cabbage, carrots, cauliflower, chicken, coleslaw, cucumbers, fish, fruit, kale, kohlrabi, lamb, lettuce, milk, parsnips, pickles, pork, potatoes, red cabbage, rutabaga, sauerkraut, tomatoes, turnips.
[g]Cruciferous vegetables: broccoli, Brussels sprouts, cabbage, cauliflower, coleslaw, kale, parsnips, turnips.
[h]β-Carotene index: dark green, leafy vegetables, carrots, yellow and red fruits, vegetables.
[i]Ten-year follow-up on 265,118 Japanese with prospective dietary data.
[j]Twenty-year follow-up of prospective study on 1954 middle-aged men.
[k]Vitamin A index: apples, bananas, beans, cabbage, carrots, cauliflower, eggs, fish, grapes, lettuce, meat, milk, oranges, peas, potatoes, rhubarb, rutabaga, tomatoes, wild berries.

cancer, while lettuce and green onions were marginally protective. Construction of various "vegetable consumption profiles" using these food items did not alter the low risks noted for individual vegetables.

Studies in Israel (Modan et al., 1974, 1975) found increased intake of fruits and vegetables to be protective against stomach and colon cancer, especially squash and eggplant for the former. The role of dietary fiber was also considered in these studies.

A study of Seventh Day Adventists (Phillips, 1975) found consumption of milk and green leafy vegetables to be protective against overall cancer rates, including colon cancer. Bjelke (1975) found consumption of carrots, eggs, and milk, and an increased "vitamin A intake index" to be protective against lung cancer. Distinguishing smokers and nonsmokers, Mettlin et al. (1979) also found carrots, milk, and vitamin A intake to be protective against lung cancer. The protective effects were greater in smokers than in nonsmokers. As in previous studies, the dietary intake index did not distinguish retinol from total carotenoid, from individual carotenoid consumption. The consumption of carrots had a lesser effect than did the total dietary intake index, and was probably associated with consumption of other green and yellow vegetables (Graham et al., 1972). The same group of investigators found carrots, cruciferous vegetables, and milk to be protective against bladder cancer (Mettlin et al., 1979). Green and yellow vegetables were also found protective against laryngeal cancer (Graham et al., 1981), as were fruits and vegetables against esophageal cancer (Mettlin et al., 1981), by this group of investigators.

MacLennan et al. (1977) investigated dietary risk factors for lung cancer in Singapore Chinese women. This Chinese population comes primarily from Southeast China and is comprised of a variety of cultural groups speaking different Chinese dialects, including Cantonese, Hokkein, and Teachew. Traditional dietary practices in these groups may be derived from the data of Anderson and Anderson (1977). Dietary questionnaires asked frequency of consumption of common dark green leafy vegetables. Univariate analysis revealed low consumption of vegetable constituents of the diet to be associated with increased lung cancer risk in women. For the multivariate analyses a dietary intake index was constructed using combinations of six common leafy vegetables, eggplant, and beans. Of these eight, an index giving equal weight to four items (mustard greens (*chai-sim*), kale (*tua-chai*), eggplant (*brin-jal*) and long beans) were as predictive of cancer as any other index using all eight.

More recently, fruits and vegetables were found protective against oral and pharyngeal cancer (Winn et al., 1984). Fresh fruits and green leafy vegetables were also examined individually and found to have protective effects. In a case-control study of prostate cancer using both hospital-based and community-based controls (Schuman et al., 1982), a series of green and yellow vegetables were found protective. Carrots and beans were protective when compared to community controls, but not hospital controls.

A study of cancer in the elderly attempted to differentiate individual food items with respect to cancer risk (Colditz et al., 1985). A strong protective effect was found for strawberries and tomatoes, and a moderate protective effect for dried fruits (apricots, raisins, prunes) and broccoli. No protective effect was found for carrots or squash, or for salads.

Ziegler et al. (1986) found that inverse associations with lung cancer risk were more pronounced for intake of vegetables, dark green vegetables, and dark yellow-orange vegetables than for vitamin A or retinol intake. They suggested one explanation for these observations: the protective agent in vegetables may not be β-carotene, but other carotenoids, vitamin C (Cameron et al., 1979), indoles (Wattenberg and Loub, 1978), plant phenols (Ames, 1983), or trace minerals, such as selenium (Willett et al., 1983). Fourteen additional diet and cancer studies shown in Table 2 are consistent with this overall pattern of foods associated with decreased risk of cancer.

DIETARY EVIDENCE ON β-CAROTENE AND CANCER

Early epidemiologic studies relating total dietary vitamin A intake to cancer (e.g., Bjelke, 1975) could not distinguish intake of specific carotenoids from intake of total carotenoids or retinol. Natural preformed vitamin A (retinol) is found only in animals, while plants contain provitamin A (α- and β-carotene) and other carotenoids with lower or absent vitamin A activity. All these studies used crude estimates of carotenoids and retinol (Shekelle et al., 1981) which did not permit differentiation of β-carotene. Most early dietary studies utilized dietary intake indices based predominantly on plant foods (Peto et al., 1981), and thus the initial epidemiologic evidence relates primarily to the effects of total carotenoids, rather than total vitamin A, or β-carotene specifically. In a prospective study where a dietary distinction was drawn between plant (carotenoid) and animal (retinol) food sources of vitamin A (Shekelle et al., 1981), plant foods, but not animal foods, were found protective against cancer.

The dietary intake studies of Graham et al. (1972, 1981) and Mettlin et al. (1979, 1981) did not generally have high specificity for individual carotenoid-containing foods. However, their broad categories of "fruits, and green and yellow vegetables" are notable for the preponderance of food items that are low or absent in β-carotene, and relatively high in other carotenoids.

One study observed increased risks of cancer with higher dietary intake of preformed vitamin A (Gregor et al., 1980). These observations may be confounded by the covariation of fat and protein intake (Armstrong and Doll, 1975) with animal products high in retinol. In one study where individual carotenoid sources were considered separately, there was no effect of β-carotene specifically (Modan et al., 1981). In their recent critical review of diet and cancer Willett and MacMahon (1984) considered it possible that constituents of green and yellow vegetables other than β-carotene may actually reduce cancer incidence. Analyses of carotenoid-containing foods substantiates this position.

RECENT COMPREHENSIVE CAROTENOID ANALYSES

Foods chosen for nutrient composition analysis, based upon the results of epidemiologic studies, are divided into two broad categories: green, leafy vegetables (e.g., broccoli, Brussels sprouts, cabbage, kale, spinach), and yellow-orange vegetables (e.g., carrots, pumpkin, red palm oil, squashes, sweet potato). The majority of the green, leafy vegetables can also be classified as cruciferous vegetables. Carotenoids can be extracted from various vegetables and separated by high performance liquid chromatography (HPLC) (Khachik et al., 1986, 1987). Extensive sampling to assess food variability has not been performed to date. Preparation of food samples for analysis is accomplished in much the same way as they are prepared for consumption with inedible parts removed. Vegetable parts are washed and drained. Large portions are reduced in size prior to homogenization (without added water). Detailed extraction, saponification, isolation, and characterization of the major carotenoids found in the green, leafy vegetables and yellow-orange vegetables are described elsewhere (Khachik et al., 1986, 1987). The abundant carotenoids of these vegetables and their corresponding HPLC peaks are identified by spectroscopy and chromatography.

The green, leafy vegetables contain (1) oxygenated carotenoids, or xanthophylls (lutein, epoxycarotenoids), (2) chlorophylls, and (3) hydrocarbon carotenoids (α- and β-carotene), while the yellow-orange vegetables contain predomiantly hydrocarbon carotenoids. Some hydrocarbon carotenoids (such as α- and β-carotene, but not lycopene) contribute to vitamin A activity, while most oxygenated carotenoids (e.g., lutein) do not. Fig. 1 shows a chromatogram of an extract from raw Brussels sprouts indicating the presence of major carotenoid and chlorophyll constituents of the green, leafy vegetables. All the green, leafy vegetables contain the same profile of carotenoids, but at varying concentrations. The total hydrocarbon carotenoid (α- and β-carotene) content of these vegetables comprises only 9–18% of the total carotenoid content. The most abundant carotenoids in the green vegetables are the oxygenated carotenoids which comprise 80–90% of the total carotenoid content, and have no vitamin A activity (Khachik et al., 1986). The quantitative distribution of the abundant carotenoids in foods found protective against human cancer in epidemiologic studies are shown in Table 3. This table contains the results of various carotenoid analyses for comparative purposes.

Table 3 indicates contents of total carotenoids, β-carotene, and xanthophylls (or oxygenated carotenoids, such as lutein). A dashed line in a column indicates that the method used in the referenced analysis did not permit speciation of the indicated carotenoid(s) or did not permit complete determination of total caro-

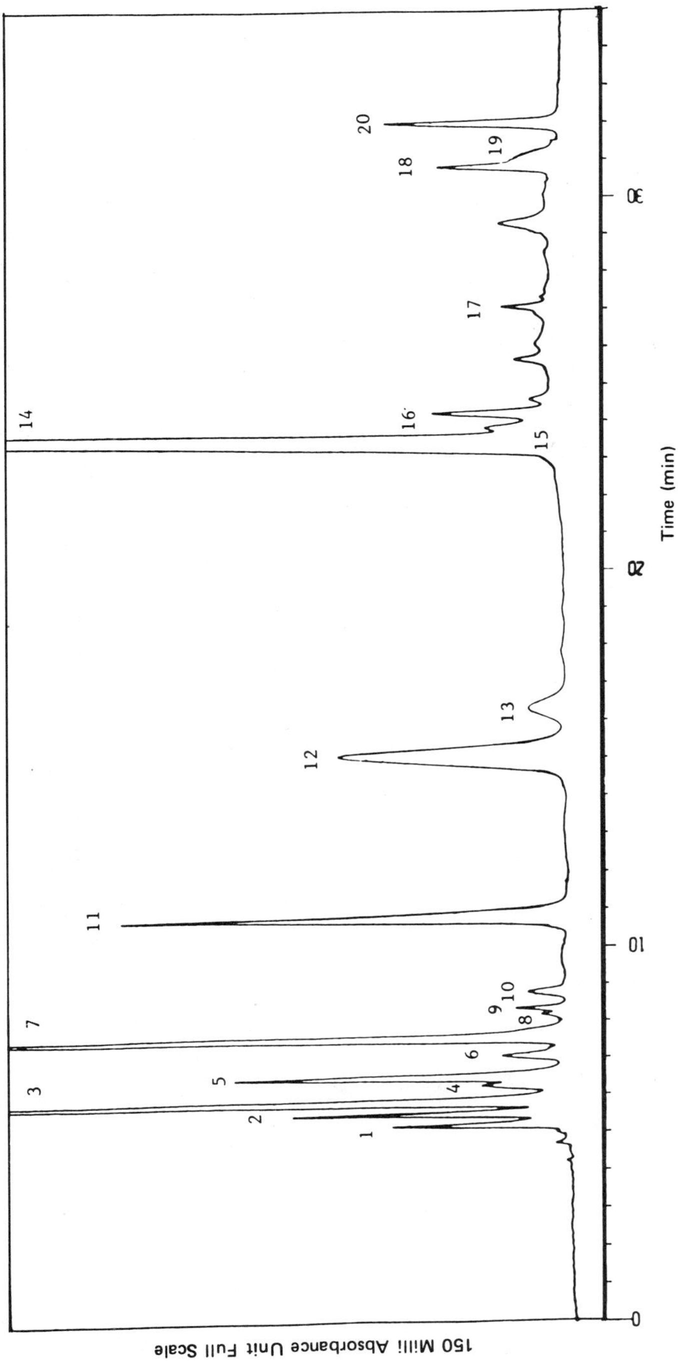

Fig. 1 The chromatogram of an extract from raw Brussels sprouts shows the presence of the major constituents of the green, leafy vegetables, which consist of three classes of compounds: (a) xanthophylls (oxygenated carotenoids, peaks 1 through 10), (b) chlorophylls and their derivatives (peaks 12 through 17), and (c) hydrocarbon carotenoids (peaks 18 and 19). β-apo-8′-carotenal (peak 11) and decapreno-β-carotene (peak 20) were employed as internal standards for the quantitative determination of xanthophylls and hydrocarbon carotenoids, respectively. The use of these internal standards assists in monitoring the losses of carotenoids that may occur as a result of extensive extraction and preparation procedures. Quantitative determination of the hydrocarbon carotenoids found in these vegetables (mainly all-trans-β-carotene and its 15,15′-*cis*-isomer) is accomplished under separate isocratic HPLC conditions. The general chromatographic profiles of the other green vegetables are very similar to that of raw Brussels sprouts.

Table 3 Carotenoid Content of Foods Associated with a Reduction in Cancer Incidence Rates

Food	Preparation	Major carotenoids (mg/100 g edible food)			References
		Total carotenoids	Hydrocarbon carotenoids	Xanthophylls	
Apricots	fresh	0.35	0.32	0.03	c
		—	0.62	0.02	b
		—	1.57	—	d
	canned	—	0.78	—	d
		—	1.3–1.7	0.27–0.30	e
	dried	3.4–6.5	—	—	k
		—	5.4–5.6	—	f
Broccoli	fresh	0.83–2.40	—	—	k
		—	0.48	3.80*	i
Beetroot	fresh	0.01–0.02	—	—	k
Brussels sprouts	fresh	0.32–0.60	—	—	k
		—	0.53	2.33*	a
Cabbage	fresh	0.02–0.07	—	—	k
		—	0.08	0.81*	i
		—	3.10	13.70*	m
Carrots	fresh	6.0–21.0	—	—	k
		—	16.4–17.9	—	g
	canned	7.2–7.4	—	—	k
Cauliflower	fresh	0.2–0.05	—	—	k
		—	0.01	—	e
Celery	fresh	0.01–0.03	—	—	k
		—	0.08	—	e

Coleslaw	fresh	—	0.38	—	e
Corn	fresh	—	6.95	6.95*	m
Cucumber	fresh	0.12–0.29	—	—	k
		—	0.03	—	e
Eggplant (Aubergine)	fresh	0.02–0.04	—	—	k
Green beans	fresh	—	0.36	—	b
Kale	fresh	0.9–7.6	—	—	k
		—	14.6	63.0*	i
	canned	3.8–3.9	—	—	l
Lettuce	fresh	0.16–1.60	—	—	k
		—	0.33	—	b
		—	2.91	7.29*	m
Lima beans	fresh	—	0.18	—	e
	cooked	—	0.22	—	e
Mustard greens	fresh	—	3.18	—	e
	cooked	—	1.82	—	e
Onions	fresh	0.01–0.05	—	—	k
	dried	0.00–0.78	—	—	k
Prunes	canned	—	0.48	—	d
	dried	—	1.19	—	d
Raisins		—	0.03	—	d
Red cabbage	fresh	0.01–0.05	—	—	k
Red palm oil		—	120.5	—	h
Rutabaga	fresh	0.00	—	—	l

Table 3 (continued)

Food	Preparation	Major carotenoids (mg/100 g edible food)			References
		Total carotenoids	Hydrocarbon carotenoids	Xanthophylls	
Spinach	fresh	3.0–5.7	–	–	k
		–	4.31	–	b
		–	6.71	29.7*	i
	canned	4.4–5.2	–	–	l
Squash		0.94–2.92	–	–	l
		1.4	–	–	k
		–	0.18	–	b
Strawberries		0.04–0.06	–	–	k
		0.064	–	–	c
		–	0.021	–	b
		–	0.23	0.062	h
Sweet potatoes	fresh, cooked	4.62	–	–	k
		–	8.61	–	b
		–	6.0–6.4	–	f
		–	15.2	–	h
	canned	–	4.6–6.6	–	l
		–	15.6–16.4	–	h

Tomatoes	fresh	0.15–2.3	—	—	k
		5.1	—	—	c
		—	0.91†	—	f
		—	7.20†	—	a
Turnip	fresh	0.00–0.19	—	—	k
Watercress	fresh	1.2–4.0	—	—	k
		—	2.83	—	e

Hydrocarbon carotenoid = primarily β-carotene, some α-carotene, both having vitamin A activity.
*Xanthophyll components consist of epoxy- and hydroxycarotenoids (mainly lutein and its stereoisomers).
†Lycophene is the major constituent in tomatoes and is also a hydrocarbon carotenoid but does not have vitamin A activity.

[a]G. Beecher et al., Int. Food Tech. Ann. Mtg., Dallas, TX, 1986.
[b]J. Bureau, R. Bushway, *J. Food Sci. 51*:128 (1986).
[c]A. Curl, *J. Food Sci. 29*:241 (1964).
[d]S. Gebhardt et al., in *Composition of Foods: Fruits and Fruit Juices*, USDA, Washington, D.C., 1982.
[e]D. Haytowitz et al., in *Composition of Foods: Vegetables and Vegetable Products*, USDA, Washington, D.C., 1984.
[f]Y. Hsieh, M. Karel, *J. Chromatogr. 259*:515 (1983).
[g]F. Khachik, G. Beecher, *J. Chromatogr. 346*:237.
[h]F. Khachik, G. Beecher, *J. Ind. Eng. Chem. Prod. Res. Dev. 25*:671.
[i]F. Khachik et al., *J. Agric. Food Chem. 34*:603 (1986).
[j]L. Posati, M. Orr, in *Composition of Foods: Dairy and Egg Products*, USDA, Washington, D.C., 1976.
[k]S. Souci et al., in *Food Composition and Nutrition Tables* 1981/82, Wissenschaftliche Verlagsgesellschaft, Stuttgart.
[l]J. Sweeney, A. Marsch, *J. Am. Dietet. Assoc. 59*:283 (1971).
[m]S. Takagi, *J. Agric. Biol. Chem. 49*:1211 (1985).

Table 4 Comparison of Carotenoid Profile with Fiber Content and Other Constituents of Foods Associated with a Reduction in Cancer Incidence Rates

Food	Carotenoid profile			Fiber content per serving	Other constituents
	Primary	Secondary	β-carotene content		
Apricots (dried)	β	xanthophylls	major	1.4	vit. C, vit. B
Broccoli	lutein	β	minor	2.2	vit. C
Brussels sprouts	lutein	β	minor	1.1	vit. C
Cabbage	lutein	β	minor	3.1	vit. C
Carrots	β	none	major	2.3	–
Cauliflower	–	–	trace	2.3	vit. C
Celery	–	–	trace	1.1	–
Cole slaw	β	–	minor	1.1	–
Corn	lutein/β	β/lutein	major	2.9	niacin
Cucumber	–	–	trace	0.4	–
Eggplant	–	–	trace		
Green beans	β	–	trace	1.6	vit. C
Green onion	–	–	trace	0.8	vit. C
Kale	lutein	β	minor	1.4	vit. C
Lettuce	lutein	β	minor	0.9	vit. C
Mustard greens	β		major		vit. C
Raisins	–	–	trace	1.3	–
Red cabbage	–	–	trace	3.3	vit. C
Rutabaga	–	–	zero		
Squash	β	–	trace	1.4	vit. C
Strawberries	β	lutein	trace	3.0	vit. C
Sweet potato	β	–	major	1.7	vit. C
Tomatoes	lycopene	–	zero	1.5	vit. C

tenoid levels. Different methods demonstrate different analytical sensitivities to carotenoids. Attention is given to relative concentrations of carotenoids in foods within a given analysis. Many foods found protective against cancer have little or no carotenoid content at all (beetroot, cauliflower, celery, cucumber, eggplant, onions, raisins, red cabbage, rutabaga, strawberries, turnips). The green, leafy vegetables (broccoli, brussels sprouts, cabbage, kale, lettuce, spinach), which are almost universally found to be protective against cancer (Table 2), are uniformly low in β-carotene, but high in xanthophyll carotenoid constituents (primarily lutein and its chemical isomers). In addition, all those vegetables with the highest total carotenoid content are relatively low in β-carotene. Vegetables which are uniquely high in β-carotene and low or absent in other carotenoid constituents (carrots, sweet potatoes) have been shown to be protective against cancer in only few studies (Table 2). In two of these earlier studies, where carrot intake was found protective against cancer, the effect was recognized to be attributable to the association of carrot consumption with the consumption of other vegetables (Graham et al., 1972). In several earlier and in most recent studies (Schuman et al., 1982, Colditz et al., 1985, Ziegler et al., 1984, 1986) a protective effect of carrots, dietary β-carotene, and /or dietary retinol intake against cancer has not been demonstrated in the general population. From Table 3 it is apparent that the preponderance of food items identified in cancer epidemiologic studies as protective against cancer are relatively low or absent in β-carotene. Many of these foods, however, appear to be abundant sources of other carotenoids, such as lutein, which in turn do not contribute to vitamin A activity.

In addition, Table 4 indicates the carotenoid profiles of foods found to be protective against cancer in relation to the fiber content per serving of those foods. Cancer protective foods are also generally high in fiber content. There is no pattern that can relate those foods highest in any particular carotenoid with those that are highest in fiber. Comparisons with other nutrient content can be carried out as well. Cancer-preventive foods are also generally high in vitamin C, even when they are not high in carotenoid content.

EFFECTS OF FOOD PROCESSING

Some epidemiologic studies have emphasized that the consumption of raw versus cooked vegetables was associated with decreased risk of cancer (Graham et al., 1972, 1978; Haenszel et al., 1972; Cook-Mozaffari et al., 1979), although raw and cooked vegetable consumption may be correlated. Other studies have not distinguished between raw versus cooked vegetable consumption, or have only indicated which vegetables are normally eaten raw or normally eaten cooked. Therefore, the effects of cooking on carotenoid content and profile in foods are examined briefly.

Vegetables are experimentally cooked by heating in a microwave oven with a small amount of water for six minutes. Comparison between the chromatographic profiles of raw and cooked vegetable extracts reveals that 60 to 68% of the total xanthophylls (oxygenated carotenoids) in cooked vegetables (Brussels sprouts and kale, respectively, are destroyed. However, losses of the hydrocarbon carotenoids in cooked Brussels sprouts and kale are only 15% and 14%, respectively. Therefore, those studies that found that cooked vegetables had less cancer-protective activity than raw vegetables (Table 2) point to the xanthophyll carotenoids (which are differentially lost with cooking), rather than the hydrocarbon carotenoids (which are relatively spared) as the cancer-protective agents.

Dried fruits, as identified recently by Colditz et al. (1985), would be expected to contain concentrated carotenoids, producing a high carotenoid-to-weight ratio in the dried fruit items. These dried fruits may therefore act as "natural" carotenoid supplements (see Table 3). However, it should be pointed out that as a result of the heat treatment in the drying process, the heat-sensitive carotenoids may undergo rearrangement, isomerization, and/or degradation.

EFFECTS OF DIGESTION ON SERUM LEVELS OF CAROTENOIDS

Epoxycarotenoids are a major xanthophyll (oxygenated carotenoid) component of vegetables. These compounds (epoxides) are extremely sensitive to traces of acids and readily subjected to rearrangement, isomerization, and degradation in low pH environment. Therefore, even if vegetables are consumed in raw form, these groups of carotenoids may be expected to undergo such structural changes owing to the presence of acids in the stomach. Among the oxygenated carotenoids (xanthophylls), lutein is by far the most stable compound and is much more resistant to heat and acid treatment than the other carotenoids of this class (Khachik et al., 1986). These observations are consistent with the profile of carotenoids seen in human plasma, where epoxycarotenoids and their rearrangement products have not been detected, while lutein is the major xanthophyll constituent (Nells and DeLeenheer, 1983).

CONCLUSION

The cancer-modifying effects of foods cited in epidemiologic studies cannot be explained primarily by the assumption that these foods are high in β-carotene or contribute significantly to vitamin A activity. These epidemiologic studies were generally not testing the protective effects of dietary β-carotene or vitamin A, but that of total carotenoids or other carotenoids without vitamin A activity, including lutein. Since dietary lutein uptake, for example, appears well reflected in serum levels (Nells and Delenheer, 1983; Brown et al., 1986), this compound may be a good candidate for a cancer-modifying agent based upon its relatively high concentration in many foods found protective against cancer. Alternatively, the preponderance of foods found protective against cancer, including the cruciferous vegetables (which are low in β-carotene, but high in lutein) may also be high in a number of other biologically active compounds, such as vitamin C, which have cancer-modifying effects (Wattenberg, 1978). The chemical composition of those foods found protective against cancer requires further analysis before definitive conclusions are drawn regarding the potential cancer-modifying effects of foods in the human diet.

SUMMARY

In 1981, it was proposed that β-carotene might be the specific dietary component of foods responsible for observed reductions of human cancer rates in studies on diet and cancer. There have been over 30 epidemiologic studies to date focusing on dietary intake of both retinol (vitamin A) and β-carotene (provitamin A). Most dietary intake indices for β-carotene and retinol were based upon incomplete or incorrect data on the nutrient composition of foods. This new analysis focuses upon *foods* (as opposed to assumed nutrients, or nutrient indices) found protective against cancer. The proponderance of food items with potential cancer modifying effects are poor sources of β-carotene but are high in other carotenoids (such as lutein), which do not have vitamin A activity, and in fiber and vitamin C.

REFERENCES

Ames, B. (1983). Dietary carcinogens and anticarcinogens. *Science 221*:1256.

Anderson, E. N., Anderson, M. L. (1977). Modern China: South. In *Food in Chinese Culture: Anthropological and Historical Perspectives*, Chang, K. C. (Ed.). Yale University Press, New Haven and London, pp. 319–382.

Armstrong, B., Doll, R. (1975). Environmental factors and cancer incidence and mortality in different countries, with special reference to dietary practices. *Int. J. Cancer 15*:617.

Atukorala, S., Basu, T. K., Dickerson, J. W. T., Donaldson, D., Sakula, A. (1979). Vitamin A, zinc and lung cancer. *British J. Cancer 40*:927.

Basu, T. K., Raven, R. W., Dickerson, J. W. T., Williams, D. C. (1974). Vitamin A nutrition and its relationship with plasma cholesterol level in the patient with cancer. *Int. J. Vit. Nutr. Res. 44*:14.

Basu, T. K., Donaldson, D., Jenner, M., Williams, D. C., Sakula, A. (1976). Plasma vitamin A in patients with bronchial carcinoma. *British J. Cancer 33*: 119.

Beecher, G., Khachik, F. (1984). Evaluation of vitamin A and carotenoid data in food composition tables. *JNCI 73*:1397.

Bjelke, E. (1975). Dietary vitamin A and human lung cancer. *Int. J. Cancer 15*: 561.

Brown, E. D., Micozzi, M., Craft, N., et al. (1986). Plasma carotenoid and retinol concentrations in healthy young males. *Fed. Proc. Abstracts 70*:592.

Byers, T., Vena, J., Mettlin, C., Swanson, M., Graham, S. (1985). Dietary vitamin A and lung cancer risk: An analysis by histologic subtypes. *Am. J. Epidemiol. 120*:769.

Cameron, E., Pauling, L., Leibovitz, B. (1979). Ascorbic acid and cancer: A review. *Cancer Res. 39*:663.

Cohen, M., Primack, A., Broder, L. E., Williams, L. R. (1977). Vitamin A serum levels and dietary vitamin A intake in lung cancer patients. *Cancer Lett. 4*:51.

Colditz, G., Branch, L., Lipnick, R., Willett, W., Rosner, B., Posner, B., Hennekens, C. (1985). Increased green and yellow vegetable intake and lowered cancer deaths in an elderly population. *Am. J. Clin. Nutr. 41*:32.

Cook-Mozaffari, P. (1979). The epidemiology of cancer of the oesophagus. *Nutrition and Cancer 1*:51.

Cook-Mozaffari, P., Azordegan, F., Day, N., Ressicaud, A., Sabai, C., Aramesh, B. (1979). Oesophageal cancer studies in the Caspian littoral of Iran: Results of a case-control study. *Br. J. Cancer 39*:293.

Doll, R., Peto, R. (1981). The causes of cancer. *JNCI 66*:1191.

Friedman, G., Blaner, W., Goodman, D., et al. (1986). Serum retinol and retinol-binding protein levels do not predict subsequent lung cancer. *Am. J. Epidemiol. 123*:781.

Graham, S., Schotz, W., Martino, P. (1972). Alimentary factors in the epidemiology of gastric cancer. *Cancer 30*:927.

Graham, S., Haughey, B., Marshall, J., Priore, R., Byers, T., Rzepka, T., Mettlin, C., Pontes, J. E. (1983). Diet in the epidemiology of carcinoma of the prostate gland. *JNCI 70*:687.

Graham, S., Dayal, H., Swanson, M., Mittelman, A., Wilkinson, G. (1978). Diet in the epidemiology of cancer of the colon and rectum. *J. Nat. Cancer Inst. 61*:709.

Graham, S., Marshall, J., Mettlin, C., Rzepka, T., Nemoto, T., Byers, T. (1982). Diet in the epidemiology of breast cancer. *Am. J. Epidemiol. 116*:68.

Graham, S., Mettlin, C., Marshall, J., Priore, R., Rzepka, T., Shedd, D. (1981). Dietary factors in the epidemiology of cancer of the larynx. *Am. J. Epidemiol. 113*:675.

Gregor, A., Lee, P., Roe, F., Wilson, M., Melton, A. (1980). Comparison of dietary histories in lung cancer cases and controls with special reference to vitamin A. *Nutrition and Cancer 2*:93.

Haenszel, W., Kurihara, M., Segi, M., Lee, R. (1972). Stomach cancer among Japanese in Hawaii. *J. Natl. Cancer Inst. 49*:969.

Haenszel, W., Kurihara, M., Locke, T., et al. (1976). Stomach cancer in Japan. *JNCI 56*:265.

Hirayama, T. (1979). Diet and cancer. *J. Nutr. Cancer 1*:67.

Ibrahim, K., Jafarey, N. A., Zuberi, S. J. (1977). Plasma vitamin A and carotene levels in squamous cell carcinoma of oral cavity and oro-pharynx. *Clinical Oncology 3*:203.

Kark, J., Smith, A., Switzer, B., Hames, C. (1981). Serum vitamin A (retinol) and cancer incidence in Evans County, Georgia. *JNCI 66*:7.

Khachik, F., Beecher, G., Whittaker, N. (1986). Separation, identification and quantification of the major carotenoids and chlorophyl constituents in extracts of several green vegetables by liquid chromatography. *J. Agric. Food Chem. 34*:603.

Khachik, F., Beecher, G. (1987). Application of a c-45-beta-carotene as an internal standard for the quantification of carotenoids in yellow/orange vegetables by liquid chromatography. *J. Agric. Food Chem. 35*:732.

Kvale, G., Bjelke, E., Gart, J. J. (1983). Dietary habits and lung cancer risk. *Int. J. Cancer 31*:397.

MacLennan, R., Da Costa, J., Day, N., Law, C., Ng, Y. K., Shanmugaratnam, K. (1977). Risk factors for lung cancer in Singapore Chinese, a population with high female incidence rates. *Int. J. Cancer 20*:854.

Menkes, M., Comstock, G. (1984). Vitamins A and E and lung cancer. *Am. J. Epidemiol. 120*:49.

Menkes, M., Comstock, G., Vuilleumier, J., Helsing, K., Rider, A., Brookmeyer, R. (1986). Serum beta-carotene, vitamins A and E, selenium and the risk of lung cancer. *NEJM 315*:1250.

Mettlin, C., Graham, S. (1979). Dietary risk factors in human bladder cancer. *Am. J. Epidemiol. 110*:255.

Mettlin, C., Graham, S., Swanson, M. (1979). Vitamin A and lung cancer. *JNCI 62*:1435.

Mettlin, C., Graham, S., Priore, R., Marshall, J., Swanson, M. (1981). Diet and cancer of the esophagus. *Nutrition and Cancer 2*:143.

Micozzi, M., Boone, C., Kelloff, G., et al. (1985). Chemoprevention of cancer: Implications for clinical pharmacology. *J. Clin. Pharmacol. 25*:164.

Micozzi, M., Beecher, M. S., Taylor, G. R., Khachik, P. R. (in press). Carotenoid analyses of selected raw and cooked foods associated with a lower risk for cancer. *JNCI.*

Modan, B., Lubin, F., Barell, V., Greenberg, R., et al. (1974). The role of starches in the etiology of gastric cancer. *Cancer 34*:2087.

Modan, B., Barell, V., Lubin, F., et al. (1975). Low-fiber intake as etiologic factor in cancer of the colon. *JNCI 55*:15.

Modan, B., Cuckle, H., Lubin, F. (1981). A note on the role of dietary retinol and carotene in human gastro-intestinal cancer. *Int. J. Cancer 28*:421.

Nells, H., DeLeenheer, A. (1983). Isocratic nonaqueous reversed-phase liquid chromatography of carotenoids. *Analyt. Chem. 55*:270.

Nomura, A., Stemmermann, C., Heilbrun, L., et al. (1985). Serum vitamin levels and the risk of cancer of specific sites in men of Japanese ancestry in Hawaii. *Cancer Res. 45*:2369.

Peleg, I., Heyden, S., Knowles, M., et al. (1984). Serum retinol and risk of subsequent cancer: Extension of the Evans county, Georgia, study. *JNCI 73*: 1455.

Peto, R., Doll, R., Buckley, J., Sporn, M. (1981). Can dietary beta-carotene materially reduce human cancer rates? *Nature* (London) *290*:201.

Phillips, R. (1975). Role of life-style and dietary habits in risk of cancer among Seventh-Day Adventists. *Cancer Res. 35*:3513.

Russell-Briefel, R., Bates, M., Kuller, L. (1985). The relationship of plasma carotenoids to health and biochemical factors in middle-aged men. *Am. J. Epidemiol. 122*:741.

Saffiotti, U., Montesano, A., Selahumur, A., Borg, S. (1967). Experimental cancer of the lung–inhibition by vitamin A. *Cancer 20*:857.

Salonen, J., Salonen, R., Lappetelainen, R. (1985). Risk of cancer in relation to serum concentrations of selenium and vitamins A and E: Matched case-control analysis of prospective data. *Br. Med. J. 290*:417.

Schuman, L., Mandel, J., Blackard, C., et al. (1977). Epidemiologic study of prostate cancer: preliminary report. *Cancer Treat. Rep. 61*:181.

Schuman, L., Mandel, J., Radke, A., et al. (1982). Some selected features of the epidemiology of prostatic cancer: Minneapolis-St. Paul, Minnesota Case Control Study, 1976–1979. In *Trends in Cancer Incidence: Causes and Practical Implications*, Magnus, K. (Ed.). Hemisphere Publishing, Washington, D.C., pp. 345–354.

Shekelle, R., Liu, S., Raynor, W., Lepper, M., Maliza, C., Rossof, A., Paul, O., Shryock, A., Stamler, J. (1981). Dietary vitamin A and risk of cancer in the Western Electric study. *Lancet 2*:1185.

Sondik, E. J., Young, J. L., Horm, J. W., Gloeckler Ries, L. A. (1985). Annual cancer statistics review. NIH Publication 86-2789 U.S. Department of Health and Human Services, Public Health Service, National Institutes of Health, National Cancer Institute,Bethesda, Md. 20892.

Sporn, M. B., Dunlop, N. M., Newton, D. L., Smith, J. M. (1976). Prevention of chemical carcinogenesis by vitamin A and its synthetic analogs (retinoids). *Fed. Proc. 35*:1332.

Sporn, M. E., Newton, D. L., Roberts, A. B., et al. (1981). Retinoids and the suppression of the effects of polypeptide transforming factors. In *Molecular Action and Targets of Cancer Chemotherapeutic Agents*, Sartorelli, A. C., Bertino, J. R., Laza, J. S. (Eds.). Academic Press, New York, pp. 541–544.

Stahelin, H., Rosel, F., Buess, E., Brubacher, G. (1984). Cancer, vitamins, and plasma lipids: Prospective Basel study. *JNCI 73*:1463.

Stehr, P., Gloninger, M., Kuller, L., et al. (1985). Dietary vitamin A deficiencies and stomach cancer. *Am. J. Epidemiol. 121*:65.

Stocks, P. (1957). Cancer incidence in North Wales and Liverpool Region in relation to habits and environment. *British Empire Cancer Campaign Thirty-fourth Annual Report* (Suppl. to Part II), pp. 51–66, 119–127.

Thompson, H., Becci, P., Grubbs, C., et al. (1981). Inhibition of urinary bladder cancer in rats and mice. *Cancer Res. 41*:933.

Tuyns, A., Pequignot, G., Jensen, O. M. (1978). Nutrition, alcol et cancer de l'oesophage. *Bulletin du Cancer 65*:59.

Wahi, P., Bodkhe, R. R., Arora, S., Srivastava, M. C. (1962). Serum vitamin A studies in leukoplakia and carcinoma of the oral cavity. *Indian J. Pathol. Bacteriol. 5*:10.

Wald, N., Idle, M., Boreham, J., Bailey, A. (1980). Low serum vitamin A and subsequent risk of cancer. *Lancet 2*:813.

Wald, N., Boreham, J., Hayward, J., Bulbrook, R., et al. (1984). Plasma retinol, beta-carotene and vitamin E levels in relation to future risk of breast cancer. *Br. J. Cancer 49*:321.

Wattenberg, L., Loub, W. (1978). Inhibition of polycyclic aromatic hydrocarbon-induced neoplasia by naturally occurring indoles. *Cancer Res. 38*:1410.

Wattenberg, L. W. (1978). Inhibitors of chemical carcinogenesis. *Adv. Cancer Res. 26*:197.

Willett, W., Polk, B., Underwood, B., et al. (1984a). Relation of serum vitamins A and E and carotenoids to the risk of cancer. *NEJM 310*:430.

Willett, W., Polk, B., Underwood, B., et al. (1984b). Hypertension detection and follow-up program study of serum retinol, retinol binding protein, total carotenoids and cancer risk: A summary. *JNCI 73*:1459.

Willett, W., Polk, B., Morris, J., et al. (1983). Pre-diagnostic serum selenium and risk of cancer. *Lancet 2*:130.

Willett, W., MacMahon, B. (1984). Diet and cancer—An overview. Part I. *NEJM 310*:633.

Winn, D., Ziegler, R., Pickle, L., Gridley, G., Blot, W., Hoover, R. (1984). Diet in the etiology of oral and pharyngeal cancer among women from the Southern United States. *Cancer Res. 44*:1216.

Wolbach, D., Howe, P. (1925). Tissue changes following deprivation of fat soluble A vitamin. *J. Exper. Med. 42*:753.

Wynder, E., Bross, I. (1961). A study of etiological factors in cancer of the esophagus. *Cancer 14*:389.

Ziegler, R., Mason, T., Stemhagen, A., et al. (1984). Dietary carotene and vitamin A and risk of lung cancer among white men in New Jersey. *JNCI 73*: 1429.

Ziegler, R., Mason, T., Stemhagen, A., et al. (1986). Carotenoid intake, vegetables, and the risk of lung cancer among white men in New Jersey. *Amer. J. Epidemiol. 123*:1080.

9
Retinoids for the Prevention of Cancer

SCOTT M. LIPPMAN* and FRANK L. MEYSKENS, JR.
The University of Arizona College of Medicine, Tucson, Arizona

INTRODUCTION

Wolbach and Howe were the first investigators to discover a relationship between vitamin A and neoplasia, i.e., dietary deficiencies in rats led to "stratified keratinizing epithelium," and restoration of vitamin A to their diet reversed the neoplastic process (Wolbach and Howe, 1925). Wolbach and Howe's classic report in 1925 followed the recognition in 1909 and naming in 1920 of the fat-soluble substance essential for normal growth we now call vitamin A. Preformed vitamin A, or the aldehyde and alcohol forms and their esters, is found mainly in animal products including milk, eggs, meat, and fish and is not synthesized by plants (Wolf, 1984). On the other hand, provitamin A, which includes β-carotene among several other carotenoids, is found in plant sources and cannot be synthesized either by humans or animals. Both forms are also commonly found in over-the-counter pharmaceutical compounds. For the most part, β-carotene is converted to retinol during absorption through the intestinal mucosa, where it and preformed vitamin A are transported in the plasma by lipoproteins. Vitamin A is then stored in the liver in lipocytes as retinyl esters.

Many subsequent studies, including that by Abels et al. in 1941, which associated vitamin A deficiency with established human malignancy, strongly supported the link between vitamin A and neoplastic disease (Lippman et al., 1987). Recognition that vitamin A deficiency leads to hyperkeratosis of the skin and to squamous metaplasia spurred an initial rush to treat cutaneous disorders with this new wonder drug; however, early excitement had to be tempered because of unacceptable toxic effects in many patients, especially on the liver. Excessive

**Current affiliation*: University of Texas System Cancer Center, Houston, Texas.

intake of retinol, or hypervitaminosis A, was first reported over 100 years ago, many years before vitamin A had even been positively identified (Korner and Vollin, 1975; Windhorst and Nigra, 1982). These reports involved the ingestion of polar bear and seal livers (5-8 mg retinol/g liver) by Eskimos and Arctic explorers. Their acute symptoms included severe headaches, drowsiness, irritability, nausea, and vomiting. Twelve to 24 hours after ingestion, erythema and desquamation of the face, trunk, palms, and soles developed. Seven to 10 days later, all symptoms resolved.

Subsequent clinical observations verified these major acute symptoms of hypervitaminosis A, which occur when the intake of retinol exceeds the liver's capacity to remove and store it and after ingestion of a dose of at least 350,000 international units (IU) of vitamin A by infants, and 1,000,000 IU by adults (Korner and Vollin, 1975; Windhorst and Nigra, 1982; Wolf, 1984; Lippman et al., 1987). Minor acute side effects are more frequent and better described and include mucocutaneous dryness and ocular, gastrointestinal, and musculoskeletal complaints such as tenderness of long bones. Specific major chronic vitamin A toxicities include abnormalities of the following: reproductive function and embryological development, serum lipids, the liver, and the skeletal system. A partial hominid (*Homo erectus*) skeleton discovered in Kenya exhibited the earliest pathologically documented changes consistent with chronic hypervitaminosis A (Lippman et al., 1987). Minor chronic side effects resemble the minor acute toxicities described above, but are more subtle.

These severe side effects, primarily the hepatotoxicity, led to the search for vitamin A derivatives with improved therapeutic ratios. New drugs began to be synthesized in the mid-1950s and were called "retinoids"—a term encompassing all the natural (excluding carotenoids) and synthetic compounds having some or all of the biological activities of vitamin A (retinol).

Retinoids have a basic molecular structure consisting of a cyclic end group, a polyene side chain, and a polar end group (see Fig. 1). By modifying any part, different therapeutic ratios can be achieved (Bollag, 1973). Chemical manipulation of the polar end group and the polyene side chain produced the first-generation synthetic retinoids, which are retinyl esters, amides, aldehydes, ethers, amines, and acids. The most widely studied of these molecules are tretinoin in vitro and 13-*cis*-retinoic acid (isotretinoin) in vivo. The retinamides (e.g., 4-HPR), a group of first-generation synthetic retinoids in which the terminal carboxyl group of retinoic acid is replaced by an N-substituted carboxyamide group, are now entering clinical trial. These drugs have a different spectrum of activity and were relatively nontoxic in phase-I trials (Lippman et al., 1987). Second-generation retinoids were developed by altering the cyclic end group. The prototype second-generation molecule is etretinate. Cyclization of the polyene side chain has produced the potent third-generation retinoids, such as the

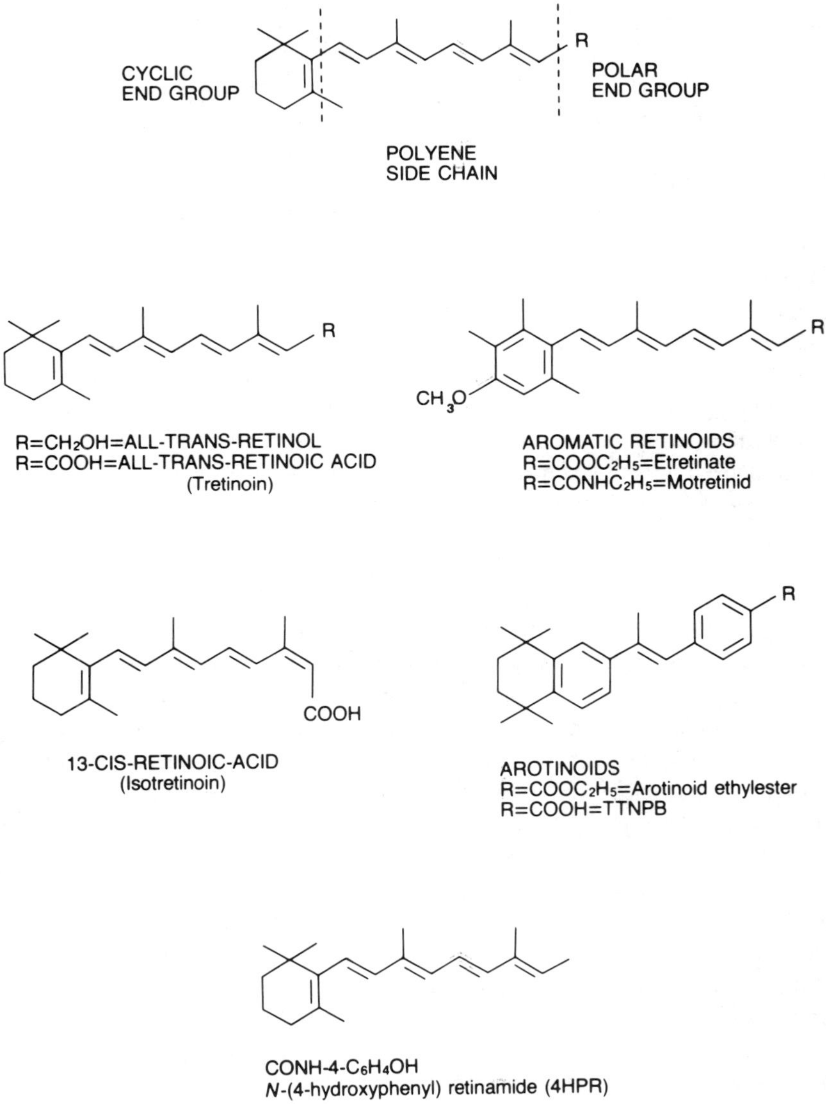

Fig. 1 Chemical structures of retinoids.

retinoidal benzoic acid derivatives (arotinoids). The arotinoid TTNPB (RO 12-7410) is less toxic and over 1000 times more potent than tretinoin and retinol in several standard screening tests and is now entering clinical trial. Although the types of side effects among retinoids have been similar (largely differing only in degree), these drugs may exhibit markedly different spectra of activity (Bollag, 1983; Lippman et al., 1987).

The accumulation of a vast amount of laboratory data has clearly demonstrated the potent differentiation-inducing and antiproliferative effects of vitamin A and many of the newer synthetic retinoids. In general, the antiproliferative activity of retinoids is cell-cycle specific, occurs in a broad range of transformed cell types, and is a reversible phenomenon (Lotan, 1980). Several studies have shown that in most cells there is a retinoic acid-sensitive G_1 restriction point (Lippman et al., 1987). In contrast to their antiproliferative effects, retinoids tend to affect differentiation in a select group of cell types and in a highly specialized, possibly irreversible way, and the mechanism(s) by which retinoids influence differentiation may differ from that affecting proliferation (Lippman et al., 1987).

Defining the structure-function relationships of retinoids through the various in vivo and in vitro assay systems has facilitated the identification of specific skeletal components of the retinoid molecules which may mediate antiproliferation and/or differentiation for a specific malignant cell type (Bollag, 1983; Lippman et al., 1987). For example, retinoic acid derivatives with a carboxyl group were significantly more active than were retinoids with a derivatized carboxyl moiety in inducing differentiation in HL-60 and F9 cell lines, in stimulating normal hematopoiesis, and in inhibiting clonal growth of leukemic cells (Tobler et al., 1986; Lippman et al., 1987). Also, the retinamide 4HPR has a high therapeutic index against chemically induced tumors of the rat mammary gland and urinary bladder and hamster trachea, however, it has limited activity in normal and malignant hematopoietic cells (Lippman et al., 1987).

The specificity of molecular components is demonstrated dramatically by the abolition of the arotinoid TTNPB's biological activity in melanoma cells resulting from moving its carboxyl group from the para to the meta position on the benzene ring (Lotan, 1980; Lippman et al., 1987). By moving the hydroxyl group of 2-hydroxypropylretinamide to the 3-position, a similar complete loss of activity was achieved in the rodent bladder carcinogenesis model (Lippman et al., 1987). In addition to providing direction to clinical study, analyses of these and other structure-activity relationships should significantly aid our understanding of the mechanism of retinoid action.

MOLECULAR MECHANISMS OF ACTION

Despite extensive investigation, the complex molecular mechanism(s) of action which causes the diverse cellular changes modulated by retinoids remains incompletely understood. Although many mechanisms have been proposed, it has only recently become possible to present a unifying hypothesis, which involves the protein kinase-C (PK-C)/phosphoinositol cascade system, to account for retinoids' varied biological effects. Several recent reviews detail the major actions of retinoids that have been hypothesized to modulate antiproliferation and differentiation (Lotan, 1980; Bollag, 1983; Jetten, 1984; Sporn and Roberts, 1984; Wolf, 1984; Sport et al., 1986; Tobler et al., 1986; Lippman et al., 1987a). Biological actions include regulation of (1) enzyme synthesis (especially of ornithine decarboxylase, transglutaminase, and the cAMP intracellular regulatory system), (2) extracellular effects, (3) membrane function, (4) growth factors (especially epidermal growth factor, or EGF), (5) binding proteins, (6) genomic, oncogenic, and postgenomic expression, (7) immunologic activity, and finally (8) the PK-C cascade system.

PK-C, the phorbol ester receptor, is a Ca^{2+}-activated, phospholipid-dependent enzyme, which plays a critical role in the carcinogenic process (Nishizuka, 1986). Recently, PK-C has been implicated in the mediation of many phorbol ester-promoted actions, such as ornithine decarboxylase (ODC) induction and EGF receptor down regulation (Jetten and Shirley, 1986). Membrane-bound activated PK-C may transmit to the nucleus a signal to increase gene (e.g., the ODC gene) transcription. PK-C may indirectly regulate gene expression by phosphorylating proteins such as histones and may also modulate oncogene (e.g., c-myc) expression. In contrast, PK-C's control of cell response to EGF is accomplished directly by the nontranscriptional actions of phosphorylating the EGF receptor and possibly by inhibiting internalization of EGF (Jetten and Shirley, 1986).

Recent research by Cope and others supports the theory that retinoids modulate PK-C activity (Cope et al., 1986). Retinoids do not directly affect phorbol ester binding to its receptor, PK-C, however, the precise way retinoids interact with PK-C at the molecular level is not known. Cope's studies of mouse-brain PK-C suggest an exciting idea of how this interaction may work. They have shown that whereas unbound retinoid-binding proteins (Apo-cRABP and Apo-cRBP) are substrates for PK-C, the holo-forms (e.g., retinoic acid-cRABP) inhibit PK-C activity. Cope also showed that the regulation of PK-C alters phosphorylation of the retinoid-binding proteins (RBPs) and other specific cytosolic and membrane substrates, which could explain the myriad reported retinoid actions, which includes their antagonism toward phorbol esters and synergistic activity with other agents, such as antiestrogens and selenium (O'Brian et al., 1986; Su et al., 1986).

ANIMAL CANCER-PREVENTION MODELS

Two-Stage Model

The best-studied model of the multistep process of chemical carcinogenesis is the two-stage carcinogenesis system first established in the mouse skin model and later shown to apply to many other model systems including bladder, lung, and mammary gland carcinogenesis in experimental animals and cell cultures (Lotan, 1980; Bollag, 1983; Bertram, 1987). The initiation phase is irreversible and occurs with only a single application of the carcinogen at a subthreshold dose. The promotion phase is a multistep process requiring repetitive promotor treatments after initiation and is initially reversible. At some point during the promotion phase, the process becomes irreversible and enters the progression phase. This two-stage system is valuable for investigating the potential effects of carcinogenesis inhibitors on both initiation and promotion. Primary prevention of neoplastic disease involves decreasing or eliminating the exposure to recognized initiating agents (e.g., cigarette smoking). The radical-trapping antioxidant action of β-carotene may act to prevent the initiation phase. Secondary prevention involves active dietary, pharmacologic, or educational intervention after an individual has been exposed to initiators or promoters but has not yet developed histologically identifiable preneoplastic changes. Tertiary prevention involves the use of dietary or pharmacologic inhibitors in situations where histologically identifiable preneoplastic changes have already developed (Bertram et al., 1987).

Unequivocally, retinoids prevent cancer in the skin, breast, bladder, lung, and other sites in experimental animals. Studies employing the mouse skin carcinogenesis model have supplied most of the preclinical evidence for retinoids' effects in the prevention of skin cancer (Lotan, 1980; Bollag, 1983; Gensler and Bowden, 1984; Boutwell et al., 1985; Bertram et al., 1987). Davies (1967) was the first investigator to show that vitamin A supplementation in mice could reduce the number and induce regression of DMBA-induced papillomas. Bollag (1979, 1983) amplified Davies' data through a series of studies in which he administered all-*trans*-retinoic acid intragastrically during the promotion phase of mouse skin carcinogenesis. He achieved a reduction of papilloma and carcinoma multiplicity and a decrease in the incidence of carcinoma. By retarding papilloma growth and enhancing its regression, Bollag inferred that retinoic acid not only prevented carcinogenesis but also had a therapeutic effect. In other experiments, he delayed administration of the natural retinoid until after the appearance of several well-established papillomas and still achieved regression, thus confirming the drugs' therapeutic activity. Bollag went on to develop the standard mouse skin assay systems for testing the therapeutic indexes of synthetic retinoids, which can be administered at pharmacological doses (Bollag, 1979, 1983).

Elaborating on work by Shamberger, Boutwell et al. (1985) pursued a large series of studies into the effects of topical synthetic and natural retinoids on skin tumor promotion. Boutwell's group demonstrated that the induction of epidermal ornithine decarboxylase (ODC) activity by tumor-promoting agents is a critical, possibly obligatory feature of skin tumor promotion and showed further that the topical application of retinoic acid 1 hour prior to applying the promotor TPA (12-0-tetradecarnoyl-phorbol-13-acetate) markedly inhibited the onset of TPA-induced ODC activity. Further tests demonstrated that several other natural and synthetic retinoids when topically applied also inhibited TPA-induced ODC activity and that this inhibition correlated with each retinoid's inhibitory effect on skin tumor promotion. Skin carcinogenesis initiated by the carcinogen DMBA (7,12-dimethylbenz[a]-anthracene) alone, however, does not respond to retinoic acid, either in inhibition of ODC induction or prevention of skin papillomas. Although the effects of retinoids on ultraviolet (UV) radiation-induced skin carcinogenesis are not clearly understood, some studies indicate that retinoic acid can enhance UV tumorigenesis (Lichti et al., 1981). What is clear, however, is that retinoic acid and other natural and synthetic retinoids inhibit two-stage phorbol ester-promoted carcinogenesis of the skin.

Many of the most salient features of retinoids' preventive effects were illustrated by Moon's studies of chemical carcinogenesis in rat mammary glands. Moon et al. (1983) initiated mammary cancer in rats with DMBA and found that those rats treated with 2.5 mg of retinyl acetate per day had 52% less cancer than those receiving a placebo diet. The authors later showed that retinoid added to the diet for a limited period of time—from two weeks before until 1 week after exposure to the initiating carcinogen (DMBA or MNU)—achieved a significant inhibition of carcinogenesis. Although continuous therapy with retinoid was needed when supplementation began after carcinogen exposure, the therapy could be delayed for 16 weeks after initiation and still retain its protective antipromoting effect. At a dietary concentration of 1 mmol/kg, retinyl acetate reduced the incidence and mean tumor number and prolonged the latency of rat mammary cancer. Delaying retinoid administration for $\geq$ 20 weeks resulted in a loss of cancer-preventive activity in this model. Subsequent studies confirmed these results and also revealed the efficacy of 4-HPR in preventing this cancer (Moon et al., 1985). Almost as effective as retinyl acetate, 4-HPR is considerably less toxic, which should be of great benefit for long-term treatment. All these retinoid effects are species specific (effective in rats but not in mice), retinoid specific (13-*cis*-retinoic-acid was ineffective), and carcinogen specific (4-HPR was more effective in DMBA-induced than in MNU-induced tumors). Tumor inhibition can be augmented when retinoid treatment is combined in this model system with other preventive modalities. Currently the most promising combined modality involves the interaction between hormonal manipulation and retinoids. Either ovariectomy or bromocriptine (a pituitary prolactin inhibitor) combined with either retinyl acetate or 4-HPR was significantly more effective than either regimen alone in rat mammary cancer prevention (Moon et al., 1985). Similarly, combining 4-HPR or retinyl acetate and the antiestrogen tamoxifen was synergistic in preventing rat mammary carcinogenesis.

Bladder carcinoma in experimental animals has been shown clearly to develop through a multistage process, which includes initiation, promotion, and propagation. In studies of bladder cancer, vitamin A deficiency causes the development of squamous metaplasia and increases susceptibility to chemical carcinogenesis. In 1977, Sport et al. were the first investigators to demonstrate the efficacy of retinoids (i.e., 13-*cis*-retinoic-acid) in decreasing the incidence and severity of bladder carcinoma. Although Sporn started 13-*cis*-retinoic-acid (13cRA) one week after completing carcinogenic exposure, Becci et al. (1979) later showed that 13cRA could be delayed up to nine weeks after carcinogenic exposure and still be efficacious. Results in this model system are analogous in several respects to results in the rat mammary model: (1) these results indicate that retinoid exposure can be effective when started within a fairly broad time spectrum during the promotion phase; (2) the retinamides, e.g., 4-HPR, had the highest therapeutic ratios; and (3) bladder studies revealed that with time, the retinoid restraint was overcome despite continued therapy, and the incidence of cancer eventually reached the same level as with controls (Hicks et al., 1985). However, treated rats had on average significantly prolonged life spans, which if extrapolated into human terms may correspond to a 5–10-year increase in symptom-free life for the patients (generally elderly) at highest risk of developing recurrent bladder cancer. Furthermore, retinoids appeared to be more effective in inhibiting tumor incidence following a higher dose of carcinogen exposure. Although most retinoids are effective in the promotion/progression phase, etretinate most effectively inhibited BBN-induced rat bladder cancer before carcinogen exposure, not during or after.

These three and many other animal carcinogenesis models clearly document in a controlled experimental setting that retinoids can be powerfully active in the prevention of cancer. A vast amount of data from in vitro work with transformed human and animal cell lines also substantiates the anticancer activity of retinoids. Both the animal model and transformed cell line studies provide a strong part of the rationale for using retinoids to treat established malignancies. Although not as clear-cut, several epidemiological studies also support retinoids for human cancer prevention.

Preclinical Screening

In addition to defining the two-stage model of carcinogenesis, animal models have been used extensively for preclinical screening. The most widely employed methods for retinoid screening are Bollag's mouse papilloma assay and Sporn's hamster tracheal organ culture system. First described in 1947, the mouse papilloma assay has undergone many subsequent variations, including Bollag's (Bollag, 1979, 1983; Lippman et al., 1987). All of the mouse assays exploit three well-studied retinoid effects on experimental skin carcinogenesis, including: (1) inhibition of the primary development of mouse skin papillomas initiated by DMBA and promoted by TPA; (2) regression of the papillomas once they have developed; and (3) suppression of the progression of benign skin papilloma to frank carcinoma. Bollag's standard assay measures the ability of retinoids to cause regression of established carcinogen-induced papillomas. Using this assay, Bollag has defined the therapeutic index of a drug in terms of the ratio between the daily intraperitoneal dose causing a defined degree of hypervitaminosis A in a 14-day study and the intraperitoneal dose causing 50% regression of all papillomas. The hamster tracheal organ culture assay measures the ability of retinoids to reverse the keratinization of the squamous metaplasia occurring in vitamin A-deficient hamster trachea (Lippman et al., 1987).

Although these screens have been predictive of efficacy for malignant epithelial disorders, additional systems are needed for screening retinoids' effects on other tissue types and disease states. It would be unfortunate if we failed to identify retinoids that could be effective in nonepithelial diseases simply because we relied exclusively on one or two epithelial-oriented screens. Therefore, many other experimental systems have been explored for retinoid activity. These include in vitro cell culture, in vitro organ culture, and in vivo approaches (Lippman et al., 1987). Interest is growing in the site-specific screening of retinoids' growth-inhibition and differentiation-inducing activity in many murine and human transformed cell lines, the most notable of which are F9, HL-60, melanoma, neuroblastoma, leukemic, and breast cell lines (Lotan, 1980; Bollag, 1983; Jetten, 1984; Sporn and Roberts, 1984; Sidell and Horn, 1985; Sporn et al., 1986; Tobler et al., 1986). These evaluate retinoids by themselves and in combination with hormones, cytotoxic agents, and/or other biological modifiers.

EPIDEMIOLOGY

Since vitamin A is critical to epithelial cell growth and differentiation in vitro and in vivo, there has been great interest in epidemiologic studies of vitamin A and cancer. An estimated 35% of U.S. cancers are due to dietary factors and over 90% of all human cancers are of epithelial origin. Evidence from several epidemiologic studies suggests the possibility that a relationship exists between dietary intake and serum levels of vitamin A and cancer risk. Unfortunately, dietary studies do not clearly distinguish between the relative protective effects of retinol and carotenoids (which the body converts in part to retinol—see introduction) (Wolf, 1984). Also, a positive risk relationship with serum retinol levels has not been uniformly reported, and some unconfirmed studies even indicate that retinoids may increase risk in some cancers. This discussion focuses on epidemiological studies of lung cancer, as this is the best-studied cancer and serves as a prototype for the limited studies of other malignancies.

There are six major types of epidemiologic studies in this area: (1) ecological dietary studies relating variations in diet to cancer rates, (2) case-control dietary studies of patients with diagnosed cancers which use "recall" or questionnaire methods to quantitate foods "rich in vitamin A," (3) prospective or cohort dietary studies, (4) dietary studies with supplementary pills with a known vitamin A content, (5) correlation between serum levels and disease in patients with established diagnoses of cancer, and (6) correlation between serum retinol levels taken from apparently healthy individuals and the subsequent development of cancer. Different ecological studies have yielded conflicting results (Rittenbaugh and Meyskens, 1986). For example, studies from Japan showed an inverse correlation between vitamin A intake and certain cancers, however, large studies from Hawaii and China failed to confirm this finding. Case-control dietary studies from England, Buffalo (NY), New Jersey, New Mexico, and Hawaii indicated an inverse correlation between vitamin A and lung cancer (Rittenbaugh and Meyskens, 1986; Bertram et al., 1987), especially in populations with marginal intake of vitamin A. The relative importance of carotenoids versus retinol is especially difficult to sort out with this retrospective study design. In 1975, Bjelke reported the first prospective study showing an inverse relationship between vitamin A intake and lung cancer. Over the succeeding 12 years, several other follow-up studies have been reported, including those conducted in Chicago (Western Electric), Boston, Norway, and Japan (Rittenbaugh and Meyskens, 1986). Several of these suggest a relatively greater protective effect with vegetables (carotenoids) than with preformed vitamin A, although this result is still questioned (Bertram et al., 1987). Dietary vitamin A supplementation (pills) may modestly increase serum retinol levels, but it remains questionable whether this effect provides protection against lung cancer, especially when the level varies only within the physiologic range.

Eleven reported series have attempted to correlate retinol levels of serum (stored samples) with the development of lung cancer many years later (Peto et al., 1981; Basu et al., 1984; Peleg et al., 1984; Willett et al., 1984; Menkes et al., 1986; Rittenbaugh and Meyskens, 1986; Bertram et al., 1987). Reported in 1980 and 1981, the first two studies were conducted in England and Evans County, Georgia, and indicated a strong inverse relationship between serum retinol and the development of lung cancer. Although highly quoted, these positive studies are supported by only two other studies. On the other hand, seven subsequent negative studies including another study from Evans County show only an insignificant trend correlating low serum retinol with lung cancer development (Peleg et al., 1984). Also negative was a study by Menkes et al. in Washington County, Maryland, (Menkes et al., 1986) in which low levels of β-carotene (but not preformed vitamin A) correlated with the development of squamous cell cancer of the lung. These conflicting results have caused some confusion (Rittenbaugh and Meyskens, 1986; Bertram et al., 1987). The differences may reflect different histologic cancer subtypes (e.g., squamous cell and adenocarcinoma), small patient numbers not allowing site-specific comparisons, other covarying micronutrients (e.g., selenium and zinc) or factors such as sex, age, and smoking. Willett et al. initially reported no association between serum retinol and the development of lung cancer, although a highly interesting follow-up publication on subgroup analysis suggested a correlation existed in patients with serum levels simultaneously low in retinol and selenium (Willett et al., 1984).

Beginning with Abels' classic report in 1941 (Abels et al., 1941), several studies, including recent comprehensive reviews of the field by Peto et al. (1981) and Basu et al. (1984), also have observed low plasma retinol levels in patients with established diagnoses of lung cancer. These studies are difficult to interpret because the effect of the malignancy on a patient's general nutritional status and the metabolism of vitamin A is unknown.

Case-control epidemiologic studies linking nutritional intake with risk of cancer suffer the difficulty of obtaining information from personal history and then trying to translate food intake into nutrients from the existing food tables, which may be quite faulty. Carcinogenic agents (e.g., smoking and dietary initiators and promotors such as saturated fats) and anticarcinogenic factors (e.g., interactive micronutrients such as selenium) are also difficult to specifically quantify in dietary studies. Some of the epidemiologic associations are supported by laboratory findings and current understanding of vitamin A metabolism, and others have no laboratory correlations as yet. For example, the mechanism controlling blood levels of vitamin A, the relation of these levels to those in target tissues, and possible cancer-induced modifications are factors only beginning to reveal themselves in laboratory studies.

Since the epidemiologic and laboratory work alone will never firmly establish this link, carefully controlled, randomized intervention trials are required to establish the direct intake-risk relationship. These trials, however, are extremely expensive and require substantial evidence from laboratory scientists and epidemiologists before they can be initiated. If the association proves out, it will have a significant impact on the public's health and on public health policy. It may become desirable to assay for serum retinol levels and serum retinol-binding protein (which corresponds strongly with serum retinol) as part of general health exams in order to identify people with higher risks of developing cancer. Establishing the positive retinol-risk association would also promote developing safe methods, which don't currently exist, for increasing serum retinol levels and would promote defining the precise mechanism of action affecting the relationship of retinol to cancer risk.

INTERACTIONS WITH OTHER MICRONUTRIENTS

At least in part, the possible anticancer effects of dietary and serum levels of vitamin A depend on interactions with other micronutrients, which also help to confound the interpretation of epidemiologic studies. Our discussion of these interactions draws upon the work of Underwood, who has reviewed much of the work in this field (1984). The principal micronutrients shown to interact with vitamin A are selenium, zinc, vitamins E and C, and iron.

Both retinoic acid and selenium are effective cancer-preventive agents in animals (Bertram et al., 1987). Their mechanisms of action may be similar, especially with respect to their recently described effects on protein kinase-C (Cope et al., 1986; Su et al., 1986). In mice, dietary selenium supplementation enhances the accumulation of retinol in DMBA-induced tumor tissue (Peng et al., 1986). In 1981, two independent groups demonstrated that selenium added to the inhibitory effect of retinyl acetate on MNU- and DMBA-induced rat mammary carcinogenesis (Ip and Ip, 1981; Thompson et al., 1981). However, the results were less clear in a recent study of the inhibitory effects of 13cRA plus selenium in DMBA-induced leukoplakia and squamous cell carcinoma of hamster tongues (Goodwin et al., 1986). Although both agents produced inhibitory effects, the results were much better with 13cRA. The addition of selenium to 13cRA did not improve its efficacy. At the dose used, however, 13cRA produced significant toxicity. Further study with lower-dose 13cRA plus selenium may yield equivalent efficacy with reduced toxicity.

Several studies have indicated interactions between zinc and vitamin A at many levels of cellular activity. Some human enzyme systems requiring zinc are directly and indirectly critical to vitamin A metabolism. Zinc reportedly influences retinaldehyde reductase, which catalyzes the irreversible oxidation of retinaldehyde to retinoic acid. Indirectly, zinc may affect vitamin A in vivo through zinc-dependent enzymes, which may be involved in the synthesis of retinol carrier and cellular binding proteins. Some information is available about dietary zinc and vitamin A interactions in tumor-bearing animals. In a study of Morris Hepatoma 7800 growth, varying levels of dietary zinc and vitamin A were achieved in research animals (Knight et al., 1983). The least number of tumors occurred in animals on a diet deficient in zinc and either deficient or excessive in vitamin A. In contrast, tumor growth was highest in animals with diets high in zinc and low in vitamin A.

In vivo research suggests potentially important interactions between both vitamins E (tocopherols) and C and vitamin A. Some investigators believe that vitamin E has only a nonspecific antioxidant role in its disputed relationship with vitamin A. Vitamin E stabilizes membranes in vivo. Vitamin E deficiency shortens the survival time of erythrocytes and accelerates the depletion rate of liver stores of vitamin A. Tocopherols provide vitamin A and carotenoids with intraluminal protection from oxidation in mixed diets. This protection results in higher levels of hepatic vitamin A and, under certain circumstances, higher circulating levels also. Microscopic studies of the retina of vitamin E-deficient rats fed vitamin A-adequate or -deficient diets indicate that vitamin E protects retinol at a cellular level as well. Vitamin E may also reduce vitamin A toxicity (Besa et al., 1987). Vitamin A deficiency and excess appear to influence the hepatic synthesis of ascorbic acid, and ascorbic acid apparently acts as an antioxidant for hepatic vitamin A when the latter is in excess. Some unconfirmed reports in rats claim to demonstrate a direct association between vitamin A deficiency and ascorbic acid synthesis.

High levels of uncomplexed iron in the intestine may contribute to destruction of precursor and preformed vitamin A-active compounds, however, no in vivo data indicate that feeding high levels of inorganic iron speeds up vitamin A deficiency in the presence of inadequate dietary vitamin A. Studies of human volunteers have revealed that vitamin A deficiency produced the gradual onset of anemia and hypoferremia that responded to vitamin A but not to medicinal iron. Nutrition surveys commonly reveal an association between anemia and inadequate dietary vitamin A.

Epidemiologic studies of children in developing countries showed a parallel increase in hemoglobin and serum iron with increasing blood levels of vitamin A. Rat studies of the interaction between iron and vitamin A showed that iron absorption is not altered by vitamin A deficiency and that vitamin A appears to help mobilize stored iron and incorporate it into erythrocytes.

CLINICAL IMPLICATIONS OF MICRONUTRIENT INTERACTIONS

The recommended daily allowance (RDA) for vitamin A is set well above the level required for most people who ingest substantial amounts of animal protein in order to compensate amply for adverse nutrient interactions that could influence levels of vitamin A (Rittenbaugh and Meyskens, 1986). One can assume that micronutrient interactions with vitamin A-active compounds are similar in effect to interactions with the synthetic analogs, or retinoids. Differences in clinical responses to retinoid therapy may reflect varying levels of interactive micronutrients in patients with the same disease, and standard medical screening of patients in the future may include serum analyses of micronutrients that affect vitamin A in the body.

Table 1 Results of Human Cancer-Prevention Trials with Retinoids

Disease	Retinoid	Form	Daily dose	No. of evaluable pts.	CR	PR	Mixed, Minor or NR	Total CR + PR (%)	References
Actinic keratosis	Retinoic acid	Topical	NS	93	46	47	0	100	Belisario, 1972
	Retinoic acid	Topical	0.1–0.3%	60	24	47	9	85	Bollag and Ott, 1975
	Etretinate	Oral	1 mg/kg	46	35	8	3	93	Grupper and Beretti, 1983
	Etretinate	Oral	75 mg	44	10	27	7	84	Moriarty et al., 1982
	Etretinate	Oral	1 mg/kg	15	14	1	0	100	Watson, 1986
	Arotinoid	Oral	1 μg/kg	16	0	10	6	62	Kingston et al., 1983
Keratoacanthoma	Etretinate	Oral	0.5–2 mg/kg	9	6	3	0	100	See text page 259
	Isotretinoin	Oral	1.5–2 mg/kg	2	1	1	0	100	
Basal cell	Isotretinoin	Oral	1–2 mg/kg	3	3,NT	0	0	100	Peck et al., 1982
Epidermodysplasia verruciformis	Etretinate	Oral	0.5–1 mg/kg	12	1	11	0	100	See text page 260
Dysplastic nevi	Tretinoin	Topical	0.05%	3	0	3	0	100	Meyskens et al., 1986
	Isotretinoin	Oral	1 mg/kg	8	0	1	7	13	Meyskens et al., 1986

Oral leukoplakia	Isotretinoin	Oral	50–100 mg	24	0	21	3	87	Koch, 1978
	Etretinate	Oral	50–100 mg	24	0	22	2	91	Koch, 1978
	Tretinoin	Oral	50–100 mg	27	0	16	11	59	Koch, 1978
	Etretinate	Oral & topical	50 mg	24	7	13	4	83	Koch, 1981
	Etretinate	Oral	75 mg	21	5	10	6	71	Koch, 1981
	Etretinate	Oral	1 mg/kg	3	1	2	0	100	Cordero et al., 1981
	Tretinoin	Topical	0.1%	5	1	4	0	100	Rague et al., 1975
	Isotretinoin	Lozenge	3–10 mg	11	3	8	0	82	Shah et al., 1983
	Isotretinoin	Oral	2 mg/kg	24	2	14	8	67	Hong et al., 1986
Bronchial metaplasia	Isotretinoin	Oral	1–2.5 mg/kg	19	0	0	19	0	Saccomanno et al., 1982
	Etretinate	Oral	25 mg	30	3	23	4	87	Mathe et al., 1982
	Etretinate	Oral	25 mg	36	4	32	0	100	Misset et al., 1986
Laryngeal papillomatosis	Isotretinoin	Oral	1–2 mg/kg	6	3	1	2	66	Alberts et al., 1986
	Etretinate	Oral	1 mg/kg	42	28	11	3	93	Bichler, 1983
Cervical dysplasia	Tretinoin	Topical	0.05–0.2%	18	2	4	NS	33	Surwit et al., 1982
	Tretinoin	Topical	0.05–0.48%	36	12	23	1	97	Weiner et al., 1986
	Tretinoin	Topical	0.372%	20	10	NS	NS	50	Graham et al., 1986
	Retinyl acetate	Topical	3–18 mg	40	NS	NS	NS	NS	Romney et al., 1985
Myelodysplastic syndromes	Isotretinoin	Oral	2–125 mg/m2	15	0	5	10	33	Gold et al., 1983
	Isotretinoin	Oral	1 mg/kg	14	0	3	11	21	Greenberg et al., 1985

Table 1 (continued)

Disease	Retinoid	Form	Daily dose	No. of evaluable pts.	CR	PR	Mixed, Minor or NR	Total CR + PR (%)	References
Myelodysplastic syndromes (cont.)	Isotretinoin	Oral	100 mg/m^2	18	2	2	14	22	Besa et al., 1985
	Isotretinoin	Oral	20 mg/m^2	6	0	4	2	25	Kerndrup et al., 1986
	Isotretinoin	Oral	2.5–4 mg/kg	15	1	8	6	60	Picozzi et al., 1986
	Isotretinoin	Oral	100 mg/m^2	1	1	0	0	100	Abrahm et al., 1986
Urinary bladder	Etretinate	Oral	25–50 mg	5	1,NT	2	NS	60	Shaerer et al., 1982
	Isotretinoin	Oral	0.5 mg/kg	22	NS	NS	NS	NS	Bonney and Prout, 1980
	Etretinate	Oral	50 mg	40	0	20	20	50	Pedersen et al., 1984
	Etretinate	Oral	25–50 mg	15	0	11	4	73	Alfthan et al., 1983
	Etretinate	Oral	25–50 mg	14	0	4	4	29	Studer et al., 1984

NS, not stated; NT, no tumor recurrence

HUMAN CANCER PREVENTION STUDIES

Oral vitamin A (retinol) intervention trials in prevention and therapy at tolerable doses with natural vitamin A are currently nonconclusive (Munoz et al., 1985; Goodman, 1986). The immediate future of vitamin A in human cancer prevention and therapy may be with the use of synthetic retinoids with higher therapeutic ratios.

Because they accumulate preferentially in the skin, retinoids were most widely used initially to manage preneoplastic skin disease (Elias and Williams, 1981). Several types of premalignant skin lesions have shown substantial responses to retinoids. These include actinic keratosis, keratoacanthoma, basal cell carcinomas, epidermodysplasia verruciformis and dysplastic nevi. Although we will discuss the actual study data only briefly, a comprehensive account of numbers of patients, dosage schedules, routes of administration, and percentages and types of responses to the various drugs employed is presented in Table 1.

About 5% of actinic keratoses lesions, which commonly occur in Caucasians exposed to high levels of ultraviolet light, annually change to nonmelanomatous skin cancer. Local destructive procedures are the current standard therapy. Both typically applied retinoic acid cream and orally administered retinoids (etretinate and the arotinoid Ro 13-6298) have produced significant results with these lesions. In the six studies reported to date (Belisario, 1972; Bollag and Ott, 1975; Moriarty et al., 1982; Grupper and Berretti, 1983; Kingston et al., 1983; Watson, 1986), complete responses of 46% to topical and 49% to oral retinoids have been achieved. The drugs were generally well tolerated, with side effects consisting mainly of chelitis and scaling. These studies clearly demonstrate that retinoids are efficacious in treating actinic keratosis, although high posttherapy relapse rates indicate that subsequent retinoid therapy may be needed to prevent disease progression.

Capable of spontaneous regression or frank malignant change (especially when multiple lesions are present), keratoacanthomas are hyperkeratotic lesions similar morphologically to squamous cell carcinoma of the skin. In studies of 11 patients (5 with multiple lesions) who had not had spontaneous regression for many years, impressive responses occurred within 2 to 3 months of retinoid treatment and have been sustained for more than one year after therapy (Grupper and Berretti, 1983; Haydey et al., 1980; Levine et al., 1984; Pichler and Fritsch, 1984; Shaw and White, 1986; Verret et al., 1985).

Isotretinoin and etretinate have prevented the development of basal cell carcinoma of the skin in a limited number of patients. Their preventive effect appeared to depend, however, on continued maintenance therapy with an average dose of 1.5 mg/kg/day (Peck et al., 1982). Begun in 1984, the Arizona Cancer Center is conducting two phase III intervention studies (to accrue 2750 patients) to evaluate the efficacy of retinoids in the prevention of cutaneous neoplasia.

Epidermodysplasia verruciformis is an unusual disorder characterized by multiple flat, wartlike lesions beginning in childhood and developing into squamous cell skin cancers. These lesions usually contain the oncogenic human papilloma virus type 5. Although limited to several isolated case reports, the use of retinoids (in particular etretinate) has produced significant clinical improvement (Guilhou et al., 1980; Edelson et al., 1981; Jablonska et al., 1981; Lutzner et al., 1981; Kanerva et al., 1985). This improvement has occurred in some cases despite the persistence of the virus in the lesions. As in the other retinoid-responsive preneoplastic diseases discussed above, relapse in these patients follows reducing or discontinuing the drug.

The dysplastic nevus syndrome may occur either familially or sporadically and frequently undergoes malignant change to melanoma. Treatment with surgical excision applies only to patients with a limited number of lesions and may be of only temporary benefit. Results with topical 5FU therapy have been variable. We treated three patients with topical tretinoin (0.05%) (Meyskens et al., 1986). After 10-12 weeks, dysplastic histologic features underwent marked reduction, a result which has never been reported to occur spontaneously. Repeated skin biopsies from treated lesions showed changes to benign nevocellular nevi without dysplasia. These results are quite exciting and require further study with more patients to assess the actual efficacy of retinoids in the resolution of the dysplastic nevi and in preventing transformation of these nevi to melanoma.

Currently, several nondermatologic premalignancies, including oral leukoplakia, bronchial metaplasia, laryngeal papillomatosis, cervical dysplasia, myelodysplastic syndromes, and urinary bladder, are receiving more attention in retinoid trials. Results of these studies are also presented comprehensively in Table 1. Table 1.

Retinyl acetate and retinol have been effective in experimental animals and in human epidemiological leukoplakia studies. Precancerous leukoplakia lesions probably do not regress spontaneously and can be safely monitored, thus presenting an excellent opportunity for the six studies with retinoids involving a total of 163 patients and producing an overall response rate of 79% (12% complete response) (Raque et al., 1975; Koch, 1978; Cordero et al., 1981; Koch, 1981; Shah et al., 1983; Hong et al., 1986). In comparing etretinate to isotretinoin and to tretinoin, Koch (1978) achieved greater results with less toxicity using etretinate (91% response rate, 50% sustained remission, 46% relapse rate, and only 4% progression rate). Relapses occurred within 1 or 2 months after completion of therapy. Koch (1981) then compared results in a second study between oral etretinate alone and oral etretinate plus topical etretinate paste. Response rates were high in both groups, with relapses again occurring within 2 months of completing therapy. Positive results were also achieved in another etretinate study by Cordero et al. (1981) and in two studies involving isotretinoin administered orally (Shah et al., 1983; Hong et al., 1986). With isotretinoin, toxicity was generally acceptable and response rates were high (100% of evaluable patients in first study, 67% of drug-treated patients in second study), but relapses with lesion progression usually occurred within 2-3 months after therapy ended.

Positive epidemiological studies and the observations that vitamin A deficiency leads to bronchial squamous metaplasia (a precursor of lung cancer) and that vitamin A and its analogs can reverse these developments (Bjelke, 1975; Basu et al., 1954; Boutwell et al., 1985; Rittenbaugh and Meyskens, 1986; Bertram et al., 1987) generated several studies in patients with high risks of developing lung cancer (Mathe et al., 1982; Saccomanno, 1982; Misset, 1986). In 1986, Misset et al. conducted a study involving 40 heavy smokers. The index of metaplasia of patients treated with etretinate for six months showed a decrease from 34.5 to 26.96%. These results, in addition to the complete resolutions of metaplasia in four patients who had ceased smoking during therapy, demonstrate that retinoids may play an active role in reversing this disease.

Laryngeal papillomatosis is a proliferation of polyploid lesions on the vocal cords, which may precede squamous cell carcinoma. Interferon controls the disease in approximately 50% of patients, but unfortunately also has significant toxicity. We have used isotretinoin 1-2 mg/kg/day to treat six patients with recurrent progressive papillomatosis of the larynx (Alberts et al., 1986; Lippman et al., 1987b). Three patients achieved a complete remission. Bichler (1983) reported similar results, using etretinate 1 mg/kg/day in 42 patients. Twenty-eight, or 67%, achieved complete resolution of their disease. These results suggest that retinoids may be an effective and relatively nontoxic alternative to interferon or surgery for the treatment of this disorder.

Along with retinoids' ability to reverse preneoplastic epithelial proliferation in other areas of the body, the epidemiologic association of dietary deficiencies of vitamin A with cervical dysplasia and carcinoma suggested these drugs for treating these disorders in situ (Romney et al., 1981; Surwit et al., 1982; Meyskens et al., 1983; Romney et al., 1985; Graham et al., 1986; Weiner et al., 1986; Bertram et al., 1987). In an initial study at the Arizona Cancer Center (ACC), a collagen sponge and standard diaphragm were used to deliver tretinoin to the affected tissues, a method resulting in unacceptable vaginal toxicity (Surwit et al., 1982). Results were promising, however, and led to a phase-I study at the same institution in which the drug was delivered by a cervical cap (Meyskens et al., 1983). Of the high- and low-dose groups, those patients in the former showed a higher response rate (complete response = 45%), clearly demonstrating the efficacy of the retinoid. Two other studies have also produced significant results, including a phase-II study at the ACC employing tretinoin in 20 patients,

10 of which achieved a complete response and 9 of which remain disease-free more than 12 months posttherapy (Weiner et al., 1986). Although their clinical use in cervical dysplasia may be limited currently by the embriopathic potential of tretinoin and the availability of other successful modalities, retinoids have produced significant results in this disorder, and newer synthetic, less toxic analogues continue to be developed. These results will have important implications for the long-term management of cervical preneoplasia.

Approximately 40% of patients with myelodysplastic syndromes (MDS) progress to acute leukemia. Vitamin A deficiency leads to anemia in humans and reduced bone marrow precursors in animals. Both abnormalities revert to normal upon vitamin A replacement. These effects, along with the in vitro antiproliferative and differentiation-inducing activities of retinoids in preleukemic and myeloid leukemic cells (Lippman et al., 1978a), led to seven clinical retinoid studies in this disorder (Gold et al., 1983; Besa et al., 1985; Greenberg et al., 1985; Abraham et al., 1986; Kerndrup et al., 1986; Picozzi et al., 1986; Clark et al., 1987). An overall response rate of 38% (1) (four complete responses) and survival prolongation in certain MDS subtypes indicate the efficacy of isotretinoin in this disorder.

Data from many studies—in vivo animal models, in vitro and epidemiologic—suggested retinoids for treating bladder cancer (Sporn et al., 1977; Becci et al., 1979; Peleg et al., 1984; Hicks et al., 1985; Rittenbaugh and Meyskens, 1986; Bertram et al., 1987). In 1972, Evard and Bollag observed a prophylactic effect of tretinoin in human bladder papilloma. Five clinical trials have involved retinoid therapy following resection of superficial bladder tumors (Bonney and Prout, 1980; Shaerer et al., 1982; Alfthan et al., 1983; Pedersen et al., 1984; Studer et al., 1984), which normally recur in approximately 40–90% of cases without drug intervention. In several studies, mucocutaneous toxicity was a significant limiting factor. In two trials, however, prolonged low-dose etretinate appeared effective and compared well to therapy with intravesical cytotoxic agents (Alfthan et al., 1983; Studer et al., 1984). These results require a cautious reading, however, due to limited patient numbers and follow-up.

THERAPEUTIC ANTICANCER ACTIVITY

In addition to retinoids' recognized preventive effects, these agents have also shown antitumor activity in several clinical studies. The growing clinical experience with retinoid therapy in established malignancies totals 476 patients and includes significant results in cutaneous basal and squamous cell carcinoma, mucosis fungoides, and acute promyelocytic leukemia. Several other malignancies, including head and neck cancer, eccrine poroma, melanoma, and several other leukemias, have also been studied for responses to retinoids (Lippman et al., 1987b; Lippman et al., 1987c; Lippman et al., 1988).

Topical and systemic retinoids have been used to treat basal cell carcinoma. A total of 49 patients were treated in several different studies of topical retinoic acid, which produced 16 complete (33%) and 32 partial responses. Bollag's (Bollag and Ott, 1975) observations that therapeutic effect occurred after 6 to 8 weeks of treatment and that a significant number of patients recurred at 10-months follow-up were characteristic of all these topical studies. Three other studies totalling 55 patients employed oral retinoids, either isotretinoin or etretinate. Data from these studies are also promising with a 51% objective response rate, although complete and partial responses required maintenance therapy to prevent recurrences. This preliminary work has not yet defined optimal preparation, dose, and treatment schedules.

Retinoid treatment for cutaneous squamous cell cancer in humans has been limited. In vivo results in animals have been promising and 4 studies involving 14 patients (Lippman et al., 1987c) with advanced squamous cell cancer of the skin have also netted significant results (71% overall response rate). The retinoids were also well tolerated by these patients. These results are very encouraging since no standard effective systemic therapy for advanced or metastatic squamous cell carcinoma of the skin currently exists.

Primarily involving the skin for most of its natural history, mycosis fungoides is an uncommon T-cell lymphoproliferative disorder. Single-agent retinoid treatment of this disease with either isotretinoin, etretinate, or arotinoids includes 92 patients and has produced impressive results (Lippman et al., 1987b) with an overall response rate of 62%. Responses in these studies generally required maintenance retinoid treatment to avoid relapse.

Acute promyelocytic leukemia (APL) is the most promising leukemic disorder to undergo clinical retinoid trial. In general, extensive human in vitro and animal in vivo data encourage the use of retinoids in leukemia. In 1983, Flynn et al. described the first APL patient treated with isotretinoin. After a 2-week course, this patient demonstrated a marked elevation of his peripheral granulocyte count. In the small total of five cases studied, remarkable responses have been documented in four of these previously refractory patients (Lippman et al., 1987b).

SIDE EFFECTS AND LIMITATIONS

Although the synthetic retinoids have higher therapeutic ratios than those of the natural vitamin A compounds, serious side effects still exist with these synthetic drugs. They have a spectrum of toxicity similar to that of natural vitamin A, with predominantly mucocutaneous and musculoskeletal side effects and the major chronic toxicities of liver, serum lipids, skeletal, and teratogenic effects (Korner and Voilin, 1975; Windhorst and Nigra, 1982; Lippman et al., 1987b).

Differences in storage, distribution, and metabolism account, in part, for the differing degrees of toxicities of various retinoids. Compared to natural vitamin A, the synthetic retinoids tend to have less central nervous system and liver side effects. In contrast to most other anticancer drugs, retinoids have no myelosuppressive toxicity. Indeed, they can stimulate normal hematopoiesis. This property makes them particularly attractive for clinical use in combination with cytotoxic drugs.

In comparison to isotretinoin, etretinate has the following effects: (1) etretinate apparently produces fewer skeletal and lipid abnormalities; (2) recent evidence suggests it produces more liver-function test abnormalities, although prospective liver biopsy studies have not revealed consistent histopathologic effects; and (3) it may have more serious potential teratogenic effects due to its long half-life (80-100 days) compared to that of isotretinoin (12-20 hours).

FUTURE DIRECTIONS

Over 60 years ago, investigators first became excited about the potential for vitamin A in treating neoplastic disorders. Several epidemiologic studies did not establish definitively the link between cancer risk and dietary or serum levels of vitamin A. Limited by dietary methods, studies need design improvements so that the suspected relationship can be either discarded or affirmed. The latter case would facilitate identifying people at high risk of developing cancers and encourage researchers in their efforts to develop safe ways to increase serum levels of retinoids in deficient or high-risk populations. Epidemiologists and laboratory workers should also focus their work on clarifying the synergistic and/or inhibitory interactions between retinoids and other micronutrients so that individuals can be evaluated for cancer risk.

Although retinoids, especially the synthetics, have shown efficacy in several premalignancies and malignancies, their clinical use lags behind the in vitro and animal in vivo work, which has unequivocally established the activity of retinoids against many malignant cell types and tumors. Recent in vitro studies are accumulating a wealth of data about the structure-function relationships of retinoids and their effects on biological and biochemical regulation. This work should further define the many diverse actions of retinoids and clarify the apparently central role of PK-C in retinoids' mechanism of action. The availability of many in vivo and in vitro assay systems, including transformed cell lines, will certainly help to focus future clinical studies by revealing the precise sensitivities of premalignancies and malignancies to specific retinoids. The need for this research is underscored by Underwood's warning that clinical advances with retinoids will be limited until the "basic science base of understanding expands" (Underwood, 1984).

Since most retinoid-responsive neoplastic processes require long-term therapy to prevent tumors, the future of retinoids may depend less on screening for efficacy than on screening for toxic effects, as investigators search for drugs with high therapeutic indexes for long-term, low-dose therapy studies. The retinamides (e.g., 4-HPR) and highly potent arotinoids, which are third-generation retinoids, are extremely promising candidates for prevention, as well as for primary treatment. Further direction to clinical research is being provided by recent in vitro studies which have documented the additive and synergistic activity of retinoids with hormones, DNA-synthesis inhibitors, radiation therapy, and other biologic modifiers and micronutrients such as interferon, vitamin D_3 and selenium (Lippman et al., 1987a,b).

Many clinical areas show special promise for future studies with retinoids. Cutaneous (e.g., actinic keratoses, and basal and squamous cell carcinomas) and noncutaneous preneoplastic disorders (e.g., MDS, bronchial metaplasia, cervical dysplasia, and urinary bladder) and established malignancies (e.g., advanced squamous cell and basal cell carcinoma of the skin, mycosis fungoides, and leukemia) all require continuing clinical trials to unequivocally establish efficacy. Another area for future clinical study involves retinoids as adjuvant therapy, especially in head and neck cancer.

Although tremendous advances have been made since Wolbach and Howe's pioneering retinoid studies, still a number of questions remain to be answered by further in vitro research, and the clinical application for single-agent and combination retinoid therapies are only beginning to be determined. Retinoids and other differentiation agents and biologic modifiers will undoubtedly reward workers in the field with many exciting future discoveries.

REFERENCES

Abels, J. C., Gorham, A. T., Pack, G. T., Rhoads, C. P. (1941). Metabolic studies in patients with cancer of the gastrointestinal tract: I. Plasma vitamin A levels in patients with malignant neoplastic disease, particularly of the gastrointestinal tract. *J. Clin. Invest. 20*:749.

Abrahm, J., Besa, E. C., Hyzinski, M., Finan, J., Nowell, P., (1986). Disappearance of cytogenetic abnormalities and clinical remission during therapy with 13-cis-retinoic acid in a patient with myelodysplastic syndrome: Inhibition of growth of the patient's malignant monocytoid clone. *Blood 67*:1323.

Alberts, D. S., Coulthard, S. W., Meyskens, F. L., Jr. (1986). Regression of aggressive laryngeal papillomatosis with 13-cis-retinoic acid (Accutane). *J. Biol. Response Mod. 5*:124.

Alfthan, O., Tarkkanen, J., Grohn, P., Heinonen, E., Pryhonen, S., Saila, K. (1983). Tigason (etretinate) in prevention of recurrence of superficial bladder tumors. *Eur. Urol. 9*:6.

Basu, T. K., Chan, U., Fields, A. (1984). Vitamin A (retinol) and epithelial cancer in man. In *Vitamins, Nutrition, and Cancer*, Prasad, K. (Ed.). Basel, Karger, pp. 35–45.

Becci, P. J., Thompson, H. J., Grubbs, C. J., Brown, C. C., Moon, R. C. (1974). Effect of delay in administration of 13-cis-retinoic-acid on the inhibition of urinary bladder carcinogenesis in the rat. *Cancer Res. 39*:3141.

Belisario, J. C. (1972). Recent advances in topical cytotoxic therapy of skin cancer and pre-cancer. In *Melanoma and Skin Cancer*, Proceedings of the International Cancer Conference, Sydney, pp. 349–365.

Bertram, J. S., Kolonel, L. N., Meyskens, F. L., Jr. (1987). Rationale and strategies for chemoprevention of cancer in humans. *Cancer Res. 47*:3012.

Besa, E. C., Hyzinski, M., Nowell, P. C., Itri, L. M., Abrahm, J. (1985). Clinical trials and in vitro evaluation of 13-cis-retinoic acid in myelodysplastic syndrome (abstr.). *Proc. Am. Soc. Clin. Oncol. 4*:841C.

Besa, E. C., Abrahm, J. L., Nowell, P. C. (1987). Increased survival in myelodysplastic syndrome (MDS) patients on high dose long term 13 cis-retinoic acid (RA); decrease of RA toxicity with alpha-tocopherol (AT). *Proc. Am. Soc. Clin. Oncol. 6*:150.

Bichler, E. (1983). The role of aromatic retinoid in treatment of laryngeal keratinizing disorders and dysplasias. In *Proceedings of the 13th International Congress of Chemotherapy*, Spitzy, K. H., Karrer, K. (Eds.). Vienna, VH Egermann, pp. 201–229.

Bjelke, E. (1975). Dietary vitamin A and human lung cancer. *Int. J. Cancer 15*: 561.

Bollag, W. (1979). Retinoids and cancer. *Cancer Chemother. Pharmacol. 3*:207.

Bollag, W. (1983). Vitamin A and retinoids: from nutrients to pharmacotherapy in dermatology and oncology. *Lancet 1*:360.

Bollag, W., Ott, F. (1975). Vitamin A acid in benign and malignant epithelial tumors of the skin. *Acta Dermatovener (Stockholm) Suppl. 74*:163.

Bonney, W. W., Prout, G. R. (1980). AUA monograph, Vol. 1. Baltimore, Williams and Wilkins, pp. 170–171.

Boutwell, R. K., Verma, A. K., Takigawa, M., Loprinzi, C. L., Carbone, P. P. (1985). Retinoids as inhibitors of tumor promotion. In *Retinoids: New Trends in Research and Therapy*, Saurat, J. H. (Ed.). Basel, Karger, pp. 83–96.

Clark, R. E., Jacobs, A., Lush, C. J., Smith, S. A. (1987). Effect of 13-cis-retinoic acid on survival of patients with myelodysplastic syndrome. *Lancet 1*:763.

Cope, P. C., Howard, B. D., Boutwell, R. K. (1986). The in vitro characterization of the inhibition of mouse brain kinase-C by retinoids and their receptors. *Experientia 42*:1023.

Cordero, A. A., Allevato, M. A. J., Barclay, C. A., Traballi, Donatti, L. B. (1981). Treatment of lichen planus and leukoplakia with the oral retinoid Ro 10-9359. In *Retinoids: Advances in Basic Research and Therapy*, Orlando, C. E., Braun-Falco, O., Farber, E. M., Grupper, C. L., Polano, M. K., Schuppli, R. (Eds.). Berling, Springer-Verlag, pp. 273–278.

Davies, R. E. (1967). Effect of vitamin A on 7,12-dimethylbenz(α) anthracene-induced papillomas in rhino mouse skin: Part 1. *Cancer Res. 27*:237.

Edelson, Y., Berretti, B., Grupper, C. (1981). Treatment of epidermodysplasia verruciformis or multiple verrucae planae by oral aromatic retinoid (Ro 10-9359-Tigason). In *Retinoids: Advances in Basic Research and Therapy*, Orfanos, C. E., Braun-Falco, O., Farber, E. M., Grupper, L. L., Polano, M. K., Schuppli, R. (Eds.). Berlin, Springer-Verlag, pp. 401–405.

Elias, P. M., Williams, M. L. (1981). Retinoids, cancer, and the skin. *Arch. Dermatol. 117*:160.

Evard, J. P., Bollag, W. (1972). Konservative Behandlung der rezidivierenden Harnblasenpapillomatose mit Vitamin A Saure. Vorlaufige mitteilung. *Schweiz. med. Wschr. 102*:1880.

Flynn, P. J., Miller, W. J., Weisdorf, D. J., Artheur, D. C., Brunning, R., Branda, R. F. (1983). Retinoic acid treatment of acute promyelocytic leukemia: in vitro and in vivo observations. *Blood 62*:1211.

Gensler, H., Bowden, G. T. (1984). Influence of 13-cis-retinoic acid on mouse skin tumor initiation and promotion. *Cancer Lett. 22*:71.

Gold, B. J., Mertelsmann, R. H., Itri, L. M., Gee, T., Arlin, Z., Kempin, S., Clarkson, B., Moore, M. A. S. (1983). Phase I clinical trial of 13-cis-retinoic acid in myelodysplastic syndromes. *Cancer Treat. Rep. 67*:981.

Goodman, G. (1986). Phase II trial of retinol in patients with advanced cancers. *Cancer Treat. Rep. 70*:1023.

Goodwin, W. J., Jr., Bordash, G. O., Huijing, F., Altman, N. (1986). Inhibition of hamster tongue carcinogenesis by selenium and retinoc acid. *Ann. Otol. Rhinol. Laryngol. 95*:162.

Graham, V., Surwit, E. S., Weiner, S., Meyskens, F. L., Jr. (1986). Phase II trials of β-all-trans retinoic acid for cervical intraepithelial neoplasia delivered via a collagen sponge and cervical cap. *West. J. Med. 145*:192.

Greenberg, B. R., Durie, B. G. M., Barnett, T. C., Meyskens, F. L., Jr. (1985). Phase I-II study of 13-cis retinoic acid in myelodysplastic syndrome. *Cancer Treat. Rep. 69*:1369.

Grupper, C. H., Berretti, B. (1983). Cutaneous neoplasia and etretinate. In *Proc. 13th International Congress of Chemotherapy*, Spitzy, K. H., Karrer, K. (Eds.). Vienna, VH Egermann, pp. 201/24–27.

Guilhou, J. J., Malbos, S., Barneon, S., Habih, A., Baldet, P., Meynadier, J. (1980). Epidermodysplasia verruciformis (2 cases). Immunological study. *Ann. Dermatol. Venereol. 107*:611.

Haydey, R. P., Reed, M. L., Dzubow, L. M., Shupack, J. L. (1980). Treatment of keratoacanthomas with oral 13-cis-retinoic acid. *N. Engl. J. Med. 303*:560.

Hicks, R. M., Thurton, J. A., Chowaniec, J., Tomlinson, C. N., Gwynne, J., Nanora, K., Chrysostomou, E., Pedrick, M. (1985). Modulation of carcinogenesis in the urinary bladder by retinoids. In *Retinoids, Differentiation and Disease*, Nugent, J., and Clark, S. (Eds.). London, Pitman, pp. 168–182.

Hong, W. K., Endicott, J., Itri, L. M., Doos, W., Batsakis, J. G., Bell, R., Fofonoff, S., Byers, S., Atkinson, N., Vaughn, C., Toth, B., Kramer, A., Dimery,

I. W., Strong, S. (1986). 13-cis-Retinoic acid in the treatment of oral leukoplakia. *N. Engl. J. Med. 315*:1501.

Ip, C., Ip, M. (1981). Chemoprevention of mammary tumorigenesis by a combined regimen of selenium and vitamin A. *Carcinogenesis 2*:915.

Jablonska, S., Obalek, S., Wolska, H., Jarzabek-Chorzelska, M. (1981). Ro 10-9359 in epidermodysplasia verruciformis. Preliminary report. In *Retinoids Advances in Basic Research and Therapy*, Orfanos, C. E., Braun-Falco, O., Farber, E. M., Grupper, C. L., Polano, M. K., Schuppli, R. (Eds.). Berlin, Springer-Verlag, pp. 401–405.

Jetten, A. M. (1984). Modulation of cell growth by retinoids and their possible mechanisms of action. *Fed. Proc. 43*:134.

Jetten, A. M., Shirley, J. E. (1986). Action of retinoic acid on the diacylglycerol-induced ornithine decarboxylase activity, reduction of EGF binding and protein kinase C activation in rat tracheal epithelial 2C5 cells. *Exp. Cell Res. 166*:519.

Kanerva, L. O., Johansson, E., Niemi, K. M., Lauharanta, J., Salo, O. P. (1985). Epidermodysplasia verriciformis. Clinical and light- electron-microscopic observations during etretinate therapy. *Arch. Dermatol. Res. 278*:153.

Kerndrup, G., Bendix-Hansen, K., Pedersen, B., Ellegaard, J., Hokland, P. (1986). Primary myelodysplastic syndrome: Treatment of 6 patients with 13-cis retinoic acid. *Scand. J.Haematol. 36*:128.

Kingston, T., Gaskell, S., Marks, R. (1983). The effects of a novel potent oral retinoid (Ro 13-6298) in the treatment of multiple solar keratoses and squamouse cell epithelioma. *Eur. J. Cancer 19*:1201.

Knight, E., Adkins, J., Knight, E., Criss, W. E. (1983). The effect of dietary zinc and vitamin A on the growth of Morris Hepatoma 7800. *J. Nutr. Growth Cancer 1*:57.

Koch, H. F. (1978). Biochemical treatment of precancerous oral lesions: the effectiveness of various analogues of retinoic acid. *J. Max. Fac. Surg. 6*:59.

Koch, H. F. (1981). Effect of retinoids on precancerous lesions of oral mucosa. In *Retinoids: Advances in Basic Research and Therapy*, Orfanos, C. E., Braun-Falco, O., Farber, E. M., Grupper, C. L., Polano, m. K., Schuppli, R. (Eds.). Berlin, Springer-Verlag, pp. 307–312.

Korner, W. F., Vollin, J. (1975). New aspects of the tolerance of retinol in humans. *Int. J. Vitamin Nutr. Res. 45*:312.

Levine, N., Miller, R. C., Meyskens, F. L., Jr. (1984). Oral isotretinoin therapy: Use in a patient with multiple cutaneous squamous cell carcinomas and keratoacanthomas. *Arch. Dermatol. 120*:1215.

Lichti, U., Patterson, E., Hennings, H., Yuspa, S. H. (1981). Differential retinoic acid inhibition of ornithine decarboxylase induction by 12-O-tetradecanoylphorbol-13-acetate and by germicidal ultraviolet light. *Cancer Res. 41*:49.

Lippman, S. M., Kessler, J. F., Meyskens, F. L., Jr. (1987a). Retinoids as preventive and therapeutic anticancer agaents. Part I. *Cancer Treat. Rep. 71*:391.

Lippman, S. M., Kessler, J. P., Meyskens, F. L., Jr. (1987b). Retinoids as preventive and therapeutic anticancer agents. Part II. *Cancer Treat. Rep. 71*:493.

Lippman, S. M., Meyskens, F. L., Jr. (1987c). Treatment of advanced squamous cell carcinoma of the skin with isotretinoin. *Ann. Intern. Med. 107*:499.
Lippman, S. M., Kessler, J. F., Al-Sarraf, M., Alberts, D. S., Itri, L. M., Mattox, D., Von Hoff, D. D., Loescher, L., Meyskens, F. L., Jr. (1988). Treatment of squamous cell carcinoma of the head and neck with isotretinoin: A phase II randomized trial. *Invest. New Drugs 6*:13.
Lotan, R. (1980). Effects of vitamin A and its analogs (retinoids) on normal and neoplastic cells. *Biochem. Biophys. Acta 605*:33.
Lutzner, M. A., Blanchet-Bardon, C., Puissant, A. (1981). Oral aromatic retinoid (Ro 10-9359) treatment of two patients suffering with severe form of epidermodysplasia verruciformis. In *Retinoids*, Orfanos, C. E., Braun-Falco, O., Farber, E. M., Grupper, C. L., Polano, M. K., Schuppli, R. (Eds.). Berlin, Springer-Verlag, pp. 407–410.
Mathe, G., Guoveia, J., Hercend, T., Gros, F., Dorval, T., Hazon, J., Misset, J. L., Schwarzenberg, L., Ribaud, P., Lemaigre, G., Santelli, G., Reizenstein, P., Homasson, J. P., Gaillard, J. P., Angebault, M., Bonniot, J. P., Lededente, A., Marsac, J., Parrot, R., Pretet, S., Gaget, H. (1982). Correlation between precancerous bronchial metaplasia and cigarette consumption, the preliminary results of retinoid treatment. *Cancer Detect. Prev. 5*:461.
Menkes, M. S., Comstock, G. W., Vuilleumier, J. P., Helsing, K. J., Rider, A. A., Brookmeyer, R. (1986). Serum beta-carotene, vitamin A and E, selenium, and the risk of lung cancer. *N. Engl. J. Med. 315*:1250.
Meyskens, F. L., Jr., Graham, V., Chvapil, M., Dorr, R. T., Alberts, D. S., Surwit, E. A. (1983). A phase I trial of β-all-trans-retinoic acid delivered via a collagen sponge and a cervical cap for mild or moderate intraepithelial cervical neoplasia. *JNCI 71*:921.
Meyskens, F. L., Jr., Edwards, L., Levine, N. (1986). Role of topical tretinoin in melanoma and dysplastic nevi. *J. Am. Acad. Dermatol. 15*:822.
Misset, J. L., Mathe, G., Santelli, G., Gouveia, J., Homasson, J. P., Suore, M. C., Gaget, H. (1986). Regression of bronchial epidermoid metaplasia in heavy smokers with etretinate. *Cancer Detect. Prev. 9*:167.
Moon, R. C., McCormick, D. L., Mehta, R. G. (1983). Inhibition of carcinogenesis by retinoids. *Cancer Res. 43*:2469.
Moon, R. C., Mehta, R. G., McCormick, D. L. (1985). Retinoids and mammary gland differentiation. In *Retinoids, Differentiation and Disease*, Nugent, J., and Clark, S. (Eds.). London, Pitman, pp. 156–167.
Moriarty, M., Dunn, J., Darragh, A., Lambe, R., Brick, I. (1982). Etretinate in treatment of actinic keratosis: a double blind crossover study. *Lancet 1*:364.
Munoz, N., Wahrendorf, J., Bang, L. J., Crespi, M., Thurnham, D. I., Day, N. E., Ji, Z. H., Grassi, A., Yan, L. W., Ling, L. G. (1985). No effect of riboflavine, retinol, and zinc on prevalence of precancerous lesions of esophagus. Randomized double-blind intervention study in high-risk population of China. *Lancet 2*:111.
Nishizuka, Y. (1986). Studies and perspectives of protein kinase C. *Science 233*: 305.

O'Brian, C. A., Liskamp, R. M., Solomon, D. H., Weinstein, I. B. (1986). Triphenylethylenes: A new class of protein kinase C inhibitors. *JNCI 76*:1243.

Peck, G. L., Gross, E. G., Butkus, D., DiGiovanna, J. J. (1982). Chemoprevention of basal cell carcinoma with isotretinoin. *J. Am. Acad. Derm. 6*:815.

Pedersen, H., Wolf, H., Jensen, S. K., Lund, F., Hansen, E., Olsen, P. R., Sorenson, B. L. (1984). Administration of a retinoid as prophylaxis of recurrent noninvasive bladder tumors. *Scand. J. Urol. Nephrol. 18*:121.

Peleg, I., Heyden, S., Knowles, M., Hames, C. G. (1984). Serum retinol and risk of subsequent cancer: extension of the Evans County, Georgia, study. *JNCI 73*:1455.

Peng, Y. M., Alberts, D. S., Xu, M. J., Watson, R. R., Gensler, H. L., Bowden, G. T. (1986). Effects of high dietary retinyl palmitate and selenium on tissue distribution of retinoids in mice exposed to tumor initiation and promotion. *J. Nutr. Growth Cancer 3*:33.

Peto, R., Doll, R., Buckley, J. D., Sporn, M. D. (1981). Can dietary beta-carotene materiall reduce human cancer rates? *Nature 290*:201.

Pichler, E., Fritsch, R. (1984). Xeroderma pigmentosum: prevention of tumors with etretinate. *Hautarzt 35*:159.

Picozzi, V. J., Swanson, G. F., Morgan, R., Hecht, F., Greenberg, P. L. (1986). 13-cis Retinoic acid treatment for myelodysplastic syndromes. *J. Clin. Oncol. 4*;589.

Raque, C. J., Biondo, R. V., Keeran, M. G., Honeycutt, W. M., Jansen, G. T. (1975). Snuff dippers keratosis (snuff-induced leukoplakia). *Southern Med. J. 68*:565.

Rittenbaugh, C. K., Meyskens, F. L., Jr. (1986). Analysis of dietary associations of vitamin A with cancer. In *1986 A Year in Nutritional Medicine*, Bland, J. (Ed.). New Canaan, Keats, pp. 264–291.

Romney, S. L., Palan, P. R., Duttagupta, C., Wassertheil-Smoller, S., Wylie, J., Miller, G., Slagle, N. S., Lucido, D. (1981). Retinoids and the prevention of cervical dysplasias. *Amer. J. Obstet. Gynecol. 141*:890.

Romney, S. L., Dwyer, A., Slagle, S., Duttagupta, C., Palan, P. R., Basu, J., Calderin, S., Kadish, A. (1985). Chemoprevention of cervix cancer: Phase I-II: A feasibility study involving the topical vaginal administration of retinyl acetate gel. *Gynecol. Oncol. 20*:109.

Saccomanno, G., Moran, P. G., Schmidt, R. D., Hartshorn, D. F., Brian, D. A., Dreher, W. H., Sowada, B. S. (1982). Effects of 13-cis retinoids on premalignant and malignant cells of lung origin. *Acta Cytol. 26*:78.

Schaerer, R., Swiercz, P., Mousseau, M., Chabert, C. (1982). Is acid aromatic vitamin A (etretinate or "Tigason") active in low grade malignant bladder carcinoma? *Cancer Chemother. Pharmacol. 9* (Suppl): 50.

Shah, J. P., Strong, E. W., DeCosse, J. J., Itri, L., Sellers, P. (1983). Effect of retinoids on oral leukoplakia. *Am. J. Surg. 146*:466.

Shaw, J. C., White, C. R. (1986). Treatment of multiple keratoacanthomas with oral isotretinoin. *J. Am. Acad. Dermatol. 15*:1079.

Sidell, N., Horn, R. (1985). Properties of human neuroblastoma cells following induction by retinoic acid. *Prog. Clin. Biol. Res. 175*:39.

Sporn, M. B., Squire, R. A., Brown, C. C., Smith, J. M., Wenk, M. L., Springer, S. (1977). 13-cis-Retinoic acid: inhibition of bladder carcinogenesis in the rat. *Science 195*:487.

Sporn, M. B., Roberts, A. B. (1984). Role of retinoids in differentiation and carcinogenesis. *JNCI 73*:1381.

Sporn, M. B., Roberts, A. B., Roche, N. S., Kagechika, H., Shudo, K. (1986). Mechanism of action of retinoids. *J. Am. Acad. Dermatol. 15*:756.

Studer, U. E., Biedermann, C., Chollet, D., Karrer, P., Kraft, R., Toggenburg, H., Vonbank, F. (1984). Prevention of recurrent superficial bladder tumors by oral etretinate: preliminary results of a randomized, double blind multicenter trial in Switzerland. *J. Urol. 131*:47.

Su, H. D., Shoji, M., Mazzei, G. J., Vogler, W. R., Koo, J. F. (1986). Effects of selenium compounds on phospholipid/Ca^{2+}-dependent protein kinase (protein kinase C) system from human leukemic cells. *Cancer Res. 46*:3584.

Surwit, E. A., Graham, V., Droegemueller, W., Alberts, D., Chvapil, M., Dorr, R. T., Davis, J. R., Meyskens, F. L. (1982). Evaluation of topically applied trans-retinoic acid in the treatment of cervical intraepithelial lesions. *Am. J. Obstet. Gynecol. 143*:821.

Thompson, J. J., Meeker, L. D., Becci, P. J. (1981). Effect of combined selenium and retinyl acetate treatment on mammary carcinogenesis. *Cancer Res. 41*:1413.

Tobler, A., Dawson, M. I., Koeffler, H. P. (1986). Retinoids: structure-function relationship in normal and leukemic hematopoiesis in vitro. *J. Clin. Invest. 78*:303.

Underwood, B. A. (1984). Summary of research needs. *JNCI 73*:1489.

Underwood, B. A. (1984b). Vitamin A in animal and human nutrition. In *The Retinoids*, Vol. 1, Sporn, M. B., Roberts, A. B., Goodman, D. S. (Eds.). New York, Academic Press, pp. 281–392.

Verret, J. L., Schnitzler, L., Anevel, M., Smulevicci, L. (1985). Etretinate and skin cancer prevention. In *Retinoids: New Trends in Research and Therapy*, Saurat, J. H. (Ed.). Basel, Karger, pp. 355–359.

Watson, A. B. (1986). Preventative effect of etretinate therapy on multiple actinic keratoses. *Cancer Detect. Prev. 9*:161.

Weiner, S. A., Surwit, E. A., Graham, V. E., Meyskens, F. L., Jr. (1986). A phase I trial of topically applied trans-retinoic acid in cervical dysplasia—clinical efficacy. *Invest. New Drugs 4*:241.

Willet, W. C., Polk, B. F., Underwood, B. A., Hames, C. G. (1984). Hypertension detection and follow-up program study of serum retinol, retinol-binding protein, total carotenoids, and cancer risk: a summary. *JNCI 73*:1459.

Windhorst, D. B., Nigra, T. (1982). General clinical toxicology of oral retinoids. *J. Am. Acad. Dermatol. 6*:675.

Wolbach, S. B., Howe, P. R. (1985). Tissue changes following deprivation of fat soluble A vitamin. *J. Exp. Med. 42*:753.

Wolf, G. (1984). Multiple functions of vitamin A. *Physiol. Rev. 64*:873.

10
β-Carotene, Canthaxanthin, and Phytoene

MICHELINE M. MATHEWS-ROTH
Harvard Medical School and Brigham and Women's Hospital, Boston, Massachusetts

Carotenoid pigments have a recognized role in the prevention of photosensitization in photosynthetic organisms, both unicellular and multicellular (Krinsky, 1968, 1971). This protective function has been utilized in the administration of carotenoid pigments to patients with the human photosensitivity disease, erythropoietic protoporphyria (EPP) (Mathews-Roth, 1982a, 1984a, 1986a); pigment administration prevents the characteristic photosensitivity reactions associated with this disease.

Reports appearing over the past 30 years in the scientific literature of the antitumor effects of vitamin A in animal models have generated interest in determining whether the precursors of vitamin A, the carotenoid pigments, have any antitumor activity of their own. In this chapter, we will review the studies dealing with carotenoids as cancer-preventive agents.

CAROTENOIDS AND CANCER PREVENTION

Animal Evidence for the Anticancer Activity of Carotenoids

In view of the success of vitamin A in suppressing tumor development in animals, it is not surprising that investigations were done to see if β-carotene, the precursor of vitamin A, had an antitumor effect. In 1973, Dorogokupla et al. induced subcutaneous tumors in rodents by injecting and topical application of 9,10-dimethyl-1,2-benzanthracene (DMBA). The authors found in both cases that animals fed a diet supplemented with "unlimited amounts of red carrots" developed tumors at a slower rate than did the animals receiving the unsupplemented diet. In that year also, Epstein (1973) reported inducing skin tumors by exposing hairless mice to ultraviolet (UV-B) radiation (290-320 nm) and found that those mice that received injections of a solution of β-carotene beadlets (Roche) developed tumors at a slower rate than did mice injected with a solution of placebo beadlets. Dorogokupla et al. (1973) proposed that the effect of β-carotene on tumor formation was due to the effect of vitamin A, which was formed from the administered β-carotene.

To determine whether or not the carotenoid molecule itself has an antitumor action, we decided to study the effects on tumor formation of two other carotenoids which have no vitamin A activity. Canthaxanthin (4,4′-diketo beta-carotene), which cannot be converted to vitamin A by mammals and which has been found to be effective in preventing photosensitization both in vitro and in vivo, and phytoene (7,8,11,12,7′,8′,11′,12′-octahydro lycopene), which we have found to have protective activity against sunbern, were studied (Mathews-Roth, 1980, 1982b). We examined the effects of these two pigments and of β-carotene on the development in hairless mice of skin tumors induced by three different methods: (1) UV-B radiation three times a week, (2) two applications of DMBA followed by twice-weekly applications of croton oil, and (3) one application of DMBA followed by UV-B radiation twice a week. We found that administration of β-carotene, canthaxanthin, or phytoene resulted in a statistically significant delay in the appearance of skin tumors induced by UV-B radiation. We also found that β-carotene and canthaxanthin had some effect in delaying the appearance of subsequent tumors when the administration of these pigments was started after one tumor had developed (Mathews-Roth, 1983). However, in the case of DMBA-croton oil tumor induction, only β-carotene was effective in delaying tumor development—canthaxanthin and phytoene had no such effect. With DMBA application and low-dose UV-B radiation, both β-carotene and canthaxanthin administration caused a delay in tumor development, but phytoene had no effect. In each case, when the administration of a given pigment caused a delay in tumor development, fewer tumors per animal were found in the pigment-treated mice as compared to the placebo-treated animals.

These experiments suggest that carotenoid pigments, irrespective of their vitamin A activity, can prevent or slow down the growth of skin tumors induced by UV-B alone. These experiments also suggest that the mechanism of tumor induction by DMBA-croton oil application must be different from that of UV-B radiation exposure. As to tumors produced by DMBA and low-dose UV-B radiation, canthaxanthin may not be able to affect initiation by DMBA but may have an effect on promotion or co-carcinogenesis by UV-B radiation. Phytoene, because of molecular differences between it and either β-carotene or canthaxanthin, may not be able to exert enough effect on the development of tumors induced by an agent other than UV-B. There are suggestions in the literature that excited species such as free radicals and singlet oxygen may be involved in the development of skin tumors induced by UV-B. It is interesting to note that β-carotene and canthaxanthin are extremely efficient quenchers of such species; phytoene is less so (Mathews-Roth et al., 1974a).

Our work has been confirmed and extended by Santamaria et al. (1983). These workers have reported that β-carotene and canthaxanthin administered orally to Swiss albino mice will delay the development of tumors induced by the application of benz(a)pyrene alone (BP) or BP plus UV-A radiation (320–400 nm). They have also found that these pigments will delay the development of skin tumors in hairless mice induced by the administration of 8-methoxy psoralen and UV-A radiation.

Seifter et al. have reported a series of experiments in which they have found that either vitamin A or β-carotene inhibits the size and/or development of transplanted tumors in mice (Rettura et al., 1982; Seifter et al., 1982, 1983). These workers also suggest that β-carotene and vitamin A administration prevent the involution of the thymus gland, which occurs when transplanted tumors take hold in the host. In addition, they have reported that administration of beta-carotene or vitamin A can decrease the incidence of DMBA-induced tumors in rats (Seifter et al., 1984). The kinds of tumors were not specified. In their studies they added β-carotene to the diet of the animals as an alcoholic solution of crystalline β-carotene. It is difficult to determine whether the added β-carotene and vitamin A survived oxidation and contributed significantly to the blood and tissue level of these substances.

In recent experiments, we have found that β-carotene or canthaxanthin at a dose of 100 mg/kg of diet, a bit higher than the 90 mg/kg of diet used by Seifter et al. (1982–1984), was not protective against tumors induced by UV-B radiation (Mathews-Roth and Krinsky, 1985). However, a dose of 3.5 mg carotenoid/5 g of diet, similar to the dose used by Santamaria et al. (1983), was protective. In all of our experiments we used β-carotene beadlets (Roche) as the source of our pigments. The beadlet formulation protects the pigments against oxidation. Indeed we could detect high levels of carotenoids in the skin of the treated animals (Mathews-Roth, 1982b, 1983, and unpublished observations). Analysis of the supplemented foods contained the specified amounts of pigments. Santamaria et al. also used Roche pigment beadlets as the source of carotenoids, as well as freshly prepared solutions of carotenoids in oil for supplemental gavage administration. In this latter case also, little deterioration of the pigments could have occurred.

The ability of carotenoid pigments to prevent the development of tumors other than skin tumors has also been studied. Alam et al. (1984) injected rats with DMBA in the submandibular salivary gland to induce tumors. The animals were divided into groups receiving β-carotene, retinoic acid, or no supplement in the diet. The authors found that the tumor incidence was "slightly lower" in the rats fed the diet supplemented with β-carotene; however, the difference was not statistically significant. Retinoic acid had no effect at all.

The experiments described to this point have been concerned with oral administration of carotenoids before and/or during tumor induction. Shamberger (1971) reported the effect of applying topical β-carotene to haired mice undergoing tumor induction with DMBA and croton oil or resin application. He found an increase of tumor formation in the animals which received β-carotene applications. It is difficult to know what happened to the β-carotene under these conditions of exposure to light and air. We have found that β-carotene applied topically to human skin bleaches quickly (Mathews-Roth et al., 1974). Shamberger's finding is also somewhat reminiscent of similar findings with topically applied vitamin A, in which some doses applied topically cause excess tumor formation and other dose levels were protective. In contrast to Shamberger's findings, a more recent report of topical application of β-carotene seems to have produced a protective effect (Suda et al., 1986). This pigment was found to significantly inhibit the formation of DMBA-induced squamous cell carcinomas of the hamster buccal pouch when applied topically on days alternate to the application of DMBA in mineral oil to the buccal pouch. The authors suggest that this action of β-carotene may be due to the induction of a tumor necrosis factor in macrophages (Schwartz et al., 1986). However, the authors have not reported that they analyzed either the tumors or the buccal pouch skin for the presence of β-carotene; thus, here again it is hard to know if β-carotene, or vitamin A, or another metabolite, or even an alteration of the DMBA by the β-carotene on the surface of the buccal pouch skin caused the inhibitory effect. Interestingly, in preliminary studies Abril et al. (1986) found that β-carotene stimulated maximal production of a tumor necrosis factor–like substance by mononuclear phagocytes in an in vitro system.

β-Carotene, canthaxanthin, and phytoene are all lipid-soluble carotenoids. Gainer et al. (1976) have been investigating the water-soluble carotenoid, crocetin, and found that this pigment, prepared by them from an extract of saffron, offered protection against DMBA-croton oil-induced tumors in haired mice. We repeated their experiments, but used hairless mice and crystalline crocetin produced synthetically. The route of administration, vehicle, and dose were those used by Gainer et al. We found only a small effect in delaying tumor development when tumors were induced with DMBA-croton oil applications. We found no effect in preventing the development of skin tumors induced by UV-B alone (Mathews-Roth, 1982c). The same amounts of radiation were used in these experiments as were used in the experiments mentioned above in which β-carotene, canthaxanthin, and phytoene had a protective effect against skin tumor formation. It is not totally clear why crocetin is not as effective as the other pigments. Perhaps the dose used was incorrect. Also, the molecular structure of crocetin differs from the other pigments, and the water solubility may affect where the pigments localize in the cell.

Lin and Wang (1986) studied a related pigment, crocin, and recently reported that this carotenoid can protect rats against the acute hepatic damage induced by the administration of aflatoxin B, and dimethylnitrosamine. Here also, the purity of the crocin, which was extracted from the fruit of *Gardenia jasminoides*, could be questioned; some other plant component might be involved in the protective effect. Their findings could be considered a sort of confirmation of those of Newberne et al. (1974), who found that β-carotene administration protected against the acute toxicity of aflatoxin and monocrotaline ingestion in the rat.

The several experiments reported here would suggest that the carotenoid molecule itself has some ability to prevent or delay the development of skin tumors induced by UV-B radiation and, in some cases, tumors induced by a chemical carcinogen (DMBA or BP) and promoted by UV-B or UV-A radiation. Certainly β-carotene should have some effect on the inhibition of tumors in organs other than skin, which have been shown to be inhibited by vitamin A. Carefully controlled experiments, where adequate dose levels of β-carotene are given, and carotenoid and vitamin A levels in the serum and target organs are measured, need to be performed to determine the antitumor spectrum of not only β-carotene but also other carotenoid pigments.

Human Studies

The reports of animal studies suggesting that vitamin A has antitumor activity have led to studies to determine whether vitamin A, or its precursor pigment in foodstuffs, β-carotene, has any such activity in human tumors.

There have been many reports in the literature of epidemiologic studies concerned with the effect of diet, particularly the ingestion of carotenoid-containing vegetables, on the incidence of cancer. The vast majority suggest that there is an inverse relationship between the ingestion of carotenoid-containing vegetables and the incidence of cancer. Most of the studies have been dietary studies. However, 12 studies analyzed the sera of cancer patients and control subjects, most finding a significantly lower level of serum carotenoids in the cancer patients. These epidemiologic studies have recently been listed and reviewed by the author (1986a), and Willett and Hunter review them in Chapter 4.

It is difficult to base conclusions of drug efficacy on dietary intake studies, because recall of specific food intake may be incomplete. Even studies examining serum levels of the compound of interest may be suspect in that control populations may not have been chosen properly. In addition, in dietary studies, there is always the possibility that the actual active compound may not be the component upon which interest is focused, but another component of the foods containing it. Even negative studies of either type do not necessarily mean that the compound of interest has no effect in preventing cancer. The compound may only be effective in certain types of cancer not yet tested or in subgroups of a population (such as people with low-normal or deficient blood levels of the compound).

The best way to determine whether a particular substance is effective in preventing human cancer is to administer it prophylactically to a large enough number of people at risk to develop the particular kind of cancer to be studied. The study population should be randomly assigned to either a group receiving the substance under study or a group receiving placebo. Indeed, the National Cancer Institute of the United States' National Institutes of Health is presently funding several studies in which β-carotene is administered in doses of 15–50 mg/day as various "beadlet" formulations to people at risk for developing certain kinds of cancer (Sestili, 1984). In each case, the study population is divided into groups receiving carotenoid and groups receiving placebo. That these intervention trials could be performed at this point in time is in part due to the findings of the studies on β-carotene administration to patients with EPP that there was no serious toxicity associated with the long-time ingestion of high doses of pure β-carotene. This fact had been inferred from observations on individuals developing carotenemia from overindulgence of carotenoid-containing fruits and vegetables, but the studies on porphyrics put this suggestion on a firm basis.

All of the β-carotene interventions are due to run for several years and may have to be extended beyond their originally planned periods, to assure that sufficient end points have been obtained. Thus it will take quite a few more years before it is definitely established whether or not β-carotene and/or vitamin A have a significant anticancer effect in humans.

Stich et al. (1984) recently reported a study in which they administered both β-carotene and retinol to betel nut and tobacco chewers. They found that this supplementation decreased the number of micronuclei in exfoliated buccal mucosa cells. Micronuclei are a measure of chromosome breaks: the numbers of micronuclei greatly increase on carcinogen administration. These workers have subsequently made a report that β-carotene alone can decrease the number of micronuclei in the buccal mucosa cells of snuff dippers and betel nut chewers (Stich et al., 1986). A long-term controlled trial should be performed to determine if carotenoid administration can prevent the development of oral cancer, an important problem in some developing countries.

A prime requirement for a cancer-prevention agent to be used in large numbers of healthy people is that it must have little or no toxicity. β-Carotene has proven to be very safe. Thus, if it is found that β-carotene is effective in preventing the development of one or more kinds of cancer, this pigment will be an extremely good candidate for use as a cancer-preventive agent in large populations. We eagerly await the results of the ongoing clinical studies described here and others which may also be undertaken in the near future.

SOME ASPECTS OF THE CLINICAL PHARMACOLOGY OF CAROTENOIDS

Role of β-Carotene in Human Nutrition

In spite of the current availability and use of synthetic vitamin A either in foods or in vitamin supplements, carotenoid vitamin A precursor-containing foods are still a very significant source of this vitamin in the diets of humans, particularly in developing countries. Diets in various parts of the world vary greatly in their content of vitamin A, either available directly in meat, fish, eggs, or dairy foods, or as the various provitamins A in vegetable sources. β-Carotene is the most important vitamin A precursor, mainly because of its prevalence in plants widely consumed by humans and livestock and because it has the greatest provitamin A activity (Thompson, 1965). In addition to availability in the diet, several factors such as severe dietary deficiency in protein, the amount, nature, and dispersion of dietary fat, and the nitrate content of the food may influence the absorption and utilization of β-carotene and other provitamins. The transformation of β-carotene to vitamin A (retinol) in the animal (plants do not contain vitamin A as such) occurs by cleavage of the carotene molecule at the central double bond (Olson, 1961; Goodman and Huang, 1966) or by cleavage of the conjugated chain adjacent to one β-ionone ring followed by sequential oxidative removal of fragments consisting of 2 to 5 carbon atoms (Glover, 1960). The activity of the enzyme carotene dioxygenase isolated from rat and human intestinal mucosa and also from liver seems to suggest that the cleavage of the molecule at the central double bond is the more important mechanism for metabolism of carotene in the mammal (Glover, 1960; Goodman, 1967, 1984).

Many studies have shown that the main point of conversion of ingested carotenoids is the intestinal mucosa. Conversion also occurs to a fairly significant degree in the liver. It was suggested that lung might also be a site of conversion, but data from heart-lung preparations have not confirmed this (Olson, 1964). Greenberg et al. suggested that sebaceous glands may convert β-carotene to vitamin A (Cornbleet and Greenberg, 1957; Greenberg et al., 1957, 1959).

Traditionally, it has been thought that only plants and bacteria can synthesize carotenoids from simple precursors (Goodwin, 1952). However, evidence has been presented that bovine corpus luteum tissue could synthesize β-carotene from acetate in vitro (Austern and Gawienowski, 1969). Further confirmation of this finding must be obtained before the present view of no carotenoid synthesis in animals can be abandoned.

The manner in which carotenoids are excreted is not clear. Hashimoto (1922) claims that none is excreted in the urine. Hess and Meyers (1919) found that urine because yellower within three quarters of an hour after giving concentrated carrot extract. Unfortunately, they did not chemically extract the urine to determine the presence of carotenoids. Almond and Logan (1942) made the same observation and attempted to chemically extract the urine. They extracted a yellow pigment, but this was found not to be β-carotene. We also looked for carotenoids in the urine of EPP patients taking carotene, and also found that the yellow pigment contained in the urine did not seem to be a carotenoid on spectrophotometric or chromatographic analysis. More work certainly needs to be done on the question of the excretion of carotenoids.

Toxicity Studies

The results of studies we have conducted on the patients with EPP treated with β-carotene and on the normal volunteers given similar doses of β-carotene for a 10-week period in our study on β-carotene and sunburn radiation (Mathews-Roth et al., 1972, 1974, 1977) have confirmed reports that the ingestion of large amounts of pure β-carotene has not led to toxic side effects (Niemann and Klein Obbink, 1954; Ostwald and Briggs, 1967). Some of our patients have been taking β-carotene for 15 years with no appearance to date of toxicity. We detected no abnormalities in blood sugar or blood urea nitrogen in either EPP patients or normal volunteers, nor have the other workers mentioned above who are using β-carotene in the treatment of EPP reported any serious toxicity attributable to β-carotene.

The complete blood count was not affected by carotene intake. Many of the patients with EPP had a mild anemia (Mathews-Roth, 1974). This was not worsened or improved by carotene intake. Leucopenia has been reported in patients who ingested large amounts of carrots (Josephs, 1944; Gjerlow, 1966). This phenomenon was found to reverse itself when the patient stops eating the abnormal amount of carrots. We found no evidence of leucopenia in any of our patients or volunteers. The absence of this finding in our study strengthens the suggestion of earlier workers that the leucopenia was probably due to substances other than β-carotene present in the carrots and that the administration of pure β-carotene did not induce leucopenia in a subject who had experienced leucopenia after eating large amounts of carrots (Niemann and Klein Obbink, 1954; Ostwald and Briggs, 1967).

Methemoglobinemia has been shown to result from the consumption of large amounts of carrot juice (Keating et al., 1973). This is another example of the toxicity of large amounts of vegetables and their products, and a reason why we do not encourage photosensitive patients to become carotenemic by ingesting large amounts of these foods.

None of our patients were found to develop abnormally high levels of serum vitamin A. This confirms what has been repeatedly reported in the literature—that individuals ingesting large amounts of β-carotene do not develop hypervitaminosis A (Hoch, 1943; Niemann and Klein Obbink, 1954; Ostwald and Briggs, 1967).

Kobza et al. (1973) report that one patient treated with β-carotene reported an increase in hay fever attacks, and another reported swelling of the tongue and face. We found no such reactions in our patients. However, it should be kept in mind that an occasional patient could be allergic to some of the other components of the beadlet preparation (gelatin, antioxidants, etc.). Perhaps such patients should be given crystalline β-carotene in vegetable oil to determine if indeed the reaction was caused by beadlet components. If the adverse reaction disappears, then the patient can continue to take the carotene in oil, if ingestion of carotene has benefitted his photosensitivity. Hannuksela and Lahti (1986) found that β-carotene administration does not precipitate urticaria or atopic dermatitis in patients who have these conditions.

Carotenoids have been found in human milk (Lesher et al., 1945; Kon and Mawson, 1950) and there are at least two reported instances of breast-fed infants becoming carotenemic on their carotenemic mothers' milk (Almond and Logan, 1942; Thomson, 1973). It also seems that carotenoids can cross the placental barrier. DeBuys (1923) reports that two children of a carotenemic mother were born carotenemic with no apparent side effects. Clausen and McCoord (1938) suggest that 1 mg of carotenoid/kg fetus/day crosses the placenta. Clausen (1931) reports the presence of some carotenoid in the cord blood at birth. After birth, the amount of carotenoid present is dependent on the child's diet.

We have studied the livers of two patients who had been taking β-carotene for photosensitivity. There was no evidence of any accumulation of large amounts of either β-carotene or vitamin A in the liver by chemical analysis, or evidence of morphological alterations attributable to carotenoids or vitamin A accumulation on light-microscopic examination (Mathews-Roth et al., 1976).

Some EPP patients taking β-carotene report transient diarrhea, nausea, or bloating, which usually disappear either spontaneously or with lowering of the dose.

The observation of local deposits of pigmented granules in the retina of some patients taking large amounts of carotenoids has recently caused concern. De-Vries-de Mol et al. (1974) had noted in a study of 39 patients that treatment with β-carotene had no effect on the patients' visual activity, dark adaptation, and color discrimination, all of these parameters being within the normal range. They found no yellow color in the lens. No mention was made of any pigmentation in the cornea. They found that most patients seemed to have "grains" in the macular region of the retina, which the authors considered not to be pathological. More recently, glistening particles have been found in the macular regions of some patients who took more than the recommended dose of canthaxanthin, which is used as an artificial suntanning agent in some countries (Cortin et al., 1982; Saraux and Laroche, 1983; Metge et al., 1984; Phillipp, 1985; Segal et al., 1985; McGuinness and Beaumont, 1985; Weber et al., 1985a,b). These granules did not seem to affect visual acuity, but had some effect on dark adaptation and electroretinogram patterns (Weber, 1985a,b). Recently, it has been found that after the patients stop taking canthaxanthin, the defects in dark adaptation and electroretinogram pattern abnormalities disappear–however, the pigment granules remain in the retina (Weber and Goerz, 1986). Poh-Fitzpatrick and Barbera (1984) examined the eyes of patients with EPP treated with β-carotene alone, and could find no granules of any kind in the macular region.

We also examined the carriage of carotenoids in the lipoprotein fractions of normal individuals taking carotene and of normal individuals on a regular diet (Mathews-Roth and Gulbrandsen, 1974). We found that the amount of carotene in each lipoprotein fraction had increased in the serum from carotenemic individuals, but that the relative increase is significant only in the LDL and HDL fractions. There was no significant difference between the cholesterol levels of each fraction of the carotenemic individuals' and noncarotenemic individuals' sera, indicating that there is no increase in serum β-lipoprotein in carotenemia. We also found, as Krinsky et al. had reported (1958), that the majority of the pigments were in the β-lipoprotein fraction of both the carotenemic and noncarotenemic volunteers.

Thus, it would seem that the only significant "side effect" from the ingestion of large amounts of β-carotene is carotenodermia, the yellowish coloration of the skin observed in many people who ingest large amounts of the pigment. As is well known, this coloration disappears several weeks after cessation of carotenoid intake. The author has reviewed carotenemia elsewhere (Mathews-Roth, 1982d).

From the results of our studies and from the data found in the literature, it would seem that there is no marked direct toxicity from the ingestion of large amounts of pure β-carotene. On the other hand, those individuals developing carotenemia and carotenodermia by means of increased intake of carotenoid-containing foods are at some risk for the development of some hematological abnormality. They also may encounter other difficulties because of the usually accompanying inadequate diet, and occasionally because of the misdiagnosis of their "jaundice" by a physician unaware of their dietary intake and unfamiliar with carotenemia.

Because of the potential dangers associated with excessive ingestion of carotenoid-containing foods, we do not recommend that patients increase their β-carotene blood levels by increasing the intake of such foods. Pure β-carotene, either as the beadlet preparation or as crystalline β-carotene for those allergic to beadlet components, is indeed the preparation to be recommended.

POSSIBLE MECHANISM OF ACTION

Studies on the action at the cellular level of carotenoids have also been performed. Mufson et al. (1979) have suggested that β-carotene can inhibit 12-O-tetradecanoyl-phorbol-13 acetate–induced arachidonic acid and prostaglandin release in chick embryo fibroblasts, but that retinoic acid has a higher activity. Dixit et al. (1983) have shown that reactive oxygen species are involved in lipid peroxide formation in rat epidermal microsomes and that β-carotene added to the cells can inhibit lipid peroxide formation. An experiment to detect lipid peroxide formation in vivo in guinea pigs as measured by pentane and ethane formation was performed by Kunert and Tappel (1983). They found that β-carotene administration as well as vitamin C administration can protect against in vivo lipid peroxidation. Okumoto et al. (1985) found that a synthetic carotenoid analog had antitumor activity against P388 leukemia in mice. Interestingly, two other polyene compounds, retinoic acid and Amphotericin B had no effect in this system.

Som et al. (1984) found that β-carotene inhibits DMBA-induced transformation of murine mammary gland cells in vitro, acting both at the initiation and promotional stages of carcinogenesis. Manoharan and Bannerjee (1985) reported that β-carotene reduces sister chromatid exchange induced either by DMBA or two nitrosamine carcinogens. These workers suggest that β-carotene can modify DNA-damaging effects of carcinogens, in this case by acting on the initiation phase of carcinogenesis. The author and Krinsky have recently found that β-carotene and canthaxanthin seem to affect the promotion phase of UV-B–induced carcinogenesis. Canthaxanthin also seemed to prevent initiation, but it could not be certain from our data whether β-carotene also had this effect.

Some recent investigations have looked at the effect of β-carotene on some immunological parameters. Leslie and Duby (1982) reported that β-carotene administration increased the cytotoxicity of natural killer cells. Bendich and Shapiro (1986) have shown that increased levels of dietary β-carotene leads to enhanced T and B lymphocyte response.

How might the carotenoids be exerting their protective action against photosensitization and against tumor development? In 1968 Krinsky outlined four possible mechanisms to explain the protective function of carotenoid pigments against photosensitization: (1) a filter system in the cell envelope to filter out potentially harmful light, (2) systems that can interact with and quench photosensitizer triplet states, (3) systems that can serve as preferred substrates for photosensitized oxidations, and (4) systems that can stabilize membranes or repair damaged membranes. Since that time, additional evidence has indicated that only the second suggested mechanism, now extended to include quenching of singlet oxygen by carotenoids, seems to be significantly associated with the pigments' protective function (Krinsky, 1971). Mechanism 1 may have some function in certain plants, although it may not be the sole explanation for the pigments' protective effects in these organisms. This mechanism is also unlikely to be involved in carotenoid protection in humans, as the amounts deposited in skin are not sufficient to act as a physical sunscreen (Lamola and Blumberg, 1976). In addition, the photoprotective effect of the carotenoids seems to be independent of the absorption spectrum. The findings in photosynthetic organisms which led to the suggestion of mechanism 3 by several groups of workers are thought to be connected with reactions involved with photosynthesis rather than with the protective function of carotenoids (Krinsky, 1971). The author and Krinsky showed that the presence of carotenoids does not seem to be involved with membrane stability in *Sarcina lutea* (Mathews-Roth and Krinsky, 1970), thus suggesting that mechanism 4 may not be of wide significance in the protective function of carotenoids.

Thus it would seem that the quenching of excited species is the most widely applicable mechanism for the carotenoids' protective effects. Since the first demonstration of the ability of carotenoids to quench the triplet state of chlorophyll (Fugimori and Tavla, 1966) and to quench singlet oxygen (Foote and Denny, 1968), many workers including ourselves have confirmed that carotenoids indeed can quench these excited species. In addition, the pigments have also been found to quench free radical reactions not involving singlet oxygen, including UV-C radiation (200-290 nm)–induced radical reactions, as well as free radical reactions independent of light (Krinsky and Deneke, 1982). The ability of carotenoids to quench excited species reactions not involving light might explain some of the anticancer actions of the pigments, as free radicals are thought to be involved in carcinogenesis, at least in some forms of cancer.

It is difficult to design an experiment to prove that reactions involving excited species actually take place in the skin of a living organism. At present, the closest approximation to the in vivo situation is to study isolated epidermis. Dubertret et al. (1982) used human epidermis soaked in a singlet oxygen/free radical trap, 1,3-diphenylbenzoisofuran (DPBF), to direct photochemical reactions in epidermis, which was also soaked in various sensitizers. These workers demonstrated the presence of these reactions in the epidermal preparations by measuring the decrease of the absorbance of the DPBF. The author applied these methods to study the ability of carotenoids to quench photochemical reactions in mice made porphyric by the administration of collidine, and also receiving either β-carotene canthaxanthin or a placebo. It was found that the decrease in absorbance of the DPBF after exposure of the isolated epidermis to light was significantly less in the epidermis prepared from porphyric mice receiving the carotenoids than it was in the mice receiving placebo, suggesting that β-carotene and canthaxanin could inhibit photochemical reactions occurring in epidermis (Mathews-Roth, 1984b). The author has also used the technique of Dubertret et al., to see if carotenoids could quench any photochemical reactions occurring in epidermis exposed to UV-B radiation (Mathews-Roth, 1986b). Here again, the decrease in abosrbance of the DPBF peak after exposure to UV-B radiation was significantly less in the epidermis of mice after having received one of the carotenoids tested (β-carotene, canthaxanthin, or phytoene) that it was in the epidermis prepared from mice receiving placebo. This suggests that carotenoids can quench excited species generated during UV-B exposure.

We cannot, of course, conclude at this time that epidermal reactions involving excited species cause the itching and burning of the skin characteristic of EPP or induce the development of UV-B-induced skin cancer. We do know that these kinds of reactions can cause cellular damage and can be prevented by the administration of carotenoids. Further research hopefully will answer this question.

SUMMARY

Carotenoid pigments, which contain 40 carbon atoms and at least 9 conjugated bonds, have been found in in vitro and in vivo systems to be able to quench excited species, such as singlet oxygen and free radicals. β-Carotene and canthaxanin are accepted by the U.S. Food and Drug Administration as food colors, and β-carotene is approved for use in the treatment of the photosensitivity associated with the genetic disease erythropoietic protoporphyria in a dosage of up to 300 mg/day. In the 11 years since its approval, no serious toxicity of β-carotene has been reported.

Because of the lack of serious toxicity, and because of some cancer-preventive activity in certain animal models, clinical trials in populations at high risk for developing certain types of cancer are already underway. The carotenoid dose employed ranges from 15 to 50 mg/day. This is much less than the usual adult dose of 180 mg/day for photosensitivity prevention. There is no way of predicting which dose will be effective in preventing cancer; the lower doses were chosen to prevent the development of marked carotenodermia. These doses will eventually cause an increase in the serum carotenoid level; whether the increase will be as great as is achieved with the higher therapeutic doses and also lead to successful protection against cancer remains to be seen.

At this time, the author feels that it is premature to make any recommendations for β-carotene or other carotenoid intake beyond encouraging people to be sure to include one or two servings of red, yellow or green vegetables in their diets each day. The most sensible course of action is to wait to find out the outcome of the ongoing clinical trials.

REFERENCES

Abril, E., Rybecki, J., Souderi, P., Watson, R. (1986). Beta-carotene stimulates mononuclear phagocytes to produce a tumor necrosis factor-like substance. *Fed. Proc. 45*:270.

Alam, B. S., Alam, S. Q., Weir, J. C., Gibson, W. A. (1984). Chemopreventive effects of beta-carotene and 13-cis retinoic acid on salivary gland tumors. *Nutr. and Cancer 6*:4.

Almond, S., Logan, R. F. L. (1942). Carotinaemia. *Brit. Med. J. II*:235.

Austern, B. M., Gawienowski, A. M. (1969). In vitro biosynthesis of beta-carotene by bovine corpus luteum tissue. *Lipids 4*:227.

Bendich, A., Shapiro, S. (1986). Effect of beta-carotene and canthaxanthin on the immune response of the rat. *Jour. Nutr. 116*:2254.

Clausen, S. W. (1931). Carotenemia and resistance to infection. *Trans. Am. Ped. Soc. 43*:27.

Clausen, S. W., McCoord, A. B. (1938). The carotenoids and vitamin A of the blood. *J. Ped. 13*:635.

Cornbleet, T., Greenberg, R. (1957). Conversion of carotene to vitamin A by sebaceous glands. *Arch. Derm. 76*:431.

Cortin, P., Corriveau, L. A., Rousseau, A. P., Tardif, Y., Malenfant, M., Biurdreault, G. (1982). Maculopathie en paillettes d'or. *Can. Jour. Ophalthmol. 17*: 103.

DeBuys, L. R. (1923). Some clinical experiences with carotenemia. *Trans. Mississippi State Med. As'sn. 56*:133.

DeVries-de Mol, E. C., Went, L. M., Volker-Dieben, H. J. (1974). Farnsworth-Munsell 100-hue results in a series of patients with long-standing therapeutic carotenemia. *Med. Prob. Ophthal. 13*:349.

Dixit, R., Mukhtar, H., Bickers, D. R. (1983). Studies on the role of reactive oxygen species in mediating lipid peroxide formation in epidermal microsomes of rat skin. *Jour. Invest. Derm. 81*:369.

Dorogokupla, A. C., Troitzkaia, E. G., Adilgireieva, L. K., Postolnikov, S. L., Chekrygina, Z. P. (1973). Effect of carotene on the development of induced tumors. *Zdravookhr. Kazakh. 10*:32.

Dubertret, L., Santus, R., Razin, M., DeSa e Melo, T. (1982). Photochemistry in human epidermis: a quantitative approach. *Photochem. Photobiol. 35*:103.

Epstein, J. H. (1973). Effects of beta-carotene on UV-induced cancer formation in the hairless mouse skin. *Photochem. Photobiol. 25*:211.

Foote, C. S., Denny, R. W. (1968). Chemistry of singlet oxygen VII. quenching by beta-carotene. *J. Am. Chem. Soc. 90*:6233.

Fugimori, E., Tavla, M. (1966). Light-induced electron transfer between chlorophyll and hydroquinone and the effect of oxygen and beta-carotene. *Photochem. Photobiol. 5*:877.

Gainer, J. L., Wallis, D. A., Jones, J. R. (1976). The effect of crocetin on skin papillomas and Rous sarcoma. *Onology 11*:222.

Gjerlow, J. (1966). Granulocytopeni som folge au karotinemi. *Tidj. Norske Legeforen. 86*:33.

Glover, J. (1960). The conversion of beta-carotene into vitamin A. *Vit. and Hormones 18*:371.

Goodman, D. S. (1967). Metabolism of beta-carotene and vitamin A. *Prog. Biochem. Pharm. 3*:487.

Goodman, D. S. (1984). Overview of current knowledge of metabolism of vitamin A and carotenoids. *Jour. Nat. Cancer Inst. 73*:1375.

Goodman, D. S., Huang, H. S. (1966). Biosynthesis of vitamin A with rat intestinal enzymes. *Science 149*:879.

Goodwin, T. W. (1952). *The Comparative Biochemistry of the Carotenoids.* Chapman and Hall, London.

Greenberg, R., Cornbleet, T., Demovsky, R. (1957). Conversion of carotene to vitamin A by sebaceous glands. *Arch. Dermatol. 76*:17.

Greenberg, R., Cornbleet, T., Jeffay, A. L. (1959). Accumulation and excretion of vitamin A-like fluorescent material by sebacceous glands after the oral feeding of various carotenoids. *Jour. Invest. Derm. 32*:599.

Hannuksela, M., Lahti, A. (1986). Peroral challenge tests with food additives in urticaria and atopic dermatitis. *Int. Jour. Derm. 25*:178.

Hashimoto, H. (1922). Carotenoid pigmentation of the skin resulting from a vegetarian diet. *Jour. Amer. Med. Assoc. 78*:1111.

Hess, A. F., Myers, V. C. (1919). Carotenemia: a new clinical picture. *Jour. Amer. Med. Assoc. 73*:1743.

Hoch, H. (1943). Effect of prolonged administration of carotene in the form of vegetables on the serum carotene and vitamin A levels in man. *Biochem. Jour. 37*:430.

Josephs, H. W. (1944). Hypervitaminosis A and carotenemia. *Amer. Jour. Dis. Child. 67*:33.

Keating, J. P., Lell, M. E., Strauss, A. W., Zarkowsky, H., Smith, G. E. (1973). Infantile methemoglobinemia caused by carrot juice. *New Eng. J. Med. 288*: 824.

Kobza, A., Ramsay, C. A., Magnus, I. A. (1973). Oral beta-carotene therapy in actinic reticuloid and solar urticaria. *Brit. Jour. Dermatol. 88*:157.

Kon, S., Mawson, M. E. (1950). Carotenoids in breast milk. *Spec. Report. Ser., Med. Res. Council*, London, No. 269.

Krinsky, N. I. (1968). The protective function of carotenoid pigments. In *Photophysiology: Current Topics*, Vol. 3, A. C. Giese, (Ed.). Academic Press, New York, pp. 123–195.

Krinsky, N. I. (1971). Function. In *Carotenoids*, Isler, O. (Ed.). Birkhauser Verlag, Basel & Stuttgart, pp. 669–716.

Krinsky, N. I., Cornwell, D. G., Oncley, J. L. (1958). Transport of vitamin A and carotene in human plasma. *Arch. Biochem. Biophys. 73*:233.

Krinsky, N. I., Deneke, S. M. (1982). Interaction of oxygen and oxy-radicals with oxygen. *Jour. Nat. Cancer Inst. 69*:205.

Kunert, K. J., Tappel, A. L. (1983). The effect of vitamin C on in vivo lipid peroxidation in guinea pigs as measured by pentane and ethane production. *Lipids 18*:271.

Lamola, A. A., Blumberg, W. E. (1976). The effectiveness of beta-carotene and phytoene as systemic sunscreens. Abstracts of the Annual Meeting of the American Society For Photobiology, Abstract No. FAM-C4.

Lesher, M., Brody, J. K., Williams, H. H., May, I. G. (1945). Human milk studies. *Amer. Jour. Dis. Child. 70*:182.

Leslie, C. A., Duby, D. P. (1982). Carotene and natural killer cell activity. *Fed. Proc. 41*:381.

Lin, J. K., Wang, C. J. (1986). Protection of crocin dyes on the acute hepatic damage induced by aflatoxin B_1 and dimethyl nitrosamine in rats. *Carcinogenesis 7*:595.

Manoharan, K., Banerjee, M. R. (1985). Beta-carotene reduces sister chromatid exchanges induced by chemical carcinogenesis in mouse mammary cells in organ culture. *Cell Biology International Reports 9*:783.

Mathews-Roth, M. M. (1974). Anemia in erythropoietic protophorphyria. *Jour. Amer. Med. Assoc. 230*:824.
Mathews-Roth, M. M. (1980). Carotenoid pigments as anti-tumor agents. In *Current Chemotherapy and Infectious Diseases*, Nelson, J. D., and Grassi, C. (Eds.). American Society for Microbiology, Washington, DC, pp. 1503–1505.
Mathews-Roth, M. M. (1982a). Photosensitization by porphyrins and prevention of photosensitization by carotenoids. *Jour. Nat. Cancer Inst. 69*:279.
Mathews-Roth, M. M. (1982b). Antitumor activity of beta-carotene, canthaxanthin, and phytoene. *Oncology 39*:33.
Mathews-Roth, M. M. (1982c). Effect of crocetin on experimental skin tumors in hairless mice. *Oncology 39*:362.
Mathews-Roth, M. M. (1982d). Beta-carotene therapy for erythropoietic protoporphyria and other photosensitivity diseases. In *The Science of Photomedicine*, J. Regan and J. Parrish (Eds.). Plenum Press, New York, pp. 409–440.
Mathews-Roth, M. M. (1983). Carotenoid pigment administration and delay in development of UV-B-induced tumors. *Photochem. Photobiol. 37*:509.
Mathews-Roth, M. M. (1984a). Carotenoid pigments and protection against photosensitization: How studies in bacteria suggested a treatment for a human disease. *Perspec. Biol. Med. 28*:127.
Mathews-Roth, M. M. (1984b). Porphyrin photosensitization and carotenoid protection in mice: in vitro and in vivo studies. *Photochem. Photobiol. 40*:63.
Mathews-Roth, M. M. (1986a). Beta-carotene therapy for erythropoietic protoporphyria and other photosensitivity diseases. *Biochimie 68*:875.
Mathews-Roth, M. M. (1986b). Carotenoids quench evolution of excited species in epidermis exposed to UV-B (290-320 nm) light. *Photochem. Photobiol. 43*:91.
Mathews-Roth, M. M., Abraham, A. A., Gabuzda, G. (1976). Beta-carotene content of certain organs from two patients receiving high doses of beta-carotene. *Clin. Chem. 22*:922.
Mathews-Roth, M. M., Gulbrandsen, C. L. (1974). Transport of beta-carotene in serum of individuals with carotenemia. *Clin. Chem. 20*:1578.
Mathews-Roth, M. M., Krinsky, N. I. (1970). Carotenoid pigments and the stability of the cell membrane of *Sarcina lutea. Biochim. Biophys. Acta 203*: 357.
Mathews-Roth, M. M., Krinsky, N. I. (1985). Carotenoid dose level and protection against UV-B induced skin tumors. *Photochem. Photobiol. 42*:35.
Mathews-Roth, M. M., Pathak, M. A., Parrish, J., Fitzpatrick, T. B., Kass, E. H., Toda, K., Clemans, W. (1972). A clinical trial of the effects of oral beta-carotene on the responses of human skin to solar radiation. *Jour. Invest. Derm. 59*:349.
Mathews-Roth, M. M., Wilson, T., Fujimori, E., Krinsky, N. I. (1974a). Carotenoid chromophore length and protection against photosensitization. *Photochem. Photobiol. 19*:217.
Mathews-Roth, M. M., Pathak, M. A., Fitzpatrick, T. B., Harber, L. C., Kass, E. H. (1974b). Beta-carotene as an oral photoprotective agent in erythropoietic protoporphyria. *Jour. Amer. Med. Assoc. 228*:1004.

Mathews-Roth, M. M., Pathak, M. A., Fitzpatrick, T. B., Harber, L. C., Kass, E. H. (1977). Beta-carotene therapy for erythropoietic protoporphyria and other photosensitivity diseases. *Arch. Dermatol. 113*:1229.

McGuinness, R., Beaumont, P. (1985). Gold dust retinopathy after the ingestion of canthaxanthine to produce skin bronzing. *Med. Jour. Austral. 143*:622.

Metge, P., Mandirac-Bonnefoy, C., Bellaube, P. (1984). Thesaurismose retinenne a la canthaxanthine. *Bull. et Mem. Soc. Franc. Ophth. 95*:547.

Mufson, R. A., DeFeo, D., Weinstein, I. B. (1979). Effect of phorbol ester tumor promoters on arachidonic acid metabolism in chick embryo fibroblasts. *Mol. Pharm. 16*:569.

Newberne, P., Chan, W-C., and Rogers, A. (1974). Influence of light, riboflavine and carotene on the response of rats to the acute toxicity of aflatoxin and monocrotaline. *Toxicol. and Appl. Pharm. 28*:200.

Niemann, C., Klein Obbink, H. J. (1954). Biochemistry and pathology of hypervitaminosis A. *Vitam. Horm. 12*:69.

Okumoto, T., Morita, N., Nakamura, I., Konishi, M., Yamaguchi, M. (1985). Activity of a novel carotenoid analog, 4,4′(3,7,12,16-tetramethyl-1,3,5,7,9,11, 13,15,17-octodeca nonaen-1,18-diyl)bis(1-ethylpyridinium)dibromide (Y-18598) on mouse leukemia P388. *Jour. Cancer Res. Clin. Oncol. 109*:257.

Olson, J. A. (1961). The absorption of beta-carotene and its conversion into vitamin A. *Amer. Jour. Clin. Nutr. 9*:1 (no. 4, part 2).

Olson, J. A. (1964). Biosynthesis and metabolism of carotenoids and related molecules. *Jour. Lipid Res 5*:281.

Ostwald, R., Briggs, G. M. (1967). Toxicity of the vitamins. In *Toxicants Occurring Naturally in Foods*, The Food Protection Commission (Eds.). National Science Foundation, Washington, DC, 1967, pp. 183–220.

Phillipp, W. (1985). Carotinoid-Einlagerungen in der Netzhaut. *Klin. Mol. Augenheilk. 187*:439.

Poh-Fitzpatrick, M. B., Barbera, L. G. (1984). Absence of crystalline retinopathy after long-term therapy with beta-carotene. *Jour. Amer. Acad. Dermatol. 11*:111.

Rettura, G., Strattford, F., Seifter, E. (1982). Prophylactic and therapeutic actions of supplemental beta-carotene in mice inoculated with C3HBA adenocarcinoma cells: lack of therapeutic action of supplemental ascorbic acid. *Jour. Nat. Cancer Inst. 69*:73.

Santamaria, L., Bianchi, A., Arnabaldi, A., Andreoni, L., Bermond, P., (1983). Dietary carotenoids block photocarcinogenic enhancement by benzo(a)-pyrene and inhibit its carcinogenesis in the dark. *Experientia 39*:1043.

Saraux, H., Laroche, L. (1983). Maculopathie a paillettes d'or apres absorption de canthaxanthine. *Bull. Soc. Ophth. France 83*:1273.

Schwartz, J., Suda, D., Light, G. (1986). Beta-carotene is associated with the regression of hamster buccal pouch carcinoma and the induction of tumor necrosis factor in macrophages. *Biochem. Biophys. Res. Comm. 136*:1130.

Segal, A., Laporte, P., Ducasse, A., S. Vidal. (1985). Un nouveau cas de thesaurismose retinenne à la canthaxanthine. *Bull. Soc. Ophth. France 85*:145.

Seifter, E., Rettura, G., Padawer, J., Levinson, S. M. (1982). Moloney murine sarcoma virus tumors in CBA/J mice: chemopreventive and chemotherapeutic actions of supplemental beta-carotene. *Jour. Nat. Cancer Inst. 68*:835.
Seifter, E., Rettura, G., Padawer, J., Strattford, F., Goodwin, P., Levinson, S. M. (1983). Regression of C3HBA mouse tumor due to x-ray therapy combined with supplementary beta-carotene or vitamin A. *Jour. Nat. Cancer Inst. 71*:409.
Seifter, E., Rettura, G., Levinson, S. M. (1984). Supplemental beta-carotene (BC): prophylactic action against 7,12 dimethylbenz(a)anthracene (DMBA) carcinogenesis. *Fed. Proc. 43*:662.
Sestili, M. A. (1984). Chemoprevention clinical trials—problems and solutions. N.I.H. Publication #85-2715.
Shamberger, R. J. (1971). Inhibitory effect of vitamin A on carcinogenesis. *Jour. Natl. Cancer Inst. 47*:667.
Som, S., Chatterjee, M., Bannerjee, M. (1984). Beta-carotene inhibition of 7, 12dimethylbenz(a)anthracene-induced transformation of murine mammary cells *in vitro. Carcinogenesis 5*:937.
Stich, H. F., Rosin, M. P., Vallejera, M. O. (1984). Reduction with vitamin A and beta-carotene administration of proportion of micronucleated buccal mucosal cells in Asian betel nut and tobacco chewers. *Lancet II* (June 2) 1204.
Stich, H. F., Rosin, M. P., Hornby, A. P., Yee, G. E. (1986). Cellular beta-carotene levels influence the clastogenic action of carcinogens in *in vivo* and *in vitro* systems. *Proc. Amer. Assoc. Cancer. Res. 27*:121.
Suda, D., Schwartz, J., Skhlar, G. (1986). Inhibition of experimental oral carcinogenesis by topical beta-carotene. *Carcinogenesis 7*:711.
Thompson, S. Y. (1965). Occurrence, distribution and absorption of provitamins. *Proc. Nutr. Soc. 24*:136.
Thomson, M. L. (1973). Carotenemia in a suckling. *Arch. Dis. Child. 18*:112.
Weber, U., Goerz, G., Hennekes, R. (1985a). Carotinoid-retinopathie. I. Morphologische und funktionelle Befunde. *Klin. Mbl. Augenheilk. 186*:351.
Weber, U., Hennekes, R., Goerz, G. (1985b). Carotinoid-retinopathie. II Elektrophysiologische Befunde bei 23 carotinoid-behandelten Patienten. *Klin. Mbl. Augenehilk. 187*:507.
Weber, U., Goerz, G. (1986). Carotinoid-retinopathie. III Reversibilitat. *Klin Mbl. Augenheilk. 188*:20.

11

Calcium, Vitamin D, and the Prevention of Gastrointestinal Cancer

MICHAEL J. WARGOVICH
The University of Texas M. D. Anderson Cancer Center, Houston, Texas

INTRODUCTION

The thesis that the diet of modern man has attained a composition that promotes gastrointestinal cancer appears to be gaining acceptance among scientifics. The evidence from human studies has been criticized because of the inaccuracies in recalling consumption of certain foods and the variability of dietary instruments used in diet-cancer studies (Block, 1982). Yet, certain patterns have emerged from many well-conducted studies in humans. It is now conjectured that the level of dietary fat, especially that from animal sources, has a direct bearing on the development of cancer of the colon. Although this suspicion is not new, concrete evidence in humans has lagged behind the substantive evidence in animals that dietary fat promotes certain forms of cancer (National Academy of Sciences, 1982), most notably colorectal cancer (Smith et al., 1985). The process of tumor promotion viewed from the perspective of cell biology is an extraordinary and complex evolution for the gastrointestinal cell. The odyssey from that of normality to the tumorigenic phenotype is a protracted process; it is estimated that a primary malignancy of the colon, for instance, may take 20 years to evolve in man (Schottenfeld and Haas, 1978). Because of the time required for a lesion in the gastrointestinal tract to become invasive, it is generally accepted that opportunities exist to alter the carcinogenic process.

Recent suggestions concerning the processes governing the cellular events underlying tumor promotion in the gastrointestinal tract have centered upon the induction of aberrant cellular proliferation by a number of purported etiologic agents including dietary lipids and fiber (Jacobs and White, 1983; Craven et al., 1986). Essential to the regulation of cellular proliferation in many tissues is the maintenance of intracellular calcium levels (Hennings et al., 1980). It is possible that reduced bioavailability of calcium or disruption in the mechanics of calcium transport may be one of the critical early events in tumor promotion (Whitfield et al., 1973). The intent of this chapter is to review the recognizable features of tumor promotion in the gastrointestinal tract and to introduce newer concepts regarding the effects of calcium and vitamin D in prevention of gastrointestinal cancer, with a specific emphasis on cancer of the colon.

TUMOR PROMOTION IN THE GASTROINTESTINAL TRACT

Cellular Proliferation in Normal and Tumor Tissue

The epithelium lining the mucosa of the gastrointestinal tract is ordinarily subject to ordered cycles of cellular replication (Deschner and Lipkin, 1976). The growth kinetics of the epithelium of the small bowel and colon have been extensively studied (Lipkin et al., 1963). It is known that proliferation in the undiseased colon is governed by diurnal pressures and availability of nutrients (Hagemann and Stragand, 1977; Hamilton, 1979). Generally, the proliferation of gastrointestinal epithelium reflects a steady state balance between production of new cells and cell loss due to age of the cell or abrasion by the passage of food (Stragand and Hagemann, 1977). Imbalances in cell loss may serve as a stimulus for cellular replication. Thus inducers of cellular proliferation, over and above the normal requisite for cell replacement, may act to augment tumor promotion. Loss of cellular control of proliferation and appearance of chaotic variations in cell kinetic patterns are harbingers of tumorigenesis.

In the gastrointestinal tumor alterations in growth kinetics have been reported (Kovacs et al., 1981). Yet the growth of the tumor is slow. It is suspected that many years are required for an adenocarcinoma to become invasive (Day, 1985). What, then, is the danger of enhanced cellular proliferation in the premalignant tissue? In the colon, enhanced cellular proliferation brings upon the cell a number of adverse consequences. Though at first inspection it might seem sensible for a colon cell mutated with a carcinogen to be rapidly eliminated, the very act may serve to fatally commit the cell to the carcinogenic sequence. Most, if not all, normal cells have the ability to repair the genetic damage induced by mutagenic chemicals (Demple et al., 1986). The process of DNA repair, however, requires time. If a cell has not completed repairs to the genome and is forced into active cycling, fixation of a mutagenic lesion may occur, commencing the tumorigenic process (Hicks, 1983). In terms of cancer prevention, several avenues of protection are available to the cell: regulation of cellular proliferation, removal of the putative promoting substance, alteration of its cellular receptors, or induction of terminal differentiation. In experimental studies, tumor promotion has been widely observed for several forms of gastrointestinal cancer, and many of the suspected agents are derived from the diet.

Suspect Tumor Promoters in the Diet

Inspired by the suggestive results from human studies linking consumption of dietary fat to increased risk for cancer of the colon, attempts to construct a laboratory model to examine the effects of diet on tumorigenesis have been made. These attempts have largely succeeded. For instance, it is possible to feed rodents diets that simulate the composition of the human diet in terms of content and calories. The advent of organ-specific carcinogens have made it possible to investigate effects of single nutrients on esophagus, stomach, and colon (Sugimura and Kawachi, 1978; Rogers and Nauss, 1985). In support of the epidemiologic evidence linking elevated risk for cancer of the colon by consumption of a diet rich in fat, studies in animals have shown that diets in excess of 30% of calories as fat strongly promote colon cancer (Reddy and Maeura, 1984). At under 30% of calories, vegetable fats are more likely than not to promote tumorigenesis; low-fat diets containing animal sources of lipids apparently do not reproducibly cause increases in tumor numbers (Reddy et al., 1977). Table 1 reflects some of the evidence in animal studies for the cancer-promoting effects of fat. Though many experiments confirm enhancement of tumorigenesis for high levels of dietary fat, few have proposed a mechanism by which the promotion occurs.

What is unique to dietary fats that could account for the biologic effect of augmenting tumor growth? One answer may be found in the chemistry of digested lipids. Dietary fat in the colon consists mainly of fatty acids and bile acids with residual di- and triglycerides that have escaped reabsorption in the small bowel (Johnston, 1977). Free bile and fatty acids are biochemically active molecules. The detergent and tissue-damaging effects of these acids have been well characterized (Vahouny et al., 1984). Secondary bile acids, such as deoxycholic acid, perturb cellular membranes and can be necrogenic to the colonic epithelium (Craven et al., 1986). Moreover, the activity of free bile or fatty acids is pH dependent; in a basic pH they are highly ionized and biochemically active, whereas in acidic pH they are less so (McJunkin et al., 1981). It is interesting to note that colonic pH itself may be a risk factor for colon cancer: vegetarians at low risk for colon cancer generally exhibit an acidic environment in the colon (Thornton, 1981). The tissue effects of ionized bile acids and fatty acids are notable including epitheliolysis, induction of diarrhea, and, subsequently, stimulation of cellular proliferation (Chadwick et al., 1976; Palmer, 1979; Bull et al., 1983). Thus, exposure of the colon mucosa to the "wounding" induced by ionized lipids may be one of the major causes of tumor promotion.

Table 1 Experimental Evidence for Promotion of Colon Cancer by Dietary Lipids

Lipid type	Biologic effect	Reference
Bile acids:		
Deoxycholate	proliferation tumorigenesis	Bull et al., 1983 Reddy et al., 1976
Lithocholate	tumorigenesis	Narisawa et al., 1974
Cholate	proliferation tumorigenesis	Weidema et al., 1985 Reddy et al., 1977
Fatty acids:		
Oleic	proliferation	Wargovich et al., 1984
Linoleic	proliferation tumorigenesis	 Sakaguchi et al., 1984
Stearic hydroperoxides	No effect on tumor load	Bull et al., 1984
Natural fats:		
Beef tallow	Incidence of tumors at 30% of diet vs. 5%	Reddy et al., 1977
Lard	Incidence of tumors at 20% of diet	Trundel et al., 1983
Corn oil	Incidence of tumors at 20–30% of diet vs. 5%	Reddy and Maeura, 1984

Other Biologic Effects of Tumor Promoters

Information on cellular and molecular effects of tumor promoters is limited to what has been gained from certain well-studied chemical promoters, such as the phorbol esters, which promote carcinogenesis at many sites, most notably the skin (Slaga and Klein-Szanto, 1983). It has been shown most recently that gastrointestinal cells in short-term culture respond to phorbol esters. Friedman et al. (1984) treated adenoma and adenocarcinomas with tetradecanoyl phorbol acetate (TPA). It was found that TPA induced release of plasminogen activator in most of the malignant tissues. Secretion of plasminogen activator in response to TPA may be linked to changes in morphology and function during malignant transformation (Davies et al., 1983). Phorbol esters are mitogens, and this has been demonstrated in a number of cell systems (Diamond et al., 1980). So far it has not been possible to separate mitogenic factors in the phorbol esters that induce proliferation from other biochemical and physical changes in the cell as the critical event in enhancing the tumorigenic process. Other secondary changes include alterations in enzyme profiles (ornithine decarboxylase, for example) and disruption of metabolic cooperation and intracellular communication (Boutwell, 1982; Trosko et al., 1983). Understanding the importance of the sequence of events that trigger tumor promotion will create opportunities to inhibit the process. A new and potentially rewarding area of research is the identification of antipromoters: substances that modify tumor promotion. Integral to many cellular processes and strongly implicated in the regulation of cellular proliferation is the level of intracellular calcium (Hennings et al., 1980). Calcium and cofactors which facilitate its transport (vitamin D) are subjects of a current investigation probing their utility as clinically promising cancer preventative agents.

INHIBITION OF GASTROINTESTINAL CANCER BY CALCIUM

Calcium figures prominently in many cellular functions. None is more important in terms of survival of the cell than the regulatory nature of this element on cellular proliferation and synthesis of DNA (Whitfield et al., 1979). Imbalances in calcium concentration have been correlated to aberrant cellular behavior, typically demonstrated by the neoplastic cell (Parson et al., 1983). From the perspective of calcium-cell interactions, there are at least two mechanisms by which ionic calcium could interfere with tumor promotion. The first, more specific for tumor promotion in the colonic epithelium, concerns the active role of dietary lipids and their chemical affinity for calcium. The second, a more generalized effect, concerns the physiological and molecular aspects of cellular proliferation.

Promotion of Colon Cancer by Lipids: Effects of Ionized Calcium

The digestion of fat yields micellular aggregates of fatty acids, monoacylglycerides, and cholesterol, intermixed with bile acids that function to solubilize these less polar compounds (Watkins et al., 1974). In the upper jejunum tri and diacylglycerols interact with pancreatic lipases to yield free and bound fatty and bile acids (Johnston, 1977). Bound lipids are largely in the form of calcium soaps that are reported to be biologically inert (Hann et al., 1970; Drenick, 1961). The behavior of the free lipids is very much dependent on pH; dihydroxy bile acids, suggested to be etiologic factors in diarrhea are tissue damaging in alkaline pH (McJunker et al., 1981; Wargovich et al., 1983). It is in this environment that unbound fatty and bile acids have a high affinity for calcium. Addition of calcium to the diet does not change serum triglyceride levels (Bhattacharyya et al., 1969), but incorporation of high levels of calcium in the diet significantly increased fecal excretion of saturated fatty acids (Fleischmann et al.,

1966). The binding affinity of calcium to colonic lipids is high and on the same order as that of EDTA (Newmark et al., 1985). Thus, with entry of dietary fat into the colonic lumen a significant loss of calcium could occur.

Loss of calcium from colonic epithelial cells could have a number of effects contributing to initiation of the tumorigenic process. Aside from the effects on cellular proliferation, calcium governs the maintenance of the microtubule network and crosslinking of membrane proteins (Lorand et al., 1978). In epidermal tissues the level of ionized calcium is suspected to regulate the balance of growth of keratinocytes and induce differentiation (Stanley and Yuspa, 1983). It is possible that these same regulatory functions are present in the colonic mucosa. In this regard it is reasonable to assume that the same molecular mechanisms for calcium regulation may be at work in the colon, mediated through the calcium-binding protein, calmodulin (Cheung, 1980).

Work in our laboratory has confirmed that the proliferative effects of ionized bile and fatty acids on mouse colon epithelium could be abrogated by pretreatment with calcium carbonate or lactate (Wargovich et al.,1983, 1984). In those studies the tissue necrosis commonly observed by instillation of ionized bile acids was notably absent, as was the compensatory induction of proliferation. Assumedly the binding of the ionized lipids irreversibly to calcium prevented tissue interactions.

Clinical Studies

That calcium could offset abnormal cellular proliferation has been tested clinically in two studies (Lipkin and Newmark, 1985; Rosen et al., 1987). In both investigations it was found that supplementation by 1250 mg of calcium/day significantly reduced mucosal proliferation in patients at high risk for large bowel cancer based on increases in the size of the colonic proliferative compartment. Epidemiologic studies support the hypothesis that a higher calcium intake reduces risk for colon cancer, though confirmation awaits the completion of other prospective studies (Garland et al., 1985). Laboratory and clinical investigations of calcium as a cancer control agent are shown in Table 2.

Addition of calcium to the diet will not be a simple solution; calcium is bound by many dietary factors, including phosphate, fiber, phytate, and oxalates (Rendelman, 1982; Kelsay, 1985; Morris and Ellis, 1985). Studies in our laboratory have shown that phytate, found in fibrous foods, stimulates colonic proliferation (Wargovich, 1987). Phytate binds with strong affinity to calcium and may lead to dietary insufficiency of this element in humans. The interplay between ionic calcium and dietary lipids is complex. As understanding of the molecular processes of tumor promotion increases, the importance of calcium as a regulatory element looms larger. Also critical are the agents that facilitate calcium transport, such as vitamin D. In terms of cancer prevention, little is

Table 2 Experimental and Clinical Evidence for Cancer Prevention by Dietary Calcium

Study	Endpoint	Ca^{++} source	Ref.
Mouse colon	^{3}HTdR uptake	$CaCO_3$	Wargovich et al., 1982
Mouse colon	^{3}HTdR uptake	Ca lactate	Wargovich et al., 1984
Mouse colon	Mitotic index	$CaHPO_4$	Bird, 1986
Rat colon	Colon cancer	Ca gluconate	Pence and Buddingh, 1987
Human colon	^{3}HTdR uptake	$CaCO_3$	Lipkin and Newmark, 1985
Human colon	^{3}HTdR uptake	$CaCO_3$	Rosen et al., 1987
Human colon	^{3}HTdR uptake	$CaCl_2$	Buset et al., 1986

known about the effects of this vitamin, yet new information leads to the exciting speculation that the compound and its metabolites may be prominent in inhibiting tumorigenesis.

CANCER-PREVENTATIVE EFFECTS OF VITAMIN D

Mechanism of Action

Basic research investigations of the anticancer properties of vitamin D have only recently appeared in the literature (Frampton et al., 1983; Homma et al., 1983). In light of the suspected regulatory effects of calcium, it is not surprising that this is so. Yet another facet of the function of vitamin D must be considered: the potential function alone as a steroid hormone (Norman, 1980). Receptors for vitamin D have been found in the small intestine, kidney, pituitary, parathyroid and bone (Haussler, 1986), all considered target organs. Through a series of hydroxylations in liver and kidney, vitamin D_3 is transformed into the active metabolite, 1,25-dihydroxyvitamin D_3, that functions in calcium and phosphorus homeostasis. It is the suggested functions in cellular growth and differentiation that distinguishes the action of the metabolite. A summary of the biological properties of vitamin D are shown in Table 3.

Anticancer Properties

Antiproliferative and differentiation effects have been reported for vitamin D in leukemic cells and in cells derived from sarcoma and melanoma (Colston et al., 1981; Do Koh et al., 1984). A high degree of receptivity for vitamin D was

Table 3 Biological Effects of Vitamin D_3 Relevant to Inhibition of Cancer

Tissue	Cellular effect	Reference
In Vitro:		
Hs695T Melanoma cells	suppressed growth	Colston et al., 1981
Breast cancer cells	suppressed growth	Eisman et al., 1979
Murine myeloid leukemia	slow growth and differentiation	Abe et al., 1981
HL 60 myeloid leukemia	slow growth and differentiation	Munker et al., 1986
In Vivo:		
TPA-promoted skin cancer	tumor inhibition	Wood et al., 1983
TPA-induced skin ODC activity	ODC inhibited	Chida et al., 1985
DMBA-induced skin cancer	increased tumor yield	Wood et al., 1985

shown in human colon tumors (Frampton et al., 1982). In our own laboratory the addition of supraphysiologic levels of 1,25-dihydroxyvitamin D_3 to the serum free medium of exponentially growing LoVo cells (a human colon cancer cell line) retarded growth and altered cellular morphology; physiologic doses did not effect growth (Lointier et al., 1987). In this study a low capacity, high affinity receptor was detected for the vitamin. It is also known that cellular levels of polyamines are subject to vitamin D regulation and that the compound has a marked effect on cellular membrane composition and the fluidity of membrane (Anonymous, 1984). Vitamin D-deficient rats undergo changes in the fatty acid composition of cellular membranes, incorporating more saturated fatty acids (Brasitus et al., 1986). Whether vitamin D has pronounced effects on the colonic epithelium remains to be confirmed. Chida et al. (1985) demonstrated that topical application of 1,25-dihydroxyvitamin D_3 inhibited ornithine decarboxylase activity in epidermal cells promoted by TPA. In our own studies, the hormonally active form of the vitamin also reduced in a dose-related manner the colonic proliferation in mice treated intrarectally with 0.1–0.5 μg of 1,25-dihydroxyvitamin D_3 (Wargovich, unpublished data). Whether the parental form of the vitamin D_3 shows the same antiproliferative effects in vivo has yet to be resolved. Also unknown is the effect of vitamin D in diminishing the mitogenic stimuli of lipids to the colonic epithelium, a cancer-promoting process with biochemical events possibly unrelated to the promoting effects of phorbol esters. Of interest is the analysis of the diets and the intensity of sunlight (and thus vitamin D levels) at various latitudes in the United States by Garland et al. (1985). In this study increased vitamin D levels were suggested to be a protective factor for cancer of the colon.

SUMMARY

The argument for supplementation of the diet with additional amounts of calcium or vitamin D has been largely derived for the suggested prevention of osteoporosis, an escalating disease in the United States (Warren, 1985). Suggestive evidence from clinical studies of the effects of calcium in the potential prevention of colon cancer concur in the suggestion that the present RDA for calcium be increased from 800 mg/day to 1500 mg/day (Newmark et al., 1984). It is premature to recommend supplementation to the public until confirmation of the benefit of added calcium has been shown more convincingly in animal models for gastrointestinal cancer. At least one study of this type has indicated an anticancer effect for calcium (see Table 2). Further preclinical testing of calcium should include the opportunity to test the effect of this element in trials featuring reduction of human mucosal proliferation or premalignant lesions of the gastrointestinal tract such as the adenoma. Human studies of the cancer prevention effects of vitamin D have yet to be developed, and nutritional supplementation must be considered only as a prospect of the future.

ACKNOWLEDGMENTS

I wish to thank Ms. Betty Harwerth for preparation of the manuscript.

REFERENCES

Abe, E., Miyaura, H., Sakagami, M., Takeda, K., Konno, T., Yamasaki, S., Yoshiki, S., Suda, T. (1981). Differentiation of mouse myeloid leukemia cells by 1, alpha 25 dihydroxyvitamin D_3. Proc. Natl. Acad. Sci. USA 78:4990.

Anonymous (1984). Altered membrane lipid composition: A possible molecular basis of vitamin D action. *Nutr. Rev. 42 (10)*:357.

Bhattacharyya, K. K., Thera, C., Anderson, J. T., Grande, F., Keys, A. (1969). Dietary calcium and fat. *Am. J. Clin. Nutr. 22(9)*:1161.

Bird, R. P. (1986). Effect of dietary components on the pathobiology of colonic epithelium: Possible relationship with colon tumorigenesis. *Lipids 21(4)*: 289.

Block, G. (1982). A review of validations of dietary assessment methods. *Amer. J. Epidemiol. 115*:492.

Brasitus, T. A., Dudija, P. K., Eby, B., Lau, K. (1986). Correction by 1-25 dihydroxycholecalciferol of the abnormal fluidity and lipid composition of enterocyte brush border membranes in vitamin D deprived rats. *J. Biol. Chem. 261(35)*:16404.

Boutwell, R. K. (1982). Inhibition of chemical carcinogenesis based on the inhibition of essential steps in the biochemical mechanisms of tumor promotion. In *New Approaches to the Design of Antineoplastic Agents*, Bardos, S. Kalman (Ed.). Elsevier, New York, pp. 261–271.

Bull, A. W., Marnett, E. J., Dawe, E. J., Nigro, N. D. (1983). Stimulation of deoxythymidine incorporation in the colon of rats treated intrarectally with bile acids and fats. *Carcinogenesis 4*:207.

Bull, A. W., Nigro, N. D., Golembieski, W. A., Crissman, J. D., Marnett, I. J. (1984). In vivo stimulation of DNA synthesis and induction of ornithine decarboxylase by fatty acid hydroperoxides, auto-oxidation products of unsaturated fatty acids. *Cancer Res. 44*:4924.

Buset, M., Lipkin, M., Winawer, S., Swaroop, S., Friedman, E. (1986). Inhibition of human colonic epithelial cell proliferation *in vivo* and *in vitro* by calcium. *Cancer Res. 46*:5426.

Chadwick, V. S., Gaginella, T. S., DeBongie, J. C., Carlson, G. L., Phillips, S. F., Hoffman, A. F. (1976). Mucosal epitheliolysis: a mechanism for increased permeability induced by dihydroxy bile acids. *Gastroenterology 17*:816.

Cheung, W. Y. (1980). Calmodulin plays a pivotal role in cellular regulation. *Science 207*:19.

Chida, K., Hashiba, H., Fukushima, M., Suda, T., Kuroki, T. (1985). Inhibition of tumour promotion in mouse skin by 1,25-dihydroxyvitamin D_3. *Cancer Res. 45*:5426.

Colson, K., Colston, M. J., Feldman, D. (1981). 1,25-dihydroxyvitamin D_3 and malignant melanoma: The presence of receptor and inhibition of cell growth in culture. *Endocrinology 108*:1083.

Craven, P. A., Pfansteil, J., DeRubrtis, F. R. (1986). Role of reactive oxygen in bile salt stimulation of colonic epithelial proliferation. *J. Clin. Invest. 77*: 850.

Davies, R. L., Rifkin, D. B., Tepper, R., Miller, A., Kucherlapati, R. (1983). A polypeptide secreted by transformed cells that modulates human plasminogen activator production. *Science 221*:171.

Day, D. W. (1985). Adenocarcinoma sequence. *Prog. Clin. Biol. Res. 186*:99.

Demple, B., Daikh, Y., Greenberg, J., Johnson, A. (1986). Alklylation and oxidative damages to DNA. Constitutive and inducible repair systems. In *Antimutagenesis and Anticarcinogenesis*, D. M. Shakel, P. E. Hartman, T. Kada, A. Hollaender (Eds.). Plenum Press, New York, pp. 205–219.

Deschner, E. E., Lipkin, M. (1976). Cell proliferation in normal, preneoplastic, and neoplastic gastrointestinal cells. *Clin. Gastroenterol. 5(3)*:545.

Diamond, L., O'Brien, T. G., Baird, W. M. (1980). Tumor promoters and the mechanism of tumour promotion. *Adv. Cancer Res. 32*:1.

Do Koh, S., Donaldson, C. A., Haussler, M. R. (1984). Influence of 1,25-dihydroxyvitamin D_3 on cultured osteogenic sarcoma: Correlation with the 1,25 dihydroxyvitamin D_3 receptor. *Cancer Res. 44*:2103.

Drenick, E. J. (1961). The influence of calcium and other soap-forming substances on fecal rat. *Gastroenterology 41*:242.

Eisman, J. A., McIntyre, I., Martin, T., Moseley, J. M. (1979). 1,25 dihydroxy-vitamin D receptors in breast cancer cells. *Lancet 2*:1335.

Fleischmann, A. I., Yacowitz, H., Hayton, T., Bierenbaum, M. L. (1966). Effects of dietary calcium upon lipid metabolism in mature rats fed beef tallow. *J. Nutr. 88*:255.

Frampton, R. J., Suva, L. J., Eisman, J. A. (1982). Presence of 1,25 dihydroxy-vitamin D_3 receptors in established human cancer cell lines in culture. *Cancer Res. 42*:1116.

Frampton, R. J., Olmond, S. A., Eisman, J. A. (1983). Inhibition of human cancer cell growth by 1,25-dihydroxyvitamin D_3 metabolites. *Cancer Res. 43*: 4443.

Friedman, E., Urmacher, C., Winawer, S. (1984). A model for human colon carcinoma evolution based on the differential response of cultured preneoplastic, premalignant and malignant cells to 12-0-tetradecanoyl phorbol-13-acetate. *Cancer Res. 44*:1568.

Garland, C., Shekelle, R. B., Barrett-Coner, E., Criqui, M. H., Rossoff, A. H., Paul, O. (1985). Dietary vitamin D and calcium and risk of colorectal cancer: A 19 year prospective study in men. *Lancet 1*:307.

Hagemann, R. F., Stragand, J. J. (1977). Fasting and refeeding: cell kinetic response of jejunum, ileiu and colon. *Cell Tissue Kinet. 10*:3.

Hamilton, E. (1979). Diurnal variations in the proliferative compartments and their relationship to cryptogenic cells in the mouse colon. *Cell Tissue Kinet. 12*:91.

Hann, F. M., Navarette, D. A., Hsu, E. (1970). Calcium fatty acid absorption in term infants fed human milk and prepared formulas stimulating human milk. *Pediatrics 45*:216.

Haussler, M. R. (1986). Vitamin D receptors: Nature and function. *Ann. Rev. Nutr. 6*:527.

Hennings, H., Michael, D., Cheng, C., Steinert, P., Holbrook, K., Yuspa, S. H. (1980). Calcium regulation of growth and differentiation of mouse epidermal cells in culture. *Cell 19*:245.

Hicks, R. M. (1983). Pathological and biochemical aspects of tumour promotion. *Carcinogenesis 4(10)*:1209.

Homma, Y., Hozumi, M., Abe, E., Konna, K., Fukushima, M., Hata, S., Nishi, Y., DeLuca, H. F., Suda, T. (1983). 1α, 25-dihydroxyvitamin D_3 and 1α, hydroxyvitamin D_3 prolong survival time of mice incoulated with myeloid leukemia cells. *Proc. Natl. Acad. Sci. USA 80*:201.

Jacobs, L. R., White, F. A. (1983). Modulation of mucosal cell proliferation in the intestine of rats fed a wheat bran diet. *Am. J. Clin. Nutr. 35*:697.

Johnston, J. M. (1977). Gastrointestinal tissue. In *Lipid Metabolism in Mammals*, F. Snyder (Ed.). Plenum Press, New York, pp. 151–189.

Kelsay, J. L. (1985). Effect of oxalic acid on calcium bioavailability. In *Nutritional Bioavailability of Calcium*, C. Kies (Ed.). American Chemical Society, Washington, DC, pp. 105–116.

Kovacs, C. J., Evans, M. J., Schenken, L. L., Burholt, D. R. (1981). Alterations in gastrointestinal steady state kinetics associated with growth of experimental tumours. *Cell Tissue Kinet. 14*:241.

Lipkin, M., Newmark, H. L. (1985). Effect of added dietary calcium on colonic epithelial-cell proliferation in subjects at high risk for familial colon cancer. *N. Engl. J. Med. 313*:1381.

Lipkin, M., Sherlock, P., Bell, B. (1963). Cell proliferation kinetics in the gastrointestinal tract. *Gastroenterology 45*:721.

Lointier, P. H., Wargovich, M. J., Saez, S., Levin, B., Wildrick, D., Boman, B. (1987). The role of vitamin D_3 in the proliferation of a human colon cancer *in vitro. Anticancer Res. 7(4)*:817.

Lorand, L, Siefring, G. E., Lowe-Kreutz, L. (1978). Formation of α-glutamyl-E-lysine bridges between membranes proteins by a Ca^{2+} regulated enzyme in intact erythrocytes. *Proc. Nat. Acad. Sci. USA 74*:3908.

McJunkin, B., Fromm, H., Sarva, R. P., Prafulla, A. (1981). Factors in the mechanism of diarrhea in bile acid malabsorption: fecal pH—a key determinant. *Gastroenterology 80*:1454.

Morris, E. R.. Ellis, R. (1985). Bioavailability of dietary calcium: Effects of phytate on adult men consuming nonvegetarian diets. In *Nutritional Bioavailability of Calcium*, C. Kies (Ed.). American Chemical Society, Washington, DC, pp. 63–173.

Munker, R., Norman, A., Koeffler, H. P. (1986). Vitamin D compounds. *J. Clin. Invest. 78*:424.

Narisawa, T., Magadia, N., Weisburger, J. H., Wynder, E. (1974). Promoting effect of bile acids on colon carcinogenesis after intrarectal instillation of N-methyl-N-nitro-N-nitrosoguanidine in rats. *JNCI 53*:1093.

National Academy of Sciences (1982). Lipids (fats and cholesterol). In *Diet, Nutrition, and Cancer*. National Academy Press, Washington, DC, pp. 73–106.

Newmark, H. L., Wargovich, M. J., Bruce, W. R. (1984). Colon cancer and dietary fat, phosphate, and calcium: A hypothesis. *JNCI 72*:1321.

Newmark, H. L., Wargovich, M. J., Bruce, W. R., Boynton, A. L., Klein, L., Whitfield, J. F., Jannson, B., Cameron, I. L. (1985). In *Large Bowel Cancer*, A. Mastromarino, M. Braittain (Eds.). Praeger Press, New York, pp. 102–130.

Norman, A. W. (1980). 1,25 $(OH)_2$-D_3 as a steroid hormone. In *Vitamin D*, A. W. Norman (Ed.). Marcel Dekker, New York, pp. 197–250.

Palmer, R. H. (1979). Bile acid heterogeneity and the gastrointestinal epithelium: from diarrhea to colon cancer. *J. Lab. Clin. Med. 94(5)*:655.

Parson, P. G., Musk, P., Goss, P. D., Leah, J. (1983). Effects of calcium depletion on human cells in vitro and anomalous behavior of the human melanoma cell line MM170. *Cancer Res. 43*:2081.

Pence, B. C., Buddingh, F. (1988). Inhibition of dietary fat promotion of colon carcinogenesis by supplemental calcium or vitamin D. *Proc. Am. Assoc. Cancer Res. Carcinogenesis 9*:187.

Reddy, B. S., Maeura, Y. (1984). Tumor promotion by dietary fat in axoxymethane-induced colon carcinogenesis in female F344 rats: Influence of amount and source of fat. *JNCI 72*:745.

Reddy, B. S., Narisawa, T., Weisburger, J. H., Wynder, E. L. (1976). Promoting effect of sodium deoxycholate on adenocarcinomas in germ-free rats. *JNCI 56*:441.

Reddy, B. S., Watanabe, K., Weisburger, J. H., Wynder, E. L. (1977). Promoting effect of bile acids in colon carcinogenesis in germ-free and conventional F344 rats. *Cancer Res. 37*:3238.

Rendelman, J. A. (1982). Cereal complexes: Binding of calcium by bran and components of bran. *Cereal Chem. 59*:302.

Rogers, A., Nauss, K. (1985). Contributions of laboratory animals studies of colon carcinogenesis. In *Large Bowel Cancer*, A. Mastromarino, M. G. Braittain (Eds.). Praeger Press, New York, pp. 1–46.

Rosen, P., Fireman, Z., Wax, Y., Ron, E. (1987). Oral calcium suppresses increased colonic mucosal proliferation of persons at risk for colorectal neoplasia. *Gastroenterology 92*:1603.

Sakaguichi, M., Hitamatsu, Y., Takada, H., Yammamura, M., Hioki, K., Saito, K., Yammamoto, M. (1984). Effect of dietary unsaturated and saturated fats on azoxymethane induced colon cancer in rats. *Cancer Res. 44*:1472.

Sauerheber, R. D., Gordon, L. M. (1975). Spin label studies on rat liver plasma membrane. *Proc. Soc. Exp. Biol. Med. 150*:28.

Schottenfeld, D., Haas, J. F. (1978). Epidemiology of colorectal cancer. In *Gastrointestinal Tract Cancer*, M. Lipkin, R. Good (Eds.). Plenum Press, New York, pp. 207–237.

Slaga, T. J., Klein-Szanto, A. J. P. (1983). Initiation-promotion versus complete skin carcinogenesis in mice: Importance of dark basal keratinocytes (stem cells). *Cancer Invest. 1(5)*:425.

Smith, A. H., Pearce, N. E., Joseph, J. G. (1985). Major colorectal cancer aetiological hypotheses do not explain mortality trends among Maori and non-Maori New Zealanders. *Int. J. Epidemiol. 14(1)*:79.

Stanley, J. R., Yuspa, S. H. (1983). Specific epidermal protein markers are modulated during calcium induced terminal differentiation. *J. Cell Biol. 96*:1809.

Stragand, J. J., Kagemann, R. F. (1977). Effect of lumenal contents on colonic cell replacement. *Am. J. Physiol. 233(3)*:E208.

Sugimura, T., Kawachi, T. (1978). Experimental stomach carcinogenesis. In *Gastrointestinal Tract Cancer*, M. Lipkin, R. Good (Eds.). Plenum Press, New York, pp. 327–337.

Thornton, J. R. (1981). High colonic pH promotes colorectal cancer. *Lancet 1*: 1081.

Trosko, J. E., Chang, C-C., Medcalf, A. (1983). Mechanisms of tumor promotion: Potential role of intercellular communication. *Clin. Invest. 1(6)*:511.

Trundel, J. L., Senterman, M. K., Brown, R. A. (1983). The fat/fiber antagonism in experimental carcinogenesis. *Surgery 94*:691.

Vahouny, G. V., Satchithanandam, S., Lightfoot, F., Grau, L., Haas-Smith, S., Kritchevsky, D., Cassidy, M. M. (1984). Morphological disruption of colonic mucosa by free or cholestyramine-bound bile acids. *Dig. Dis. Sci. 29(5)*:432.

Wargovich, M. J. (1987). Phytic acid, a calcium chelating agent in fiber rich cereals stimulates colonic cellular proliferation. *Gastroenterology*.

Wargovich, M. J., Eng, V. W. S., Newmark, H. L., Bruce, W. R. (1983). Calcium ameliorates the toxic effects of deoxycholic acid on colonic epithelium. *Carcinogenesis 4(9)*:1205.

Wargovich, M. J., Eng, V. W. S., Newmark, H. L. (1984). Calcium inhibits the damaging and compensatory proliferative effects of fatty acids on mouse colon epithelium. *Cancer Lett. 23*:253.

Warren, R. A. (1985). Osteoporosis. *Contemporary Nutr. 10(1)*. (pamphlet)

Watkins, J. B., Bliss, C. M., Donaldson, R. M., Lester, R. (1974). Characterization of newborn fecal lipid. *Pediatrics 43(4)*:511.

Weidema, W. F., Deschner, E. E., Cohen, B. I., DeCosse, J. J. (1985). Acute effects of dietary cholic acid and methylazoxymethanol acetate on colon epithelial cell proliferation; metabolism of bile salts and neutral sterols in conventional and germ free SD in rats. *JNCI 74*:665.

Whitfield, J. F., MacManus, J. P., Gilan, D. J. (1973). Calcium dependent stimulation by phorbol ester (PMA) of thymic lymphoblast DNA synthesis and proliferation. *J. Cell Physiol. 82*:151.

Whitfield, J. F., Boynton, A. L., MacManus, J. P., Sikorska, M., Tsang, B. K. (1979). The regulation of cell proliferation by calcium and cyclic AMP. *Mol. Cell Biochem. 27*:155.

Wood, A. W., Chang, R. L., Huang, M-T., Uskokovic, M., Conney, A. H. (1983). 1 α,25 dihydroxyvitamin D_3 inhibits phorbol ester dependent chemical carcinogenesis in mouse skin. *Biochem. Biophys. Res. Commun. 116(2)*:605.

Wood, A. W., Chang, R. L., Huang, M. T., Baggiolini, E., Partridge, J. J., Uskokovic, M., Conney, A. H. (1985). Stimulatory effect of 1α, 25 dihydroxyvitamin D_3 on the formation of skin tumors in mice treated chronically with 7,12 dimethylbenzanthracene. *Biochem. Biophys. Res. Commun. 130(2)*: 924.

12
α-Tocopherols (Vitamin E)

WILLIAM J. MERGENS and HEMMIGE N. BHAGAVAN
Hoffman-La Roche Inc., Nutley, New Jersey

INTRODUCTION

In 1922, Evans and Bishop started a series of investigations on the influence of nutrition on reproduction in the rat that eventually led to the establishment of vitamin E as an essential micronutrient for animals and humans (see Evans, 1962). Following the decades of exploration since these original studies, it is now well established that vitamin E deficiency can result in pathology of the vascular, nervous, and reproductive systems and tissues such as liver (Mason, 1954; Nelson, 1980). In some species, vitamin E alone is not effective to correct the deficiency symptoms if the diet is also low in selenium. Rats maintained on low vitamin E diets high in linoleate will die prematurely (Machlin et al., 1977). In adult humans, chronic ingestion of a low vitamin E diet leads to a decrease in red blood cell survival times. Hemolytic anemia and thrombocythemia have been observed in premature infants with low plasma vitamin E levels. Cystic fibrosis patients have low plasma vitamin E levels and decreased red blood cell survival times, and myopathy, cardiomyopathy, and testicular degeneration have been observed in some patients with cystic fibrosis.

Frank vitamin E deficiency secondary to lipid malabsorption has now been well documented in humans and is correlated with the occurrence of specific neurological and neuromuscular symptoms. The condition can be corrected by vitamin E treatment if started promptly (Sokol et al., 1983).

While scientific and technological advances have brought prospects of a longer life span, they have also caused increased exposure to environmental pollutants and the associated risk for diseases, such as cancer. Most people can fully expect to live well into their 70s; at the same time, cancer has been identified as the second leading cause of mortality in many Western countries. More than 800,000 new cases of cancer occur each year in the United States, and are responsible for over 20% of the approximately 2 million annual deaths. The search for the causes of cancer and possible control remains intense. At the same time, however, the potential role of dietary factors in the etiology and prevention of cancer has gained considerable attention (Palmer, 1986). Since Doll and Peto (1981) raised the possibility that a high dietary intake of β-carotene might decrease the risk of human cancer, considerable interest has been focused on micronutrients and cancer prevention. These investigators provided a wide range of estimates (10-70%) for the proportion of deaths from cancer that could be reduced by practical dietary means, concluding that dietary modification might eventually result in a 35% reduction in cancer mortality in the United States.

In 1982, the National Research Council Committee on Diet, Nutrition, and Cancer, part of the National Academy of Sciences, conducted an in-depth review of the literature and concluded that cancers of most major sites are influenced by dietary patterns (National Research Council, 1982). However, the data were found to be insufficient to quantitate the contribution of diet to overall cancer risk or to determine the percent reduction in risk that might be achieved by dietary modification. The data in the literature on vitamin E were found not to be sufficient to draw any firm conclusions about its relationship to human cancer. However, since the NRC review, many new studies have appeared in the literature. This chapter, then, summarizes the animal and human evidence on the role of vitamin E in human cancer with particular reference to the possible mechanisms of action involved, pharmacokinetic factors, dose and formulation of vitamin E, and the dietary considerations in relation to other foods and nutrients. In this context, the potential role of vitamin E to be explored is clearly not one related to deficiency states but, rather, an optimal nutritional intake that is likely to reduce the risk of cancer.

ORIGINS OF CANCER

Considerable effort has been devoted to studying the influence of environmental factors on the incidence of cancer (Miller and Miller, 1977). These include ultraviolet radiation, toxic substances in the air and water, occupational exposure, lifestyle, in addition to the foods we eat. Modern technology and industrial research has led to the development of a number of food additives, pesticides, insecticides, and industrial chemicals being introduced during the last several decades. Some of these compounds have been specifically identified as human carcinogens (Doll and Peto, 1981). Chemical carcinogens, believed to account for most human cancers, have been classified into eight categories, which in turn belong to two main groups. The first, genotoxic carcinogens, includes direct-acting carcinogens, procarcinogens, and inorganic carcinogens. The other main group operates through epigenetic mechanisms and includes solid state carcinogens, hormones, immunosuppressors, cocarcinogens, and promoters (Weisburger and Horn, 1982).

Cancer is not a single disease entity, and a multiple of chemical carcinogens and dietary factors affect the development of cancers in different ways. In recet years, new knowledge of the mechanisms of carcinogenesis has emerged. In spite of the multiplicity of causative factors, most cancers develop through a series of defined steps. An understanding of these progressive stages in cancer development has provided the possibility of intervening at selected points in the process so as to prevent, arrest, or even reverse neoplastic growth.

The sequence of stages progressing from the molecular to the tissue level of biological organization has been identified in vivo and in vitro using cultures of both animal and human cell lines (Pitot, 1978). In the first stage, *initiation* occurs at the molecular level and involves an irreversible alteration of a genetically important macromolecule (e.g., DNA). This event does not necessarily result in aberrant cell growth but, rather, "fixes" the potential for aberrant growth in the memory of the cell. The second stage, called *promotion*, triggers the transformation of normal cells to tumor cells by affecting cell differentiation and phenotypic expression and increases cell proliferation. This critical stage may be reversed by deactivating mechanisms. Various aspects of promotion and subsequent events have been reviewed in detail (Miller and Miller, 1977; Sugimura et al., 1981). When cell proliferation proceeds uncontrolled (*progression*), transformed cells accumulate and eventually lead to manifestation of the biological entity called cancer.

Newel (1981) has summarized a number of generally accepted facts concerning cancer.

1. Carcinogenesis is dose dependent, with dose being a function of both carcinogen concentration and exposure time.
2. There is a long latent period between carcinogen exposure and tumor development. In humans, this period could be 5-30 years.
3. There is no testable evidence of a threshold dose below which there is no risk of cancer.
4. Carcinogens can act transplacentally and can cause tumors in offspring.
5. Transformation of normal cells to cancer cells is a multistep process with initiating agents enhanced by promoting agents, hormonal agents, and other cofactors.
6. Cells with a rapid proliferation rate (high turnover) are more susceptible.
7. There is antigenic diversity to the same chemical stimulus, and immune responses differ.
8. The same chemicals can cause different types of tumors.

STUDIES ON THE INHIBITION OF CARCINOGENESIS BY α-TOCOPHEROL

Wattenberg (1978, 1983) has classified inhibitors of carcinogenesis into three categories dependent upon their mechanistic stage of action. They include compounds that (1) prevent the formation of carcinogens from precursors; (2) inhibit carcinogens from reaching or reacting with target sites (blocking agents); and (3) suppress the expression of neoplasia by exposed cells (suppressive agents).

α-Tocopherol has been studied in many model systems which reflect these potential inhibitory roles.

In Vitro Studies

There are a number of studies that reflect an active role for α-tocopherol in blocking initiation-related events. The binding of metabolically activated ^{14}C-benzo(a)pyrene (BP) to rat liver nuclei was studied by Matsuura et al. (1979). The nuclear framework structure, termed the nuclear matrix, was found to bind BP preferably. α-Tocopherol inhibited the binding of BP to nuclear macromolecules in the presence of phenobarbitol (PB)-induced microsomes. α-Tocopherol decreased the level of BP metabolites in nuclei but did not inhibit the activation of BP by PB-induced microsomes. α-Tocopherol inhibited benzopyrene-induced chromosomal damage to mammalian cells grown in culture (Smalls and Patterson, 1982). Shamberger et al. (1973) observed that vitamin E reduced the in vitro DMBA-induced mutagenesis of human lymphocytes.

Patterson, Smalls, and Lyn-Cook (1981) reported on the reduction of dimethylsulfoxide (DMSO)-induced chromosomal alterations in mammalian cells by vitamin E. Chinese hamster ovary (CHO) cells were exposed to 3% DMSO for 24 hours and graded levels (25–150 μg/ml) of α-tocopherol for 48 hours. Experimental cultures treated with 3% DMSO contained 19% total aberrations, while those with added tocopherol (25 μg/ml) had a total of 10% total aberrations. Increasing levels of tocopherol further reduced the level of aberrations, but not totally to the control levels (4%). In further studies, vitamin E was found to reduce the sister chromatid exchange frequencies to near control levels for CHO cells exposed to 1-2% DMSO.

Beckman, Roy, and Sproule (1982) found that vitamin E could modify the radiation-induced, sex-linked recessive lethal mutation frequency in *Drosophila*. Their data suggested that the vitamin might be exerting a beneficial effect on the DNA repair process. Russo et al. (1984) found that vitamin E induced an increased alkaline elution rate of liver DNA in rats and suggested that this might mean that the vitamin can modify patterns of gene expression. Konings and Trieling (1977) observed, however, an enhanced inhibition of [^{3}H]-thymidine incorporation into DNA of vitamin E-depleted lymphosarcoma cells.

Similarly, α-tocopherol has been shown to be effective in inhibiting promotion-related events (suppressive agent). Perchellet et al. (1985) reported that the constituent amino acids of reduced glutathione (GSH), GSH itself, and α-tocopherol inhibited 12-0-tetradecanoylphorbyl-13-acetate (TPA)-induced ornithine decarboxylase (ODC,L-ornithine carboxylase; EC 4.1.1.17) activity in mouse epidermis in vivo and in vitro. The inhibitory effects of cysteine, GSH, and α-tocopherol on ODC induction were proportional to their abilities to decrease the incidence of skin tumors in an initiation-promotion protocol. The in vivo inhibitory effect of α-tocopherol (40 μmol) on TPA (8.5 nmol)-induced ODC activity was approximately 70%. These results suggest that GSH level–raising agents and other antioxidants might inhibit by diverse means the effects of TPA on GSH metabolism and skin tumor promotion. Kozumbo, Seed, and Kensler (1983) reported that the in vivo ID_{50} on ODC activity for α-tocopherol was 25 μmol in mice treated with TPA at 17 nmol. The results demonstrate an early and direct inhibition of TPA-induced ODC activity by antioxidants and suggest a role for reactive oxygen and/or free radical species in tumor production.

Protection mechanisms related to postinitiation events do not only include antipromoter effects but also increases in immune response. Two major functions of the immune system are to protect the host from infections and the proliferation of precancerous and tumor-forming cells. Recent data based upon in vitro and in vivo studies indicate that vitamin E is an important micronutrient for the immune system. (The animal data will be discussed later in this chapter.) When lymphocytes from vitamin E-deficient animals are cultured with synthetic antioxidants, the vitamin E-deficient cells do not under go proliferation responses at the level found with lymphocytes from animals given vitamin E. These studies indicate that vitamin E must be present during the synthesis of all the cellular components of lymphocytes for these cells to function optimally. Low levels of dietary vitamin E are insufficient to enhance lymphocyte proliferative responses, even though the diet contains all other nutrients at the recommended levels (Bendich, Gabriel, and Machlin, 1986). When lymphocytes from mice containing normal levels of vitamin E are exposed to substances which could induce peroxidative damage throught the generation of free radicals, proliferative responses and antibody formation are significantly inhibited. When supplemental vitamin E or other antioxidants are added to these cultures, the immunosuppression is overcome (Hoffeld, 1981, 1983). Agents that block membrane lipid peroxidation enhance mouse spleen cell immune activities in vitro.

The phenomenon of differentiation of tumor cells is important not only from the prevention point of view but also from the perspective of treatment. Vitamin E (as the succinate ester) was found to enhance the effect of gamma irradiation and heat on neuroblastoma cells in culture. Vitamin E succinate, which by itself inhibited the growth of cells, enhanced the effect of heat or gamma irradiation. All three agents inhibited the growth of neuroblastoma cells (Rama,

Detsch, and Prasad, 1984). Vitamin E succinate has also been reported to induce irreversible morphological changes and growth inhibition in mouse melanoma (B-16) cells in culture (Prasad and Edwards-Prasad, 1982). Antitumor activity of α-tocopheryl succinate against human neuroblastoma in vitro and in nude mice has also been reported (Helson, Verma, and Helson, 1982). The greater potency of vitamin E succinate over vitamin E acetate and α-tocopherol in these studies may be due to the fact that the tumor cells pick up this form of the vitamin more readily. A recent study has shown that α-tocopherol induces morphological differentiation in mouse myeloid leukemia cells in culture without affecting the growth rate (Sakagami et al., 1981).

The role of α-tocopherol in preventing the formation of carcinogens from precursors has also been studied. A class of carcinogenic compounds that has received considerable attention by researchers since the late 1960s is N-nitroso compounds (i.e., nitrosamines and nitrosamides), which includes members with remarkable carcinogenic properties. It has been suggested that because of their potency and the fact that they have been found in many foods and elsewhere in our environment, the N-nitroso compounds could represent a major group of human carcinogens, at least in the gastrointestinal system. Today, it is recognized that nitrosamines can be produced from the reaction of either primary, secondary, and even tertiary amines with a nitrosating agent. The inhibiting role of α-tocopherol is one of competing with an amine or amide for the nitrosating agent, particularly in a lipid environment, to prevent N-nitroso compound formation. Ascorbic acid has been shown to behave analagously in the aqueous phase. The chemistry of these reactions has been studied (Tannenbaum and Mergens, 1980). In reacting with a nitrosating agent, α-tocopherol is converted (oxidized) to α-tocopherylquinone (Kamm et al., 1977), an irreversible reaction that is also the first step in the normal metabolism of α-tocopherol (Csallany, Draper, and Shah, 1962; Weber and Wiss, 1964) and a known oxidation product formed by loss of tocopherol in foods (Bauernfeind, 1977). In a lipid system, α-tocopherol has been shown to be an effective inhibitor of nitrosamine formation from precursor molecules in food and model gastrointestinal systems (Mergens et al., 1978; Mergens, Chau, and Newmark, 1980). In fact, α-tocopherol has been recently approved by FDA and USDA as a nitrosamine inhibitor for use in pump cured bacon at a level of 500 ppm in the final product (Federal Register, 1985).

Vitamin E has been shown to be a very effective blocker of nitrosamine formation both in vitro and in vivo (Kamm et al., 1977; Fiddler et al., 1978; Mergens et al., 1978; Newmark and Mergens, 1981). These studies also demonstrate the importance of employing the proper form of the vitamin E molecule (i.e., free tocopherol) in order to achieve effective results. The esterified forms of the molecule as well as its first oxidation product (α-tocopherylquinone) are unable to complete with the nitrite ion to inhibit nitrosamine/nitrosamide formation resulting from the respective amine/amide nitrite reaction.

Animal Studies (Precancer Models)

The possibility that α-tocopherol could inhibit the formation of nitrosomorpholine in vivo was investigated in mice injected i.p. with 2 mg morpholine and subsubsequently exposed to 47 ppm of NO_2 in an inhalation chamber for 2 hours. Pretreatment of these animals with oral doses of α-tocopherol (2.5-100 mg/kg b.w.) once daily for 6 days significantly decreased nitrosomorpholine formation in vivo during exposure to nitrogen dioxide. Whole body α-tocopherol levels increased in mice over the 6-day period in a dose-dependent manner. In this system, a maximal 50-70% inhibition of nitrosamine formation occurred at total body levels of α-tocopherol of 5 μg/kg b.w. (Norkus et al., 1986). One of the important observations from these studies, which represent extended work on earlier studies with this model (Iqbal, Dahl, and Epstein, 1980; Epstein, Iqbal, and Johnson, 1980; Van Stee et al., 1983; Mirvish, Issenberg, and Sams, 1981; Mirvish, Sams, and Issenberg, 1983; Norkus et al., 1984), was to demonstrate that body levels of α-tocopherol, rather than dietary intake, correlated more precisely with inhibition effects.

For the carcinogen dimethylnitrosamine (DMN), Skaare and Nafstad (1978) suggested and Dashman and Kamm (1979) have demonstrated that the administration of relatively high doses of vitamin E (55 mg/kg per day, i.m.) to rats for 3 days resulted in a significant decrease in acute hepatoxocity of DMN. The decrease in toxicity was apparently associated with a decrease in hepatic metabolism of DMN. Since the metabolism of DMN is mediated by the liver microsomal mixed-function oxidase (MFO), these latter authors suggested that DMN demethylase and ethylmorphine demethylase activities and cytochrome P-450 activities were decreased in animals pretreated with 45-100 mg/kg of vitamin E administered i.m.

Ohshima and Bartsch (1981) provided the first conclusive demonstration that nitrosamines can be produced endogenously in humans using a nitrate-proline regimen. The noncarcinogenic nitrosoproline molecule is quantitatively excreted in the urine. The aqueous phase nitrosation reaction in the stomach was inhibited 81% by the water-soluble vitamin C and 57% by the fat-soluble vitamin E when administered as an emulsion. Several comprehensive reports on the usefulness of vitamin E as well as vitamin C to inhibit nitrosation reactions have been written (Mirvish, 1981; Newmark and Mergens, 1981). Overall, the effectiveness of vitamin E in these examples is very much dependent on the molecule being present at the right time and place depending on the experimental model.

Animal Studies (Cancer Models)

Animal studies on the effect of α-tocopherol on carcinogenesis date back to the earliest days of vitamin E chemistry and have continued to appear in the literature with a notable increase in frequency since the 1982 NRC Report on Diet, Nutrition, and Cancer. Generally, these reports have dealt with ultraviolet light (UVL)-induced and chemically induced cancers. Overall, these studies have revealed an inhibitory effect of α-tocopherol but not without some inconsistencies.

Ultraviolet Light-induced Carcinogenesis

Black and Chan (1975) found that a dietary antioxidant mixture consisting of 2% (w/w) additives (1.2% ascorbic acid, 0.5% butylated hydroxyanisole, 0.2% α-tocopherol, and 0.1% reduced glutathione) was effective in reducing the number and severity of direct UVL-induced squamous cell carcinomas in skin of hairless mice. However, Pauling et al. (1982) were not able to reproduce these results when they evaluated α-tocopheryl acetate alone in the diet.

Later reports (Black et al., 1983b, 1985), using this same antioxidant mixture, have continued to explore the hairless mice-UVL model. They have concluded that (a) dietary lipid level has a direct effect upon the carcinogenic response to UVL both in regard to tumor latency and tumor multiplicity; (b) antioxidants produce an inhibitory effect almost equal to the degree of exacerbation of carcinogenesis evoked by increasing lipid levels, at least in the ranges that were studied; and (c) dietary antioxidants inhibit the formation of epidermal thiobarbituric acid-reacting materials. These data strongly imply that free radical reactions, specifically lipid peroxides, play a role in at least part of the photocarcinogenic response.

This same group has reported that the degree of saturation of dietary lipids markedly influenced the UVL carcinogenic response. Unsaturated lipids enhanced UVL carcinogenesis both with respect to latency and multiplicity, and it was suggested that unsaturated lipids might be required in photocarcinogenesis just as in the case for certain chemically induced cancers. In addition, the level of unsaturated lipids appeared to affect both the direction and magnitude of antioxidant-mediated modification of photocarcinogensis (Black et al., 1983a; Black, 1983).

Tumor Growth Studies (Transplanted/Established Tumors)

The influence of α-tocopherol (5 mg/100 g b.w. i.m.) on the effect of local irradiation on transplanted tumors (20 methylcholanthrene-induced) in the rat under normal and temporary hypoxic conditions was studied (Kagerud et al., 1978). α-Tocopherol significantly enhanced the toxic effect of irradiation on the tumor. This is in contrast to the tumor-protecting effect previously reported with large doses of α-tocopherol (Sakamoto and Sakka, 1973). The latter study employed α-tocopherol (100 mg/100 g b.w.) given i.p. 0.5 hours before irradiation, whereas Kagerud et al. (1978) noted that the most pronounced effect of tocopherol was observed when the vitamin was administered in a single dose of 5 mg/100 g b.w. 7 days before irradiation. Plasma, muscle, and tumor levels of tocopherol were examined. Maximum concentrations were found 1 day, 3 days, and 3–14 days after administration, respectively. The correlation of cellular radiosensitivity to local tissue oxygenation might suggest that a moderate dose of tocopherol increases the sensitivity of radioresistent hypoxic tumor cells to irradiation, while the radioprotecting property of tocopherol might be more pronounced at the higher tissue concentration of α-tocopherol. Timing, dosage, and route of administration all appear to play a role in the potentiating or protective effect of tocopherol with respect to irradiation (Kagerud, Lund, and Peterson, 1981).

Sadek (1984) found that vitamin E increased the regression of established skin papillomas in the Egyptian toad. DMBA was applied to the dorsal skin of toads for 3 months. The α-tocopherol–treated group then received 500 mg/kg/day (as tocopheryl acetate) for 2 weeks by injection into the dorsal lymph sac. Tumor regression in the treated group was 54% vs. 10%in the control group. Kurek and Corwin (1982) reported that mice fed 0.5 g tocopheryl acetate/kg in a semipurified diet demonstrated decreased incidence and rate of appearance of tumors produced by transplanted sarcoma cells compared to the control groups fed diets without vitamin supplement. Protection was dependent on the degree of unsaturation of dietary fat and on the size of the tumor cell challenge. The 0.5 g/kg inhibitor level was protective against tumor growth when hydrogenated coconut oil was the dietary fat source but not when corn oil was used (at a 2000 sarcoma cell/animal challenge). The 0.5 g tocopheryl acetate/kg level plus corn oil combination, however, became increasingly protective as the tumor cell load was reduced from 2000/animal to 500/animal. Interestingly enough, when the tocopheryl acetate dose was raised to 5 g/kg of diet, the protective effect against tumor growth was completely lost. The loss of vitamin E antitumor activity at extremely high inhibitor dose levels has been observed in several models employing polycyclic aromatic hydrocarbons as well; these are presented in the following section.

Polynuclear Aromatic Hydrocarbons (PAH)

Many polynuclear aromatic hydrocarbons exert their carcinogenic action by metabolism to an arene oxide, hydration to a dihydrodiol, and additional oxidation to a diol epoxide. A comprehensive review of structure, chemistry, metabolism and relative carcinogenicity has been written (Dipple, Moschel, and Bigger, 1984). Studies evaluating the potential antitumor effect of α-tocopherol reflect a number of carcinogenesis models, including variations on initiation and promotion.

Jaffe (1946) reported a 50% reduction in the incidence of sarcomas arising from the intraperitoneal injection of 3-methylcholanthrene when mice were supplemented with wheat germ oil, although no explanation of the mechanism of the protective effect was given. A concomitant marked reduction in the toxicity of 3-methylcholanthrene was also observed in the supplemented mice.

Chan and Black (1977) also found reduced frequency of premalignant lesions and their subsequent development into tumors in mice fed an antioxidant mixture of 1.2% ascorbic acid, 0.5% BHT, 0.2% α-tocopherol, and 0.1% reduced glutathione (2% w/w in the diet) when their dorsal median was painted with 3-methylcholanthrene followed by weekly applications of 0.5% croton oil for 15 weeks. At 33 weeks after treatment, tumor frequency in the control group was twice that of the antioxidant-supplemented group.

Haber and Wissler (1962), using female mice receiving 30–100 times the normal dietary intake of α-tocopherol and injected subcutaneously with 3-methylcholanthrene (100 μg/ml) in mineral oil, found that only about half as many sarcomas appeared in the group on the vitamin E-enriched diet than in the nonsupplemented controls. An additional experiment on black male C57 mice also showed a 50% reduction in sarcoma incidence in the mice fed α-tocopherol (7 g/kg) in the diet. However, Epstein et al. (1967) reported that vitamin E (tocopheryl acetate 2.5 and 5.0% of diet) did not suppress subcutaneous sarcoma induction in mice given 3,4,9,10-dibenzpyrene by injection.

Swick and Baumann (1951) reported that in rats, hepatomas induced by 3′-methyl-4-dimethylaminoazobenzene (3′-MeDAB) accumulated dietary α-tocopherol more rapidly than did adjacent liver tissue. In depletion experiments, hepatoms held α-tocopherol more tenaciously than normal tissue. The Jensen sarcoma, the Walker carcinoma, and the Flexner-Jobling carcinoma also absorbed tocopherol more rapidly than liver or muscle. It has been suggested that in later stages of the tumorigenic process accumulation of vitamin E in malignant tissue might put it at an advantage compared to surrounding tissue because of decreased autooxidantion (Burton et al., 1983).

Vitamin E (1 g/kg of diet with 5% corn oil) decreased the incidence of hepatomas when fed after the 8-week dose regimen of 3′-MeDAB was completed. The vitamin increased tumor incidence slightly when fed between two periods of dye feeding. Variations in intake during the time the carcinogen was fed had little effect on final tumor incidence (Swick and Bauman, 1951). Harr et al. (1972) found that the combination of selenite supplementation of vitamin E-adequate diets substantially decreased the effect of cancer induction by N-2-fluorenylacetamide (FAA). Narayan (1970) observed that vitamin E-deficient diets did not accelerate the induction of rat liver tumors induced by the same carcinogen.

Bonmassar, Dallavalle, and Giuliani (1968) injected mice subcutaneously with benzo[a]pyrene dissolved in ethyl oleate (100 μg/day for 20 days) and found that α-tocopherol (300 μg/day) administered simultaneously with the carcinogen for 20 days shortened the time of appearance of the tumors, but most tumors in the vitamin E-treated animals disappeared a few weeks later; consequently, mortality was largely reduced.

A study by Shamberger and Rudolph (1966) used the initiator 7,12-dimethylbenz[a]-anthracene (DMBA) in combination with croton oil in the mouse model. The roles of several antioxidant compounds were evaluated in preventing tumor growth. The authors found that the incorporation of 0.25% α-tocopheryl acetate with the promoter resulted in a 62% suppression in tumor response over a 16-week period. Shamberger (1970) also conducted a series of mouse skin tumor promotion studies where the α-tocopherol (325 μg/mouse/day) application times were varied. When applied after DMBA administration but before croton oil, vitamin E significantly reduced the tumor incidence in one of three experiments. In the other two experiments, there were fewer papillomas per mouse. When applied concomitantly with phenol (1.25 mg/mouse/day) as the promoter, vitamin E also significantly decreased the number of papillomas. Vitamin E (325 μg/mouse/day), when applied topically with 25 μg methylcholanthrene for 19 weeks, had no effect on the number of mice with cancers after 30 weeks. It was not clear whether α-tocopherol or α-tocopheryl acetate was the source of vitamin E in any of these studies. α-Tocopherol (43 μg/mouse) applied topically 5 minutes prior to DMBA (25 μg/mouse) application did not inhibit epidermal neoplasia in mice when subsequently promoted (1/week) with croton oil (800 μg/mouse) (Wattenberg, 1972).

Perchellet et al. (1985) evaluated the effectiveness of α-tocopherol in the DMBA-TPA initiation-promotion mouse skin model. The topical application of α-tocopherol (40 μmol) at least 5 minutes before each promotion with TPA inhibited the tumor-promoting ability of TPA by 74% at 22 weeks. Since α-tocopherol did not alter directly the intracellular ratio of GSH/GSSH, the authors suggested that the 83% inhibition of TPA-induced ODC activity elicited by this antioxidant in vitro is not related to the replenishment of intracellular GSH in TPA-treated cells but, rather, the inhibition of some earlier events responsible for the decline in the ratio of GSH/GSSH during TPA treatment. Thus, the anitoxidant mechanisms by which α-tocopherol and GSH level–raising agents inhibit the tumor promoting ability of TPA are likely to be different, and a combination of these treatments should produce a greater therapeutic effect.

Nakadate et al. (1984) reported that the inhibitory effects of flavinoids and antioxidants (including α-tocopherol) on TPA-ODC induction and tumor promotion were roughly parallel with their activities of lipoxygenase inhibition. α-Tocopherol was found to inhibit significantly TPA-induced ODC induction but not affect TPA-caused DNA synthesis. TPA-induced skin tumor promotion was slightly inhibited by α-tocopherol.

The carcinogen DMBA has been evaluated in several other models. Shklar (1982) and Weerapradist and Shklar (1982) reported that α-tocopherol inhibited oral carcinogenesis in hamsters. In their standard model for hamster buccal pouch oral cancer, using a 0.5% solution of 7,12-DMBA, it was shown that α-tocopherol (10 mg on alternate days) inhibited carcinogenesis when administered systemically by mouth. With a less potent carcinogen (0.1% DMBA), α-tocopherol was shown to prevent tumor development (Trickler and Shklar, 1987). Odukoya, Hawach, and Shklar (1984) found similar results with vitamin E administered topically to the buccal pouch. Mechanistically, Schwartz et al. (1985) reported that vitamin E administration in addition to DMBA treatment resulted in a less dramatic decrease in Langerhan cell density in hamster cheek epithelium. Since vitamin E has been shown to retard experimental oral cancer in this model, it may act by maintaining the number of Langerhan cells.

The balance of DMBA studies include a mouse forestomach and a number of rat mammary model investigations. Wattenberg (1972) found that α-tocopherol (10 g/kg diet) fed along with DMBA (50 mg/kg diet) only slightly inhibited (-41%) the number of forestomach tumors in mice.

Diverse results have been reported from studies on the effect of α-tocopherol on the induction of mammary tumors in rats by DMBA. Wattenberg (1972) initially treated rats with α-tocopherol (200 mg/rat), followed 1 hour later with DMBA (12 mg/rat) and monitored them for 25 weeks. At the end of this period, the α-tocopherol–treated rats exhibited a 30% lower incidence of tumors, but the results were not statistically significant. King and McCay (1983) found that vitamin E was ineffective against DMBA (10 mg/rat)-induced mammary tumorigenesis. In this experiment, vitamin E was added to the semisynthetic diet at 2 g/kg. However, Harman (1969) reported that vitamin E supplementation (at 50 and 200 mg/kg) into a 20% corn oil semisynthetic diet decreased the number of tumor-bearing, DMBA-treated (10 mg i.g.) rats by 25% and 60%, respectively. Lee and Chen (1979) reported that rats fed vitamin E-deficient diets had an increased incidence of DMBA-induced mammary tumors.

The effect of α-tocopherol on this model has been reported to depend on the concentration of polyunsaturated fat in the diet (Ip, 1982; King and McCay, 1983). Rats fed a high corn oil diet showed a marked increase in tumor incidence when the vitamin E intake was low (Ip, 1982). Vitamin E intake, however, had little effect on tumor incidence on rats fed a low corn oil diet. In a further study, Horvath and Ip (1983) found that the vitamin E by itself was ineffective in inhibiting the development of DMBA- or N-nitrosomethyl urea (NMU)-induced mammary tumors, whereas vitamin E (2000 IU/kg diet) potentiated the tumor inhibitory effect of selenium (2.5 mg/kg diet) when fed throughout the study.

Other Models

Cook and McNamara (1980) reported that mice fed a low vitamin E diet (10 mg/kg) had significantly more dimethylhydrazine-induced colonic tumors than those fed a high vitamin E diet (600 mg/kg); however, Toth and Patil (1983) reported that vitamin E enhanced the intestinal tumor-producing ability of dimethylhydrazine in mice. The latter study employed substantially higher levels of vitamin E in the diet (4%), and the animals were allowed to live until term vs. 38 weeks in the Cook and McNamara study. Toth and Patil could not explain their unusual findings except to speculate that, perhaps, the antioxidant could prevent and enhance cancer formation depending upon the experimental design.

Certain antineoplastic agents have been recognized as potential carcinogens for a number of years (Adamson and Sieber, 1977; Schmahl and Habs, 1978). Wang (1982) has shown that vitamin E can protect against the cancer-inducing effect of one such compound, Daunomycin.

Review of Animal Studies

Positive results have been observed for α-tocopherol inhibition of tumor formation in all the classes of animal studies reported here. Similar results have been obtained in the in vitro models. There is experimental evidence to support the role of α-tocopherol inhibiting (a) the formation of carcinogens; (b) the initiation of carcinogenic-related events; and (c) the expression of tumorigenesis. The results, however, have not been consistent. Ranges of effectiveness, in the various experimental models for which quantitative data are readily available, vary widely. One possible explanation is that α-tocopherol is simply not effective against certain specific chemical carcinogens. This might prove to be true as more environmental cancer-causing agents are identified and/or evaluated in animals models; but for the studies currently appearing in the literature, α-tocopherol has been found to inhibit tumor formation to a lesser or greater degree in the *same* model. This would appear to point more toward variations in experimental design, dose regimen, and route of administration as influencing factors.

Recently, Mirvish (1986) has made the following observations regarding animal studies. "An inhibitor of carcinogenesis can be regarded as raising the effective dose of a carcinogen [S. S. Mirvish, 1987, personal communication]. Such an effect is best observed when the dose of the carcinogen is near the top of the steepest section of the usually S-shaped dose-response curve (response being the tumor yield). An inhibitor will have little effect if the carcinogen dose is excessive (on the flat upper section of the S). Hence, dose-response levels should be constructed before inhibition experiments are performed. This consideration may help explain the negative results in some tests [e.g., Epstein et al., 1967]. Toth and Patil (1983) observed an enhancement of tumor yield by vitamin E, but the dose (4% in diet) seems excessive. The same comment applied to the Epstein study." Two other studies presented in the tumor growth studies section also used very high doses of inhibitor with null effects (Sakamoto and Sakka, 1973; Kurek and Corwin, 1982), whereas similar experimental protocols using lower doses showed positive effects. While the reasons for this are not entirely clear, in the Kurek and Corwin (1982) study, exposure of the tumor cell to excessive levels of the vitamin depressed the ability to induce a cytotoxic response. Whether this is due to increased exposure of antigens, thereby increasing the induction of suppressor cells, or whether excess vitamin actually depressed antigen exposure has yet to be determined.

Composition of the diet has been found to be another factor which influences the effectiveness of α-tocopherol as an antitumor agent, particularly unsaturated fat. The effective of α-tocopherol in the mouse mammary model depended on the concentration of PUFA in the diet (Ip, 1982). Dependence upon dietary fat type and amount as well as the composition of laboratory diets as being undefined chows or semipurified diets has been studied by King and McCay (1983). It has been fairly well established that the intake of dietary fat, especially polyunsaturated fat, must be accompanied by an elevated level of antioxidant to prevent pathological tissue damage (Horwitt, 1970). However, when the combination of stress factors (e.g., carcinogenic agent plus unsaturated fat) becomes too high, inhibitory effects of α-tocopherol are overridden. The Kurek and Corwin (1982) study is a clearly described example of this effect. The relevance of this finding to the human experience relates directly to an understanding of how well animal experiments approximate human exposure to carcinogens and promoters as well as composition of the diet. The importance of the latter has recently been addressed by Newmark (1987) in terms of nutrient density as an experimental variable.

Timing of the inhibitor dose also has been shown to be an influencing factor. In the mouse (DMBA) skin model, addition of α-tocopherol just prior to or along with each promotion consistently yields an inhibitory effect. Similarly, in the hamster-buccal model, all the studies reported demonstrate a consistent inhibitory effect whether fed orally on alternate days or topically applied to the buccal pouch. The mouse mammary model, on the other hand, seems to be the most complex of all.

In the mammary model, all of the studies incorporated vitamin E as part of the diet regimen except one in which it was shown that intragastric administration of α-tocopherol inhibited tumor induction by 41% (Wattenberg, 1972). While the timing of vitamin E administration in these mammary studies was essentially consistent, the results were not. It appears as if the influence of diet fat content and selenium play a dominant role in this model. A point that should not be overlooked, however, is the lack of information on the distribution and concentration of α-tocopherol in mammary tissue. Perhaps, optimal dietary feeding levels could be calculated more carefully with such information. Continued, systematic examination of this model is warranted.

An equally important finding reported in several of the models is the data suggesting that α-tocopherol and selenium act together to inhibit tumor formation. This is an interesting observation regarding tumor inhibition but not a surprising association in light of the known need for and complimentary roles these two micronutrients play as cellular antioxidants. It raises the question: Are these the only micronutrients that can act in symphony to optimize the body's antioxidant defense system against cancer induction?

In summary, animal studies indicate that α-tocopherol does exhibit antitumor properties. Its role in cancer prevention is probably not a solitary one but likely related to its synergy with other key molecules that contribute to the body's antioxidant defense system.

POSSIBLE MECHANISMS OF ACTION

The major interest in α-tocopherol as a cancer-preventive agent is predicated on its well-recognized antioxidant free radical scavenging property. On an experimental level, it is sometimes difficult to dissociate antioxidant function from an observed effect of α-tocopherol on enzyme activity, an alkylating agent, differentiation, tumor growth, etc., since all of these events either generate or are associated with free radicals. One approach to a discussion of possible mechanisms of action is to address the observed effects of α-tocopherol by arena of activity, which fall into the categories of exogenous, host-mediated, and cellular effects.

Exogenous Effects

The protective role of vitamin E on an exogenous level is, perhaps, most quantitatively described in the studies on inhibiting nitrosamine formation. Here, the vitamin must be free α-tocopherol (not esters), and there is a direct inhibitory relationship between the quantities of vitamin E present in the system and the amount of nitrosating agent plus reactive amine. The chemistry is strictly one of competitive kinetics. α-Tocopherol participates in a redox reaction with the nitrosating agent and is stoichiometrically oxidized to α-tocopherylquinone.

The role of α-tocopherol as a food antioxidant is to protect unsaturated fats against peroxidation. In many of the animal studies reported herein, investigators employed tocopherol acetate as the dietary source of vitamin E. While this form of vitamin E is biologically available to the animal, it should be noted that it will not impart any protective effect to the unsaturated fats in the diet, particularly stripped oils. This is in contrast to other compounds, such as BHT, BHA, propyl gallate, etc., which do not need de-esterification to become active antioxidants. Some of the oxidation products of fat may be potentially harmful to the host. It has been shown, for instance, that malonaldehyde as well as a number of monohydroperoxides, dihydroperoxides, and hydroperoxyendoperoxides derived from methyl linoleate and methyl linolenate are mutagenic (Shamberger et al., 1979; MacGregor et al., 1985). Sugai et al. (1962), for example, demonstrated that the polymeric fraction of heated fat accelerates the induction of tumors in rats.

In as much as these and other undesirable exogenous reactions contribute to the ingestion of preformed carcinogens or promoters of cancer, vitamin E has been shown to exhibit a protective role. The mechanism of action of α-tocopherol on an exogenous level is clearly one of an antioxidant free radical scavenger.

Host-Mediated Effects

Two major functions of the immune system are to protect the host from infections and to recognize and destroy precancerous and cancer cells. Some of the studies reported here, especially on transplanted tumors, suggest immunostimulation as one of the mechanisms for vitamin E action. The data on vitamin E and immune responses from animal studies consistently demonstrate the need for vitamin E for optimal activities of lymphocytes and mononuclear cells. Tengerdy et al. (1981) has summarized the role of vitamin E in disease resistance and immune response in animals.

Vitamin E may exert its effect on the immune system by modulating the release of arachidonic acid from membrane phosphatide and/or affecting prostaglandin synthesis and lipoxygenase activity. Both biosynthetic pathways proceed via free radical mechanisms (Carpenter, 1986). The mechanism of the immunoenhancing of vitamin E appears to be related to its antioxidant activity.

At least one study on immunostimulation in humans has appeared in the literature. Black et al. (1984) reported on the stimulation of prognostically favorable cell-mediated immunity of breast cancer patients by high doses of vitamin A and vitamin E. The dose of vitamin E was 1200 IU/day for 18 days and longer, and this was found to be beneficial with respect to recurrence of breast cancer. This work needs to be confirmed and extended. The relevance of immunostimulatory approaches to cancer prevention using pharmacological doses of vitamin E appears to have merit and, therefore, needs to be explored further.

Cellular Effects

The cellular oxidant state is of importance in cellular protection against the oncogenic potential of radiation and chemicals, both in the initiation and promotion phases of transformation. This has been studied extensively by a number of investigators and underscores the idea that free radicals play a role in carcinogenesis.

By far the most studied animal system has been DMBA, followed by methylcholanthrene and DMH. Mechanistically, in DMBA systems, Slaga and Brackern

(1977) found that vitamin E as well as other antioxidants were effective inhibitors of DMBA tumor initiation and attributed their activity to their ability to prevent in vivo activation of PAHs to carcinogenic epoxides and other reactive intermediates. Perchelet et al. (1985) reported that the tocopherol effect on the DMBA-TPA system was not a replenishment of GSH level and concluded that the mechanism by which tocopherol and GSH level–raising agents inhibit the tumor-promoting ability of TPA are likely to be different and that a combination of these treatments should produce greater therapeutic effects. Mirvish (1986) reported that the primary effect of vitamin E may be on promotion, since application of this compound to the skin inhibited tumor promotion by TPA in a mouse model and prevented this agent from increasing ornithine decarboxylase levels and reducing the intracellular ratio of free glutathione to glutathione disulfide (both of which are events linked with promotion).

Kahl (1986), in a comprehensive review of the dual role of antioxidants in the modification of chemical carcinogenesis, observed that most attempts to explain the antitumorigenic action of an antioxidant have centered on initiation mechanisms. In a significant number of the studies, however, the experimental design precluded discrimination of initiation or postinitiation events because the antioxidant was either administered for life or continued for days or weeks after the onset of carcinogen treatment. Kahl (1986) notes that mouse skin studies initiated with DMBA and promoted with croton oil or TPA point to an antipromoter effect since the vitamin was administered only shortly before the application of promoter. King and McCay (1983) concluded that, in spite of the rational associations of many known sources of oxidative stress in tissues, there was no clear-cut evidence that it is the antioxidant property of antioxidants that is crucial to tumor inhibition. At present, antioxidant properties of inhibitors is a plausible working hypothesis, but the lack of a consistent effect of closely related antioxidants (McCay, King, and Pitha, 1981) suggests that this hypothesis may not be correct or that it applies only to certain carcinogens that require the formation of reactive radicals.

The available evidence supports the role of α-tocopherol as an antipromoter, but the exact mechanism by which it exhibits this effect remains to be elucidated.

HUMAN STUDIES: VITAMIN E INTAKE AND CANCER RISK

Epidemiologic Studies

There is some epidemiologic evidence to support the role of vitamin E in preventing human cancer. Vitamin E is present in a wide variety of foods of both plant and animal origin, and although this makes it difficult to identify large population groups with vastly different intakes, recent findings are suggestive of relatively low vitamin E status being associated with increased risk for certain types of cancer.

Recently, however, Tuyns, Riboli, and Doornbos (1985) reported the results of a case-control epidemiological study (n = 723) on the incidence of esphogeal cancer in Calvados, France. Alcohol and tobacco were the major risk factors. A systematic analysis of nutrients, corrected for alcohol and tobacco consumption, revealed a clear protective effect for nicotinic acid, vitamin C, and vitamin E, with sizably reduced risks in high consumers. The relative risk for vitamin E at the high consumption level was 0.27.

In the Melbourne Colorectal Cancer (CRC) Study, which is a case-control study and part of a large-scale investigation of CRC incidence, etiology, and survival, Kune, Kune, and Watson (1987) found that the use of vitamin supplements, which included vitamin E, was a protective factor.

Prospective Cancer Studies

Most studies in the literature have attempted to relate serum vitamin E levels to be the subsequent development of cancer. Some of the studies have found that low serum vitamin E correlates with an elevated risk of cancer.

Breast

A prospective epidemiological study of breast cancer has been conducted (Wald et al., 1984). Blood from 5000 women in the Channel Islands, England, was stored deep-frozen for up to 14 years. During this time, 39 subjects developed breast cancer. The original serum level of vitamin E and β-carotene was compared with the serum levels in two matched controls (i.e., subjects who did not develop cancer). Significantly lower serum concentrations of vitamin E were found in cancer cases than in controls, consistently in all age groups. Those subjects who had the lowest serum levels (less than 3.3 mg/L, first quintile) had an incidence of breast cancer 5 times higher than those with the higher serum levels of vitamin E (greater than 5 mg/L, 3-5th quintile). The results thus show that a relatively high serum level of vitamin E is protective with respect to breast cancer. The long interval between the time when blood samples were collected and when breast cancer was diagnosed (5 years average) makes it unlikely that cancer caused the decrease in serum vitamin E levels.

Lung

Menkes et al. (1986) identified 99 cases of lung cancer from the Washington County, Maryland, cancer registry of the approximately 26,000 participants in 1974. Serum levels of β-carotene and α-tocopherol were both significantly higher (13.7% and 11.8%, respectively) in the controls than in the cases. The upper tail of the vitamin E plasma level distribution curve was composed *entirely* of values from the control subjects. These data support the association between low levels of serum vitamin E and the risk for all types of lung cancer. The apparent lack of difference in their preliminary report may be attributed to data analysis on a limited number of samples.

Although the magnitude of the effects reported by Menkes et al. (1986) were large, the confidence limits were wide and reportedly compatible with the small to moderate reduction in the risk for cancer attributable to the micronutrients that seem most plausible. It was suggested that a clinical trial could more reliably detect small to moderate effects and determine if the relationship is a causal one (Hennekens, 1986).

Gastric

As part of an ongoing cohort study of gastric cancer precursors in Narino, Columbia, blood levels of ascorbic acid, α-tocopherol, retinol, prealbumin, RBP, and carotenoids were measured and correlated with histopathologic findings of gastric biopsies (Haenszel et al., 1985). The data show that circulating carotene levels in both sexes and vitamin E in males were significantly lower in subjects with gastric dysplasia than in subjects with normal mucosa or subjects with less advanced gastric lesions.

Ovarian

Heinonen, Koskinen, and Tuimala (1985) found no significant differences in vitamin E levels between women with and without ovarian tumors.

All Sites

Nomura et al. (1985) found no association between serum vitamin E levels and subsequent development of lung, colon, rectum, stomach, or bladder cancer in men of Japanese ancestry living in Hawaii.

Wald et al. (1987) recently summarized the results of the BUPA (British United Provident Association) study. In progress for 10 years, this prospective etiological study of adult male cancer involves about 22,000 men aged 35-64. An inverse relation between vitamin E status and cancer incidence was found. However, it was suggested that this association was a consequence of early cancer rather than the low plasma vitamin E levels being a cause. These authors added that the extent to which this (early cancer) offers a complete explanation of the results from all prospective studies awaits the results of examining data from other studies according to the interval between blood collection and the point of cancer diagnosis.

Gey, Brubacher, and Stahelin (1987) reported on the 7-year follow-up in the prospective Basel study on cardiovascular and peripheral arterial diseases. Cancers of the lung, stomach, large bowel, and all other sites were treated separately.

The absolute plasma level of age-standardized mean α-tocopherol was significantly lower at baseline in subjects who later died from combined gastrointestinal cancers (stomach and colorectal).

CIAVIT is a new concept introduced by these authors and is defined as a normalized cumulative index of the antioxidant vitamins obtained by multiplying the micromolar levels of β-carotene, vitamin C, and standardized vitamin E. The age-standardized mean value of CIAVIT is reported to be a more sensitive index for cancer risk than the individual antioxidants.

In the same Basel study, Gey, Brubacher, and Stahelin (1987) found that relative risk (RR) for combined gastrointestinal cancers using age-standardized α-tocopherol mean values was RR ($< 30\ \mu M$) = 1.7 and RR ($> 30\ \mu M$) = 0.75. Using the CIAVIT index, the following was reported: CIAVIT > 100, RR = 2.0; CIAVIT (100–400), RR = 1.2; CIAVIT (> 400), RR = 0.7.

Serum vitamin E levels in subjects (n = 111) in the Hypertension Detection and Follow-up Program who later developed cancer were lower than those of controls (n = 210) matched for age, sex, race, and time of blood collection (Willett et al., 1984). Serum vitamin E levels were lower in subjects who later had cancer as compared with controls: 1.16 and 1.26 mg/dl. When adjusted for serum cholesterol levels (lipid levels), the case-control difference was -0.05 mg/dl. Although the data in this particular study do not support the hypothesis relating intake or serum levels of vitamin E to a reduced risk of cancer, the study design has come under criticism.

The observations of Menkes et al. (1986) that vitamin E is inversely related to lung cancer prompted an analysis of 10,532 subjects in The Netherlands (Kok et al., 1987). In the nine years since the study commenced, 114 subjects have died of cancer. Risk analysis according to quintile showed a strong negative trend for vitamin E, suggesting an increased risk of all cancers associated with lower serum levels of vitamin E. The relative risk was in the lowest quintile for serum vitamin E was 4.4 when the highest quintile was used as the reference category. At this intermediate point, the results of this 1975 prospective study do not support the Menkes study for lung cancer alone but become statistically significant when *all* cancers are considered. The authors report that the number of lung cancer cases was probably too small to make the 9% difference in mean serum levels of vitamin E between cases and controls significant.

Salonen et al. (1985) determined the independent and joint association of serum selenium, retinol, and α-tocopherol concentrations with the risk of death from cancer using the Eastern Finland Heart Survey data of 1977. The adjusted risk of fatal cancer was 5.8-fold (95% confidence interval 1.2–29.0) among subjects in the lowest tertile of selenium concentrations compared to those with higher values. Subjects with both low selenium and low α-tocopherol concentrations in serum had an 11.4-fold adjusted risk. Among smoking men with cancer, serum retinol concentrations were 26% lower than in smoking controls (p =

0.002). These data suggest that dietary selenium deficiency is associated with an increased risk of fatal cancer, that low vitamin E intake may enhance this effect, and that decreased vitamin A or provitamin A intake contributes to the risk of lung cancer among smoking men with a low selenium intake. In contrast, the recent report by Menkes et al. (1986) found an interaction of high serum selenium levels with low serum α-tocopherol levels in association with an increased risk of lung cancer. The authors addressed the possibility that serum concentrations may merely be indicators of other measures which might be the real or more important protective factors.

Review of Human Data

Data from several prospective studies support an association of lower plasma α-tocopherol levels with an increased risk of cancer, particularly lung, breast, and gastrointestinal. While the data are encouraging, they are not conclusive. Additional work is needed to confirm these findings. There are a few reports where no significant associations were found, and this can be attributed to relatively small numbers of cancer deaths observed.

In spite of the preliminary nature and limitations, the data are informative in a number of ways. The importance of reporting standardized vitamin E plasma levels has been a critical factor regarding data interpretation. It is interesting to note the variations in the mean plasma or serum vitamin E values of control subjects in several of these studies (e.g., Menkes, Kok, Willett, and Gey studies). Whether this means that risk varies substantially between populations is not clear.

The association of selenium and vitamin E is in keeping with data from animal cancer studies. In addition, the new concept of CIAVIT appears to be an important and a useful approach to explore the potential for synergy among all the antioxidant vitamins. It would, therefore, seem logical to include selenium and other antioxidant micronutrients as part of these measurements in future studies. Given the multitude of potential causes for cancers, it is not surprising that the potential exists for synergistic effect of all the micronutrients that contribute to the body's antioxidant defense system.

Epidemiologic evidence alone is not adequate to prove a direct relationship between vitamin E (and other antioxidants) and cancer. The proof of these associations can only be expected from properly designed intervention trials.

CLINICAL TRIALS

Years of laboratory and epidemiologic research have yielded encouraging results. Both the animal experiments and epidemiologic data have provided significant leads as to the importance of nutrition and specific dietary components as risk

Table 1 Clinical Trials Related to Vitamin E and Cancer Prevention

Target site	Target group	Cancer-Preventive agents in addition to vitamin E
Colon	Familial polyposis	Vitamin C, bran
Colon	Adenomatous polyps	β-Carotene, vitamin C
Colon	Normal subjects	Vitamin C
Esophagus	Dysplasia	Multiple vitamins and minerals
Esophagus	High-risk population	Multiple vitamins and minerals
Lung	Smokers (male)	β-Carotene
Skin	Basal cell carcinoma	β-Carotene, vitamin C
All sites	Normal (nurses)	Vitamin A, vitamin C, vitamin B_6, selenium

Source: Adapted from DeWys et al., 1986.

factors for cancer. The primary reasons for conducting the clinical trials are to determine the specificity of the epidemiologic findings and the clinical relevance of experimental data. The objectives are to prevent/reverse precursor lesions; prevent progression to malignancy; reduce incidence of malignancy; and, finally, reduce mortality. A range of inhibitory agents are being examined, among them a number of micronutrients including key antioxidants. A list of studies involving vitamin E are shown in Table 1. In many of the trials, serum levels of the micronutrients are also being analyzed so that correlations can be made with subsequent development of cancer. The next few years should be exciting as preliminary data from the chemoprevention program will begin to emerge, and should the results continue to show promise, large-scale trials could then be undertaken to document the efficacy of the micronutrients.

α-TOCOPHEROL: PHARMACOKINETICS—ANIMAL AND HUMAN TISSUE RESPONSE

Absorption

α-Tocopherol, the principle form of vitamin E, is a fat-soluble compound. As such, the absorption of this substance as well as related compounds follows the course of fat digestion and is dependent on an individual's ability to absorb fat. Studies in animals have shown that bile is essential for absorption (Gallo-Torres, 1970; McMahon and Thompson, 1970). The main site of absorption of α-tocopherol in the rat is the jejunum (Gallo-Torres, 1980).

Absorption of vitamin E in humans is maximal in the median portion of the small intestine. Although not proven, vitamin E is apparently absorbed as a lipid-bile micelle together with free fatty acids, monoglycerides, and other fat-soluble vitamins by penetrating the epithelial cells through the plasma membrane of the absorptive cells in the brush border. Tocopheryl acetate, a major stabilized ester form of vitamin E, is almost completely hydrolyzed prior to absorption (Mathias et al., 1981). There is no absorption of the unhydrolyzed ester. Unlike vitamin A, α-tocopherol is not reesterified during absorption. The efficiency of absorption is dependent upon several factors. As the dose increases, the percentage of absorption decreases. Schmandke, Sima, and Manne (1967) evaluated the absorption of α-tocopherol in humans over a dose range of 10 to 2000 mg. The percent absorbed over a 24-hour period ranged from 97% to 55%, respectively. Dietary lipids can modulate the efficiency of absorption of the vitamin. Medium chain triglycerides enhance absorption, and polyunsaturated fatty acids are inhibitory (Brin and Gallo-Torres, 1974). Generally, in animals, it has been observed that vitamin E is absorbed twice as well from aqueous emulsions as from oil solutions (Schmandke and Schmidt, 1965).

Transport

α-Tocopherol is transported from the intestine into the lymph in chylomicrons, which rapidly equilibrate with other lipoproteins. The majority of vitamin E is distributed in the low density lipoproteins. There is some evidence that lipoprotein distribution is different in males vs. females (Behrens, Thompson, and Madere, 1982). The level of plasma tocopherol is correlated rather well with total plasma lipids, total plasma cholesterol, as well as low density lipoprotein (Rubinstein, Dietz, and Srinivasan, 1969).

Tissue Levels

In animals, the tissue uptake of tocopherol increases linearly with the logarithm of the dose (Kayden, Chow, and Bjornson, 1973; Gallo-Torres, 1980; Behrens, Thompson, and Madere, 1982). In therapeutic terms, a 10-fold increase in tocopherol intake would approximately double plasma levels with a similar or smaller increase occurring in the tissues. Tissues vary in their concentration of vitamin E with the adrenal and pituitary glands, testes, and platelets exhibiting the highest vitamin E concentrations (see Table 2). α-Tocopherol has been found to be most concentrated in cell fractions rich in membranelike mitochondria and microsomes. Recent reports have demonstrated the existence of cytosol-binding proteins which apparently are involved in the transport of the vitamin into mitochondrial (Mowri, et al., 1981) and microsomal membranes (Murphy and Mavis, 1981).

Table 2 α-Tocopherol Content of Human Tissues

Tissue	μ/g tissue	mg/g lipid
Plasma	9.5	1.4
Erythrocytes	2.3	0.5
Platelets	30.0	1.3
Adipose tissue	150.0	0.2
Kidney	7.0	0.3
Liver	13.0	0.3
Muscle	19.0	0.4
Ovary	11.0	0.6
Uterus	9.0	0.7
Heart	20.0	0.7
Adrenal	132.0	0.7
Testis	40.0	1.0
Pituitary	40.0	1.2

Source: Adapted from Machlin, 1984.

Metabolism

Vitamin E undergoes very little metabolism. The major route of excretion is fecal elimination of the unabsorbed vitamin, which differs widely depending on the administered dose and composition of the preparation. Tocopherol excretion into the feces can also be from secretion from the intestinal mucosal cells back into the lumen, desquamation of intestinal epithelial cell, and biliary excretion. Usually, less than 1% of the dose is excreted in the urine, largely as tocopheronic acid or tocopheronolactone (Simon's metabolites). It is not known whether vitamin E (or its metabolite) undergoes enterohepatic circulation. An excellent discussion of the biochemistry of vitamin E has been written by Gallo-Torres (1980).

SIDE EFFECTS

Both acute and chronic studies with several species of animals have demonstrated that high doses of vitamin E are relatively nontoxic. Vitamin E has also been found to be nonmutagenic, nonteratogenic, and noncarcinogenic (Anonymous 1975).

An interesting interaction has been observed between vitamin E and vitamin K in both animals and humans (Corrigan, 1982). Administration of large doses of vitamin E to vitamin K-deficient animals and also humans can exacerbate the coagulation defect due to vitamin K deficiency. This is also true in subjects on anticoagulant therapy. In this situation, one could either stop the vitamin E supplementation or reduce the dosage of the anticoagulant. It is important to note that in individuals with normal vitamin K status, ingestion of large doses of vitamin E has no effect on the coagulant system.

In humans, there are scattered reports of a few side effects of high-dose vitamin E ingestion, but these are largely subjective and based upon uncontrolled observation. Transient gastrointestinal disturbance has been more commonly mentioned. Roberts (1981), based upon experience in his own practice, reported a relationship between thrombophlebitis and ingestion of large doses of vitamin E. However, this anecdotal finding has not been confirmed.

Salkeld (1979) has made an exhaustive review of side effects of vitamin E reported in over 10,000 cases. These subjects were ingesting over 200 IU of vitamin E per day orally on a chronic basis and, of these, 5000 were taking in excess of 1000 IU per day. In all these, incidence of side effects of a minor nature (GI symptoms, etc.) were reported by only 0.8% of the subjects. This degree of side effects would be expected in any normal population; thus, the current evidence documents the safety of vitamin E.

DOSE AND FORMULATION

The "vitamin E" of commerce is a loose term that includes several different tocopherol moieties, principally the unesterified forms of the molecules as well as the acetic and succinic esters. All of these molecules have three asymmetric centers at positions 2′, 4′, and 8′ in the phytol chain, which appear to have some effect on the biological activity. The biological activity is based upon animal bioassays; and, consequently, the activity of the various forms is given in units of activity and not milligrams. The generally accepted values for these activities in international units (IU/mg) are as follows: dl-α-tocopheryl acetate (all racemic), 1.00; dl-α-tocopherol (all racemic), 1.10; d-α-tocopheryl acetate (RRR), 1.36; d-α-tocopherol (RRR), 1.49; dl-α-tocopheryl acid succinate (all racemic), 0.89; d-α-tocopheryl acid succinate (RRR), 1.21.

Most commercially available forms of vitamin E are the esters, particularly the acetate. The hemisuccinate form is less popular. These esters are not naturally occurring but were developed as a means of stabilizing the tocopherol molecule for use in foods and pharmaceuticals that present processing and long-term stability problems. It is important to recognize that these esters of vitamin E are not active per se as antioxidants or free radical scavengers. This is a significant distinction since exogenous applications involving inhibition of lipid peroxidation, nitroso compound formation, etc. require the free tocopherol molecule. This is also true of studies seeking to evaluate the activity of α-tocopherol in the upper portion of the GI tract (stomach, duodenum, etc.) because little or no hydrolysis of these esters can be expected to occur in these regions.

All of these forms of the vitamin E molecule are either oils or, at best, low melting solids. Their use in solid dosage forms requires that these physical properties be altered to yield forms that can withstand the rigors of a tabletting press and not affect the desired physical properties of the tablet. Similarly, hard shell gelatin capsule formulations generally also require a solid material. Successfully marketed forms of vitamin E accomplish this goal by employing microencapsulation techniques using a number of substrates as a matrix (e.g., gelatin, starch, gums, etc.). This approach not only addresses the physical need but also produces vitamin E forms with enhanced absorption. The latter is the result of emulsifying and subdividing the pure material in a range of particle sizes (1-3 μm) that aids the absorption process in the lower GI tract. The same approach has been used to develop oily forms of vitamin E for use in applications such as soft elastic gelatin capsules. The proper use of emulsifying agents and carefully selected triglycerides will facilitate disperson of these oily forms in the GI tract providing optimum absorption efficiency.

As data emerge from the many prospective studies underway on the relationship of vitamin E to cancer in humans, a more definitive picture should develop on target plasma levels. Dosage forms and regimens to achieve these targets can readily be met with the currently available commercial forms of vitamin E and th formulation technology at hand.

DIETARY CONSIDERATIONS FOR α-TOCOPHEROL

Vitamin E occurs widely in nature in foods of animal and plant origin as well as vegetable oils. While estimates of dietary intake are theoretically possible to calculate from food tables, in practice, a poor correlation is found because of the many influences (seasonal, age, processing, etc.) on the factual content of many foods (Bauernfeind, 1980; Bright-See, 1984). A typical "well-balanced" U.S. diet is expected to provide about 15 IU of vitamin E daily, and the current RDA for vitamin E is, in fact, based on this premise. In a normal adult American not taking any supplements, serum plasma levels of vitamin E are generally in the range of 0.8-1.0 mg/dl. This is quite adequate with respect to preventing deficiency, and the current data indicate that plasma levels below 0.5 mg/dl will lead to deficiency symptoms as assessed by the RBC hemolysis test. The definition of adequacy with respect to preventing deficiency states will not necessarily apply to optimal plasma levels to reduce risk for cancer. This type of data will only become available from the prospective studies, some of which are currently underway. There is some preliminary data that does suggest that for lowering the risk for intestinal cancer, for instance, plasma vitamin E level would have to be greater than 1.29 mg/dl. This would mean an intake of 60–100 IU (Gey, Brubacher, and Stahelin, 1987).

MACRONUTRIENT INTERACTIONS

Polyunsaturated fatty acids (PUFA) represent the primary macronutrients having an impact on vitamin E status, and there is a direct relationship between the PUFA content of diet and vitamin E needs. Approximate requirements for vitamin E in terms of PUFA intake have been calculated and the generally accepted vitamin E/PUFA ratio (mg α-tocopherol/g of PUFA) is 0.4 (Food and Nutrition Board, 1980). The source of dietary fat with reference to P:S ratio, therefore, has an effect on vitamin E needs.

SUMMARY AND CONCLUSIONS

Insight into the mechanisms of cancer induction has provided the framework to evaluate the potential role of vitamin E in cancer prevention. Evidence presented in this chapter reflect the role of α-tocopherol in preventing the formation of carcinogens, inhibiting carcinogens from reaching target sites, and suppressing the expression of neoplasia. The inhibition of N-nitroso compound formation is a good example of the role of α-tocopherol in blocking the formation of carcinogens. This has now been well documented in both in vitro and in vivo studies. α-Tocopherol has also been shown to inhibit initiation-related events, e.g., binding of metabolically activated carcinogens to DNA, carcinogen-induced chromosomal damage, and sister-chromatid exchanges. Similarly, α-tocopherol has been shown to be effective in inhibiting promotion-related events such as TPA-caused ODC induction. The stimulatory effect of α-tocopherol on the immune system represents another important function in cancer prevention.

Animal studies have mainly employed UV-induced and chemically induced cancer. In these more complex models, the cancer inhibitory effect of α-tocopherol is less clear-cut. α-Tocopherol exhibits a consistent effect as an inhibitor of promotion, particularly croton oil and TPA in two-stage skin models. In DMBA-induced oral cancer in hamsters, α-tocopherol has again been found to be consistently effective. In the mammary tumor model, however, the effectiveness of α-tocopherol is very much influenced by changes in dietary composition and other micronutrients such as selenium. Similar influences have been reported in UVL-skin and DMBA-skin models. It is, therefore, not surprising to find that the combination of more than one micronutrient (i.e., selenium and α-tocopherol) may be consistently more effective in certain experimental models.

The data from human prospective studies exploring the association of elevated serum α-tocopherol with lower cancer risk also are encouraging but by no means conclusive. As data from these prospective studies and others become available, a more definitive conclusion on the relationship between plasma tocopherol levels and cancer risk can be made. As in the case of animal models, evidence of synergy between selected micronutrients is also emerging. In this context, the concept of CIAVIT (cumulative antioxidant index), developed by Gey and his colleagues, is attractive and relevant and, therefore, should be taken into account in future prospective studies. This would mean optimizing the antioxidant potential of the individual by appropriate intake of all the antioxidant micronutrients so as to reduce the risk for cancer. It is possible that the promise of vitamin E for cancer prevention may be much greater when considered in association with other key antioxidants.

ACKNOWLEDGMENTS

The authors wish to thank Ms. Carol Piascik for her excellent and dedicated efforts in the preparation of this manuscript and Professors A. H. Conney and H. L. Newmark for their valuable suggestions.

REFERENCES

Adamson, R. H., Sieber, S. M. (1977). Antineoplastic agents as potential carcinogens. In *Origins of Human Cancer*, H. H. Hiatt, J. D. Watson, and J. A. Winston (Eds.). Cold Spring Harbor Laboratory, New York, pp. 429–443.

Anonymous. (1975). Evaluations of the health aspects of tocopherols and alpha-tocopheryl acetate as food ingredients. Report No. PB262653 prepared for the RDA by the Federation of the American Societies for Experimental Biology, Bethesda, MD.

Bauernfeind, J. C. (1977). The tocopherol content of food and influencing factors. *CRC Crit. Rev. Food Sci. Nutr. 8*(4):337.

Bauernfeind, J. C. (1980). Tocopherols in foods. In *Vitamin E: A Comprehensive Treatise*, L. J. Machlin (Ed.). Marcel Dekker, New York, pp. 99–168.

Beckman, C., Roy, R. M., Sproule, A. (1982). Modification of radiation induced sex linked recessive lethal mutation frequency by tocopherol. *Mutation Res. 105*:73.

Behrens, W. A., Thompson, J. N., Madere, R. (1982). Distribution of alpha-tocopherol in human plasma lipoproteins. *Am. J. Clin. Nutr. 35*:691.

Bendich, A., Gabriel, E., Machlin, L. J. (1986). Dietary vitamin E requirement for optimum immune response in the rat. *J. Nutr. 116*:675.

Black, H. S. (1983). Utility of the skin/UV-carcinogenesis model for evaluating the role of nutritional lipids in cancer. In *Diet, Nutrition, and Cancer: From Basic Research to Policy Implications*, D. A. Roe (Ed.). Alan R. Liss Inc., New York, pp. 49–60.

Black, H. S., Chan, J. T. (1975). Suppression of ultraviolet light-induced tumor formation by dietary antioxidants. *J. Invest. Dermatol. 65*:412.

Black, H. S., Lenger, W., Phelps, A. W., Thornby, J. I. (1983a). Influence of dietary lipid upon ultra-violet light carcinogenesis. *Nutr. Cancer 5*:59.

Black, H. S., Lenger, W. A., McCann, V., Thornby, J. I. (1983b). Relation of UV dose to antioxidant modification of photocarcinogenesis. *J. Amer. College of Tox. 2*:201.

Black, M. M., Zachrau, R. E., Dion, A. S., Katz, M. (1984). Stimulation of prognostically favorable cell-mediated immunity of breast cancer patients by high dose vitamin A and vitamin E. In *Vitamins, Cancer, and Nutrition*, K. N. Prasad (Ed.). Karger, Basel, pp. 134–146.

Black, H. S., Lenger, W. A., Gergius, J., Thornby, J. I. (1985). Relation of antioxidants and level of dietary lipid to epidermal lipid peroxidation and ultraviolet carcinogenesis. *Cancer Res. 45*:6254.

Bonmassar, E., Dallavalle, R., Giuliani, G. (1968). Influsso della vitamina E e del gallato di propile sulla cancerogenesi da benzopirene nel toppo. *Arch. Ital. Patol. Clin. Tumori 11*:245.

Bright-See, E. (1984). Role of vitamins C and E in the etiology of human cancer. In *Vitamins, Nutrition, and Cancer,* K. N. Prasad (Ed.). Karger, Basel, pp. 68–75.

Brin, M., Gallo-Torres, H. E. (1974). Effect of medium chain triglycerides on the intestinal absorption, tissue distribution and urinary excretion of vitamin E. *Fed. Proc. 33*:671.

Burton, G. W., Cheeseman, K. H., Doba, T., Ingold, K. A., Slater, T. F. (1983). Vitamin E as an antioxidant *in vitro* and *in vivo*. In *Biology of Vitamin E*, R. Porter and J. Whelan (Eds.). Petman, London, pp. 4–18.

Carpenter, M. P. (1986). Effects of vitamin E on the immune system. In *Vitamins and Cancer*, F. L. Meyskens and K. N. Prasad (Eds.). Humana Press, Clifton, NJ, pp. 199–211.

Chan, J. T., Black, H. S. (1977). The mitigating effects of dietary antioxidants on chemically-induced carcinogenesis. *Experientia 34*:110.

Cook, M. G., McNamara, P. (1980). Effect of dietary vitamin E on dimethylhydrazine-induced colonic tumors in mice. *Cancer Res. 40*:1329.

Corrigan, Jr., J. J. (1982). The effect of vitamin E on warfarin-induced vitamin K deficiency. *Ann. N.Y. Acad. Sci. 393*:361.

Csallany, A. S., Draper, H. H., Shah, S. N. (1962). Conversion of alpha-tocopherol C^{14} to tocopheryl-p-quinone *in vivo*. *Arch. Biochem. Biophys. 98*:142.

Dashman, T., Kamm, J. J. (1979). Effects of high doses of vitamin E on dimethylnitrosamine hepatotoxicity and drug metabolism in the rat. *Biochem. Pharmacol. 28*:1485.

DeWys, W. D., Malone, W. F., Butrum, R. R., Sestili, M. A. (1986). Clinical trials in cancer prevention. *Cancer 58*:1954.

Dipple, A., Moschel, R. C., Bigger, C. A. H. (1984). Polynuclear aromatic carcinogens. In *Chemical Carcinogens*, 2 ed., Vol. I (ACS Monograph 182), C. E. Searle (Ed.). American Chemical Society, Washington, D.C., pp. 41–163.

Doll, R., Peto, R. (1981). The causes of cancer: Quantitative estimates of avoidable risks of cancer in the United States today. *J. Nat. Cancer Inst. 66*:1192.

Epstein, S. S., Iqbal, Z. M., Johnson, M. D. (1980). *In vivo* nitrosation of morpholine in mice by inhaled NO_2. In *N-Nitroso Compounds: Analysis, Formation, and Occurrence*, E. A. Walker, L. Griciute, M. Castegnaro, and M. Borzsonyi (Eds.). International Agency for Research on Cancer, Lyon, pp. 195–206.

Epstein, S. S., Joshi, S., Andrea, J., Forsyth, J., Mantel, N. (1967). The null effect of antioxidants on the carcinogencity of 3,4,9,10-dibenzpyrene to mice. *Life Sci. 6*:225.

Evans, H. E. (1962). The pioneer history of vitamin E. *Vitamin Horm. 20*:379.

Federal Register. (1985). *50*(129):27,573–575.

Food and Nutrition Board. (1980). In *Recommended Dietary Allowances*, National Academy of Sciences, Washington, D.C., pp. 63–69.

Fiddler, W., Pensabene, J. W., Piotrowski, E. G., Phillips, J. G., Keating, J., Mergens, W. J., Newmark, H. L. (1978). Inhibition of formation of volatile nitrosamines in fried bacon by the use of cure-solubilized alpha-tocopherol. *J. Ag. Food Chem. 26*:653.

Gallo-Torres, H. E. (1970). Obligatory role of bile for the intestinal absorption of vitamin E. *Lipid 5*:379.

Gallo-Torres, H. E. (1980). Absorption, transport and metabolism. In *Vitamin E: A Comprehensive Treatise*, L. J. Machlin (Ed.). Marcel Dekker, New York, pp. 170–267.

Gey, K. F., Brubacher, G. B., Stahelin, H. B. (1987). Plasma levels of antioxidant vitamins in relation to ischemic heart disease and cancer. *Am. J. Clin. Nutr. 45*:1368.

Haber, S. L., Wissler, R. W. (1962). Effect of vitamin E on the carcinogenicity of methylcholanthrene. *Proc. Soc. Exp. Biol. Med. 111*:774.

Haenszel, W., Correa, P., Lopez, A., Cuello, C., Zarama, G., Zavala, D., Fontham, E. (1985). Serum micronutrient levels in relation to gastric pathology. *Int. J. Cancer 36*:43.

Harman, D. (1969). Dimethylbenzanthrene-induced cancer: Inhibitory effect of dietary vitamin E. *Clin. Res. 17*:125.

Harr, J. R., Exon, J. H., Whanger, P. D., Weswig, P. H. (1972). Effects of dietary selenium on N-2-fluorenzyl-acetamide (FAA)-induced cancer in vitamin E supplemented, selenium depleted rats. *Clin. Toxicol. 5*(2):187.

Heinonen, P. K., Koskinen, T., Tuilmala, R. (1985). Serum levels of vitamins A and E in women with ovarian cancer. *Arch. Gynecol. 237*:37.

Helson, L., Verma, M., Helson, C. (1982). Vitamin E and human neuroblastoma. *Ann. N.Y. Acad. Sci. 393*:226.

Hennekens, C. H. (1986). Micronutrients and cancer prevention. *New England J. Med. 315*(20):1288.

Hoffeld, J. T. (1981). Agents which block membrane lipid peroxidation enhance mouse spleen cell immune activities *in vitro*: Relationship to enhancing activity of 2-mercaptoethanol. *Eur. J. Immunol. 11*:371.

Hoffeld, J. T. (1983). Inhibition of lymphocyte proliferation and antibody promotion *in vitro* by silica, talc, bentonite, or corynebacterium parvam:

Involvement of peroxidative process. *Eur. J. Immunol. 13*:364.

Horvath, P. M., Ip, C. (1983). Synergistic effect of vitamin E and selenium in the chemoprevention of mammary carcinogenesis in rats. *Cancer Res. 43*:5335.

Horwitt, M. K. (1970). Tocopherol and polyunsaturated fatty acid relationships. In *International Symposium on Vitamin E*, N. Shimazono and Y. Takagi (Eds.). Kyoritsu Chuppan Co. Ltd., Tokoyo, p. 45.

Ip, C. (1982). Dietary vitamin E intake and mammary carcinogenesis in rats. *Carcinogenesis 3*(12):1453.

Iqbal, Z. M., Dahl, K., Epstein, S. S. (1980). Role of nitrogen dioxide in the biosynthesis of nitrosamines in mice. *Science 207*:1475.

Jaffe, W. (1946). The influence of wheat germ oil on the production of tumors in rats by methylcholanthrene. *Exptl. Med. Surg. 4*:278.

Kagerud, A., Holm, G., Larsson, H., Peterson, H. I. (1978). Tocopherol and local x-ray irradiation of two transplanted rat tumors. *Cancer Letters 5*:123.

Kagerud, A., Lund, N., Peterson, H. I. (1981). Tocopherol in irradiation of temporary hypoxic tumors. *Acta Radiologica 20*:1.

Kahl, R. (1986). The dual role of antioxidants in the modification of chemical carcinogenesis. *J. Environ. Sci. Health C4*(1):47.

Kamm, J. J., Dashman, T., Newmark, H. L., Mergens, W. J. (1977). Inhibition of amine-nitrite hepatotoxicity by alpha-tocopherol. *Toxicol. Appl. Pharmacol. 41*(3):575.

Kayden, H. J., Chow, C. K., Bjornson, L. K. (1973). Spectrophotometric method for the determination of tocopherol in red blood cells. *J. Lipid Res. 14*: 533.

King, M. M., McCay, P. B. (1983). Modulation of tumor incidence and possible mechanism of mammary carcinogenesis by dietary antioxidants. *Cancer Res. (Suppl.) 43*:2485s.

Kok, F. J., Van Duijn, C. M., Hofman, A., Vermeeren, R., De Bruijn, A. M., Valkenburg, H. A. (1987). Micronutrients and the risk of lung cancer (Letter to the Editor). *New England J. Med. 316*:1416.

Konings, A. W. T., Trieling, W. B. (1977). The inhibition of DNA synthesis in vitamin E depleted lymphosarcoma cells by X-rays and cytostatics. *Int. J. Radiation Biol. 31*:397.

Kozumbo, W. J., Seed, J. L., Kensler, T. W. (1983). Inhibition by 2(3)tert-butyl-4-hydroxyanisole and other antioxidants of epidermal ornithine decarboxylase activity induced by 12-0-tetradecanoyl-phorbyl-13-acetate. *Cancer Res. 43*:2555.

Kune, S., Kune, G. A., Watson, L. F. (1987). Case-control study of dietary etiological factors: The Melbourne Colorectal Cancer Study. *Nutrition and Cancer 9*(1):21.

Kurek, M. P., Corwin, L. M. (1982). Vitamin E protection against tumor formation by transplanted murine Sarcoma cells. *Nutr. Cancer 4*:128.

Lee, C., Chen, C. (1979). Enhancement of mammary tumorigenesis in rats by vitamin E deficiency. *Proc. Am. Assoc. Cancer Res. Am. Soc. Clin. Oncol. 20*:132.

MacGregor, J. T., Wilson, R. E., Neff, W. E., Frankel, E. N. (1985). Mutagenicity tests of lipid peroxidation products in *Salmonella Typhimurium*: Monohydroperoxides and secondary oxidation products of methyl linoleate and methyl linolenate. *Fd. Chem. Toxic. 23*:1041.

Machlin, L. J., Filipski, R. J., Nelson, J., Horn, L., Brin, M. (1977). Effects of a prolonged vitamin E deficiency in the rat. *J. Nutr. 107*:1200.

Machlin, L. J., ed. (1984). In *Handbook of Vitamins*. Marcel Dekker, New York.

Mason, K. (1954). Effects of deficiency. In *The Vitamins*, Part III, Vol. 3, W. H. Sebrell and R. S. Harris (Eds.). Academic Press, New York, pp. 514–562.

Mathias, P. M., Harries, J. T., Peters, T. J., Muller, D. P. R. (1981). Studies on the *in vivo* absorption of micellar solutions of tocopherol and tocopheryl acetate in the rat: Demonstration and partial characterization of a mucosal esterase localized to the endoplasmic reticulum of the enterocyte. *J. Lipid Res. 22*:829.

Matsuura, T., Ueyama, H., Nomi, S., Ueda, K. (1979). Effect of alpha-tocopherol on the binding of benzo(A)pyrene to nuclear macromolecules. *J. Nutr. Sci. Vitaminol. 25*:495.

McCay, P. B., King, M. M., Pitha, J. V. (1981). Evidence that the effectiveness of antioxidants as inhibitors of 7,12-DMBA-induced mammary tumors is a function of dietary fat composition. *Cancer Res. 41*:3745.

McMahon, M. T., Thompson, G. R. (1970). Comparison of the absorption of a polar lipid, oleic acid, and a non-polar lipid, alpha-tocopherol, from mixed micellar solution and emulsions. *Eur. J. Clin. Investigation 1*:161.

Menkes, M. S., Comstock, G. W., Vuilleumier, J. P., Helsing, K. J., Rider, A. A., Brookmeyer, R. (1986). Serum beta-carotene, vitamins A and E, selenium and the risk of lung cancer. *New England J. Med. 315*(20):1250.

Mergens, W. J., Kamm, J. J., Newmark, H. L., Fiddler, W., Pensabene, J. (1978). alpha-Tocopherol: Uses in preventing nitrosamine formation. In *Environmental Aspects of N-Nitroso Compounds*, E. A. Walker, M. Castegnaro, L. Griciuite, and R. E. Lyle (Eds.). International Agency for Research on Cancer, Lyon, pp. 199–212.

Mergens, W. J., Chau, J., Newmark, H. L. (1980). The influence of ascorbic acid and dl-alpha-tocopherol on the formation of nitrosamines in an *in vitro* gastrointestinal model system. In *N-Nitroso Compounds: Analysis, Formation, and Occurrence*, E. A. Walker, M. Castegnaro, L. Griciute, and M. Borzsonyi (Eds.). International Agency for Research on Cancer, Lyon, pp. 259–267.

Miller, J. A., Miller, E. C. (1977). Ultimate chemical carcinogens as reactive mutagenic electrophiles. In *Origins of Human Cancer, Book B: Mechanisms of carcinogenesis*, H. H. Hiatt, J. D. Watson, and J. A. Winsten (Eds.). Cold Spring Harbor Laboratory, New York, pp. 605–629.

Mirvish, S. S. (1981). Ascorbic acid inhibition of N-nitroso compound formation in chemical, food, and biological systems. In *Inhibition of Tumor Induction and Development*, M. S. Zedeck and M. Lipkin (Eds.). Plenum Press, New York, pp. 101–126.

Mirvish, S. S. (1986). Effect of vitamins C and E on N-nitroso compound formation, carcinogenesis, and cancer. *Cancer 58*(8):1842.

Mirvish, S. S., Issenberg, P., Sams, J. P. (1981). N-Nitroso-morpholine synthesis in rodents exposed to NO_2 and morpholine. In *N-Nitroso Compounds* (ACS Symposium Series 174), R. A. Scanlan and S. R. Tannenbaum (Eds.). American Chemical Society, Washington, D.C., pp. 181–193.

Mirvish, S. S., Sams, J. P., Issenberg, P. (1983). The nitrosating agent in mice exposed to nitrogen dioxide: Improved extraction method and localization in the skin. *Cancer Res. 43*:2550.

Mowri, H., Nakagawa, Y., Inove, K., Nojima, S. (1981). Enhancement of the transfer of alpha-tocopherol between liposomes and mitochondria by rat liver protein(s). *Eur. J. Biochem. 117*:537.

Murphy, D. J., Mavis, R. D. (1981). Membrane transfer of alpha-tocopherol. *J. Biol. Chem. 256*:10,464–468.

Nakadate, T., Yamamoto, S., Aizu, E., Kato, R. (1984). Effects of flavinoids and antioxidants on 12-0-tetradecanoylphorbol-13-acetate caused by epidermal ornithine decarboxylase induction on tumor promotion in relation to lipoxygenase inhibition by these compounds. *GANN 75*:214.

Narayan, K. A. (1970). Vitamin E deficiency and chemical carcinogenesis. *Experientia 26*:840.

National Research Council. (1982). *Diet, nutrition, and cancer*. Commission on Life Sciences, National Academy of Sciences, National Research Council, Washington, D.C.

Nelson, J. (1980). Pathology of vitamin E deficiency. In *Vitamin E: A Comprehensive Treatise*, L. J. Machlin (Ed.). Marcel Dekker, New York, pp. 397–428.

Newel, G. R. (1981). General mechanisms of carcinogenesis. In *Nutrition and Cancer: Etiology and Treatment, Progress in Cancer Research and Therapy*, Vol. 17, G. R. Newel and N. M. Ellison (Eds.). Raven Press, New York, pp. 49–58.

Newmark, H. L., Mergens, W. J. (1981). alpha-Tocopherol (vitamin E) and its relationship to tumor induction and development. In *Inhibition of Tumor Induction and Development*, M. S. Zedeck and M. Lipkin (Eds.). Plenum Publishing Corp., New York, pp. 127–168.

Newmark, H. L. (1987). Nutrient density: an important and useful tool for laboratory animals studies. *Carcinogenesis 8*:871.

Nomura, A. M. Y., Stemmerman, G. N., Heilbrun, L. K., Salkeld, R. M., Vuillemier, J. P. (1985). Serum vitamin levels and the risk of cancer of specific sites in men of Japanese ancestry in Hawaii. *Cancer Res. 45*:2369.

Norkus, E. P., Boyle, S., Kuenzig, W., Mergens, W. J. (1984). Formation of N-nitrosomorpholine in mice treated with morpholine and exposed to nitrogen dioxide. *Carcinogenesis 5*(5):549.

Norkus, E. P., Kuenzig, W. A., Chau, J., Mergens, W. J., Conney, A. H. (1986). Inhibitory effect of alpha-tocopherol on the formation of nitrosomorpholine in mice treated with morpholine and exposed to nitrogen dioxide. *Carcinogenesis 7*(3):357.

Odukoya, O., Hawach, F., Shklar, G. (1984). Retardation of experimental oral cancer by topical vitamin E. *Nutr. Cancer 6*:98.

Ohshima, H., Bartsch, H. (1981). Quantitative estimation of endogeneous nitrosation in humans by monitoring N-nitrosoproline excreted in the urine. *Cancer Res. 41*:3658.

Palmer, S. (1986). Dietary considerations for risk reduction. *Cancer 58*:1949.

Patterson, R. M., Smalls, E., Lyn-Cook, B. D. (1981). Reduction of DMSO induced chromasomal alterations by vitamin E. *J. Cell Biol. 91*:60a.

Pauling, L., Willowghby, R., Reynolds, R., Blaesdell, B. E., Lawson, S. (1982). Incidence of squamous cell carcinoma in hairless mice irradiated with UV light in relation to intake of ascorbic acid and dl-alpha-tocopheryl acetate. *Int. J. Nutr. Res. Suppl. 23*:53.

Perchellet, J. P., Owen, M. D., Posey, T. D., Orten, D. K., Schneider, B. A. (1985). Inhibitory effects of glutathione level raising agents and d-alpha-tocopherol on ornithine decarboxylase induction and mouse skin tumor promotion by 12-0-tetradecanoylphorbal-13-acetate. *Carcinogenesis 6*:567.

Pitot, H. C. (1978). Interactions in the natural history of aging and carcinogenesis. *Fed. Proc. 37*:2841.

Prasad, K. N., Edwards-Prasad, J. (1982). Effects of tocopheryl acid succinate on morpholigical alterations and growth inhibition in melanoma cells in culture. *Cancer Res. 42*:550.

Rama, B. N., Detsch, R. M., Prasad, K. N. (1984). Combined effect of dl-alpha-tocopheryl succinate gamma irradiation and hyperthermia on neuroblastoma cells in culture. *J. Amer. Clin. Nutr. 3*:252. (Abstract)

Roberts, H. J. (1981). Perspective on vitamin E therapy. *JAMA 246*(2):129.

Rubinstein, H. M., Dietz, A. A., Srinivasan, R. (1969). Relation of vitamin E and serum lipids. *Clin. Chimica Acta. 23*:1.

Russo, P., Pala, M., Parodi, S., Ghiara, C., Ferrari, N., Vidali, G. (1984). Effects of vitamin E on liver DNA. *Cancer Lett. 25*:163.

Sadek, I. (1984). Vitamin E and its effect on skin papilloma. In *Vitamins, Nutrition, and Cancer*, K. N. Prasad (Ed.). Karger, Basel, pp. 118–122.

Sakagami, H., Asaka, K., Abe, E., Miyaura, C., Suda, T., Konno, K. (1981). Effect of dl-alpha-tocopherol (vitamin E) on the differentiation of mouse myeloid leukemia cells. *J. Nutr. Sci. Vitaminol. 27*:291.

Sakamoto, K., Sakka, M. (1973). Reduced effect of irradiation on normal and malignant cells irradiated *in vivo* in mice pretreated with vitamin E. *Brit. J. Radiol. 46*:538.

Salkeld, R. M. (1979). *Fed. Register 44*:16,172–176.

Salonen, J. T., Salonen, R., Lappetelainen, R., Maenpaa, P. H., Alfthan, G., Puska, P. (1985). Risk of cancer in relation to serum concentrations of selenium and vitamins A and E: Matched case-control analysis of prospective data. *Brit. Med. J. 290*:417.

Schmahl, D., Habs, M. (1978). Experimental carcinogencity of antitumor drugs. *Cancer Treatment Rev. 5*:175.

Schmandke, H., Schmidt, G. (1965). Absorption of alpha-tocopherol from oily and aqueous solutions. *Int. J. Vit. Nutr. Res. 35*:138.

Schmandke, H., Sima, C., Manne, R. (1967). Die Absorbierung über alpha-Tocopherol bein Menschen. *Int. Z. Vitam. Forsch. 39*:296.

Schwartz, J., Odukoya, O., Stoufi, E., Shklar, G. (1985). alpha-Tocopherol alters the distribution of Langerhans cells in DMBA-treated hamster cheek epithelium. *J. Dent. Res. 64*(2):117.

Shamberger, R. J., Rudolph, G. (1966). Protection against carcinogenesis by antioxidants. *Experientia 22*:116.

Shamberger, R. J. (1970). Relationship of selenium to cancer. I. Inhibitory effect of selenium on carcinogenesis. *J. Nat. Cancer Inst. 44*:931.

Shamberger, R., Baughman, F. F., Kalchert, S. S., Willis, C. E. (1973). Carcinogen-induced chromasomal breakage decreased by antioxidants. *Proc. Nat. Acad. Sci. USA 70*:1461.

Shamberger, R. J., Corlett, C. L., Beaman, K. D., Kasten, B. L. (1979). Antioxidants reduce the mutagenic effect of malonaldehyde and beta-propiolactone. *Mutation Res. 66*:349.

Shklar, G. (1982). Oral mucosal carcinogenesis in hamsters: Inhibition by vitamin E. *J. Nat. Cancer Inst. 68*(5):791.

Skaare, J. U., Nafstad, I. (1978). Interaction of vitamin E and selenium with the hepatoxic agent dimethylnitrosamine. *Acta Pharmacol. Toxicol. 43*:119.

Slaga, T. J., Bracken, W. M. (1977). The effects of antioxidants on skin tumor initiation promotion and aryl hydrocarbon hydroxylase. *Cancer Res. 37*: 1631.

Smalls, E., Patterson, R. M. (1982). Reduction of benzo[a] pyrene induced chromosomal aberrations by dl-alpha-tocopherol. *Eur. J. Cell Biol. 28*:92.

Sokol, R. J., Bove, K. E., Heubi, J. E., Iannaccone, S. T. (1983). Vitamin E deficiency during chronic childhood cholestasis: Presence of sural nerve lesion prior to 2 1/2 years of age. *J. Pediatrics 103*:197.

Sugai, M., Witting, L. A., Tsuchiyama, H., Kummerow, F. A. (1962). The effect of heated fat on the carcinogenic activity of 2-acetylaminofluorene. *Cancer Res. 22*:510.

Sugimura, T., Kawachi, T., Nagao, M., Yahagi, T. (1981). Mutagens in foods as causes of cancer. In *Nutrition and Cancer: Etiology and Treatment, Progress in Cancer Research and Therapy*, Vol. 17, G. R. Newell and N. M. Ellison (Eds.). Raven Press, New York, pp. 59–71.

Swick, R. W., Bauman, C. A. (1951). Tocopherol in tumor tissues and effects of tocopherol on the development of liver tumors. *Cancer Res. 11*(12):948.

Tannenbaum, S. R., Mergens, W. J. (1980). Reaction of nitrite with vitamins C and E. *Ann. N.Y. Acad. Sci. 355*:267.

Tengerdy, R. P., Mathias, M. M., Nockels, C. F. (1981). Vitamin E: Immunity and disease resistance. *Adv. Exp. Med. Biol. 135*:27.

Toth, B., Patil, K. (1983). Enhancing effect of vitamin E on murine intestinal tumorigenesis by 1,2 dimethylhydrazine dihydrochloride. *J. Nat. Cancer Inst. 70*:1107.

Trickler, D., Shklar, G. (1987). Prevention by vitamin E of experimental carcinogenesis. *J. Nat. Cancer Inst. 78*(1):165.

Tuyns, A. J., Riboli, E., Doornbos, G. (1985). Nutrition and cancer of the esophagus. In *Diet and Human Carcinogenesis*. J. V. Joossens, M. J. Hill, J. Geboers (Eds.). Excerpta Medica Elsevier, Amsterdam, pp. 71–79.

Van Stee, E. W., Sloane, R. A., Simmons, J. E., Brunnemann, K. D. (1983). *In vivo* formation of N-nitrosomorpholine in CD-1 mice exposed by inhalation to nitrogen dioxide and gavaged with morpholine. *J. Nat. Cancer Inst. 70*: 375.

Wald, N. J., Boreham, J., Hayward, J. L., Bulbrook, R. D. (1984). Plasma retinol, beta-carotene, and vitamin E levels in relation to the future risk of breast cancer. *Brit. J. Cancer 49*:321.

Wald, N. J., Thompson, S. G., Densen, J., Boreham, J., Bailey, A. (1987). Serum vitamin E and human cancer. In *Clinical and Nutritional Aspects of Vitamin E*, O. Hayaishi, M. Mino (Eds.), Elsevier, Amsterdam, pp. 73–82.

Wang, Y-M., Howell, S. K., Kimball, J. C., Tsai, C. C., Sato, J., Gleiser, C. A. (1982). Alpha-Tocopherol as a potential modifier of daunomyein carcinogenicity in Sprague-Dawley rats. In *Molecular Interrelations of Nutrition and Cancer*, Arnott, M. S., VanEys, J., Wang, Y-M. (Eds.), Raven Press, pp. 369–379.

Wattenberg, L. W. (1972). Inhibition of carcinogenic and toxic effects of polycyclic hydrocarbons by phenolic antioxidants and ethoxyquin. *J. Nat. Cancer Inst. 48*:1425.

Wattenberg, L. W. (1978). Inhibition of chemical carcinogenesis. *J. Nat. Cancer Inst. 60*:11.

Wattenberg, L. W. (1983). Inhibition of neoplasia by minor dietary constituents. *Cancer Res.* (Suppl.). *43*:2448S.

Weber, F., Wiss, O. (1964). Synergism of d- and l-alpha-tocopherol during absorption. *Biochem. Biophys. Res. Commun. 14*:186.

Weerapradist, W., Shklar, G. (1982). Vitamin E inhibition of hamster buccal pouch carcinogenesis: A gross histologic and ultrastructural study. *Oral Surg. 54*:304.

Weisburger, J. H., and Horn, C. (1982). Nutrition and cancer: Mechanisms of genotoxic and epigenetic carcinogens in nutritional and carcinogenesis. *Bull. NY Acad. Sci. 58*:296.

Willett, W. C., Polk, F., Underwood, B. A., Stampfer, M. J., Pressel, S., Rosner, B., Taylor, J. O., Schneider, K., Hames, C. G. (1984). Relation of serum vitamins A and E and carotenoids to the risk of cancer. *New England J. Med. 310*:430.

13

Ascorbic Acid in Cancer Prevention

GLADYS BLOCK and MARILYN MENKES
National Cancer Institute, National Institutes of Health, Bethesda, Maryland
MARILYN MENKES*
The Johns Hopkins School of Hygiene and Public Health, Baltimore, Maryland

Ascorbic acid, long known for its role in the prevention of scurvy, is becoming increasingly recognized as an important biochemical factor in many physiologic and biochemical systems. It is used in the synthesis of collagen, the most abundant protein in the body; in the synthesis of hormones and neurotransmitters including norepinephrine, epinephrine, and serotonin; and in hydrogen-ion transfer and regulation of the proper oxidation state of biologically important metal ions such as iron and copper. An antioxidant and free radical scavenger, it is an effective detoxifier of various poisons and carcinogens, and is thought to protect other important antioxidants such as vitamin E, vitamin A, BHA, and glutathione (Hodges, 1980; Sauberlich, 1984).

These and other functions, as well as laboratory and animal studies of the role of ascorbic acid in carcinogenesis, are discussed below. Epidemiologic evidence for a role in human cancer as well as human requirements, dosage, and toxicity are also discussed.

STRUCTURE, SYNTHESIS, AND DISTRIBUTION

Structure and Synthesis

Ascorbic acid is a six-carbon molecule only a few biosynthetic steps removed from glucose (or galactose) (Fig. 1). It is synthesized by amphibians, reptiles, some birds, and most mammals. Among mammals, vitamin C does not appear to be synthesized by guinea pigs, fruit bats, and most primates, including humans (Chatterjee et al., 1975). This is considered further below.

**Current affiliation:* University of Texas System Cancer Center, Houston, Texas.

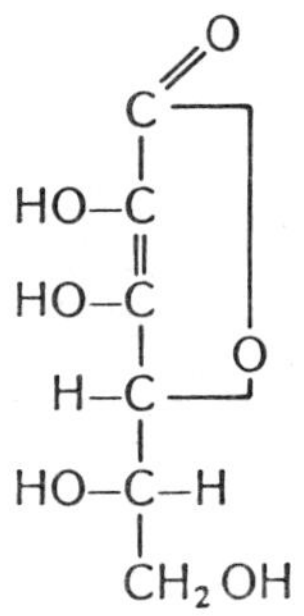

Fig. 1 Structure of ascorbic acid.

In mammals, the vitamin is synthesized in the liver. While microsomal enzymes appear to be responsible for most of the activity, some evidence (Burns and Evans, 1956) suggests that mitochondria may be responsible for as much as 25% of the activity in rats. Since mitochondria are self-replicative (Guyton, 1976), contain their own DNA (distinct from that in the nucleus), and are transmitted by maternal inheritance only, their participation in ascorbate biosynthesis deserves further exploration.

Animal data suggest that in animals that fail to synthesize the vitamin, the deficiency is in one or all of three enzymes: uronolactonase, glucuronolactone reductase, or gulonolactone oxidase. It has been suggested (Burns et al., 1956; Chatterjee et al., 1975) that the deficiency is a result of a mutation involving a gene deletion. Several lines of evidence, however, suggest that this may not be the case. First, the same gene deletion would have had to occur several times, since the biosynthetic ability is lacking in several branches of the evolutionary tree, in some but not all bats, birds, and primates. While multiple occurrences of the same mutation are not impossible, it is reasonable to examine alternative mechanisms.

Evidence against an actual gene deletion is contained in work by DeFabro (1967) and Zloch and Ginter (1984). DeFabro found that one of the "missing" enzymes, L-gulonolactone oxidase, was active in the livers (the site of ascorbate synthesis) of guinea pig embryos. The enzyme activity was absent in other organs of the embryos and was absent in the liver of the adult guinea pigs. This suggests that there may not be an actual gene deletion, but rather repression of the expression of an existing gene at some point during embryonic development. This alternative to the gene-deletion hypothesis raises the possibility of individual variability in the degree to which various suppressor or competitor proteins may be expressed. Such variability in expression is well established for other genes (Sutton, 1975). For example, heterozygotes for the sickle cell gene vary considerably in the degree to which they are affected by oxygen deprivation. And, indeed, Gross (quoted in Chatterjee et al., 1985, p. 46) describes reports of finding gulonolactone oxidase in the liver of some guinea pigs, and indicates that in a large group of guinea pigs it is possible to find some which will not become scorbutic. Yew (1975) gives several references suggesting variability in synthesis, requirement, and metabolism in both humans and guinea pigs.

Finally, Zloch and Ginter (1984) examined a group of guinea pigs bred in a region from which the authors had observed some guinea pigs to be resistant to scurvy. Ten of the twelve animals showed no ascorbic acid-producing enzymes in their liver microsomes, and on an ascorbic acid-free diet, their serum levels fell to 0.05 mg/dl. An eleventh animal also had no enzyme activity, but the serum level fell only to 0.55 mg/dl, presumably reflecting a marked difference in catabolism. The twelfth animal had a level of microsomal enzyme production comparable to that of healthy young rats (an ascorbic acid-synthesizing species) and had serum levels of 0.99 mg/dl. These data demonstrate the presence and physiologically adequate level of biosynthetic activity in some individuals of this species.

Thus, although it is usually stated that humans and guinea pigs completely lack the ability to synthesize ascorbic acid, there are data indicating the possibility of varying levels of synthesis. It would be of interest to study in vivo biosynthesis in human studies with larger numbers and diverse genetic backgrounds. The question cannot be answered in studies of three or even 30 individuals.

Distribution in the Body

Ascorbic acid is transported against a concentration gradient to numerous tissues. The highest levels are found in the adrenal and pituitary glands, where concentrations are 50–100 times the plasma levels in humans. Very high uptake and concentrations, 30–50 times the plasma levels, are also found in the central nervous system, spleen, testes, salivary glands, eye lens, bone marrow, and leukocytes, leading Hornig (1975) to suggest that "a distinct role of ascorbic acid in these tissues seems to be implied."

POTENTIAL ANTITUMOR ACTIONS

Evidence exists to support several mechanisms by which ascorbic acid may act in cancer prevention. Such mechanisms include blocking the formation of a carcinogen or tumor promoter, converting it to a less harmful metabolite, or enhancing host resistance to progression and dissemination. These are discussed below.

Blocking and Detoxifying Carcinogens

Nitrosamines and Other Chemical Carcinogens

Because of the known carcinogenicity of nitrosamines, considerable interest has focused on the nitrosation reaction. The first step in the formation of nitrosamines and nitrosamides is the conversion of nitrates to nitrites. While there are many dietary sources of nitrates (White, 1975), those same sources (cabbage, green leafy vegetables) are good sources of ascorbic acid as well. Ranieri and Weisburger (1975) showed in vitro that in foods incubated at 25°C there was a natural conversion of nitrates to nitrites. By addition of ascorbic acid at 4:1 molar ratios, however, this conversion could be reduced to 57% of the level found in the ascorbic acid-free preparation.

The next step in nitrosation is the combining of nitrite with amines and amides found in proteins to form nitrosamines. This step is also prevented by ascorbic acid. Ranieri and Weisburger (1975) added labeled N-methylurea and nitrite to food samples prior to incubation and examined the levels of methylnitrosourea formed. With ascorbic acid at a 4:1 molar ratio (ascorbate:nitrite), there was a 93% inhibition in nitrosamine formation. There is general agreement, after the work of these investigators and others discussed below, that ascorbic acid is effective in reducing or preventing the formation of nitrosamines.

Several workers have investigated whether these antinitrosation functions of ascorbic acid are associated with clinically relevant effects on acute toxicity, mutagenicity, and carcinogenicity. Kamm et al. (1973, 1975) and others (Cardesa et al., 1974; Mirvish and Shubik, 1974) found that ascorbate completely prevented the *acute effects* of liver toxicity caused by administration of aminopyrine and sodium nitrite. No protective effect is observed when ascorbate is administered with preformed dimethylnitrosamine.

The *mutagenicity* of various foods common in the diet of countries with high and low incidence of gastric cancer was studied by Marquardt et al. (1977), using the Ames test. American hot dogs and beef containing nitrite produced only 6 and 15 His+ revertant colonies per plate, respectively. However, Japanese raw fish with nitrite produced 297 such colonies. When ascorbic acid was added in a 2:1 molar ratio (ascorbate:nitrite), only 7 His+ revertant colonies were produced by the Japanese raw fish. The authors conclude that "vitamin C and foods rich in this essential micronutrient may be useful as an easily available means of prevention of (gastric) cancer."

Other investigators (Schlegel et al., 1969a,b; Mirvish et al., 1973; Mirvish, 1975) have focused on the *carcinogenicity* of nitrites plus amines and the possible protective effect of ascorbic acid. Mirvish et al. (1973, 1975) found a significant dose-related protective effect against lung adenomas induced by administration of piperazine plus nitrite to mice. Schlegel et al. (1969a,b) found significantly fewer 3-hydroxyanthranilic acid-induced bladder tumors in mice that received ascorbic acid in their drinking water.

Weisburger et al. (1980) demonstrated that nitrite-incubated fish was a cancer initiator, inducing tumors in rats after a brief exposure in youth, even if the carcinogenic diet was followed by 18 months on a noncarcinogenic diet. The experiment thus simulated human exposure in youth to dietary nitrosamines, followed by an adult diet with no such exposure. Since Weisburger and others had previously shown that addition of ascorbic acid almost completely blocked formation of nitrosamine in nitrite-incubated fish, the authors suggest that inclusion of vitamin C sources with every meal from childhood onwards may be important to block cancer initiation.

Although the prevention of the formation of nitrosamines is the best-known effect of the reducing capacity of ascorbic acid, other chemical carcinogens are also blocked by this antioxidant action. Warren (1943) found that anthracene and 3,4-benzpyrene, two known carcinogens, are oxidized in vitro in the presence of ascorbic acid to anthranol and 5-hydroxy-3,4-benzpyrene, respectively. Street and Chadwick (1975) found that ascorbic acid detoxified organochlorine pesticides such as DDT, Dieldrin, and Lindane. Fox (1975) found protective effects against heavy metal toxicity.

Free Radical and Antioxidant Actions

There is considerable evidence to suggest that free radicals play a role in carcinogenesis (Pryor, 1977; Ts'o et al., 1977). Reactive oxygen species such as the superoxide anion radical ($O_2\ \cdot$) and the hydroperoxy radical ($HO_2\ \cdot$) are generated during normal cellular metabolism as well as during exposures to oxidant gases, to radiation, and to chemical carcinogens. Vitamin C is among a number of dietary factors which function to inhibit free radical reactions and may thereby prevent oxidant damage to DNA macromolecules and other vital cellular components.

Ascorbic acid is necessary for hydroxylations carried out by the cytochrome P_{450}-dependent mixed function oxidase system (Zannoni and Sato, 1975; Hodges, 1980) and is required for the optimal function of a number of other mixed-function oxidases. It has been shown to function synergistically with two other antioxidants, glutathione and vitamin E, in protecting tissues from free radical-mediated injury. Forni and Willson (1983) demonstrated that the repair activity of ascorbate in quenching carbon-centered free radicals such as those located on nucleic acid sugar residues or lipid membranes is enhanced by glutathione. Ascorbic acid reconstitutes reduced glutathione, and thus both are required for optimal quenching. Ascorbic acid has also been shown to participate in the electron transport chain of mammalian microsomes (Levine, 1986).

Vitamin C is also thought to function synergistically with the antioxidant α-tocopherol (vitamin E) in the removal of singlet electrons via coupled redox reactions (Tappel, 1962; Menzel, 1970). Packer et al. (1979) have directly observed the rapid sequential formation of the free radical intermediates of vitamins C and E in vitro. Free radical autoxidation of micelles containing linoleic acid and methyl linoleate was found to be more effectively inhibited in the presence of both ascorbic acid and α-tocopherol than when α-tocopherol was used alone (Barclay et al., 1983). Chen et al. (1978, 1980) showed that ascorbic acid supplementation of weanling rats significantly increased plasma α-tocopherol levels and may spare the metabolism of this micronutrient. Further evidence for the interaction of vitamins C and E is provided by Hatch et al. (1986), who reported that ascorbic acid deficiency in guinea pigs was accompanied by lowered α-tocopherol levels in the lung (74% of control), and enhanced pulmonary toxicity of nitrogen dioxide.

Enhancing Host Resistance

In contrast to humans, whose serum and leukocyte vitamin C levels are extremely low during chronic disease and cancer, animals that can synthesize ascorbic acid do so at a greatly increased rate in response to physiologic insult (Bodansky et al., 1951, 1952; Schlegel et al., 1969a,b; Pipkin et al., 1969; Cameron and Pauling, 1973; Kamm et al., 1975). Several authors have found increased synthesis in rats and mice in response to a variety of chemical agents, including carcinogenic agents. Burns et al. (1960) found that methylcholanthrene, benzpyrene, and various other cyclic hydrocarbons greatly increased synthesis. Boyland et al. (1961) found similar results, and Schmidt et al. (1963) found a great increase in ascorbic acid synthesis in tumor-bearing rats.

While the mechanisms are unknown, several functions of vitamin C could be involved in this increased synthesis in response to chemical or physiologic stress: enhancement of c-AMP through phosphodiesterase inhibition (Moffat et al., 1972; Buck and Zadunaisky, 1975; Friedman, 1976; Lyko and Hartman, 1980); biosynthesis of epinephrine and norepinephrine (Stone and Townsley, 1973; Deana et al., 1975); effects on microsomal drug metabolism (Zannoni and Sato, 1975); quenching of reactive oxygen and other free radical species generated either by the carcinogen or by the leukocyte response to it (Krinsky, 1974; Markert and Frei, 1982; Babior, 1982; Demopoulos et al., 1983); synergism with glutathione and mixed function oxidases (Zannoni and Sato, 1975; Forni and Willson, 1983); enhancement of leukocyte activity (Shilotri, 1977a,b); hyaluronidase and collagenase inhibition (McCormick, 1959; Cameron, 1966; Cameron and Pauling, 1974; Clayson and David, 1975). Although these mechanisms cannot be presented in detail, a few are discussed below.

Immunological Enhancement

Leukocytes have a very high concentration of ascorbic acid, and since circulating lymphocytes have been shown to be effective in destroying some cancer cells, it has been suggested that ascorbic acid concentration may play a role in the effectiveness of immunological surveillance (Good and Fisher, 1972; Laroye, 1974). A deficiency of this vitamin in guinea pigs has been associated with reduced immunocompetence as shown by their prolonged tolerance of allografts (Kalden and Guthy, 1972). The addition of vitamin C to the drinking water of mice or to the culture medium of human lymphocytes significantly increased T-lymphocyte responses to the mitogen concanavalin A (Siegel and Morton, 1977; Delafuente and Panush, 1979). Ganguly et al. (1976) examined peritoneal exudate cells from normal and from progressively more ascorbic acid-deficient guinea pigs. Although they observed no decrease in phagocytic activity in cells from deficient animals, they did find a 25% reduction in the number of phagocytic cells and a 55–65% reduction in the migration ability of these cells. Addition of ascorbic acid to such cells in vitro enhanced leukocyte migration ability, essential to cytotoxic action. Others have also observed significant increases in neutrophil chemotaxis and migration with vitamin C both in vitro (Goetzl et al., 1974; Boxer et al., 1976, 1979; Anderson and Theron, 1979) and in vivo (Anderson et al., 1980). With regard to the effect of ascorbic acid on numoral immunity, some studies show increases in serum levels of IgA, IgG, IgM, and complement component C3 (Vallance 1975, 1977; Prinz et al., 1977), while others find no effect or reductions in immunoglobulins (Siegel and Morton, 1977; Dobias et al., 1986).

Mechanical Barriers to Invasion and Growth of Tumors

Ascorbic acid is required for the production of collagen, the major structural protein of basement membranes, which constitute the first barrier to tumor invasiveness and micrometastatic penetration of blood vessels and tissues. It may also increase host resistance to tumor cell invasiveness by increasing the viscosity of the interstitial substance between cells, through stimulation of enzymes involved in chondroitin sulfate synthesis (Weiss and Greep, 1977) or by regulating the action of hyaluronidase and collagenase (Cameron, 1966).

Animal Evidence Regarding Antitumor Effect

Space does not permit a comprehensive review of the animal data. A few studies are described below. Evidence for an antitumorigenic role for ascorbic acid is seen in many but not all animal models and dosage regimens. The administration of ascorbic acid was found to inhibit the development of metaplastic and neoplastic lesions of the respiratory tract of mice exposed to fiberglass dust (Morrison et al., 1981) and of rats exposed to plutonium dioxide particles (Sanders and Mahaffey, 1983) and to protect hamster lung cultures that were subjected repeatedly to cigarette smoke against abnormal growth and malignant transformation (Leuchtenberger and Leuchtenberger, 1977). Harada et al. (1985) found that high doses of vitamin C appeared to inhibit tumor induction by diethylnitrosamine and exposure to cigarette smoke in the hamster nasal cavity. While tracheal tumors were significantly greater in the ascorbate group at 32 and 36 weeks, overall there was neither a protective nor carcinogen enhancing effect of ascorbic acid on tracheal and laryngeal tumors. Ascorbic acid supplementation prevented the initiation of skin tumors induced by chemical carcinogens (Slaga and Bracken, 1977) and ultraviolet light (Dunham et al., 1982). However, consistent with the nitrosamine discussion above, it failed to reduce the incidences of preformed N-nitrosoguanidine-induced gastric cancer (Kawasaki et al., 1982), although it did produce a marked reduction in the histologic grade of the gastric lesion.

Reddy and Hirota (1979) found that sodium ascorbate, fed ad libitum in the diet, completely prevented 1,2-dimethylhydrazine-induced colon tumors in rats and reduced DMH-induced kidney tumors. Logue and Frommer (1980) found that high-dose vitamin C administered three times per week significantly reduced DMH-incuded colorectal tumors in mice. Using a slightly larger carcinogen dose, Jones et al. (1981) observed no effect of ascorbic acid alone against DMH-induced colon neoplasms, although it did synergistically enhance the antitumor effect of BHA (butylated hydroxyanisole), another reducing agent.

Studies of the therapeutic action of supplemental ascrobic acid or its metabolites on the establishment and growth of transplanted tumor cells have yielded inconsistent results (Yagashita et al., 1976; Rettura et al., 1982; Poydock et al., 1982).

In vitro studies of cancer cells indicate a potentally important effect of ascorbic acid. Park et al. (1980) found that vitamin C, at physiologic concentrations, suppressed the in vitro growth of leukemic cells from 25% of patients with acute nonlymphocytic leukemia. The authors note that "profound suppression of leukemic cells can be achieved without any damage to normal myeloid precursor cells."

Benedict et al. (1980) studied C3H/10T½ mouse embryo cells exposed to the carcinogen, 3-methylcholanthrene (MCA). Addition of ascorbic acid at physiologic concentrations completely prevented malignant transformation of these cells, even when added as late as 23 days after MCA exposure. In addition, in 80% of cultures transformed cells actually reverted to a normal morphological appearance when ascorbic acid was added. While reversion to normal phenotype has been observed with other agents such as the retinoids, the reversion produced by ascorbic acid was distinctive in that under some circumstances it appeared to be irreversible.

EPIDEMIOLOGIC EVIDENCE REGARDING ASCORBIC ACID IN CANCER PREVENTION

Before turning to a discussion of the human studies, it is important to consider some limitations and problems in the interpretation of such studies.

Limitations of Ecological or Correlation Studies

In ecological studies, the incidence or mortality rate of a disease in several countries or regions is correlated with their average food availability or group mean values of food intake. The difficulties in interpreting such data have been discussed elsewhere (Block and Hartman, 1983). Such studies are best used to suggest hypotheses, not to test them (Lilienfeld and Lilienfeld, 1980). Only three such studies are reported below.

Problems of Interpretation and Analysis of Dietary Studies

Misclassification

This subject has been discussed extensively elsewhere (Chapter 6) and will only be summarized briefly here. Diet studies rely upon three general types of dietary data, 24-hour recall, multiple-day records, and food frequency or diet history. Since a person's intake varies considerably from day to day, methods based on one-day or few-day data result in such misclassification in the estimate of the individual's long-term intake that only very powerful effects can usually be detected. The required sample size is greatly magnified (Walker and Blettner, 1985), and the observed risk would be substantially lower than the true risk. Frequency questionnaires or diet histories avoid the problem of nonrepresentativeness of short-term diet. However, they may be limited by the adequacy of the food list. Some food lists may not represent important dietary sources of vitamin C or may combine them to such an extent as to make frequency or content estimation very imprecise. Others may include so many separate sources of vitamin C that the overall estimate is too high and probably imprecise as well. A substantial degree of over- or understimation increases concern that imprecision in ranking may also have been introduced, and therefore the absolute values of the estimates should always be examined to assess whether they fall within a reasonable range.

Thus, all dietary assessment methods–whether questionnaires, food records or replicate meal analysis–produce some misclassification of an individual's true usual intake. This results in an attenuation of the observable relative risk and a weakening of power to detect a significant effect. In studies which nevertheless show an effect in the face of this, the true relative risk is likely to be even stronger than the observed risk.

Homogeneity

Studies conducted within a single population group may be limited in their ability to detect a nutrient effect, if the population is quite homogeneous with respect to intake of that nutrient. If most members of a study group are either well nourished or very poorly nourished with regard to a micronutrient, little or no light can be shed on the effect of low vs. high intake. For example, if a very high-risk population is studied in a case-control design, the control group as well as the case group may have a high level of exposure to a carcinogenic agent. Thus, consideration should always be given to the absolute value of the nutrient intake or serum levels reported, so that the study population's place in the whole spectrum of intake can be evaluated. Without such a consideration, the meaning of negative findings may be difficult to interpret.

Disentangling the Effects of Other Nutrients

People do not eat "ascorbic acid." Rather they eat *foods*, which invariably contain not one but many well-established nutrients and scores of other elements not commonly specified as nutrients, such as rutins, indoles, and others, which may play a role in human health. Thus, the consumption of one nutrient is always positively associated with other nutrients in the same foods, associations which are often so close as to make it impossible to determine which factor is in fact responsible for an effect. For nutrients which are very highly correlated, attempts to "control" for one of them by including them in multivariate models are largely illusory.

Moreover, the consumption of one nutrient or food group is often negatively associated with another. Individuals with low percent of caloric intake derived from fat usually have a high intake of carbohydrate foods, since protein intake tends to be quite stable. As a result, their diets may often contain large amounts of dietary fiber and micronutrients. It is no easier to "control" for strong negative correlations than strong positive correlations, making it difficult to determine which of the factors may be influencing disease incidence.

Most of the studies reported below have studied *foods*; in some instances they have computed a vitamin C index or other nutrient indices based on those foods, but it is well to keep in mind that the raw data consist of information on frequency of consumption of foods, and usually a limited list of foods. The particular nutrient index that is reported reflects the interest of the investigator and at best can only partially reflect the complexity of dietary exposure. Even if results appear to support current hypotheses, it is always essential to consider seriously that the apparent agent may be only a surrogate for the true effective agent.

Epidemiologic Studies

Most studies of diet and cancer have not examined the role of vitamin C. Many have used food lists designed to assess only macronutrients such as fats. Others have used lists that included some vegetables, but which were not designed to assess vitamin C adequately. Such studies shed little or no light on the role of vitamin C and cancer. The studies reported below are those which have explicitly reported on a vitamin C index or on the apparent role of fruits or vegetables that are important sources of vitamin C. These studies are summarized in Appendix A.

Lung Cancer

Mettlin et al. (1979) examined 292 lung cancer patients and 801 controls, all of whom had completed a dietary interview prior to diagnosis. While a significant effect was found for vitamin A index, none was found for vitamin C. Byers et al. (1984) examined a set of patients, which included many of the same cases and controls, and found no significant trend for any histologic subtype. It is important to note, for these and other studies reported below, that the adequacy of this particular food list for vitamin C assessment can be questioned. The Roswell Park instrument (Graham et al., 1967), although reflecting an early and foresightful interest in dietary epidemiology, contained only five items which represented important vitamin C sources in the U.S. diet (Block et al., 1985). A single item combined all citrus fruits and juices, and another item combined apples (relatively low in vitamin C) with other fresh fruit, making actual vitamin C estimation difficult.

In 1987 Byers et al. reported the results of a large case-control study of lung cancer, using not the 1967 "Roswell Park" questionnaire but a newly developed 129-item diet history questionnaire. No effect was seen for vitamin C. Because of illness or death, only one-fourth of the eligible cases were interviewed, raising the possibility that a nutrient effect could be missed if low intake increased the severity or progression of the disease. Significant protective effects were seen, however, for fiber in males and for carotenes in nonsmokers.

Kvale et al. (1983) reported no apparent protective effect of vitamin C among 16,713 respondents followed for 11 years, whereas they did find a significant effect for a vitamin A index. However, of the two foods which approach significance by themselves, one is tomatoes, a poor source of β-carotene but a good source of vitamin C.

Hinds et al. (1984) examined 364 lung cancer patients and 627 matched population controls. The diet history method asked about use of 84 food items in a "usual week," and the authors estimate that this represented 85% of vitamin A and 78% of vitamin C intake. The vitamin C analyses were controlled for vitamin A intake, but vitamin A analyses were apparently not controlled for vitamin C. For vitamin A, a significant elevation in risk was found among males, but not females, at the lowest intake level. For vitamin C, a similar direction of effect was seen, but the risk (1.6 among males) was lower than that seen for vitamin A, and was not statistically significant.

Shekelle et al. (1981) followed 1954 men for 19 years, and observed a total of 33 lung cancer cases. Because the original diet data had been lost, the vitamin C results were reported only in terms of group means among cases and noncases.

The mean daily intake at baseline was 91.8 mg among the 33 persons who subsequently developed lung cancer, while among noncases the mean was 101.0 mg. Given the small number of cases, the p value of 0.20 may be considered suggestive.

A 1,000,000-person prospective study initiated by the American Cancer Society was analyzed by Long-de and Hammond (1985) for the role of fruit consumption in subsequent lung cancer, among white male cigarette smokers aged 40–75 years. In each of six age groups a protective effect was seen for frequent fruit consumption, with a consistent dose response. Over all age groups, the mortality ratio was 1.75 for those who ate fruit 0–2 times per week, compared with those who ate it 5–7 times per week.

Several studies have examined diet in relation to lung cancer but have not reported specifically on the role of vitamin C (MacLennan et al., 1977; Gregor et al., 1980; Bjelke et al., 1982; Ziegler et al., 1984), in some cases clearly because the dietary interview was not intended to assess vitamin C. One of these, MacLennan (1979), found a reduced risk associated with high consumption of three leafy green vegetables, typically good sources of vitamin C as well as provitamin A and folate.

Because of limitations in assessment methods or analysis, the available data provide ambiguous evidence regarding an effect of vitamin C in the prevention of lung cancer. In summary, one retrospective and three prospective studies offer some suggestion of a protective effect, while two retrospective studies found no effect. Additional prospective studies are needed which are large enough to ensure adequate numbers of lung cancer outcomes, and with dietary methods capable of assessing vitamin C as well as other nutrients such as carotenoids, folate, and vitamin E.

Cancer of the Larynx

Only one published report was found which examined the role of diet in cancer of the larynx. Graham et al. (1981) studied 374 patients and 381 controls, using the Roswell Park instrument described above. Highly significant effects were found for both vitamin A and vitamin C. After control for the effects of cigarettes and alcohol, a low intake of vitamin C was associated with a relative risk of 2.49, $p < 0.005$, with a clear dose-response relationship.

Oral Cancer

Marshall et al. (1982) examined 427 white male oral cancer patients at Roswell Park and 558 controls with nonneoplastic diseases of other sites. After control for smoking, alcohol, and age, vitamin C was associated with a significant risk trend, with an odds ratio of 1.7 for lowest to highest intake. A somewhat stronger association was observed for the vitamin A index, OR = 2.0. The authors note, however, that "the difference in the estimated effects of vitamin A and vitamin C could also be the result of differential measurement error; the scale measuring vitamin A in the diet may be more accurate than the vitamin C scale. If the effects of these substances were equal, with vitamin A measured more accurately than vitamin C, it would be estimated that the effect of vitamin A is stronger than that of vitamin C." (Marshall et al., 1982, p. 149). As noted above, the Roswell Park instrument used in the collection of these data in 1958–1965 certainly resulted in considerable misclassification with respect to vitamin C intake, with consequent reduction in power to detect an effect.

Winn et al. (1984) conducted a study of 227 female oral cancer patients and 405 matched controls, using a 21-food-item frequency questionnaire for the dietary assessment. A highly significant protective effect was found for frequent (once a day or more) consumption of fresh fruit (OR = 0.6). Green leafy vegetables and other vegetables also had an effect in the protective direction, although nonsignificant.

Finally, preliminary analyses have been conducted at the National Cancer Institute of a case-control study of dietary factors in oral cancer. A strongly protective effect for both fruit and supplemental vitamin C intake was observed. (Dr. Joseph McLaughlin, 1987, personal communication.)

Cancer of the Esophagus

Mettlin et al. (1980) examined 147 esophageal cancer patients and 264 controls, using the same Roswell Park dietary instrument mentioned above in Marshall's study of oral cancer. Significant results were found for vitamin A, and an even stronger effect for vitamin C. After adjustment for smoking and alcohol consumption, the relative risk for low vitamin C consumption was 2.41 with respect to the high-intake category, with a Chi-square for trend significant at $p = 0.004$.

Ziegler et al. (1981) examined the role of nutrition in esophageal cancer among black men. Vitamin C was the only statistically significant micronutrient, with relative risks for low intake of 2.1 and 1.8, respectively, before and after control for alcohol intake. No relationship was seen between esophageal cancer and nitrite-containing foods, suggesting that the protective effect of vitamin C may take place through a mechanism other than that of prevention or nitrosation. Slightly stronger effects were seen when risk estimates were based on the foods themselves, rather than the nutrient indices derived from them. After control for alcohol, fruits had a relative risk of 2.0, vegetables 1.6, and fresh or frozen meats or fish, 2.2. Poor nutrition in general, rather than deficiency of a single nutrient, may be significant in this and other cancer sites.

Cook-Mozaffari et al. (1979) conducted a case-control study of esophageal cancer in northern Iran. Frequent consumption of oranges was the most highly statistically significant dietary factor in both males and females. Consumption of fruits in general, and of raw green vegetables, was also significantly protective in both sexes. These relationships remained significant even after adjustment for socioeconomic and other factors.

For esophageal cancer, the data are reasonably persuasive that vitamin C, or some factor in vitamin C–containing foods, plays a protective role in the etiology of this disease.

Stomach Cancer

An ecological study was conducted by Kolonel et al. (1981). They estimated the stomach cancer incidence of Japanese and Caucasian Hawaiians by place of birth; they then interviewed healthy persons of those four race-birthplace groups and estimated their dietary intake. There was a lower intake of vitamin C among males in the higher-risk subgroup. The pattern was also consistent among females when supplement use of vitamin C was included.

In a similar ecologic study of gastric cancer, Correa et al. (1983) studied families' average dietary intake in four Colombian villages, one at low and one at high risk of gastric cancer, and two with intermediate risks. The village with the low incidence rate consumed significantly more oranges, cabbages, tomatoes, plantain, achrote (a fresh vegetable), lettuce, and carrots. When quantitative nutrient estimates were calculated form the data, however, all villages appeared to be consuming more than the WHO-recommended level of ascorbic acid.

The same group of investigators, Haenszel et al. (1985), studied the relationship between a precursor lesion, atrophic gastritis, or dysplasia, and serum levels of six micronutrients in a Colombian population at extremely high risk of gastric cancer. Serum was prepared on site and shipped on dry ice to New Orleans for analysis within three weeks of collection. The authors report significant differences between the mean serum levels of the 47 dysplasia cases and 464 persons with normal or superficial gastritis for carotene but not for vitamin C. However, it is notable that the entire range of both cases and controls for serum ascorbic acid, 1.25 mg/dl, appears to be above normal, "well-nourished" levels. From the stated standard error it can be calculated that at least 95% of both cases and controls are above 0.70 mg/dl. For comparison, Hodges (1980) states that low levels are between 0.1–0.39 mg/100 ml, and well-nourished are above 0.60 mg/100 ml; and Goodman and Gilman (1980) indicat that "adequate" ingestion is associated with concentrations over 0.5 mg/dl. Thus, it would appear that either virtually everyone in this population has very good vitamin C nutriture, or there may have been some inaccuracy in the serum measurements. In either event, the possible effect of poor vitamin C nutriture cannot be estimated in this study.

Graham et al. (1967) examined dietary factors among 188 stomach cancer patients and 800 controls, using the Roswell Park dietary instrument. No significant differences were observed between cases and controls in the frequency of eating citrus fruits/juices, or other fruits.

Haenszel et al. (1972) examined frequency of consumption of various foods among Japanese-Americans with and without stomach cancer in Hawaii. Several vegetables showed protective effects in one group or another. Only tomatoes (an important source of vitamin C) showed a statistically significant protective effect in both first generation (Issei) and second generation Japanese American (Nisei). No effects were observed for fruit.

Other investigators have, however, found a significant protective role for vitamin C in stomach cancer. Correa et al. (1985) studied 391 gastric cancer cases and an equal number of controls in south Louisiana, a high-risk area for gastric cancer. Dietary factors were categorized into quartiles based on the control distribution. Even after adjusting for several risk factors, a significant trend for vitamin C intake was observed, the odds ratio for the highest vs. lowest quartrile being 0.50 for whites and 0.33 for blacks. For carotenoids, a nonsignificant risk reduction to 0.68 was observed for whites, but no risk reduction (OR = 1.08) was seen for blacks. The protective effect of carotenoids disappeared when vitamin C was controlled, but "the strong protective effect from vitamin C remains after controlling for confounding and other risk factors, including carotenoid intake" (Correa et al., 1985, p. 651).

Bjelke (1971, 1973) studied 228 stomach cancer cases and 1394 controls, in Norway. He found the vitamin C index to be "the dietary variable which discriminated most strongly between the total group of stomach cancer cases . . . and the controls" (Bjelke, 1973, p. 302). The same significantly protective result was obtained when analysis was restricted to those subjects for whom the food consumption estimates given by spouses for subjects' intake was concordant with the subjects' estimates themselves (a subset with presumably more accurate diet responses.) In the latter subset the relative odds for a high intake (approximately upper quartrile) of the vitamin A index was 0.87, and for a vitamin C index, 0.64 (more protective). The relative odds among all subjects for high- vs. low-intake groups were 0.6 for those aged 60 or older, and 0.3 for those under age 60.

Cancer of the Colon and Rectum

A protective effect of ascorbic acid in colorectal carcinogenesis could take place by its prevention of fecal N-nitrosamines (Bruce et al., 1977) or against other fecal mutagens (Dion et al., 1982). In addition, a mechanism has been proposed whereby ascorbate increases c-AMP levels by competing for the active sites of c-AMP-phosphodiesterase (PDE) (Moffat et al., 1972; Buck and Zadunaisky, 1975; Lewin, 1976; Lyko and Hartman, 1980, p. 68). This inhibits PDE destruction of c-AMP, thereby increasing c-AMP levels, which in turn inhibits DNA synthesis and proliferation of preneoplastic cells at the crypt surface

(Friedman, 1976). Administration of ascorbate has been shown to produce a 30 to 40% increase in c-AMP and c-GMP serum levels in the baboon (Van Wyk and Kotze, 1975).

Studies of the precursor lesion, rectal polyps, among familial polyposis patients support the possibility of a protective effect of vitamin C in polyp formation, and thus possibly in colorectal cancer. Decosse et al. (1975) reported a regression of rectal adenomas in four of five patients with 3 g/day intake of ascorbic acid. In a randomized trial of ascorbic acid in polyposis patients (Bussey, 1982), there was a statistically significant difference between the treatment and control groups, at eight months, in the number of patients with reduced rectal polyp area, and nonsignificant differences in the same direction at 12 and 15 months. While the study was limited by small sample size (17 treatment and 14 control patients at 18 months), the differences in polyp area were notable: the treatment group had a reduction in polyp area from 61 mm^2 at baseline to 23 mm^2 at 18 months; the control group actually had a small increase, from 46 mm^2 at baseline to 49 mm^2 at 18 months. There was also a reduction in thymidine uptake at 18 months in the treatment group, indicating a reduction in colonic cell proliferation.

McKeown-Eyssen et al. (1987) administered 400 mg of vitamins C and E to patients following polypectomy. After two years, the polyp recurrence data rate was reduced approximately 20% in the treatment group, although not statistically significantly. Polyp area was not reported.

Studies of the fecal mutagen, fecapentaene, provide evidence of a different mechanism for a protective effect of ascorbic acid. Dion (1982) administered vitamins C and E and observed a reduced level of mutagens in stool. Wilkins (1981) failed to replicate this, in an examination of five individuals.

However, a recent study of diet and fecapentaene levels conducted at the National Cancer Institute found a strong negative association between fecapentaene levels and both usual dietary vitamin C intake and supplemental vitamin C (Schiffman, 1987). Strong negative associations with citrus fruit and with vitamin E were also observed. Consumption of citrus fruit and supplemented vitamin C were two of only four factors significantly correlated with fecal mutagen levels in both study groups. The other two factors were supplemental vitamin E, negatively correlated, and consumption of butter/margarine, positively correlated. Thus, if fecal mutagens play a role in colon carcinogenesis, there is evidence that ascorbic acid may function, either independently or synergistically with vitamin E, in preventing or detoxifying the carcinogen.

Jain et al. (1980) examined colon and rectum cancer cases and hospital and neighborhood controls using an extensive list-based diet history questionnaire. Use of supplemental vitamin C was not included. They found no significant difference in mean vitamin C intake between cases and either control group, nor were relative risks consistent after multiple logistic regression. Estimates of mean dietary intake were high for both cases and controls (163 mg/day for male and 156 mg/day for female colon cancer cases). This raises the possibility that either the assessment instrument was imprecise or that the average intake in this Canadian population was too high to identify a risk at lower levels.

Others have, however, found significant protective effects for vitamin C, particularly for rectal cancer. Tuyns (1986), in reporting preliminary results of a large case-control study in Belgium, found a statistically significant protective effect of vitamin C for both colon cancer (RR = 0.74) and rectal cancer (RR = 0.68). Risks are expressed for "heavy" vs. "light" consumers.

Potter and McMichael (1986) examined 419 colon and rectal cancer cases and 732 controls in Australia. For colon cancer, no consistent results were seen for vitamin C (nor for β-carotene or retinol). A high fiber intake was associated with a significantly *elevated* risk in female colon cancer, which on closer inspection was found to be associated solely with cereal fiber; vegetable fiber was not associated with excess risk.

For rectal cancer, however, vitamin C was associated with a reduced risk in both sexes, significantly so in females (OR = 0.3). Neither carotene nor retinol was protective against rectal cancer; cereal fiber, but not vegetable fiber, was associated with a high and significant excess risk.

Bjelke (1970, 1973) investigated 162 colon and 116 rectal cancer cases and 1394 controls. He found a reduced risk associated with consumption of vegetables, and particularly for a vitamin A index, when colon and rectum cancer were considered together. Among a subset of subjects whose dietary data were probably more reliable (as evidenced by concordance with spouse reports of the subjects' diet), the relative odds were 0.43 for a high score on vitamin A index and 0.66 for vitamin C. The vegetable index discriminated most strongly between colorectal cancer cases and controls. For colon cancer the data indicate a stronger protective effect for vitamin A than for vitamin C. For rectal cancer, however, the author states that "patients with cancer of the rectum . . . differed from the colonic cancer patients by having a lower consumption of fruits and berries and, in particular, of vitamin C." These results are consistent with those of Potter and McMichael for rectal cancer, and with those of Tuyns, and suggest a protective role for vitamin C in rectal cancer.

Several studies have examined the relationship between diet and colon cancer by constructing fiber indices, without estimating the vitamin C content of the foods considered. Stocks (1957), Phillips (1975), Graham et al. (1978), and Haenszel et al. (1980) reported reduced risks with various vegetable foods. In 1975 Modan et al. (1975) reported a reduced risk with a "fiber" item. However, the item consisted of 73 foods, most of which were vegetable rather than cereal. Indeed, two of four foods consumed significantly *more* by cases than by controls (thus suggesting an *elevated* risk) were cereals. In 1981, Modan et al. studied 406 GI cancer patients, including patients with cancer of the stomach, colon, rectum, and other GI sites. No significant trend was noted for carrots and pumpkin, rich sources of carotene but not of vitamin C. In contrast, oranges, tomatoes and green peppers had the most highly significant trends, $p < 0.0002$; these foods are rich sources of vitamin C but rather poor sources of β-carotene. (Tomatoes, for example, contain primarily lycopene, not β-carotene.)

An ecologic study by Bingham et al. (1979), which was initially interpreted as showing a strong negative correlation for the fiber fraction pentose, revealed, upon reanalysis (1985), no relationship with pentose and a stronger correlation for vitamin C (-0.84) than for total dietary fiber (-0.72). As with any ecologic correlation many factors could affect the correlation and its significance, but these results do suggest that vitamin C (or something else in vegetables and fruits) could be as important or more important than dietary fiber in this population.

Thus, it appears possible that what some have interpreted to be a protective effect of fiber may be instead an effect of something else in fruits and vegetables. Although international correlation data are often interpreted as implicating dietary fiber, other legitimate candidates include vitamin C, carotenoids, folate, vitamin E, or other factors and their interactions. The evidence for a protective role for vitamin C is inconclusive but suggestive, particularly for rectal cancer.

Cancer of the Pancreas

A case-control study of 99 patients with pancreatic cancer, 138 population controls, and 163 hospital controls was conducted by Norell et al. (1986). Dietary information was collected by means of a food frequency questionnaire. Marginally significant elevations in risk were found for frequent use of fatty foods, margarine, and fried or grilled meat, although the latter were based on very small numbers of exposed persons. A statistically significant protective effect was observed, for both hospital and population controls, for frequent consumption of carrots and of citrus fruits. Citrus fruits are important sources of vitamin C and unimportant as sources of carotenoids. The relative risk associated with daily consumption of citrus fruits was 0.3 using hospital controls and 0.5 using population controls. Inclusion of both foods in a logistic regression model did not apparently weaken the association of either one.

Thus, this study is consistent with the hypothesis of a protective role of vitamin C in pancreatic cancer.

Cancer of the Bladder

Kolonel et al. (1985) reported preliminary results of a case-control study of 164 bladder cancer patients and 314 controls. No difference in vitamin C consumption (including supplements) was seen for Japanese males, but in the remaining three ethnic-sex groups consumption among controls was greater than among cases, suggesting a protective effect. For females these differences were substantial (318 vs. 634 mg/day among Caucasian females, for example), but the numbers were small (18 Caucasian female cases and 32 controls).

Cancer of the Prostate

Graham et al. (1983) conducted a case-control study of diet and prostate cancer using the Roswell Park dietary questionnaire described earlier. A statistically significant *increased* risk was seen for the vitamin C index among men 70 years of age or older. A similar increased risk in this age group was also seen for increased consumption of vitamin A.

Kolonel et al. (1985) studied 418 patients with prostate cancer and 771 controls using a frequency-based diet history questionnaire, with photographs to aid in portion size assessment. They found no evidence of either increased or reduced risk associated with vitamin C intake.

Heshmat et al. (1985) conducted a study of 181 black patients with prostate cancer and matched hospital controls. A frequency questionnaire was used to estimate, retrospectively, the patients' nutrient intake between the ages of 30–49 and 50+. Results were expressed per 1000 calories, an imprecise approach for micronutrients. Elevated risk was found for total vitamin A but neither an increased nor reduced risk was associated with vitamin C consumption.

Cancer of the Cervix

Marshall et al. (1983) examined 513 cervical cancer patients and 490 hospital controls using the Roswell Park dietary questionnaire described above under Mettlin's study of lung cancer. No relationship was found for vitamin C.

On the other hand, Wassertheil-Smoller et al. (1981) and Romney et al. (1985) examined ascorbic acid in relation to the precancerous condition cervical dysplasia and found evidence to support a protective effect. As Haenszel et al. (1985, p. 118) indicated in their study of gastric dysplasia, examination of precursor conditions is useful because "it makes less tenable the interpretation that the serum levels are a consequence of the disease." Romney et al. (1985) examined 46 cases, defined as women who had either two consecutive suspicious (Class III) or one positive (Class IV) Papanicolaou smear in a 12-month period. The 34 control women had negative smears and negative colposcopic examination. Plasma vitamin C levels were 0.75 mg/dl in controls and 0.36 mg/dl in cases, $p < 0.0001$. The authors conclude that "multivariate analysis, controlling for other confounding variables known to be important epidemiologic factors in cervical cancer, such as early onset of sexual activity, multiple partners, and multiple pregnancy, established vitamin C as an independent risk factor in all degrees of dysplasia and carcinoma in site. This relationship held in both lower and higher socioeconomic groups."

Whereas Romney et al. examined plasma vitamin C, Wassertheil-Smoller (1981) examined dietary intake in 87 cases and 82 controls recruited from subjects who came to a free walk-in screening clinic. Case definitions were similar to those of Romney et al. Mean intake of vitamin C by 3-day record and 24-hour recall was significantly lower in cases than controls, for blacks and whites separately and overall. Within each race, the median intake among controls was about twice as high as among cases. By 3-day food record, the median intake for controls was 104 mg/day (mean, 107 mg/day), while in cases it was 67 mg/day (mean, 80 mg/day). The odds ratio associated with being below the overall case-control median of 76 mg/day was 4.35. For those below 30 mg/day (50% of the RDA), the odds ratio was 6.66; 23% of cases had an intake below 30 mg/day, as measured by three-day food record. The same results were seen in both lower and higher income groups. Multiple logistic regression analyses indicated that vitamin C was a significant independent contributor to risk, even when age and sexual activity were controlled.

Preliminary analyses of a case-control study of cervical cancer conducted in Australia (Brock, 1987) indicate a clearly protective effect of dietary vitamin C and a modest effect of dietary carotene. Plasma carotene was associated with a strongly protective effect; plasma vitamin C was not measured.

While further study is warranted, these studies present strong preliminary evidence of an important protective effect for vitamin C in cervical cancer.

Childhood Brain Tumors

A study of environmental factors and childhood brain tumors was conducted in Ohio by John R. Wilkins III and Thomas Sinks, Jr. (personal communication, 1987). Parents of 100 cases and 200 controls were interviewed regarding diet during pregnancy, as well as other factors. High maternal intake of ascorbic acid during pregnancy was associated with a statistically significant protective effect, with an odds ratio of 0.34. The effect remained after adjustment for other factors.

Cancer of All Sites

In a prospective study of 1271 persons 66 years of age or older, five-year mortality was examined by Colditz et al. (1985). There were 42 deaths due to cancer. A green and yellow fruit and vegetable score was constructed based on the frequency of consumption of six foods. The overall score produced a statistically significant trend when divided into quintiles, with the highest quintile having a relative risk of 0.3 in relation to the lowest intake quintile. When the six foods comprising the score are examined individually for significance, however, carrots, squash, salads, broccoli, and dried fruits have nonsignificant relative risks; only strawberries and tomatoes have significantly low relative risks, of RR = 0.3

and RR = 0.5, respectively. These two items are significantly more important contributors of vitamin C than of provitamin A.

Thus, these data are consistent with the possibility of a role for vitamin C in the prevention of the unspecified cancers seen in this study.

Treatment and Palliation Effects

Since the topic of this book is prevention, the relevant treatment studies will not be discussed in detail. Prolongation of survival has been reported (Cameron and Campbell, 1974; Cameron et al., 1975; Cameron and Pauling, 1976), discussed (Jaffey, 1982), and not replicated (Moertel, 1985). For the present discussion it is only important to note that treatment studies in patients with advanced cancer for whom traditional therapy has failed or whose physical condition is too poor to permit cytotoxic regimens (Moertel et al., 1985, p. 687) have no bearing on cancer prevention. As discussed earlier, cancer *prevention* must take place at the early stages of initiation or promotion, or involve immune surveillance and control of early phases of micrometastasis and proliferation.

REQUIREMENTS, DOSAGE, AND TOXICITY

Human Requirements

Diets for nonhuman primates and guinea pigs, two other species which typically do not synthesize ascorbic acid, are formulated at concentrations providing 16–35 mg per kilogram body weight, equivalent to approximately 1000-2000 mg per day for a 60-kg man (National Research Council, 1978a,b). For humans, estimates of requirement depend on the criteria used to define adequacy. As little as 10 mg/day can alleviate the clinical symptoms of scurvy, but allow no reserves (Hodges et al., 1969, 1971). Approximately 60 mg/day will raise serum ascorbate in healthy adults to levels which are "adequate to protect against clinical signs of scurvy in the adult male for at least one month" (Sauberlich, 1984, p. 263). Little is known regarding requirements in the adult female (Food and Nutrition Board, 1980, p. 75), but there is some evidence of physiological differences in retention or requirements between the two sexes (Dodds, 1969; Milne et al., 1971; Burr et al., 1974).

Various physiologic and environmental factors increase the requirement for vitamin C. Smokers have lower blood levels than nonsmokers, and ascorbic acid metabolism in smokers is markedly increased (Pelletier, 1975, 1977; Kallner et al., 1982). Pelletier suggests that "smokers would need about twice as much vitamin C as nonsmokers to maintain comparable levels." Use of oral contraceptives is found by most but not all investigators to lower plasma levels (Briggs and Briggs, 1972; Prasad et al., 1975; Rivers, 1975; Rivers and Devine, 1975). Aspirin consumption lowers blood ascorbate levels by increasing its urinary excretion (Spitzer and Shapiro, 1948; Sahud and Cohen, 1971). More important, aspirin dramatically inhibits ascorbate absorption by leukocytes, lowering leukocyte ascorbate to just above scorbutic levels and raising the possibility of impaired leukocyte function (Loh et al., 1973). During pregnancy the placenta transmits ascorbic acid to the fetus against a concentration gradient, resulting in fetal levels 50% higher than maternal at term (Hamil et al., 1947; Kattab et al., 1970). This apparent fetal need is associated with lower maternal levels during pregnancy (Vobecky et al., 1974; Morse et al., 1975; Rivers and Devine, 1975). The elderly are frequently found to have lower serum ascorbate levels, which can be raised by supplementation (Brook and Grimshaw, 1968; Salvatore et al., 1969; Roine et al., 1972; Burr et al., 1974). Persons subjected to stresses such as heat, cold, surgery, or other trauma require higher intake to maintain normal serum levels than do healthy unstressed volunteers (Sauberlich and Baker, 1967; Visagie et al., 1974; Bondarev et al., 1975; Vallance, 1975; Visagie et al., 1975). For example, South African mine workers were found to require 200-250 mg/day to achieve serum levels which, in healthy young volunteers, are normally achieved by 60-75 mg/day (Dodds and MacLeod, 1947; Hodges et al., 1971; Sauberlich, 1975; Visagie et al., 1975).

The Recommended Daily Allowance (RDA) set by the Food and Nutrition Board is 60 mg/day, a level which "will protect against overt signs of scurvy in the adult male for a period of 30-45 days" (Food and Nutrition Board, 1980), as observed in studies among healthy young adult male volunteers (Hodges et al., 1971).

Physiologic Levels

The level constituting a "normal" serum ascorbate concentration varies with different authors: 0.5 mg/dl (Gilman et al., 1980; p. 1578), 0.6 mg/dl (Hodges, 1980), 0.75 mg/dl (Food and Nutrition Board, 1980, p. 73), 1.0 mg/dl (Cameron and Pauling, 1979). Serum levels below approximately 0.2 mg/dl are very poor and may be associated with clinical symptoms of scurvy. (Among U.S. black males over 45, 12-18% have serum levels at or below this level, according to the NHANES II serum data) (National Cancer Center for Health Statistics, 1982; Block and Sorenson, 1987). Levels which might be relevant to cancer risk are unknown.

Active transport of ascorbic acid against a concentration gradient occurs in many tissues (Lewin, 1976, pp. 119-122). Thus, it would appear that blood is primarily a transport vehicle, and it would be more relevant to examine actual tissue levels whenever possible. Leukocytes represent an accessible and relevant tissue, where concentrations are much higher than in serum. Buffy coat concentrations above 16 mg/10^8 cells reflect a well-nourished status, while those below 10mg/10^8 cells reflect low or deficient states according to Hodges, 1980). However, the technique is not simple, and values may vary among investigators. Cameron and Pauling (1979, p. 124), for example, found a mean among 100 healthy individuals of 32 mg/10^8 cells, with saturation levels of 60-70 mg/10_8 WBC attanable among healthy volunteers who consumed 10 g of ascorbic acid per day in four divided doses.

Ascorbic acid may be administered orally or by intravenous injection (Gilman et al., 1980). Oral administration should be in divided doses. The more divided doses, the higher the proportion of a given daily amount which will be absorbed. Timed-release tablets would seem to be appealing; however, they should be viewed with caution, as timed-release tablets have been observed to pass through the gut completely unabsorbed. Regardless of the administration, the blood (and leukocyte, if possible) levels of study participants should be monitored routinely to confirm that administered doses are in fact being absorbed.

Toxicity

Ascorbic acid is remarkably nontoxic at levels many times the RDA. In studies on guinea pigs, Demole found that "the animals tolerate 500–1000 times the therapeutic dose of ascorbic acid daily without ill effects" (1934, p. 771). Studies in humans on prolonged high dosage have also found no toxic effects (Lowry et al., 1953). A review of ascorbic acid toxicity may be found in a paper by Sestili (1983). Several effects have been observed or proposed.

Gastrointestinal Upset

The most commonly suggested adverse effects of high doses of ascorbic acid are gastrointestinal disturbances, particularly loose bowels but also flatulence and nausea and vomiting (Goldsmith, 1971; Hoffer, 1971; Hume and Weyers, 1973; Cameron and Campbell, 1974), primarily in healthy volunteers. None of the above studies included a placebo control. On the other hand, in a placebo-controlled clinical trial in advanced cancer patients receiving 10 g/day (Creagan et al., 1979) there were no significant differences in nausea and vomiting between the placebo and ascorbic acid groups. In a subsequent study by the same group (Moertel, 1985), the authors found that patients tolerated the 10 g/day very well. Two of 51 ascorbate patients reduced the dose and one of 49 placebo patients withdrew from the study because of unacceptable gastrointestinal symptoms.

It seems clear that some individuals do experience gastrointestinal symptoms at high doses, although it is equally clear that many do not. This may be due simply to biologic variability in metabolism; however, the above data also raise the possibility that cancer patients, or others with severe biological stress, may be more tolerant of high doses than are healthy volunteers. Indeed, it has been suggested (Cathcart, 1981) that bowel tolerance may be a fairly reliable indicator of requirement.

Interference with Diagnostic Tests

Presence of high ascorbate may produce false negatives in occult blood tests, and persons should stop taking vitamin C 48-72 hours before such tests (Jaffe et al., 1975; Garrick et al., 1977). When ascorbic acid is added to samples at 2 to 40 times the concentration attainable in blood, there is interference with colorimetric tests for SGOT, SGPT, LDH, bilirubin, uric acid, and glucose. At physiologic levels, however, interference is negligible (Caraway and Kammeyer, 1972; Heinegard and Tiderstrom, 1973; Katz and Di Silvio, 1973; Spiegel and Pinili, 1974; Nahata and McLeod, 1978).

Interference with Medications

One case report (Rosenthal, 1971) as well as an animal study (Sigell and Flessa, 1940) suggest that ascorbic acid may shorten prothrombin time in individuals receiving warfarin anticoagulants. It would seem prudent to avoid high doses under such conditions.

Excess Iron Absorption

Vitamin C substantially increases nonheme iron absorption (Hallberg, 1981). Thus, high levels of vitamin C could produce iron overload in individuals with the inborn error of iron metabolism, hemochromatosis, or in persons for whom iron overload is a problem for other reasons, such as those with β-thalassemia who must receive regular blood transfusion.

Interference with Vitamin B_{12} Metabolism

Herbert and Jacob (1974) reported an in vitro study suggesting that vitamin B_{12} in a meal could be destroyed by the presence of 100-500 mg of vitamin C. However, replication using an analytic method which protected the vitamin B_{12} from destruction by heat found much less loss of the vitamin (Newmark et al., 1979), and subsequent studies have found no destruction of B_{12} if the analytic method included cyanide, the anionic group of cyanocobalamin, to prevent B_{12} destruction (Marcus et al., 1980; Marcus, 1981). In vivo studies by DeCosse et al. (1975) and others (Afroz et al., 1975; Hogenkamp, 1980) found no reduction in serum B_{12} levels in patients undergoing long-term administration of 3-4 grams per day of ascorbic acid.

Formation of Calcium Oxalate Kidney Stones

This has been hypothesized as a possible adverse effect of high doses of ascorbic acid, because one of the catabolic pathways results in the production of oxalic acid. Studies of urinary oxalate excretion after administration of ascorbic acid have been variable, one finding increased urinary oxlate after 1-9 g/day but no evidence of a dose response (Hughes et al., 1981); another finding large elevations in 3 of 67 volunteers (Briggs, 1976); and others finding no statistically significant increase after 3-4 g/day for up to six months (Lamden and Chrystowski, 1954; Takiguchi et al., 1966). However, it is unclear that oxalate excretion is a useful indicator for risk of kidney stones. When 50 normal subjects and 75 patients with kidney stones were tested, their urinary oxalate was virtually identical (Tiselius, 1977).

Finally, actual evidence of stone formation associated with use of ascorbic acid is minimal. Only three case reports were found of individuals who presented with kidney stones and who also had consumed ascorbic acid (Briggs, 1973; Smith, 1974). As with any case report, these can do no more than suggest possible hypotheses, since there is no comparison with vitamin consumption in a control group who did not present with stones, nor incidence data among those who did and did not consume vitamin C. Of several clinical trials in which large doses of ascorbic acid (up to 10 g/day) were administered to cancer patients for periods of up to two years (Cameron and Campbell, 1974; Creagan et al., 1979; Moertel et al., 1985), there were no reports of kidney stones. Several researchers who have regularly prescribed large daily doses have reported no instances of kidney stones (Klenner, 1971; Poser, 1972).

Only epidemiologic studies on the relationship between kidney stones (not urinary oxalate) and ascorbate intake could resolve the question. However, given the absence of reports of kidney stones in the several large-scale clinical studies which have administered vitamin C, this is very unlikely to be a notable problem.

Rebound Effects

A few case reports exist of persons who developed clinical symptoms when they suddenly discontinued high doses of ascorbic acid (Schrauzer and Rhead, 1973; Schrauzer, 1979; Siegel et al., 1982). Studies in guinea pigs both support (Norkus and Rosso, 1975) and refute (Hornig et al., 1973; Alleva et al., 1976) the induction of a deficiency state after suddenly discontinuing high doses. It is commonly recommended that users taper off rather than stopping dosage suddenly. A few case reports also exist regarding rebound scurvy in newborn infants whose mothers had taken high levels of vitamin C during their pregnancy (Cochrane, 1965). Prudence would suggest moderating dosage during pregnancy and alerting the pediatrician to the possible effect.

Tumor Hemorrhage and Necrosis

In the Vale of Leven studies (Cameron and Campbell, 1974; Cameron and Pauling, 1976), 10 g of ascorbic acid per day was administered to patients with advanced cancer. Three of 50 patients, described by the authors as "terminal but not moribund," suffered rapid deterioration and death within days after initiation of ascorbic acid therapy. All had massive tumor burden, extensive metastatic disease, and aggressive, rapidly dividing tumors. The authors concluded that death was caused by tumor hemorrhage and the toxic effects of massive tumor necrosis. These observations would suggest caution in the use of high-dose ascorbic acid in patients with massive aggressive metastatic disease.

CONCLUSIONS AND DIRECTIONS FOR FUTURE RESEARCH

Conclusions

The biological functions of ascorbic acid are significantly more diverse and more complex than the now generally recognized one of preventing the formation of nitrosamines. It is required in the synthesis of an array of major biomolecules, including collagen, norepinephrine, and carnitine. In its role as a reducing agent and free radical quencher, it can prevent the formation of carcinogens and reduce the toxic or carcinogenic effects of numerous chemical and radiologic agents. It plays an important role in many enzyme-mediated reactions which require metal ions to be in the reduced state for full activity. And it may enhance host resistance in a variety of ways.

The current evidence for a cancer prevention role in humans was presented above. For cancers of the esophagus, oral cavity, and uterine cervix the evidence appears quite strong. For cancers of the stomach and rectum the evidence is mixed, but some studies suggest a strong protective effect. Cancer of the larynx was examined by only one study, but the results indicated a significant protective effect. Bladder and pancreatic cancer were also examined by a single study, with suggestive results. For lung cancer the current evidence is weak for vitamin C but very strong for carotenoids. For prostate cancer there is currently no evidence for a protective effect of vitamin C, as measured by the study designs and assessment methods used thus far.

The existence of such laboratory and human evidence of major biologic functions and cancer-preventive actions would seem to justify considerable further research on ascorbic acid, both at the biochemical and epidemiologic levels.

Future Research

Some experimental epidemiology is currently under way, sponsored by the National Cancer Institute. Dr. Jerome DeCosse, of the Cornell University Medical College, is conducting a clinical trial of ascorbic acid in conjunction with vitamin E and dietary fiber in preventing the recurrence of rectal polyps. Dr. Robert Greenberg of the Norris Cotton Cancer Center in Hanover, New Hampshire, is also examining the prevention of polyps, using vitamin C, vitamin E, and β-carotene. Dr. Bijan Safai of the Memorial Hospital for Cancer and Allied Diseases in New York City is conducting a clinical trial of vitamin C, vitamin E, and β-carotene in the prevention of basal cell skin carcinomas.

Other high priority clinical trials could be envisioned, such as the prevention of progression of early-stage dysplasias or precursor conditions of cervical, oral, and esophageal cancer, or the prevention of recurrences of cancers detected and treated in early stages. In addition, clinical trials involving other sites and agents should include a dietary assessment which would permit the analyses of differential treatment effects in those with good or poor vitamin C nutriture. And in view of possible variability in metabolism and synthesis, both clinical trials and analytic epidemiologic studies should measure blood levels whenever possible.

Finally, analytic epidemiology has barely begun to make the contribution it can make to an understanding of the role of diet in disease prevention. Many diseases and cancer sites have not been studied at all with regard to dietary factors. Many studies have been carried out with dietary methods which are poor estimators of vitamin C and other nutrients in individuals' diets and would benefit from reexamination with better methods. In addition to improved assessment methods, future epidemiologic studies should consider smoking, aspirin, or alcohol use, and chronic disease or stress, which can reduce the proportion of ingested vitamin C which is actually available to have an effect on the disease under study. And future studies should assess not one or two nutrients but the whole range of dietary and supplement intake, so as to be able to examine the effect of nutrients acting in synergy rather than independently.

With few exceptions, it is highly unlikely that nutrients act singly and without regard to the level and action of other nutrients. For example, ascorbic acid provides electron and hydrogen atom transfer in the reconstitution of active forms of vitamin E, vitamin A, and glutathione. Moreover, numerous free radical-generating or -oxidizing reactions in the body may be preferentially scavenged by different agents; since many of these reactions are linked in cascades or interrelated processes, any single agent may be less effective alone than in combination with complementary agents (Demopoulos, 1973).

Several potentially important protective effects of vitamin C have been described above, and further biochemical and epidemiologic research is clearly warranted. The nature of its role in cancer prevention, both as an independent agent and in concert with other factors, can be clarified with the help of better assessment methods and a recognition of the complexities of dietary physiology.

APPENDIX A Summary of Epidemiologic Studies

	Reference	Population	Assessment method	Results	Comments
Lung	Mettlin et al., 1979	292 cases, 801 Controls, New York	Roswell Park Questionnaire	No effect for vit. C index	Effect was seen for vitamin A index
	Byers et al., 1984	Most of same population as above	Roswell Park Questionnaire	No effect for vit. C index	Effect was seen for vitamin A index
	Byers et al., 1987	450 cases, 902 controls, New York	129-item interview	No effect for vit. C index	Effect was seen for carotenoids
	Kvale et al., 1983	16,713 Danes followed for 11 years	Food frequency questionnaire	No effect for vit. C index. Tomatoes one of two foods significant	Effect was seen for vitamin A index
	Hinds et al., 1984	364 cases, 627 controls	Freq. of use of 84 items in a "usual week"	OR = 1.6 for low vit. C intake, among males. $p > 0.05$	Effect was seen for vitamin A index Prospective study.
	Shekelle et al., 1981	1,954 men followed for 19 years. 33 lung cancers	Mean intake at baseline, among those who did and did not develop lung cancer By 24-hr recall.	Among 33 who developed lung cancer 91.8 mg/day. Among the rest, 101.0 mg/day, $p = 0.20$	Effect was seen for vitamin A index Prospective study.
	Long-de et al., 1985	White male cigarette smokers, U.S.	Frequency of fruit consumption	Mortality ratio = 1.75 for infrequent fruit consumption.	Prospective study.

	MacLennan et al., 1977	233 cases, 300 controls, Singapore Chinese	Frequency interview	Reduced risk with increased consumption of 3 leafy green veg.	
Larynx	Graham et al., 1981	374 cases, 381 controls, New York	Roswell Park Questionnaire	OR = 2.49 for low intake of vitamin C, $p < 0.005$.	Effect was seen for vitamin A index
Oral	Marshall et al., 1982	427 white male cases, New York	Roswell Park Questionnaire	OR = 1.7 for low intake of vitamin C, trend significant, even after control for smoking, age and alcohol	Effect was seen for vitamin A index
	Winn et al., 1984	227 female cases, 405 controls, U.S. South	21-item frequency questionnaire	Daily consumption of fresh fruit highly significant, OR = 0.6	Green leafy vegetables in protective direction, but not significant
	McLaughlin et al. (in preparation)	Oral cancer cases and controls	Extensive frequency interviews including portion size	Strongly protective effect of dietary and supplemental vitamin C	
Esophagus	Mettlin et al., 1980	147 cases, 264 controls New York	Roswell Park Questionnaire	OR = 2.41 for low intake of vitamin C, p for trend = 0.004, even after control for smoking and alcohol	Effect was seen for vitamin A index, slightly weaker than for vitamin C but significant

	Reference	Population	Assessment method	Results	Comments
	Cook-Mozaffari, 1979	344 cases, 688 controls, Iran	Diet interview	Frequent consumption of oranges the most highly significant factor. Fruits and raw vegetables significantly protective	
	Ziegler et al., 1981	120 black male cases, 250 controls	31-item frequency interview	OR = 1.8 for low vitamin C index, after control alcohol. OR = 2.0 for low consumption of fruits	Poor nutrition overall may be important
Stomach	Kolonel et al., 1981	Japanese and Caucasians in Hawaii	Group mean values	Lower intake of vitamin C in the high-risk subgroup	Ecologic study.
	Correa et al., 1983	Four Colombian villages	Group mean values	Higher consumption of oranges, cabbage, tomatoes in village with low cancer incidence	Ecologic study. All villages appeared to be consuming more than WHO recommendation for vitamin C

	Haenszel et al., 1985	Columbia. 47 persons with gastric dysplasia, 464 controls	Serum ascorbate	No difference in mean serum ascorbate in dysplasia cases and controls	All serum levels appear to be in the well-nourished range for vitamin C
	Graham et al., 1967	188 cases, 800 controls, New York	Roswell Park Questionnaire	No difference in frequency of eating citrus fruits/juices	
	Haenszel et al., 1972	220 cases, 440 controls. Japanese in Hawaii	Frequency questionnaire	Only tomatoes showed significant protective effect on both Issei and Nisei, OR = 0.5. No effect for fruit	
	Correa et al., 1985	391 cases, 391 controls, Louisiana	Frequency interview	OR = 0.50 for white, 0.33 for blacks, for high intakes of vitamin C	Weaker and nonsignificant effect for carotenoids
	Bjelke, 1971, 1973	228 cases, 1394 controls	Frequency questionnaire	OR = 0.6 for age 60+. OR = 0.3 for age < 60, for high take of vitamin C	Weaker effect for vitamin A
Colon, rectum	Decosse et al., 1975	5 patients with rectal adenomas	Intervention study on polyp regression	Regression of polyps in 4 of 5 patients	Small sample size

Reference	Population	Assessment method	Results	Comments
Bussey et al., 1982	17 treatment, 14 control patients at 18 months	Intervention study on polyp number and area	Reduction in polyp area, significant at 8 months	Small sample size. Timed-release tablets
McKeown-Eyssen et al., 1987	200 patients after polypectomy	Intervention study on polyp recurrence	Recurrence after polypectomy reduced 20% in treatment group, $p > 0.05$	Polyp area not reported
Dion et al., 1982	20 volunteers	Intervention study on fecal mutagens	Reduction in fecal mutagens in group receiving vitamins C and E	Small sample size
Wilkins et al., 1981	5 volunteers	Intervention study on fecal mutagens	No effect observed for vitamins C and E	Small sample size
Schiffman, 1987	80 subjects with non-GI or benign GI disorders	Block diet history interview	Strong negative assoc. between both dietary and and supplemental vitamin C and fecal mutagens	Vitamin E also negatively associated
Jain et al., 1980	542 cases of colon and rectum cancer combined, 1077 controls, Canada	Extensive diet history interview	No effect of vitamin C	Very high estimated intake (2.5 × RDA) among both cases and controls

Tuyns, 1986	679 colon, 528 rectal cases, 3531 controls, Belgium	157-item frequency questionnaire, "usual week"	OR = 0.74 for colon cancer, 0.68 for rectal cancer, for high intake of vitamin C	
Potter and McMichael, 1986	419 colon/rectal cases, 732 controls, Australia	141-item self-administered frequency questionnaire	Colon cancer: no effect. Rectal cancer: OR = 0.3 in females, significant, OR = 0.6 in males, NS, for high intake of vitamin C	No effect for carotenoids
Bjelke, 1973	162 colon, 116 rectal cases, 1394 controls	Frequency questionnaire	Rectal cancer: OR = 0.66 for high intake of vitamin C, among spouse-concordant respondents	For colon cancer, stronger effect for vitamin A, vegetable index
Modan et al., 1981	406 patients with GI cancer, 812 controls, Israel	Frequency questionnaire	Strong significant effect for oranges, tomatoes, green peppers	Colon and rectal cases combined
Bingham et al., 1979, 1985	9 geographic regions, England	Household food survey	Negative correlation (−0.84) between mean vitamin C intake and colorectal cancer incidence	Ecologic study

	Reference	Population	Assessment method	Results	Comments
Pancreas	Norell et al., 1986	99 cases, 301 controls	Food frequency questionnaire	Consumption of citrus fruits protective, OR = 0.3 using hospital controls, significant	Carrots also protective
Bladder	Kolonel et al., 1985	164 cases, 314 controls	Frequency-based diet history questionnaire	Vitamin C protective in 3 of 4 ethnic-sex groups	
Prostate	Graham et al., 1983	311 cases, 294 controls	Roswell Park Questionnaire	Elevated risk with increased vitamin C, significant in men over age 70	Elevated risk for vitamin A intake, also
	Kolonel et al., 1985	418 cases, 771 controls	Frequency-based diet history questionnaire	No effect	

	Heshmat et al., 1985	181 black cases, matched controls	Frequency questionnaire, diet at age 30–49 and 50+	No effect of vitamin C	Elevated risk for vitamin A intake
Cervix	Marshall et al., 1983	513 cases, 490 controls	Roswell Park Questionnaire	No effect	
	Romney et al., 1985	46 cases with class III or IV Pap smear, 34 controls	Serum ascorbate	0.75 mg/dl in controls, 0.36 mg/dl in cases, $p < 0.0001$	Controlled for confounders
	Wassertheil-Smoller et al., 1981	87 cases with Class III or IV Pap smear, 82 controls	Three-day diet record, and 24-hour recall	OR = 4.35 for those below the case-control median of 76 mg vitamin C per day	Controlled for confounders
"All sites"	Colditz et al., 1985	1271 persons followed for 5 years	6-item frequency questionnaire	Strawberries, tomatoes significant, RR = 0.3, 0.5	Prospective study

REFERENCES

Afroz M., Bhothinard B, Etzkorn, J. R., et al. (1975). Vitamins C and B12. *JAMA 232*:246.

Alleva, F. R., Alleva, J. J., Balazs, T. (1976). Effect of large daily doses of ascorbic acid on pregnancy in guinea pigs, rats and hamsters. *Toxicol. Applied Pharm. 35*:393.

Anderson, R., Theron, A. (1979). Effects of ascorbate on leucocytes. III. In vitro and in vivo stimulation of abnormal neutrophil motility by ascorbate. *So. Afr. Med. J. 56*:429.

Anderson, R., Oosthuizen, R., Maritz, R., Theron, A., Van Rensburg, A. J. (1980). The effects of increasing weekly doses of ascorbate on certain cellular and humoral immune functions in normal volunteers. *Am. J. Clin. Nutr. 33*:71.

Babior, B. M. (1982). The enzymatic basis for O_2 production by human neutrophils. *Can. J. Physiol. Pharmacol. 60*:1353.

Barclay, L. R. C., Locke, S. J., MacNeil, J. M. (1983). The autoxidation of unsaturated lipids in micelles. Synergism of inhibitors vitamin C and E. *Can. J. Chem. 61*:1288.

Benedict, W. F., Wheatley, W. L., Jones, P. A. (1980). Inhibition of chemically induced morphological transformation and reversion of the transformed phenotype by ascorbic acid in C3H/10T 1/2 cells. *Cancer Res. 40*:2796.

Bingham, S., Williams, D. R. R., Cole, T. J., James, P. T. (1979). Dietary fibre and regional large-bowel cancer mortality in Britain. *Br. J. Cancer 40*:456.

Bingham, S. A., Williams, D. R. R., Cummings, J. H. (1985). Dietary fibre consumption in Britain: new estimates and their relation to large bowel cancer mortality. *Br. J. Cancer 52*:399.

Bjelke, E. (1971). Case-control study of cancer of the stomach, colon and rectum. In Oncology 1970. Clark R. L., Cumley, R. W., McCay, J. E., Copeland, M. M. (eds.). Proceedings of the 10th International Cancer Congress, Yearbook Medical Publishers, Chicago, pp. 320–334.

Bjelke, E. (1973). Epidemiologic studies of cancer of the stomach, colon, and rectum; With special emphasis on the role of diet. Vols. I–IV. Doctoral dissertation. University Microfilms, Ann Arbor, Michigan.

Bjelke, E., et al. (1982). Dietary factors and lung cancer mortality. The Lutheran Brotherhood study 1966–77. Proc 13th International Cancer Congress, Seattle.

Block, G., Hartman, A. M. (1983). Understanding the results of epidemiologic studies. *Seminars in Oncology 3*:257.

Block, G., Dresser, C. M., Hartman, A. M., Carroll, M. D. (1985). Nutrient sources in the American diet: Quantitative data from the NHANES II survey. I. Vitamins and Minerals. *Am. J. Epidemiol. 122*:13.

Block, G., Sorenson, A. (1987). Vitamin C intake and dietary sources by demographic characteristics. *Nutr. Cancer 10*:53.

Bodansky, O., Wroblewski, F., Markardt, B. (1951). Concentrations of ascorbic acid in plasma and white cells of patients with cancer and noncancerous chronic disease. *Cancer Res. 11*:238 (Abstract).

Bodansky, O., Wroblewski, F., Markardt, B. (1952). Concentrations of ascorbic acid in plasma and white blood cells of patients with cancer and noncancerous chronic disease. *Cancer 5*:678.

Bondarev, G. I., Golikov, K. K., Laricheva, K. A. (1975). Vitamin C allowance for sailors against the background of qualitatively differing nutrition. *Vopr. Pitan. 1*:11.

Boxer, L. A., Watanabe, A. M., Rister, M., Besch, H. R., Allen, J., Baehner, R. L. (1976). Correction of leukocyte function in Chediak-Higashi syndrome by ascorbate. *N. Engl. J. Med. 295*:1041.

Boxer, L. A., Vanderbilt, B., Bonsib, S., Jersild, R., Yang, H., Baehner, R. L. (1979). Enhancement of chemotactic response and microtubule assembly in human leukocytes by ascorbic acid. *J. Cellular Physiol. 100*:119.

Boyland, E., Grover, P. L. (1961). Stimulation of ascorbic acid synthesis and excretion by carcinogenic and other foreign compounds. *Biochem. J. 81*: 163.

Briggs, M., Briggs, M. (1972). Vitamin C requirements and oral contraceptives. *Nature 238*:277.

Briggs, M. (1973). Side effects of vitamin C. *Lancet II*:1439.

Briggs, M. (1976). Vitamin C induced hyperoxaluria. *Lancet 1*:154.

Brock, K. E., Berry, G., Mock, P. A., MacLennan, R., Truswell, A. S., Brinton, L. A. (1988). Nutrients in diet and plasma and risk of in situ cervical cancer. *JNCI*. In press.

Brook, M., Grimshaw, J. J. (1968). Vitamin C concentration of plasma and leukocytes as related to smoking habit, age, and sex of humans. *Am. J. Clin. Nutr. 21*:1254.

Bruce, W. R., Varghese, A. J., Furrer, R., Eng, Z., Land, T. C. (1977). A mutagen in the feces of normal humans. In *Origins of Human Cancer*, Hiatt, H. H., Watson, J. D., Weinsten, J. A. (Eds.). Cold Spring Harbor Laboratory, Cold Spring Harbor, New York, pp. 1641–1646.

Buck, M. G., Zadunaisky, J. A. (1975). Stimulation of ion transport by ascorbic acid through inhibition of 3′:5′-cyclic-AMP phosphodiesterase in the corneal epithelium and other tissues. *Biochem. Biophys. Acta 389*:251.

Burns, J. J., Evans, C. (1956). The synthesis of L-ascorbic acid in the rat from D-glucuronolactone and L-gulonolactone. *J. Biol. Chem. 223*:897.

Burns, J. J., Peyser, P., Moltz, A. (1956). Missing step in guinea pigs required for the biosynthesis of L-ascorbic acid. *Science 124*:1148.

Burns, J. J., Conney, A. H., Peter, G. D., Evans, C., Martin, G. R., Taller, D. (1960). Observations on the drug-induced synthesis of D-glucuronic, L-gulonic, and L-ascorbic acids in rats. *J. Pharmacol. Exptl. Therap. 129*:132.

Burr, M. L., Elwood, P. C., Holes, D. J., Hurley, R. J., Hughes, R. E. (1974). Plasma and leukocyte ascorbic acid levels in the elderly. *Am. J. Clin. Nutr. 27*:144.

Bussey, H. J. R., DeCosse, J. J., Deschner, E. E., et al. (1982). A randomized trial of ascorbic acid in polyposis coli. *Cancer 50*:1434.

Byers, T. E., Vena, J., Mettlin, C., et al. (1984). Dietary vitamin A and lung cancer risk: An analysis by histologic subtypes. *Am. J. Epidemiol. 120*:769.

Byers, T. E., Graham, S., Haughey, B. P., Marshall, J. R., Swanson, M. K. (1987). Diet and lung cancer: Findings from the Western New York diet study. *Am. J. Epidemiol. 125*:351.

Cameron, E. (1966). *Hyaluronidase and Cancer.* Pergamon Press, London.

Cameron, E., Pauling, L. (1973). Ascorbic acid and the glycosaminoglycans. *Oncology 27*:181.

Cameron, E., Campbell, A. (1974). The orthomolecular treatment of cancer. II. Clinical trial of high-dose ascorbic acid supplements in advanced human cancer. *Chem. Biol. Interact. 9*:285.

Cameron, E., Pauling, L. (1974). The orthomolecular treatment of cancer. I. The role of ascorbic acid in host resistance. *Chemico-Biol. Interact. 9*:273.

Cameron, E., Campbell, A., Jack, T. (1975). The orthomolecular treatment of cancer. III. Reticulum cell sarcoma: Double complete regression induced by high-dose ascorbic acid therapy. *Chemico-Biol. Interact. 11*:387.

Cameron, E., Pauling, L. (1976). Supplemental ascorbate in the supportive treatment of cancer: Prolongation of survival times in human cancer. *Proc. Nat. Acad. Sci. USA 73*:3685.

Cameron, E., Pauling, L. (1979). *Cancer and Vitamin C.* Linus Pauling Institute of Science and Medicine, Menlo Park, Cal.

Caraway, W. T., Kammeyer, C. W. (1972). Chemical interference by drugs and other substances with clinical laboratory test procedures. *Clin. Chim. Acta 41*:395.

Cardesa, A., Mirvish, S. S., Haven, G. T., Shubik, P. (1974). Inhibitory effect of ascorbic acid on the acute toxicity of dimethylamine plus nitrite in the rat. *Proc. Soc. Exptl. Biol. Med. 145*:124.

Cathcart, R. F., III (1981). The method of determining proper doses of vitamin C for treatment of disease by titrating to bowel tolerance. *J. Orthomolecular Psychiatry 10*:125.

Chatterjee, I. B., Majumder, A. K., Nandi, B. K., Subramanian, N. (1975). Synthesis and some major functions of vitamin C in animals. *Ann. NY Acad. Sci. 258*:24.

Chen, L. H., Chang, M. L. (1978). Effect of dietary vitamin E and vitamin C on respiration and swelling of guinea pig liver mitochondria. *J. Nutr. 108*:1616.

Chen, L. H., Lee, M. S., Hsing, W. F., Chen, S. H. (1980). Effect of vitamin C on tissue antioxidant status of vitamin E deficient rats. *Internat. J. Vit. Nutr. Res. 50*:156.

Clayson, D., David, B. (1975). Nutrition and experimental carcinogenesis: A review. *Cancer Res. 35*:3292.

Cochrane, W. (1965). Overnutrition in prenatal and neonatal life: A problem? *Can. Med. Assoc. J. 93*:893.

Colditz, G. A., Branch, L. G., Lipnick, R. J., et al. (1985). Increased green and yellow vegetable intake and lowered cancer deaths in an elderly population. *Am. J. Clin. Nutr. 41*:32.

Cook-Mozaffari, P. J., Azordegan, F., Day, N.E., et al. (1979). Oesophageal cancer studies in the Caspian littoral of Iran: Results of a case-control study. *Br. J. Cancer 39*:293.

Correa, P., Cuello, C., Fajardo, L. F., Haenszel, W., Bolanos, O., de Ramirez, B. (1983). Diet and gastric cancer: Nutrition survey in a high-risk area. *JNCI 70*: 673.

Correa, P., Fontham, E., Pickle, L. W. (1985). Dietary determinants of gastric cancer in south Louisiana inhabitants. *JNCI 75*:645.

Creagan, E. T., Moertel, C. G., O'Fallon, J. R. (1979). Failure of high-dose vitamin C (ascorbic acid) therapy to benefit patients with advanced cancer. *New Engl. J. Med. 301*:687.

Deana, R., Bharaj, B. S., Verjee, Z. H., Galzigna, L. (1975). Changes relevant to catecholamine metabolism in liver and brain of ascorbic acid deficient guinea pigs. *Int. J. Vit. Nutr. Res. 45*:175.

DeCosse, J. J., Adams, M. B., Kuzma, J. F. (1975). Effect of ascorbic acid on rectal polyps of patients with familial polyposis. *Surgery 78*:608.

DeFabro, S. P. (1967). Activite de la gulone-lactone-oxydase chez l'embryon de cobaye. *Comptes Rendu des Seances de la Soc. Biol. Filiales 162*:284.

Delafuente, J. C., Panush, R. S. (1979). Modulation of certain immunologic responses by vitamin C. *Internat. J. Vit. Nutr. Res. 50*:44.

Demole, V. (1934). On the physiological action of ascorbic acid and some related compounds. *Biochemical Journal 28*:770.

Demopoulos, H. B. (1973). Control of free radicals in biological systems. *Fed. Proc. 32*:1903.

Demopoulos, H. B., Pietronigro, D. D., Seligman, M. L. (1983). The development of secondary pathology with free radical reactions as a threshold mechanism. *J. Am. Col. Toxicol. 2*:173.

Dion, P. W., Bright-See, E. B., Smith, C. C., Furrer, R., Eng, Z., Bruce, W. R. (1982). The effect of dietary ascorbic acid and alpha-tocopherol on fecal mutagenicity. *Mutat. Res. 102*:27.

Dobias, L., Lochman, I., Machalek, J. (1986). Effect of ascorbic acid on humoral and other factors of immunity in coal-tar exposed workers. *J. Appl. Toxicol. 6*:9.

Dodd, M. J., MacLeod, F. L. (1947). Blood plasma ascorbic acid levels on controlled intakes of ascorbic acid. *Science 106*:67.

Dodds, M. L. (1969). Sex as a factor in blood levels of ascorbic acid. *J. Am. Diet. Assoc. 54*:32.

Dunham, W. B., Zuckerkandl, E., Reynolds, R., Willoughby, R., Marcuson, R., Barth, R., Pauling, L., (1982). Effect of intake of L-ascorbic acid on the incidence of dermal neoplasms induced in mice by ultraviolet light. *Proc. Natl. Acad. Sci. USA 79*:7532.

Food and Nutrition Board (1980). *Recommended Dietary Allowances*. National Academy of Sciences, Washington, D.C.

Forni, L. G., Willson, R. L. (1983). Vitamin C and consecutive hydrogen atom and electron transfer reactions in free radical protection: A novel catalytic role for glutathione. In *Protective Agents in Cancer*, McBrien, D. C. H., and Slater, T. F. (Eds.). Academic Press, London, pp. 169–173.

Fox, M. R. S. (1975). Protective effects of ascorbic acid against toxicity of heavy metals. *Ann. NY Acad. Sci. 258*:144.

Friedman, D. L. (1976). Role of cyclic nucleotides in cell growth and differentiation. *Physiol. Rev. 56*:652.

Ganguly, R., Durieux, M-F., Waldman, R. H. (1976). Macrophage function in vitamin C-deficient guinea pigs. *Am. J. Clin. Nutr. 29*:762.

Garrick, D. P., Close, J. R., McMurray, W. (1977). Detection of occult blood in faeces. *Lancet 2*:820.

Gilman, A. G., Goodman, L. S., Gilman, A. (eds.) (1980). *Goodman and Gilman's The Pharmacological Basis of Therapeutics*. MacMillan Publishing Company, New York.

Goetzl, E. J., Wasserman, S. I., Gigli, I., Austen, K. F. (1974). Enhancement of random migration and chemotactic response of human leukocytes by ascorbic acid. *J. Clin. Invest. 53*:813.

Goldsmith, G. A. (1971). Common cold: Prevention and treatment with ascorbic acid not effective. *J. Amer. Med. Assoc. 216*:337.

Good, R. A., Fisher, D. W. (eds.) (1972). *Immunobiology*. Sinauer Associates, Stanford, Conn.

Graham, S., Lilienfeld, A. M., Tidings, J. E. (1967). Dietary and purgation factors in the epidemiology of gastric cancer. *Cancer 20*:2224.

Graham, S., Dayal, H., Swanson, M., et al. (1978). Diet in the epidemiology of cancer of the colon and rectum. *JNCI 61*:709.

Graham, S., Mettlin, C., Marshall, J., et al. (1981). Dietary factors in the epidemiology of cancer of the larynx. *Am. J. Epidemiol. 113*:675.

Graham, S., Haughey, B., Marshall, J., Priore, R., Byers, T., Rzepka, T., Mettlin, C., and Pontes, J. E. (1983). Diet in the epidemiology of carcinoma of the prostate gland. *JNCI 70*:687.

Gregor, A., Lee, P. N., Roe, F. J. C., Wilson, M. J., Melton, A. (1980). Comparison of dietary histories in lung cancer cases and controls with special reference to vitamin A. *Nutrition and Cancer 2*:93.

Guyton, A. C. (1976). *Textbook of Medical Physiology*. W. B. Saunders Company, Philadelphia.

Haenszel, W., Kurihara, M., Segi, M., Lee, R. K. C. (1972). Stomach cancer among Japanese in Hawaii. *JNCI 49*:969.

Haenszel, W., Locke, F. B., Segi, M. (1980). A case-control study of larger bowel cancer in Japan. *JNCI 64*:17.

Haenszel, W., Cuello, C., Correa, P., et al. (1985) Correlations of values of micronutrients in sera with gastric pathology. *Natl. Cancer Inst. Monogr. 69*: 115.

Hallberg, L. (1981). Effect of vitamin C on the bioavailability of iron from food. In *Vitamin C (ascorbic acid)*, Counsel, J. N., Hornig, D. H. (eds.). New Jersey, Applied Science Publishers, p. 49.

Hamil, B. M., Munks, B., Moyer, E. Z., Kaucher, M., Williams, H. H. (1947). Vitamin C in the blood and urine of the newborn and in the cord and maternal blood. *Am. J. Dis. Child. 74*:417.

Harada, T., Kitazawa, T., Maita, K., Shirasu, Y. (1985). Effects of vitamin C on tumor induction by diethylnitrosamine in the respiratory tract of hamsters exposed to cigarette smoke. *Cancer Lett. 26*:163.

Hatch, G. E., Slade, R., Selgrade, M. K., Stead, A. G. (1986). Nitrogen dioxide exposure and lung antioxidants in ascorbic acid-deficient guinea pigs. *Toxicol. Appl. Pharmac. 82*:351.

Heinegard, D., Tiderstrom, G. (1973). Determination of serum creatinine by a direct colorimetric method. *Clin. Chim. Acta 43*:305.

Herbert, V., Jacob, E. (1974). Destruction of vitamin B12 by ascorbic acid. *J. Amer. Med. Assoc. 230*:241.

Heshmat, M. Y., Kaul, L., Kovi, J., et al. (1985). Nutrition and prostate cancer: A case-control study. *Prostate 6*:7.

Hinds, M. W., Kolonel, L. N., Hankin, J. H., et al. (1984). Dietary vitamin A, carotene, vitamin C and risk of lung cancer in Hawaii. *Am. J. Epidemiol. 119*:227.

Hodges, R. E., Baker, E. M., Hood, J., Sauberlich, H. E., March, S. C. (1969). Experimental scurvy in man. *Am. J. Clin. Nutr. 22*:535.

Hodges, R. E., Hood, J., Canham, J. E. Sauberlich, H. E., Baker, E. M. (1971). Clinical manifestations of ascorbic acid deficiency in man. *Am. J. Clin. Nutr. 24*:432.

Hodges, R. E. (1980). Ascorbic acid. In *Modern Nutrition in Health and Disease*, Sixth Edition. Goodhart, R. S. and Shils, M. E. (Eds.). Lea and Febiger, Philadelphia.

Hoffer, A. (1971). Ascorbic acid and toxicity. *N. Engl. J. Med. 285*:635.

Hogenkamp, H. P. C. (1980). The interaction between vitamin B12 and vitamin C. *Am. J. Clin. Nutr. 33*:1.

Hornig, D., Weiser, H., Weber, F., Wiss, O. (1973). Effect of massive doses of ascorbic acid on its catabolism in guinea pigs. *Int. J. Vitamin Nutr. Res. 43*: 28.

Hornig, D. (1975). Distribution of ascorbic acid, metabolites and analogues in man and animals. *Ann. NY Acad. Sci. 258*:103.

Hughes, C., Dutton, S., Truswell, A. S. (1981). High intakes of ascorbic acid and urinary oxalate. *J. Hum. Nutr. 35*:274.

Hume, R., Weyers, E. (1973). Changes in leucocyte ascorbic acid during the common cold. *Scot. Med. 18*:3.

Jaffe, R. M., Kasten, B., Young, D. S., MacLowry, J. D. (1975). False-negative stool occult blood tests caused by ingestion of ascorbic acid (vitamin C). *Ann. Int. Med. 83*:824.

Jaffey, M. (1982). Vitamin C and cancer: Examination of the Vale of Leven trial results using broad inductive reasoning. *Med. Hypoth. 8*:49.

Jain, M., Cook, G. M., Davis, F. G., et al. (1980). A case-control study of diet and colo-rectal cancer. *Int. J. Cancer 26*:757.

Jones, F. E., Komorowski, R. A., Condon, R. E. (1981). Chemoprevention of 1,2-dimethylhyrazine-induced large bowel neoplasms. *Surgical Forum 32*: 435.

Kalden, J. R., Guthy, E. A. (1972). Prolonged skin allograft survived in vitamin C-deficient guinea-pigs. *Europ. Surg. Res. 4*:114.

Kallner, A., Hornig, D., Hartman, D. (1982). In *Advances in Chemistry Series*, No. 200. American Chemical Society, Washington, D.C., pp. 335–348.
Kamm, J. J., Dashman, T., Conney, A. H., Burns, J. J. (1973). Protective effect of ascorbic acid on hepatotoxicity caused by sodium nitrite plus aminopyrine. *Proc. Nat. Acad. Sci. 70*:747.
Kamm, J. J., Dashman, T., Conney, A. H., Burns, J. J. (1971). Effect of ascorbic acid on amine-nitrite toxicity. *Ann. NY Acad. Sci. 258*:169.
Kattab, A. K., Al Nagdy, S. A., Mourad, K. A. H., El Azghal, H. I. (1970). Foetal maternal ascorbic acid gradient in normal Egyptian subjects. *J. Trop. Pediatr. 16*:112.
Katz, S. M., Di Silvio, T. V. (1973). Ascorbic acid effects on serum glucose values. *JAMA 224*:628.
Kawasaki, H., Morishige, F., Tanaka, H., Kimoto, E. (1982). Influence of oral supplementation of ascorbate upon the induction of N-methyl-N′-nitro-N-nitrosoguanidine. *Cancer Lett. 16*:57–63.
Klenner, F. R. (1971). Observations on the dose and administration of ascorbic acid when employed beyond the range of a vitamin in human pathology. *J. Applied Nutrition 23*:61.
Kolonel, L. N., Nomura, A. M. Y., Hirohata, T., et al. (1981). Association of diet and place of birth with stomach cancer incidence in Hawaii Japanese and Caucasians. *Am. J. Clin. Nutr. 34*:2478.
Kolonel, L. N., Hinds, M. W., Nomura, A. M. Y., et al. (1985). Relationship of dietary vitamin A and ascorbic acid intake to the risk for cancers of the lung, bladder, and prostate in Hawaii. *Natl. Cancer Inst. Monogr. 69*:137.
Krinsky, N. I. (1974). Single excited oxygen as a mediator of the antibacterial action of leukocytes. *Science 186*:363.
Kvale, G., Bjelke, E., Gart, J. J. (1983). Dietary habits and lung cancer risk. *Int. J. Cancer 31*:397.
Lamden, M. P., Chrystowski, G. A. (1954). Urinary oxalate excretion by man following ascorbic acid ingestion. *Proc. Soc. Exptl. Biol. Med. 85*:190.
Laroye, G. J. (1974). How efficient is immunological surveillance against cancer and why does it fail? *Lancet 1*:1097.
Leuchtenberger, C., Leuchtenberger, R. (1977). Protection of hamster lung cultures by L-cysteine or vitamin C against carcinogenic effects of fresh smoke from tobacco or marihuana cigarettes. *Br. J. Exp. Path. 58*:625.
Levine, M. (1986). New concepts in the biology and biochemistry of ascorbic acid. *NEJM 314*:892.
Lewin, S. (1976). *Vitamin C: Its Molecular Biology and Medical Potential*. Academic Press, London.
Lilienfeld, A. M., Lilienfeld, D. E. (1980). *Foundations of Epidemiology*. Oxford University Press, New York, pp. 14, 291.
Logue, T., Frommer, D. (1980). The influence of oral vitamin C supplements on experimental colorectal tumour induction. *Aust. NZ J. Med. 10*:588.
Loh, H. S., Watters, D. C. H. K., Wilson, C. W. M. (1973). The effects of aspirin on the metabolic availability of ascorbic acid in human beings. *J. Clin. Pharmacol.* :480.

Long-de, W., Hammond, E. C. (1985). Lung cancer, fruit, green salad and vitamin pills. *Chinese Med. J. 98*:206.

Lowry, O. H., Bessey, O. A., Burch, H. B. (1953). Effects of prolonged high dosage with ascorbic acid. *Public Health Research Inst.* 361.

Lyko, H. C., Hartman, J. X. (1980). Ascorbate, cyclic nucleotides, citrus and a model for preventing large bowel cancer. *J. Theor. Biol. 83*:675.

MacLennan, R., DaCosta, J., Day, N. E., et al. (1977). Risk factors for lung cancer in Singapore Chinese, a population with high female incidence rates. *Int. J. Cancer 20*:854.

Marcus, M., Prabhudesai, M., Wassef, S. (1980). Stability of vitamin B12 in the presence of ascorbic acid in food and serum. Restoration by cyanide of apparent loss. *Am. J. Clin. Nutr. 33*:137.

Marcus, M. (1981). Vitamin B12. Response to Dr. Herbert. *Am. J. Clin. Nutr. 34*:1622.

Markert, M., Frei, J. (1982). The respiratory burst in human polymorphonuclear leukocytes stimulated by particles. In *Biochemistry and Functions of Phagocytes*, F. Rossi, P. Patriarca (Eds.). Plenum Press, New York, p. 383.

Marquardt, H., Rufino, F., Weisburger, J. H. (1977). Mutagenic activity of nitrite-treated foods: Human stomach cancer may be related to dietary factors. *Science 196*:1000.

Marshall, J., Graham, S., Mettlin, C., et al. (1982). Diet in the epidemiology of oral cancer. *Nutrition and Cancer 3*:145.

Marshall, J. R., Graham, S., Byers, T., et al. (1983). Diet and smoking in the epidemiology of cancer of the cervix. *JNCI 70*:847.

McCormick, W. J. (1959). Cancer: A collagen disease, secondary to a nutritional deficiency? *Arch. Pediat. 76*:166.

McKeown-Eyssen, G. E., Holloway, C., Jazmaji, V., et al. (1987). A randomized trial of vitamin C and E supplementation in the prevention of recurrence of colorectal polyps. Abstract, Eleventh Annual Meeting of the American Society of Preventive Oncology. San Francisco, March 11–13.

Menzel, D. B. (1970). Toxicity of ozone, oxygen and radiation. *Ann. Rev. Pharmacol. 10*:379.

Mettlin, C., Graham, S., Swanson, M. (1979). Vitamin A and lung cancer. *JNCI 62*:1435.

Mettlin, C., Graham, S., Priore, R., et al. (1980). Diet and cancer of the esophagus. *Nutrition and Cancer 2*:143.

Milne, J. S., Lonergan, M. E., Williamson, J., Moor, F. L. M., McMaster, Percy, N. (1971). Leucocyte ascorbic acid levels and vitamin C intake in older people. *Br. Med. J. 4*:383.

Mirvish, S. S., Cardesa, A., Wallcave, L., Shubik, P. (1973). Effect of sodium ascorbate on lung adenoma induction by amines plus nitrite. *Proc. Am. Assoc. Cancer Res. 14*:102.

Mirvish, S. S., Shubik, P. (1974). Ascorbic acid and nitrosamine. *Nature 250*: 684.

Mirvish, S. S. (1975). Blocking the formation of N-nitroso compounds with ascorbic acid in vitro and in vivo. *Ann. NY Acad. Sci. 258*:175.

Modan, B., Barell, V., Lubin, F., Modan, M., Greenberg, R. A., Graham, S. (1975). Low-fibre intake as an etiologic factor in cancer of the colon. *JNCI 55*:15.

Modan, B., Cuckle, H., Lubin, F. (1981). A note on the role of dietary retinol and carotene in human gastro-intestinal cancer. *Int. J. Cancer 28*:421.

Moertel, C. G., Fleming, T. R., Creagan, E. T., Rubin, J., O'Connell, M. J., Ames, M. M. (1985). High-dose vitamin C versus placebo in the treatment of patients with advanced cancer who have had no prior chemotherapy. *New Engl. J. Med. 312*:137.

Moffat, A. C., Patterson, D. A., Currey, A. S., Owen, P. (1972). Inhibition in vitro of cyclic 3′,5′ nucleotide phosphodiesterase activity by drugs. *European J. Toxicol. 5*:160.

Morrison, D. G., Daniel, J., Lynd, F. T., Moyer, M. P., Esparza, R. J., Moyer, R. C., Rogers, W. (1981). *Nutr. Cancer 3*:81.

Morse, E. H., Clarke, R. P., Keyser, D. E., Merrow, S. B., Bee. (1975). Comparison of the nutritional status of pregnant adolescents with adult pregnant women. I. Biochemical findings. *Am. J. Clin. Nutr. 28*:1000.

Nahata, M. C., McLeod, D. C. (1978). Noneffect of oral ascorbic acid on urinary copper reduction glucose test. *Diabetes Care 1*:34.

National Center for Health Statistics, R. Fullwood, C. L. Johnson, J. D. Bryner, and others (1982). Hematological and nutritional biochemistry reference data for persons 6 months-74 years of age: United States, 1976–80. Vital and Health Statistics. Series 11-No. 232. DHHS Pub. No. (PHS) 83-1682. Public Health Service. U.S. Government Printing Office, Washington, D.C.

National Research Council. (1978a). Committee on Animal Nutrition. Nutrient Requirements of Nonhuman Primates. National Academy of Sciences, Washington, D.C.

National Research Council. (1978b). Committee on Animal Nutrition. Nutrient Requirements of Laboratory Animals. National Academy of Sciences, Washington, D.C.

Newmark, H. L., Scheiner, J. M., Marcus, M., et al. (1979). Ascorbic acid and vitamin B12. *J. Amer. Med. Assoc. 242*:2319.

Norell, S. E., Ahlbom, A., Erwald, R., et al. (1986). Diet and pancreatic cancer: A case-control study. *Am. J. Epidemiol. 124*:894.

Norkus, E. P., Rosso, P. (1975). Changes in ascorbic acid metabolism of the offspring following high maternal intake of this vitamin in the pregnant guinea pig. *Ann. NY Acad. Sci. 258*:401.

Packer, J. E., Slater, T. F., Willson, R. L. (1979). Direct observation of a free radical interaction between vitamin E and vitamin C. *Nature 278*:737.

Park, C. H., Amare, M., Savin, M. A., Hoogstraten, B. (1980). Growth suppression of human leukemic cells in vitro by L-ascorbic acid. *Cancer Res. 40*: 1062.

Pelletier, O. (1975). Vitamin C and cigarette smokers. *Ann. NY Acad. Sci. 258*: 156.

Pelletier, O. (1977). Vitamin C and tobacco. *Int. J. Vit. Nutr. Res. 16*:147.

Phillips, R. (1975). Role of life-style and dietary habits in risk of cancer among Seventh-Day Adventists. *Cancer Res. 35*:3513.

Pipkin, G. E., Schlegel, J. U., Nishimura, R., Shultz, G. N. (1969). Inhibitory effect of L-ascorbate on tumor formation in urinary bladders implanted with 3-hydroxyanthranilic acid. *Proc. Soc. Exptl. Biol. Med. 131*:522.

Poser, E. (1972). Large ascorbic acid intake. *New Engl. J. Med. 287*:412.

Potter, J. D., McMichael, A. J. (1986). Diet and cancer of the colon and rectum: A case-control study. *JNCI 76*:557.

Poydock, M. E., Reikert, D., Rice, J., Aleandri, L. (1982). Inhibiting effect of dehydroascorbic acid on cell division in ascites tumors in mice. *Expl. Cell Biol. 50*:34.

Prasad, A. S., Lei, K. Y., Oberleas, D., Moghissi, O. S., Stryker, J. C. (1975). Effect of oral contraceptive agents on nutrients: Vitamins. *Am. J. Clin. Nutr. 28*:385.

Prinz, W., Bortz, R., Bregin, B., Hersch, M. (1977). The effect of ascorbic acid supplementation on some parameters of the human immunological defence system. *Internat. J. Vit. Nutr. Res. 47*:248.

Pryor, W. A. (ed.). (1977). *Free Radicals in Biology* Vol. I. Academic Press, New York.

Ranieri, R., Weisburger, J. H. (1975). Reduction of carcinogens with ascorbic acid. *Ann. NY Acad. Sci. 258*:181.

Reddy, B. S., Hirota, N. (1979). Effect of dietary ascorbic acid on 1,2-dimethylhydrazine-induced colon cancer in rats. *Fed. Proc. 38*:714.

Rettura, G., Stratford, F., Levenson, S. M., Seifter, E. (1982). Prophylactic and therapeutic actions of supplemental beta-carotene in mice inoculated with C3HBA adenocarcinoma cells: Lack of therapeutic action of supplemental ascorbic acid. *JNCI 69*:73.

Rivers, J. M. (1975). Oral contraceptives and ascorbic acid. *Am. J. Clin. Nutr. 28*:50.

Rivers, J. M., Devine, M. M. (1975). Relationships of ascorbic acid to pregnancy and oral contraceptive steroids. *Ann. NY Acad. Sci. 258*:465.

Roine, P., Koivula, L., Pekkarinen, M. (1972). Plasma vitamin C level and erythrocyte transketolase activity compared with vitamin intakes among old people in Finland, Vol. 4. In Proceedings, 9th International Congress on Nutrition, Mexico, S. Karger, Basel, pp. 116–120.

Romney, S. L., Duttagupta, C., Basu, J., et al. (1985). Plasma vitamin C and uterine cervical dysplasia. *Am. J. Obstet. Gynecol. 151*:976.

Rosenthal, G. (1971). Interaction of ascorbic acid and warfarin. *J. Amer. Med. Assoc. 215*:1671.

Sahud, M. A., Cohen, R. J. (1971). Effect of aspirin ingestion on ascorbic acid levels in rheumatoid arthritis. *Lancet 1*:937.

Salvatore, J. E., Vinton, P. W., Rapuano, J. A. (1969). Nutrition in the aged: review of the literature. *J. Am. Geriatr. Soc. 17*:790.

Sanders, C. L., Mahaffey, J. A. (1983). Action of vitamin C on pulmonary carcinogenesis from inhaled $^{239}PuO_2$. *Health Phys. 43*:794.

Sauberlich, H. E., Baker, E. M. (1967). Studies in human nutrition. In Annual Research Progress Report, U.S. Army Medical Research and Nutrition Laboratory, 30 June, San Francisco, pp. 180–7.

Sauberlich, H. E. (1975). Vitamin C status: methods and findings. *Ann. NY Acad. Sci. 258*:438.

Sauberlich, H. E. (1984). Ascorbic acid. In Nutrition Review's *Present Knowledge in Nutrition*. The Nutrition Foundation, Washington, D.C.

Schiffman, M. H. (1987). Diet and fecal genotoxicity. Cancer Surveys.

Schlegel, J. U., Pipkin, G. E., Nishimura, R., Duke, G. A. (1969). Studies in the etiology and prevention of bladder carcinoma. *J. Urol. 101*:317.

Schlegel, J. U., Pipkin, G. E., Nishimura, R., Schultz, G. N. (1969). The role of ascorbic acid in the prevention of bladder tumor formation. *Transact. Amer. Assoc. Genito-Urinary Surg. 61*:85.

Schmidt, F., Schmandte, H., Gassman, B. (1963). Vitamin C und Krebs. *Z. Arztl. Fortbild. 57*:1315.

Schrauzer, G. N., Rhead, W. J. (1973). Ascorbic acid abuse: Effects of long-term ingestion of excessive amounts on blood levels and urinary excretion. *Int. J. Vitamin Nutr. Res. 43*:201.

Schrauzer, G. N. (1979). Vitamin C: Conservative human requirements and aspects of overdosage. *Internal Rev. of Biochem, Biochem of Nutr. 27*:167.

Sestili, M. A. (1983). Possible adverse health effects of vitamin C and ascorbic acid. *Seminars in Oncology 10*:299.

Shekelle, R. B., Lepper, M., Liu, S., et al. (1981). Dietary vitamin A and risk of cancer in the Western Electric study. *Lancet 2*:1185.

Shilotri, P. G. (1977a). Glycolytic, hexose monophosphate shunt and bactericidal activities of leukocytes in ascorbic acid deficient guinea pigs. *J. Nutr. 107*: 1507.

Shilotri, P. G. (1977b). Phagocytosis and leukocyte enzymes in ascorbic acid deficient guinea pigs. *J. Nutr. 107*:1513.

Siegel, B. V., Morton, J. I. (1977). Vitamin C and the immune response. *Experientia 33*:393.

Siegel, C. Barker, B., Kundstadter, M. (1982). Conditioned oral scurvy due to megavitamin C withdrawal. *J. Periodontology 53*:453.

Sigell, L. T., Flessa, H. C. (1940). Drug interactions with anticoagulants. *J. Amer. Med. Assoc. 214*:2035.

Slaga, T. J., Bracken, W. M. (1977). The effects of antioxidants on skin tumor initiation and aryl hydrocarbon hydroxylase. *Cancer Res. 37*:1631.

Smith, L. H. (1974). Medical evaluation of urolithiasis: Etiologic aspects and diagnostic evaluation. *Urol. Clin. North Am. 1*:241.

Spiegel, H. E., Pinili, E. (1974). Effect of vitamin C on SGOT, SGPT, LDH, and bilirubin. *Med. J. Austral. 2*:265.

Spitzer, J. M., Shapiro, S. (1948). The effect of salicylate medication upon the urinary excretion of vitamin C. *Am. J. Digestive Dis. 15*:80.

Stocks, P. (1957). Cancer incidence in North Wales and Liverpool region in relation to habits and environment. In *British Empire Cancer Campaign*. 35th annual report, Suppl. to part 2, p. 1.

Stone, K. J., Townsley, B. H. (1973). The effect of L-ascorbate on catecholamine biosynthesis. *Biochem. J. 131*:611.

Street, J. C., Chadwick, W. R. (1975). Ascorbic acid requirements and metabolism in relation to organochlorine pesticides. *Ann. NY Acad. Sci. 258*:132.

Sutton, H. E. (1975). *An introduction to human genetics*. Holt, Rinehart and Winston, New York.

Takiguchi, H., Furuyama, S., Shimazono, N. (1966). Urinary oxalic excretion by man following ingestion of large amounts of ascorbic acid. *J. Vitaminol. 12*:307.

Tappel, A. L. (1962). Vitamin E as the biological lipid antioxidant. *Vitamins Hormones 20*:493.

Tiselius, H. G. (1977). Excretion of 4-pyridoxic acid and oxalic acid in patients with urinary calculi. *Invest. Urology 15*:5.

Ts'o, P., Caspary, W. J., Lorentzen, R. J. (1977). The involvement of free radicals in chemical carcinogenesis. In *Free Radicals in Biology*, Vol. III, W. A. Pryor (Ed.). Academic Press, New York, pp. 251–303.

Tuyns, A. J. (1986). A case-control study on colorectal cancer in Belgium. Preliminary results. *Sozial- and Praventivmedizin 31*:81.

Vallance, S. (1975). Vitamin C nutrition on a British Antarctic survey base. *Br. Antarct. Surv. Bull. 41, 42*:139.

Vallance, S. (1977). Relationships between ascorbic acid and serum proteins of the immune system. *Brit. Med. J. 2*:437.

Van Wyk, C. P., Kotze, J. P. (1975). Effect of ascorbic acid on plasma adenosine 3′,5′-cyclic monophosphate level in the baboon, Papio Ursinus. *South African J. of Science 71*:28.

Visagie, M. E., DuPlessis, J. P., Groothof, G., Alberts, A., Laubscher, N. F. (1974). Change in vitamin A and C levels in black mine-workers. *S. Afr. Med. J. 48*:2502.

Visagie, M. E., DuPlessis, J. P., Laubscher, N. F. (1975). Effect of vitamin C supplementation on black mine-workers. *S. Afr. Med. J. 49*:889.

Vobecky, J. S., Vobecky, J., Shapcott, D., Muman, L. (1974). Vitamin C and outcome of pregnancy. *Lancet 1*: 630.

Walker, A. M., Blettner, M. (1985). Comparing imperfect measures of exposure. *Am. J. Epidemiol. 121*:783.

Warren, F. L. (1943). Aerobic oxidation of aromatic hydrocarbons in the presence of ascorbic acid. *Biochem. J. 37*:338.

Wassertheil-Smoller, S., Romney, S. L., Wylie-Rosett, J., et al. (1981). Dietary vitamin C and uterine cervical dysplasia. *Am. J. Epidemiol. 114*:714.

Weisburger, J. H., Ranieri, R. (1975). Dietarv factors and the etiology of gastric cancer. *Cancer Res. 35*:3469.

Weisburger, J. H., Marquardt, H., Mower, H. F., et al. (1980). Inhibition of carcinogenesis: Vitamin C and the prevention of gastric cancer. *Prev. Med. 9*: 352.

Weiss, L., Greep, R. O. (eds.) (1977). *Histology*. McGraw-Hill Book Company, New York.

White, J. W. (1975). Relative significance of dietary sources of nitrate and nitrite. *J. Agric. Food Chem. 23*:886.

Wilkins, T., et al. (1981). Banbury Report #7, pp. 205–226.

Winn, D. M., Ziegler, R. G., Pickle, L. W., et al. (1984). Diet in the etiology of oral and pharyngeal cancer among women from the Southern United States. *Cancer Res. 44*:1216.

Yagashita, K., Takahashi, N., Yamamoto, H., Jinnouchi, H., Hiyoshi, S., Miyakawa, T. (1976). Effects of tetraacetyl-bis-dehydroascorbic acid, a derivative of ascorbic acid, on Ehrlich cells and HeLa cells (human carcinoma cells). *J. Nutr. Sci. Vitaminol. 22*:419.

Yews, M-L. S. (1975). Biological variation in ascorbic acid needs. *Ann. NY Acad. Sci. 258*:451.

Zannoni, V. G., Sato, P. H. (1975). Effects of ascorbic acid on microsomal drug metabolism. *Ann. NY Acad. Sci. 258*:119.

Ziegler, R. G., Morris, L. E., Blot, W. J., et al. (1981). Esophageal cancer among Black men in Washington, D. C. II. Role of nutrition. *JNCI 67*:1199.

Ziegler, R. G., Mason, T. J., Stemhagen, A., Hoover, R., Schoenberg, J. B., Gridley, G., Virgo, P. W., Altman, R., Fraumeni, J. F. (1984). Dietary carotene and vitamin A and risk of lung cancer among White men in New Jersey. *JNCI*: 1429.

Zloch, Z., Ginter, E. (1984). Experimentally proved biosynthesis of vitamin C in a guinea pig. *Naturwissenschaften 71*:533.

14
Selenium

GERALD F. COMBS, JR.
Cornell University, Ithaca, New York

HISTORIC BACKGROUND FOR CONSIDERING A RELATIONSHIP BETWEEN SELENIUM AND CARCINOGENESIS

Questions were first raised concerning the possibility of a relationship between selenium (Se) and carcinogenesis some 40 years ago with the apparently discrepant reports of Nelson et al. (1943) and Clayton and Bauman (1949). The former report suggested that relatively high dietary levels of Se (i.e., several parts per million) could produce liver cell adenoma or low-grade carcinoma in rats that first developed cirrhosis. The latter report, however, indicated that high levels of Se protected against azo dye*-induced hepatic tumors in rats. Thus, a decade before the discoveries that low levels of Se are important in the nutrition of experimental animals (Patterson et al., 1957; Schwartz and Foltz, 1957; Schwartz et al., 1957), it was unclear whether the element could be carcinogenic or anticarcinogenic.

In the latter part of the 1950s, the independent studies of Schwarz et al. (1957) and Patterson et al. (1957) showed that Se prevents necrotic liver degeneration in the vitamin E-deficient rat and exudative diathesis in the vitamin E-deficient chick, thus demonstrating for this element a nutritional role related to that of vitamin E. It was not until 1970 that Se was found to have a nutritional activity beyond that of vitamin E, i.e., that it prevents the degeneration of the acinar pancreas in the vitamin E-fed chick (Thompson and Scott, 1970); this

*Dimethylaminoazobenzene.

discovery established Se as an essential nutrient. And so, by the 1970s, Se was recognized as having nutritional activity, much but not all of which related to vitamin E in a variety of species. This recognition and consideration of the use of Se compounds as nutritional supplements to formulated animal feeds again put focus on the possibility of a relationship of Se and carcinogenesis (Scott, 1973), particularly on the results reported by Nelson et al. (1943).

At about the same time, Shamberger and Frost (1969) reported that cancer mortality rates in the United States were inversely associated with the geographic distribution of Se, as indicated by the Se contents of forage crops (Kubota et al., 1967). When Allaway et al. (1968) showed that the levels of Se in selected urban blood bank samples showed geographic variations similar to those of forage crop Se, Shamberger and Willis (1971) presented calculations that showed the cancer mortality rate to be correlated negatively with blood Se level in the same communities. When large-scale chronic studies with rats (Harr et al., 1967; Tinsley et al., 1967; Volgarev and Tscherkes, 1967; Schroeder and Mitchner, 1971) were unable to confirm the results of Nelson et al. (1943), the notion that Se might be carcinogenic became discredited as the product of likely incorrect histological interpretations (Scott, 1973); it was abandoned in favor of the hypothesis that, in addition to its known nutritional role, Se might function in some way to reduce cancer risk. In 1973, when Rotruck et al. (1973) discovered a biochemical basis for the nutritional action of Se, i.e., that it is an essential constituent of the hydroperoxide-metabolizing enzyme glutathione peroxidase (E.C. 1.11.1.9) (now called Se-dependent glutathione peroxidase, SeGSHpx), it became possible to consider mechanistic hypotheses for the roles of Se that had been documented in nutrition and proposed in carcinogenesis.

In the nearly 15 years since the recognition of SeGSHpx, a substantial body of research has yielded insight into the function of Se both in normal health and in carcinogenesis. Still, much remains to be elucidated concerning the role of nutritional Se status and cancer risk. Various aspects of this information have been reviewed recently (Jansson et al., 1978; Cowgill, 1983; Clark, 1985; Milner, 1986; Salonen, 1986; Thompson et al., 1986; Watson and Leonard, 1986; Willett and Stampfer, 1986); the entire subject was summarized in some detail by Combs and Combs (1986). The purpose of this chapter is to build upon these reviews, paying particular attention to the results of the most recent research reports and presenting the major issues relevant to the possible consideration of Se compounds in cancer prevention.

EPIDEMIOLOGY OF SELENIUM AND CANCER

Ecological Associations

The Se status of a population tends to be determined in large part by the geochemical environment of the primary areas of food production, which, in most countries, is local to the population (see Combs and Combs, 1986). That is, human populations tend to show indices of Se status (e.g., blood or hair Se contents) that correspond to the Se contents of locally produced plant crops. Therefore, the results of geographical studies of the relationship of Se status and cancer incidence in human populations have been of interest. Several such studies have been conducted; each has indicated an inverse association of Se status and cancer mortality (Shamberger and Frost, 1969; Shamberger and Willis, 1971; Shamberger et al., 1974; Shamberger et al., 1976; Schrauzer et al., 1977a,b; Yu et al., 1985). An example is the study of Shamberger and Willis (1971); it found that mortality due to lymphomas and cancers of the gastrointestinal tract, peritoneum, lung, and breast were lower for both males and females residing in areas of the United States that can be classified, on the basis of the Se contents of local forage crops, as being either moderate (i.e., 0.06–0.10 ppm Se, air dry basis) or high (i.e., $>$ 0.10 ppm Se) in the element. Another example is the study of Schrauzer et al. (1977), which found that, over 27 developed countries, the overall cancer mortality rate as well as age-corrected mortality rates due to leukemia and cancers of the colon, rectum, breast, ovary, and lung correlated inversely with the authors' rough estimates of the average per capita intakes of Se in those countries. Schrauzer et al. (1977a) also reported that age-adjusted mortality rates within the United States for cancers of the breast, colon, rectum, and lung were inversely related to whole blood Se concentrations as estimated on the basis of average values obtained from blood bank samples. Similar results were reported by Yu et al. (1985) from mainland China; in a study conducted in 24 locations in a total of eight provinces in that country, they found a significantly negative correlation between age-adjusted total cancer mortality rate and whole blood Se concentration. Further, in a county with a particularly high incidence of hepatoma (Qidong County, Jiangsu Province), Yu et al. (1985) found that the geographic distribution of liver cancer incidence was inversely related to either blood Se level or to the Se contents of locally available food grains.

Clark (1985) has pointed out that, due to a number of methodological considerations, the interpretation of the results of these ecological studies, particularly the earlier ones, is not as clear as has generally been presented by those authors. These methodological concerns include the use of mortality rates that were not age-adjusted; the exclusion of a number of locations from particular analyses; the use of estimates of national per capita Se intake that were based on rather ill-defined "typical" Se contents of foods (i.e., not actual analyses) and on national average food consumption data;* the use of state-level (instead

*This approach, in the view of the present author, is almost certain to yield estimates with little relevance to actual levels of Se intake.

of county-level) Se-exposure and cancer mortality data; the failure to adjust mortality rates for differences in degree of urbanization; and the failure to use weighted least-squares regression analyses in the evaluation of the data.

With these concerns for methodology, Clark reevaluated the ecological relationship of Se status and cancer mortality in the mainland U.S. population. This analysis, described in his review (1985), involved the association of major site- and sex-specific cancers (using the U.S. cancer mortality data for 1950–1969 (Mason and McKay, 1975) and forage crop Se levels (estimated from the original data of Kubota et al. (1967). County-based data were used in the analysis to reduce misclassification of Se exposure that might otherwise result in the cases of states containing both high- and low-Se areas. The confounding effects of urbanization were also minimized by limiting the analysis to counties with populations of less than 50,000 (by the 1960 census data). An adjustment for regional differences in cancer mortality was made by considering the United States in four broad geographic regions, each of which was defined arbitrarily to include low-, moderate- and high-Se areas. Further adjustments were made for ethnicity, the presence of chemical industries, and mean annual sunlight. The analysis was a least-squares regression weighted in inverse proportion to the variance of the site- and sex-specific cancer mortality rate. The results of Clark's analysis indicated that mortality rates were significantly lower in intermediate- and high-Se counties, in comparison to low-Se counties, for cancers in both sexes at all sites combined as well as for cancers of the lung, colon, rectum, bladder, esophagus, and pancreas. Inverse associations of Se exposure were also found for females with cancers of the breast, ovary, and cervix. In contrast, cancers of the liver and stomach, Hodgkin's disease, and leukemia were positively correlated with Se exposure in both sexes.

In consideration of the limitations inherent in ecological correlational studies, it is clear from the studies described above only that the hypothesis that Se status may be related to cancer risk in humans is plausible. The testing of this hypothesis necessitates the use of more sophisticated epidemiologic approaches and the development of a supporting basic understanding of the role(s) of Se in metabolism in carcinogenesis.

Case-Control Studies

Quite a number of case-control studies have been conducted to examine the hypothesis that Se status is related to cancer risk in human populations.* Most of these have been cross-sectional in nature; their value is in challenging the plausibility of the hypothesis and not in testing the hypothesis itself. The results

*The reader is referred to the recent volume by Combs and Combs (1986c) for a compilation of the results of those studies published before 1985.

of these studies would appear to support the hypothesis that low Se status can increase cancer risk; they indicate that cancer patients are generally of lower Se status, as indicated by tissue Se levels, than healthy controls. However, the careful evaluation of these types of results necessitates determining whether the controls were actually drawn from the same population as the cancer cases, and whether the indices of Se status may have been affected by the process of carcinogenesis. For example, because many cancer patients, particularly those with late-stage and debilitating conditions, are likely to have patterns of food intake that are different from those of healthy controls, case-control studies that assess the Se status of prevalent cases may easily yield associations that do not discriminate between effects resulting from carcinogenesis and those causing it. The difficulty in making this distinction for the majority of these published studies limits their usefulness in determining whether Se status can affect cancer risk. Some case-control studies, however, have been designed in such ways as to avoid problems with confounding effects and, hence, are useful tests of the hypothesis that Se status may be related to cancer risk. These are the studies of Clark et al. (1984), Salonen et al. (1984, 1985), Willett et al. (1983), Peleg et al. (1985), Menkes et al. (1986), Schober (1986), and Kok et al. (1987).

Clark et al. (1984) studied the relationship of Se status, as indicated by plasma Se concentration, and the incidence of nonmelanomous skin cancer in a free-living population of eastern North Carolina. The selection of skin cancer offered the advantages of ready confirmation of diagnosis by histological examinations, multiple endpoints, and very low morbidity and mortality rates. The authors also felt that the nature of nonmelanomous skin cancer (i.e., basal cell epitheliomas and squamous cell carcinomas) is not likely to affect the patient's food habits or general metabolism, either of which might affect Se status secondarily. The subjects of the study (192 prevalent cases and 60 current clinic controls) were stratified by decile of plasma Se level; risk to developing skin cancer was compared between deciles. Adjustments were made for the effects of age, gender, degree of cumulative sun damage to the skin, and plasma levels of retinol and total carotenoids. Their logistic estimates of the odds ratios for the lowest (mean plasma Se: 84 ppb) versus the highest (mean plasma Se: 221 ppb) deciles were 3.91 ($p < 0.05$) for patients with basal cell epitheliomas and 3.03 ($p < 0.05$) for all nonmelanomous skin cancers combined. The unadjusted observed odds ratios were similar to these logistic estimates. Stratification of cases and controls on plasma retinol and total carotenoids (i.e., low versus high) indicated that low plasma Se was associated with significant increases in the risk of nonmelanomous skin cancer in patients low in each of these variables.

Salonen et al. (1984) conducted a prospective case-control study to evaluate the relationship of serum Se concentration and total cancer mortality in a random population sample of 8113 residents of two counties in eastern Finland.

The subjects were among a larger population that was examined in 1972; those persons free of cancer at that time were entered into the study in which they were followed for a period of six years. During that period, each cancer mortality that occurred was paired with a control matched for age, gender, tobacco use, and serum cholesterol level on the basis of data obtained at entry to the study. The analysis of 128 such matched pairs revealed that mean serum Se concentration was significantly lower in cancer cases than in controls (50.5 ± 1.1 ppb vs. 54.3 ± 1.0 ppb, $p = 0.012$), with a logistic estimate of the adjusted odds ratio of 3.1 ($p < 0.01$).

Another prospective case-control study by Salonen et al. (1985) showed that 51 terminal cancer cases from the same cohort had a mean serum Se that was 12% lower than controls matched for age, gender, and tobacco use (i.e., 53.7 ppb vs. 60.9 ppb, $p < 0.05$). The adjusted relative risk to cancer-related death was 5.8 for subjects in the low versus high tertiles of serum Se level. A significant interactive effect of Se and vitamin E status was detected: subjects in the low tertiles for both serum Se level and serum α-tocopherol level had an adjusted relative risk of fatal cancer of 11.4 when compared to subjects in the high tertiles with respect to these parameters.

Willett et al. (1983) conducted a retrospective case-control study that was nested in the Hypertension Detection and Follow-Up program (HDFP). That cohort consisted of over 11,000 cancer-free hypertensives followed over a 5-year period. A total of 111 cancer cases that were diagnosed after entry to the study were matched with 210 controls. Sera collected at entry and held frozen were subsequently analyzed for individuals in each group. The results showed a relative risk of 2.0 for cancer in subjects in the lowest versus highest quintiles of serum Se level (i.e., mean serum Se: < 115 ppb vs. > 154 ppb). Some evidence was also found for increased relative risks among low-Se subjects associated with low serum levels of retinol and α-tocopherol; however, firm conclusions were not possible due to the small sizes of some of the multifactor subgroupings.

Peleg et al. (1985) conducted another retrospective case-control study; it, too, used the Evans County HDFP cohort (Cassel, 1971) but had no subjects in common with the study of Willett et al. (1983). In their analysis, no significant differences were detected in serum Se levels between 130 cancer cases and an equal number of controls matched for age, gender, and race (the mean serum Se level for all of which was 116 ppb). In interpreting the discrepant results from those of Willett et al. (1983), Peleg et al. (1985) pointed out that none of the matched controls from the latter study came from the Evans County HDFP center, thus raising the possibility of different environmental confounders between the two studies.

Menkes et al. (1986) conducted a retrospective case-control study of the relationship of Se, vitamins A and E, and β-carotene status to the risk of lung cancer in the Washington County, Maryland, cohort. This cohort consisted of 25,802 subjects followed from 1975–1983, during which time a total of 99 subjects were diagnosed with primary lung cancer, having had no histories of cancer at entry into the study. These cases were compared with 196 controls matched for age, gender, race, month of blood donation, and tobacco use. Menkes et al. (1986) found inverse associations of serum β-carotene and α-tocopherol levels and risk of lung cancer; but no significant differences in serum Se levels between cases and controls (i.e., mean values: 113 ppb vs. 110 ppb). On the basis of histological examinations of 93 cases, they found the risk of squamous cell carcinoma of the lung to be increased among subjects in the high tertile of serum Se and the low tertile of serum α-tocopherol.

Schober (1986) also used a retrospective case-control design to study the relationship of Se and vitamin A and E status to risk of colon cancer in the Washington County cohort. A comparison of 72 cases and 143 matched controls revealed no significant independent or interactive effects of serum levels of Se, retinol, β-carotene, or α-tocopherol on risk of colon cancer.

Recently, Kok et al. (1987) reported the results of a prospective case-control study involving 10,532 residents of the Dutch town of Zoetermeer. This study entailed the collection and archiving of sera from subjects at entry to the study in 1975, and follow-up for a period of eight years. A total of 69 cancer deaths, which occurred at least one year after entry to the study, were compared to 164 controls matched for age, gender, and tobacco use. The results showed that among males the mean serum Se level of cases was significantly less than that of controls (i.e., for $n = 40$: 116.7 ± 4.0 ppb vs. 126.4 ± 3.1 ppb, $p < 0.05$); whereas among females the mean levels of cases and controls were similar (i.e., for $n = 29$: 130.6 ± 6.0 ppb vs. 129.3 ± 4.3, $p = 0.83$). For males in the lowest quintile of serum Se level compared to the other quintiles, the adjusted (by a multiple logistic model) relative risk of cancer death was 2.7 ($p = 0.05$).

The studies discussed above would support the hypothesis that Se status, as indicated by blood Se level, can be related to the risk to at least some kinds of cancer in human populations. Most of the well-designed prospective and retrospective case-control studies to date indicate an association of relatively low Se status with increased cancer risk. That all such studies have not demonstrated such a relationship (e.g., those of Peleg et al. (1985), Menkes et al. (1986), and Schober (1986) may indicate only that the role of low-Se status in the epidemiology of cancer may be that of a risk modifier rather than an effector per se of carcinogenesis. With this in mind, objections, such as those raised by Robinson et al. (1979), that such low-Se areas as New Zealand should be expected to (but do not) have cancer rates that are appreciably different from other parts of the world, can be understood as reflecting a supposition that is not supported by available data, i.e., that Se deficiency causes cancer. Indeed, the effect of a risk modifier would, by definition, be influenced by levels of exposure to the primary carcinogenic agents as well as to other risk modifiers. The results of several studies suggest that such a role of Se may relate to other factors including antioxidant nutrient status (vitamins A, C, and E, and the trace elements zinc, copper, and manganese (Clark et al. (1984), Salonen et al. (1985), Willett et al. (1983)) and, perhaps, gender (Kok et al. (1987). In the opinion of the present author, present information demonstrates the plausibility of, and provides limited support for, the hypothesis that Se status can be related to cancer risk (i.e., Se status may be a risk modifier) in human populations. Nevertheless, the actual testing of this hypothesis requires both a basic understanding of the potential actions of Se in carcinogenesis and, ultimately, the execution of well-designed intervention trials with appropriate forms of the element.

ANIMAL TUMOR MODEL STUDIES OF SELENIUM AND CARCINOGENESIS

The consideration of any hypothetical involvement of Se in experimental tumorigenesis using animal models differs in a fundamental way from the consideration of Se status as a risk factor for cancer in humans. That difference concerns the chemical nature of Se relevant to each case.

In the case of human epidemiologic studies, excluding for the moment Se-intervention trials, the Se of relevance is almost always that measurable in some tissue accessible for biopsy, usually blood or hair. The ultimate origin of this Se is quite obviously environmental; most, if not all, can be safely assumed to be derived from the diet and drinking water. Whereas most Se in drinking water is likely to be in inorganic oxidized forms, water samples are generally low in the element; hence, they are usually much less important as sources of environmental Se than are foods. The total amounts of Se in many foods have been determined,* but the chemical forms of Se in these sources are largely unknown other than that most, if not all, is associated with protein and that much is likely to be in the form of selenoaminoacids (i.e., selenomethionine, selenocysteine) or in selenotrisulfide bridges of polypeptides wherein the element is found in the same oxidation state (i.e., Se^{-2}) in which it occurs in human and animal tissues.

Anticarcinogenic Effects of High Levels of Selenium

In the case of the animal tumor model study, the Se of relevance, i.e., that to which animals are exposed experimentally, is nearly always well defined according to chemical form and route and level of exposure. For reasons of practicality as well as convention, the form of Se used in the great majority of animal tumor

*The reader is referred to Combs and Combs (1986) for an exhaustive documented collation of available analytical data concerning the Se contents of foods and animal feedstuffs.

model studies has been the inorganic oxidized salt, sodium selenite (Na_2SeO_3). This form requires reduction from its Se^{+4} state to the Se^{-2} state in which it is found in animal tissues and, presumably, is active metabolically. At high levels, this form and the more oxidized one, selenate (i.e., Se^{+6}), can be reduced through a mechanism involving thiol attack and resulting in the formation of such intermediates as selenodiglutathione (GSSeSG), glutathione selenopersulfide (GSSeH), and, probably, hydrogen selenide (see review by Combs and Combs (1986a)). Thus, it is probable that the use of high levels of such forms of Se in animal tumor model studies may result in the production, in addition to the Se-dependent factors familiar in normal metabolism (e.g., SeGSHpx and other selenoproteins), of certain Se metabolites that are not produced appreciably by humans with typical Se intakes. Some of these metabolites have been implicated in the anticarcinogenic action of Se. Therefore, the effects of high levels of Se in animal tumor models may involve different metabolic mechanisms than any relating to the putative relationship of low Se status and cancer risk in humans; responses in the former case may have little metabolic relevance to the association apparent in the latter one.

Selenium compounds have been found capable of inhibiting and/or retarding tumorigenesis in a variety of experimental animal models. These studies have been reviewed recently by Combs and Combs (1986b). Table 1 presents in summary the results of these studies, which are cited according to major finding regarding the effects of high levels of Se exposure on tumor production. Of the 77 available studies in which tumor production and/or preneoplastic changes have been monitored (in more than two dozen animal models), 48 have presented results indicative of reduction of tumor incidence and/or numbers of tumors per tumor-bearing animal*. Further, in half of these studies (24 reports), dramatic reduction (i.e., by 50% or more) in tumorigenesis was produced. Only one-fifth of these studies do not indicate Se to affect tumorigenesis; two of these (Shamberger, 1970; Johnston, 1974) employed levels of Se exposure that are within or only slightly above the nutritional range.

The few animal model studies that have measured histological parameters of preneoplastic change (e.g., esophageal dysplasia in the methylbenzylnitrosamine-treated rat, formation of γ-glytamyl transpeptidase [GGT]-positive staining foci in livers or pancreases of carcinogen-treated rats) rather than or in addition to frank tumor expression have yielded less consistent results concerning high level exposure. Half of the available studies indicate that Se may retard or inhibit early stages of tumorigenesis (Le Boeuf et al., 1985; Milks et al., 1985; Baldwin and Parker, 1986), whereas half have failed to detect significant effects of Se

*Reductions of at least 20% from responses of controls judged by the present author as likely to be nutritionally adequate in Se.

Table 1 Summary of Animal Tumor Model Studies of Effects of High Levels[a] of Se Compounds on Tumorigenesis

	Model		References, by major finding re Se		
Tumor site	Species	Agent	No effect	Antitumorigenic[b]	Tumorigenic
Colon	rat	1,2-dimethylhydrazine	Jacobs et al., 1981;[c] Jacobs, 1983[c]	Jacobs et al., 1977[c]	Jacobs, 1977[c]
		methylazoxymethanol		Jacobs et al., 1977[c]	Jacobs, 1977[c]
		bix-(2-oxypropyl)nitrosamine		Birt et al., 1982[c]	
Esophagus	rat	methylbenzylnitrosamine		Boyden et al., 1986[c]	
Intestine	rat	azoxymethane		Souillier et al., 1981[c]	Nigro et al., 1983[c]
		1,2-dimethylhydrazine		Daoud and Griffin, 1980[c,o]	Daoud and Griffin, 1980[c]
		N-methyl-N-nitro-N-nitro-soguanidine		Kobayashi, 1986[c]	
Kidney	rat	diethylnitrosamine			Dorado et al., 1985[c]
Liver	rat	2-acetylaminofluorene	Johnston, 1974;[c] Harr et al., 1972;[c] Daoud and Griffin, 1980[c]	Harr et al., 1972[c]	Marshall et al., 1979[c]
		azoxymethane	Daoud and Griffin, 1980[c]	Tanaka et al., 1985[d]	
		diethylnitrosamine		Dorado et al., 1985[c]	
		3-methyl-4-dimethylaminobenzene		Clayton and Bauman, 1949;[c] Griffin and Jacobs, 1977[e]	
Lung	rat	bis-(2-oxypropyl)nitrosamine		Birt et al., 1982[c]	

Mammary	mouse	7,12-dimethylbenz(a)anthracene		Shamberger, 1970;[c] Medina and Shepard, 1981, 1984;[c] Welsch et al., 1981;[c] Medina and Lane, 1983;[c] Lane and Medina, 1985;[c] Lane et al., 1987[c]	
		virus		Schrauzer et al., 1976, 1980a,b;[c] Medina and Shepard, 1980;[c] Thompson and Becci, 1985[c]	
		transplants	Medina and Shepard, 1980[c]	Ip et al., 1981;[c] Watrach et al., 1982[c,h]	
	rat	2-acetylaminofluorene	Harr et al., 1972[c]	Harr et al., 1973[c]	
		7,12-dimethylbenz(a)anthracene	Thompson et al., 1981;[c] Ip and Daniel, 1985[c]	Thompson and Tagliaferro, 1980;[c] Ip, 1981;[c] Ip and Ip, 1981;[c] Ip and Sinha, 1981;[c] Thompson et al., 1982;[c] Horvath and Ip, 1983;[c] Ip, 1985[c]	
		N-methyl-N-nitrosourea	Thompson et al., 1984[c,f]	Thompson et al., 1981a[c]	
		virus			Ankerst and Sjoegren, 1982[c]

Table 1 (continued)

	Model		References, by major finding re Se		
Tumor site	Species	Agent	No effect	Antitumorigenic[b]	Tumorigenic
Pancreas	hamster	bis(2-oxopropyl)nitrosamine	Birt et al., 1986[g]	Birt et al., 1986[c,i]	
Skin	mouse	benzo(a)pyrene		Wilt et al., 1979[c]	
		7,12-dimethylbenz(a)anthracene	Perchellet et al., 1987[c,h]	Shamberger, 1970[j,k]	Perchellet et al., 1987[c,h,l]
Stomach	mouse	benzo(a)pyrene	El-Bayoumy, 1985[n]	El-Bayoumy, 1985[d,m]	
Tongue	hamster	9,10-dimethyl-1-2-benzanthracene		Goodwin et al., 1985[c], 1986[j]	
Trachea	hamster	N-methyl-N-nitrosourea	Thompson and Becci, 1979[c]		
Ehrlich ascites	mouse	transplants	Poiriev and Milner, 1983[c,h]	Poirier and Milner, 1979;[c,h] Greeder and Milner, 1980; Milner, 1984[c,h]	

[a]i.e., >0.5 ppm Se (diet level equivalent), oral exposure unless otherwise indicated; in all cases except (Shamberger, 1970, Johnston, 1974, and Shrauzer et al., 1980) levels used were >1 ppm.
[b]i.e., apparent reduction by at least 20% in tumor incidence or number of tumors per tumor-bearing animal.
[c]Se provided as Na_2SeO_3.
[d]Se provided as p-methoxybenzeneselenol.
[e]Se provided as a Se-enriched yeast.
[f]Se provided as DL-selenomethionine.
[g]Males only.
[h]Se administered by injection.
[i]Females only.
[j]Se provided as Na_2Se.
[k]Se administered topically.
[l]Low carcinogen dose.
[m]Se provided as benzylselnocyanate.
[n]Se provided as phenoselenazine.
[o]Large intestine only.
[p]Small intestine only.

(Le Boeuf et al., 1985; O'Connor, 1985; Bogden et al., 1986) in various animal tumor models. It should be noted that none have shown high levels of Se to enhance the process.

Four animal tumor model studies have shown high levels of the element to enhance tumorigenesis. Dorado et al. (1985) found that dietary exposure of either 4 or 6 ppm Se (as Na_2SeO_3) to rats treated with diethylnitrosamine after partial hepatectomy and later promoted with phenobarbital produced modest reductions in the incidence of hepatic tumors, but nearly doubled the incidence of renal tumors. Perchellet et al. (1987) found that when Se (i.e., 40 μg Na_2SeO_3) was administered with α-tocopherol (40 μmols) intraperitoneally to mice treated topically with 7,12-dimethylbenz[a]anthracene (DMBA), the Se + vitamin E treatment did not affect skin tumor outcome resulting from a single high dose of the carcinogen; however, the same treatment nearly doubled the incidence of papillomas among mice given smaller multiple doses of DMBA. Ankerst and Sjoegren (1982) found Se treatment of rats to increase the incidence of 1,2-dimethylhydrazine-induced tumors of the small intestine, while decreasing the incidence of tumors of the large intestine. Those authors also found Se treatment to increase the incidence of virally induced mammary tumors in the rat.

With the exceptions of the four cases cited above, the preponderance of available information from controlled animal tumor model studies involving the induction of tumors by chemical or viral agents and by transplantation indicates that high level exposure to at least some Se compounds can be antitumorigenic. It should be noted that almost all of these studies have involved Na_2SeO_3 as the source of Se; the extent to which these effects can be extended to other sources of the element is open to question. Combs and Combs (1986b) noted that while reduction in tumorigenesis by Se in animal tumor model systems has, in most cases, been demonstrated at apparently subtoxic (i.e., not growth-depressing) levels of exposure to the element, the effectiveness of Se appears to occur only at high supranutritional levels, i.e., greater than ca. 1 ppm in the diet or ca. 0.7 ppm in drinking water.* Because these near-toxic levels of Se exposure are considerably higher than those experienced by almost all free-living people, it is appropriate to consider the specific effects of Se exposures more closely approximating those of human populations, i.e., nutritional levels of the element.

Effects of Selenium Deficiency on Carcinogenesis

Relatively few studies have been conducted in such a manner as to test the hypothesis that nutritionally limiting levels of Se can effect tumorigenesis. Table 2

---

*The dietary requirements of most species for Se are estimated to be in the range of 0.1–0.2 ppm; those of humans are probably 50–60 μg/day.

summarizes the published studies that have addressed this hypothesis using animal tumor models. It shows that, of the two dozen studies that have employed low-Se (i.e., < 0.05 ppm) semipurified diets in some 13 animal tumor models, comparisons of the tumor responses of animals fed the unsupplemented diet to those of animals treated with supplemental Se (in every case this has been Na_2SeO_3) have yielded much less consistent results than those involving high levels of Se. Ten of these studies indicate that nutritional Se deficiency can enhance tumorigenicity; seven of these have involved models of mammary carcinogenesis. In contrast, five studies have found Se deficiency to reduce tumorigenesis, although this effect has not been observed in mammary tumor models. Nine studies have failed to demonstrate any effects of Se deficiency.

In addition to the tumor model studies referenced above, four others have tested the effect of nutritional Se deficiency on the appearance of preneoplastic histological signs, i.e., the formation of GGT-positive foci in the livers (Milks et al., 1985; Baldwin and Parker, 1986, 1987) or pancreases (O'Connor, 1985) of aflatoxin B_1-treated rats. Three of these (Milks et al., 1985; O'Connor, 1985; Baldwin and Parker, 1987) show no effects of low-Se status on this indicator of tumorigenesis, whereas the report of Baldwin and Parker (1986) indicates that Se deficiency enhanced this indicator in animals fed diets very high in unsaturated fat (i.e., 20% corn oil).

The present evidence concerning the effects of nutritionally deficient levels of Se are compatible with the hypothesis generated in human epidemiological studied, i.e., that low-Se status can increase cancer risk. However, in the opinion of this author, the results of animal tumor model studies to date, in and of themselves, do not compel such a conclusion.

Hypotheses for the Mechanisms of Anticarcinogenic Actions of Selenium

Several mechanisms may be proposed as hypotheses for the inhibition of tumorigenesis by high levels of Se. Some that have been presented are the alteration in carcinogen metabolism by Se, the protection against oxidative damage by Se, and the cytotoxicity of intermediates formed under high-Se conditions.

Several studies have examined the effect of Se on various aspects of carcinogen metabolism (see review by Combs and Combs (1986b)). Some indicate that under some circumstances the constitutive activities of cytochrome P_{450} and at least certain hepatic mixed-function oxygenases (e.g., aryl hydrocarbon hydroxylase) may be enhanced by Se (Capel et al., 1980; Chow and Gairola, 1984); however, there is little evidence to suggest that induced activities are affected (Gairola and Chow, 1982; Chow and Gairola, 1984; Thompson, 1984). Studies of carcinogen metabolism per se have yielded varying results concerning the effects of Se. For example, comparable dietary levels of Se (2 ppm as Na_2SeO_3)

Table 2 Summary of Animal Tumor Model Studies of Effects of Nutritionally Limiting Levels[a] of Se on Tumorigenesis

	Model		References, by major finding re Se deficiency		
Tumor site	Species	Agent	No effect	Antitumorigenic	Tumorigenic
Colon	rat	azoxymethane	Reddy and Tanaka, 1986[d,e]	Ready and Tanaka, 1986[d,f]	
		1,2-dimethylhydrazine	Pence and Buddingh, 1985[d]		
Intestine	rat	azoxymethane			Reddy and Tanaka, 1986[d,e,f]
Liver	rat	2-acetylaminofluorene	Harr et al., 1973[d]	Harr et al., 1972[d]	
Mammary	mouse	7,12-dimethybenz(a)anthracene	Shamberger, 1970[d]		Shamberger, 1970[d]
		virus	Schrauzer et al., 1976[d]		
	rat	2-acetylaminofluorene	Harr et al., 1972[d]		
		7,12-dimethylbenz(a)anthracene	Thompson et al., 1981[b], 1982[d]		Ip, 1981;[d] Ip and Sinha, 1981b;[d] Thompson et al., 1986, 1982;[d] Ip and Daniel, 1985[d]

		N-methyl-N-nitrosourea			Thompson and Becci, 1985[d]
		transplants	Ip et al., 1981[d]		
Pancreas	hamster	bis (2-oxopropyl)nitrosamine		Birt et al., 1986[d,h]	Birt et al., 1986[d,g]
Skin	mouse	benzo(a)pyrene		Shamberger, 1970[d]	Wilt et al., 1979[d]
		7,12-dimethylbenz(a)anthracene		Shamberger, 1970[d]	

[a] i.e., exposure <0.1 ppm, dietary basis.
[b] Apparant effect of Se treatment within 20% of control rates of incidence of tumors or numbers of tumors per tumor-bearing animal.
[c] Apparent effect of Se treatment >20% of control.
[d] Se provided as Na_2SeO_3.
[e] High-lard diet.
[f] High-corn oil diet.
[g] Females only.
[h] Males only.

reduced the formation of covalent adducts of aflatoxin B_1 metabolites and DNA in the chick (Chen et al., 1982) but increased the process in the rat (Chen et al., 1982a). Treatment with Se has been shown to shift the metabolism of 2-acetylaminofluorene (2-AAF) away from N-hydroxylation towards ring-hydroxylation, thus reducing its activation to the carcinogenic form. Studies using Ames-type Salmonella tester systems have shown Se supplementation of rats from which hepatic microsomal preparations are made to reduce the production of mutagenic metabolites of several carcinogens: N,N-dimethylanaline (Olsson et al., 1984), DMBA (Tsen and Tappel, 1958; Jacobs et al., 1977; Schiallaci et al., 1982; Grunau and Milner, 1983; Martin and Schillaci, 1984), 2-AAF (Gairola and Chow, 1982; Chow and Gairola, 1984) and benzo(a)pyrene (Teel and Kain, 1984). These reports indicate that, while high level Se supplementation can affect carcinogen metabolism, this effect is not universal with respect to either carcinogen or host species.

In view of the findings that Se can be inhibitory to both chemically induced and viral-induced tumors, that its inhibition appears to involve postinitiation events as well as those associated with the initiation phase, and that the effects of Se appear to be reversible, Medina (1986) suggested that the antitumorigenic effects of Se result from cellular responses based upon endocrine and/or immune systems. While there is no evidence for involvement of Se in hormone production or action, there is some basis for considering Se as an affector of immune function (see review by Combs and Combs (1986d). This includes findings of impaired humoral immune responses in Se-deficient animals; but, because such responses are dependent upon the function of T-cells and macrophages in addition to B-cells, it is possible that they indicate secondary effects on the cells of the first and/or second types, which have also been documented. While it is possible that at least some of the effects of Se on tumorigenesis may be mediated by immune systems, the scant information presently available concerning the action of Se in such systems does not permit a critical evaluation of this hypothesis.

Griffin (1979) suggested that Se may have anticarcinogenic activity through its role as an essential component of SeGSHpx, which is important in the metabolic protection from oxidant stress. Support for this hypothesis comes from the finding by Shamberger et al. (1979) of the mutagenicity and carcinogenicity of malonyldialdehyde, a product of the peroxidative degradation of linoleic acid, which is presumed to be formed in conditions of Se (hence, SeGSHpx) deficiency. Also, the similar protection afforded by Se or the antioxidant factors vitamin E and superoxide dismutase against the mitogenic effects of several tumor promoters (Romano et al., 1986) is consistent with a SeGSHpx-mediated response. However, whereas correction of cellular SeGSHpx deficiencies would account for the action of Se supplements to deficient animals, it should be noted that most studies that have examined tumor responses to Se in this range have not produced positive results. A SeGSHpx response is not relevant to the case of the responses to supplemental Se by animals fed Se-adequate diets; such animals show plateaued tissue activities of the selenoenzyme at levels of Se intake above ca. 0.2 ppm (dietary basis). Further, the findings that antitumorigenic amounts of Se reduced tissue lipid peroxidation potential only slightly (Lane and Medina, 1985) or not at all (Horvath and Ip, 1983) suggest that the antitumorigenic effect of Se is independent of the known nutritional function of the element via SeGSHpx in cellular antioxidant systems.

It is likely that the antitumorigenic effect of Se, at least at high exposure levels, involves the perturbation of normal metabolism and/or production of cytotoxic metabolites due to the presence of large amounts of Se-compounds. Le Boeuf and Hoekstra (1983, 1985) proposed that high levels of Se, achieved by giving selenite in the majority of the animal tumor model studies, may perturb intracellular levels of reduced (GSH) and oxidized (GSSG) glutathione by the catalytic oxidation of GSH by selenite. They showed that chronic feeding of a high-Se diet (6 ppm as Na_2SeO_3) to rats resulted in increased hepatic concentrations of both GSH and GSSG with an decrease in the GSH:GSSG ratio (Le Boeuf and Hoekstra, 1983). The same high-Se treatment produced increases in the hepatic activities of glutathione reductase and glucose-6-phosphate dehydrogenase which the authors interpreted as adaptive responses to selenite-induced GSH oxidation. The authors observed similar biochemical changes in cultured hepatoma cells treated with high levels of selenite and found the Se-treatment to retard the doubling time of the cultured cells. In consideration of these results, Le Boeuf and Hoekstra (1985) suggested that the Se-induced increase in GSSG affected the process of protein synthesis. They pointed out that GSSG is known to activate a protein kinase which inactivates, through phosphorylation, eukaryotic initiation factor 2 (Jacobs et al., 1977b; Ernst et al., 1978), which Safer et al. (1980) found to be inactivated by selenite.

Several studies have shown high levels of Se to inhibit cell proliferation in ways apparently related to effects on protein synthesis (Vernie et al., 1974, 1975, 1980, 1981; Gruenwedel and Cruikshank, 1979; Le Boeuf and Hoekstra, 1983, 1985; Vernie, 1987). The studies of Vernie et al. (Vernie et al., 1974, 1975, 1980, 1981; Vernie, 1987) and Poirier and Milner (1983) suggest that such effects may be mediated by an intermediate similar to GSSG, i.e., the metabolic product of the reduction of selenite by GSH, GSSeSG. Vernie et al. (1974) found that GSSeSG very effective in specifically inhibiting eukaryotic elongation factor 2. The same group found that this inhibition corresponds to inhibition by GSSeSG of tumor growth in mice implanted with malignant lymphoblasts (Vernie et al., 1981), and Poirier and Milner (1983) found GSSeSG to be more effective in inhibiting the growth of Ehrlich ascites tumors in mice than either sodium selenite, sodium selenide, dimethyl selenide, selenocystine, or selenomethionine. These results suggest that, under conditions of excessive selenite exposure, abnormally high levels of the reductive metabolite, GSSeSG, are produced which inhibit protein synthesis, presumably preferentially affecting the proliferative response, thus mediating the antitumorigenic effect associated with high-level selenite treatment in animal tumor models. However, this hypothesis is subject to the concern that GSSeSG is unstable; at physiological GSSG:GSH ratios, i.e., less than 1:4 (which, even with high selenite treatment, are not achieved (Le Boeur and Hoekstra, 1985), it breaks down to GSSeH and H_2Se. Thus, Le Boeuf and Hoekstra (1985) concluded that it is unlikely that intracellular concentrations of GSSeSG are ever great enough to affect protein synthesis.

The anticarcinogenicity of high levels of Se may also involve the formation of other more stable selenotrisulfides, such as those of proteins, which impair tumor cell metabolism. Evidence for such an effect comes from the studies of Ganther and Corcoran (1969) who showed Se to inhibit bovine pancreatic ribonuclease by forming an intramolecular selenotrisulfide bridge in the place of the normal disulfide one. A similar effect was shown by Donaldson (1977), i.e., selenotrisulfide formation involving the sulfhydryl groups of chick hepatic fatty acid synthase and resulting in the inhibition of the enzymatic activity of the enzyme. These results, as well as findings of inhibition by selenite of Na,-K-ATPase (Bunce et al., 1984; Bergad and Rathburn, 1986), suggest that the antitumorigenic effects of high levels of selenite may involve the inhibition of important sulfhydryl-sensitive enzymes.

In summary, it is possible that the antitumorigenic action of Se may be mediated through one of more of several mechanisms which have been shown experimentally to be plausible. At the present time, however, it is not clear which, if any, of these possibilities relate to the antitumorigenic effect that have been demonstrated in animal tumor models. Further, the extent to which any of these possibilities may be generalized to include forms of Se other than Na_2SeO_3 is also not clear. What is apparent, however, is that high levels of at least some forms of Se can impair metabolism in several fundamental ways, each of which would be expected to have greatest effects on proliferating cells.

CONSIDERING SELENIUM COMPOUNDS AS POTENTIAL CANCER PREVENTIVE OR CHEMOTHERAPUETIC AGENTS

Despite early claims of the value of Se in cancer chemotherapy (Walker and Klein, 1915), most animal tumor model studies have evaluated Se as a cancer-preventative agent. Those that have tested the chemotherapeutic efficacy of

Se have yielded mixed results. Several studies with transplanted tumors have shown high levels of Se to retard tumor growth (Greeder and Milner, 1980; Ip, 1981; Milner and Hsu, 1982; Watrach et al., 1982), while others have failed to demonstrate significant effects of Se (Schrauzer et al., 1980b; Medina and Lane, 1983). Therefore, while the potential for Se to be useful in cancer chemotherapy would appear clear, many questions remain concerning the types of tumors that may be affected, the compounds of Se that may be effective, and the dose regimens that may be appropriate.

As discussed in the previous sections, the case for considering Se compounds as possible cancer-preventative agents is much stronger by virtue of the results of quite a number of studies both with animal tumor models and of basic metabolism. Nevertheless, evidence has yet to be presented concerning the effects of Se supplementation on cancer incidence in human populations; such information must await the completion of double blind Se-intervention clinical trials with free-living of humans, several of which are currently underway. Clark and Combs (1986) presented some of the major issues relating to the design of such intervention trials: the selection of appropriate dose levels and chemical forms of Se, and the period of time appropriate for follow up. Each of these issues involves questions of Se toxicity which cannot be resolved readily on the basis of present information (information concerning the toxicity of Se for humans is particularly scant). Therefore, those authors suggested the use in intervention trials of food forms of Se (e.g., selenoaminoacids, high-Se wheat, Se-enriched yeasts) roughly comparable to those within the normal dietary experiences of human populations, and at levels similar to the Se intakes of healthy populations residing in regions of the world naturally high in the element (e.g., parts of Venezuela, Colombia, and the People's Republic of China).

Determining whether Se has a role in human carcinogenesis will necessitate, in addition to the conduct of intervention trials, the prosecution of more extensive studies of the metabolism and toxicology of various chemical forms of the element. Several practical questions must be answered: how to interpret differences in serum/plasma Se levels (raised recently by Burk (1986)? which of the available parameters is most appropriate for assessing Se status (which may vary according to Se source)? which responses are characteristic of the element per se and which are characteristic of particular Se compounds? what clinical and biochemical signs can be used to detect Se toxicity? In general, the information to date is encouraging that at least some compounds of Se may be found to be useful in reducing cancer risk; however, the dose levels at which these compounds appear to be effective are uncomfortably close to the apparent toxic range of the element. Therefore, the questions raised above must be addressed in order to determine whether Se may be useful in cancer prevention or therapy.

REFERENCES

Allaway, W. H., Kubota, J., Losee, F., Roth, M. (1968). Selenium, molybdenum and vanadium in human blood. *Arch. Environ. Health 16*:342.

Ankerst, J., Sjoegren, H. O. (1982). Effect of selenium on the induction of breast fibroadenomas by adenovirus type 9 and 1,2-dimethylhydrazine-induced bowel carcinogenesis in rats. *Int. J. Cancer 29*:707.

Baldwin, S., Parker, R. S. (1987). The effects of dietary fat and selenium on the development of preneoplastic lesions in rat liver. *Nutr. Cancer 8*:273.

Baldwin, S., Parker, R. S. (1986). Influence of dietary fat and selenium in initiation and promotion of aflatoxin B_1-induced preneoplastic foci in rat liver. *Carcinogen 8*:101.

Bergad, P. L., Rathbun, W. B. (1986). Inhibition of Na,K-ATPase by sodium selenite and reversal by glutathione. *Curr. Eye Res. 5*:919.

Besbris, H. J., Wortzman, M. S., Cohen, A. M. (1982). Effect of dietary selenium on the metabolism and excretion of 2-acetylaminofluorene in the rat. *J. Toxicol. Environ. Health 9*:63.

Birt, D. F., Julius, A. D., Runice, C. E., Salmasi, S. (1986). Effects of dietary selenium on bis(2-oxopropyl)nitrosamine-induced carcinogenesis in Syrian Golden Hamsters. *J. Nat. Cancer Inst. 6*:1281.

Birt, D. F., Lawson, T. A., Julius, A. D., Runice, C. E., Salmasi, S. (1982). Inhibition by dietary selenium of colon cancer induced in the rat by bis(2-oxypropyl)nitrosamine. *Cancer Res. 42*:4455.

Bogden, J. D., Chung, H. B., Kemp, F. W., Holding, K., Bruening, K. S., Naveh, Y. (1986). Effect of selenium and molybdenum on methylbenzylnitrosamine-induced esophageal lesions and tissue trace metals in the rat. *J. Nutr. 116*: 2432.

Broghamer, W. L., Jr., McConnell, K. P., Grimaldi, M., Blotcky, A. J. (1978). Serum selenium and reticuloendothelial tumors. *Cancer 41*:1462.

Broghamer, W. L., Jr., McConnell, K. P., Blotcky, A. J. (1976). Relationship between serum selenium levels and patients with carcinoma. *Cancer 37*:1384.

Bunce, G. E., Hess, J. L., Batra, L. (1984). Lens calcium and selenite-induced cataract. *Curr. Eye Res. 3*:315.

Burguera, J. A., Edds, G. T., Osuna, O. (1983). Influence of selenium on aflatoxin B_1 or crotalaria toxicity in turkey poults. *Am. J. Vet. Res. 44*:1714.

Burk, R. F. (1986). Selenium and cancer: Meaning of serum selenium levels. *J. Nutr. 116*:1584.

Calautti, P., Moschini, G., Stievano, B. M., Tomio, L., Clazavara, F., Perona, G. (1980). Serum selenium levels in malignant lymphoproliferative diseases. *Scand. J. Haematol. 24*:63.

Capel, I. D., Jenner, M., Darrell, H. M., Williams, D. C. (1980). The influence of selenium on some hepatic carcinogen metabolizing enzymes of rats. *IRCS Med. Sci. Libr. Compend. 8*:382.

Cassel, J. C. (1971). The Evans County Cardiovascular and Cerebrovascular Epidemiological Study. *Ach. Intern. Med. 128*:883.

Chen, J., Goetchius, M. P., Cambell, C., Combs, G. F., Jr. (1982a). Effects of dietary selenium and vitamin E on hepatic mixed-function oxidase activities and in vivo covalent binding of aflatoxin B_1 in rats. *J. Nutr. 112*:324.

Chen, J., Goetchius, M. P., Combs, G. F., Jr., Cambell, C. T. (1982b). Effects of dietary selenium and vitamin E on covalent binding of aflatoxin to chick liver cell macromolecules. *J. Nutr. 112*:350.

Chow, C. K., Gairola, G. C. (1984). Influence of dietary vitamin E and selenium on metabolic activation of chemicals to mutagens. *J. Agric. Food Chem. 32*: 443.

Chu, Y. J., Liu, Q. Y., Hou, Co., Yu, S. Y. (1984). Blood selenium concentration in residents of areas in China having a high incidence of lung cancer. *Biol. Trace Elem. Res. 6*:133.

Clark, L. C. (1985). The epidemiology of selenium and cancer. *Federation Proc. 44*:2584.

Clark, L. C., Combs, G. F., Jr. (1986). Selenium compounds and the prevention of cancer: Research needs and public health implications. *J. Nutr. 116*:170.

Clark, L. C., Graham, G. F., Crounse, R. G., Grimson, R., Hulka, B., Shy, C. M. (1984). Plasma selenium and skin neoplasma: A case-control study. *Nutr. Cancer 6*:13.

Clayton, C. C., Bauman, C. A. (1949). Diet and azo dye tumors: effect of diet during a period when the dye is not fed. *Cancer Res. 9*:575.

Combs, G. F., Jr., Combs, S. B. (1986a). Absorption, excretion, and metabolism of selenium. In *The Role of Selenium in Nutrition*. Academic Press, New York, p. 179.

Combs, G. F., Jr., Combs, S. B. (1986b). Selenium and cancer. In *The Role of Selenium in Nutrition*. Academic Press, New York, p. 413.

Combs, G. F., Jr., Combs, S. B. (1986c). Selenium in foods and feeds. In *The Role of Selenium in Nutrition*. Academic Press, New York, p. 41.

Combs, G. F., Jr., Combs, S. B. (1986d). Selenium in immunity and infection. In *The Role of Selenium in Nutrition*. Academic Press, New York, p. 401.

Cowgill, V. M. (1983). The distribution of selenium and cancer mortality in the continental U.S. *Biol. Trace Elem. Res. 5*:345.

Daoud, A. H., Griffin, A. C. (1980). Effect of retinoic acid, butylated hydroxytoluene, selenium and sorbic acid on azo-dye hepatocarcinogenesis. *Cancer Lett. 9*:299.

Das, N. P., Ma, C. W., Salmon, Y. M. (1986). Serum selenium concentrations in ovarian cancer patients using a simplified fluorimetric procedure. *Biol. Trace Elem. Res. 10*:215.

Donaldson, W. E. (1977). Selenium inhibition of avian fatty acid synthase complex. *Chem.-Biol. Interact. 17*:313.

Dorado, R. D., Porta, E. A., Aquino, T. M. (1985). Effects of dietary selenium on hepatic and renal tumorigenesis induced in rats by diethylnitrosamine. *Hepatol. 5*:1201.

El-Bayoumy, K. (1985). Effects of organoselenium compounds on induction of mouse forestomach tumors by benzo(a)pyrene. *Cancer Res. 45*:3631.

El-Yazigi, A., Al-Saleh, I., Al-Mefty, O. Concentration of Ag, Al, Au, Bi, Cd, Cu, Pb, Sb and Se in cerebrospinal fluid of patients with cerebral neoplasms. *Clin. Chem. 30*:1358.

Ernst, V., Levin, D. H., London, I. M. (1978). Inhibition of protein synthesis initiation by oxidized glutathione: Activation of a protein kinase that phosphorylates the subunit of eukaryotic initiation factor 2. *Proc. Nat. Acad. Sci. USA 75*:4110.

Gairola, C., Chow, C. K. (1982). Dietary selenium, hepatic arylhydrocarbon hydroxylase and mutagenic activation of benzo(a)pyrene, 2-aminoanthracene and 2-aminofluorene. *Toxicol. Lett. 11*:281.

Ganther, H. E., Corcoran, C. (1969). Selenotrisulfides. II. Cross-linking of reduced pancreatic ribonuclease with selenium. *Biochem. 8*:2557.

Gerhardsson, L., Brune, D., Nordberg, I. G. F., Wester, P. O. (1986). Selenium and other trace elements in lung tissue in smelter workers. Relationship to the occurrence of lung cancer. *Acta Physiol. Toxicol. 59*(suppl. 7):256.

Gerhardsson, L., Brune, D., Nordberg, I. G. F., Wester, P. O. (1985). Protective effect of selenium on lung cancer in smelter workers. *Brit. J. Indust. Med. 42*: 617.

Goodwin, W. J., Jr., Huijing, F., Bordash, G. D., Altman, N. (1986). Inhibition of hamster tongue carcinogenesis by selenium and retinoic acid. *Ann. Otol. Rhinol. Larynol. 95*:162.

Goodwin, W. J., Bordash, G. D., Xue, J. W., Huijing, F., Altman, N. (1985). Selenium inhibition of chemical carcinogenesis in the upper aerodigestive tract of hamsters. *Otolryngol. Head Neck Surg. 93*:373.

Goodwin, W. J., Lane, H. W., Bradford, K., Marshall, M. V., Griffin, A. C., Geopfert, H., Jesse, R. H. (1983). Selenium and glutathione peroxidase levels in patients with epidermoid carcinoma in the oral cavity and oropharynx. *Cancer 51*:110.

Greeder, G. A., Milner, J. A. (1980). Factors influencing the inhibitory effect of selenium on mice inoculated with Ehrlich ascites tumor cells. *Science 209*: 825.

Griffin, A. C. (1979). Role of selenium in the chemoprevention of cancer. *Adv. Cancer Res. 29*:419.

Griffin, A. C., Jacobs, M. M. (1977). Effects of selenium on azo dye hepatocarcinogenesis. *Cancer Lett. 4*:177.

Gruenwedel, D. W., Cruikshank, M. K. (1979). The influence of sodium selenite on the viability and intracellular synthetic activity (DNA, RNA and protein synthesis) of HeLa S3 cells. *Tox. Appl. Pharmacol. 50*:1.

Grunau, J. A., Milner, J. A. (1983). Selenium modification of 7,12-dimethylbenz(a)anthracene metabolism. *Federation Proc. 42*:928 (abstract).

Harr, J. R., Exon, J. H., Weswig, P. H., Whanger, P. D. (1973). Relationship of dietary selenium concentration, chemical cancer induction and tissue concentration of selenium in rats. *Clin. Toxicol. 6*:487.

Harr, J. R., Exon, J. H., Whanger, P. D., Weswig, P. H. (1972). Effect of dietary selenium on N-2-fluorenyl acetamide(FFA)-induced cancer in vitamin E-supplemented, selenium-depleted rats. *Clin. Toxicol. 5*:187.

Harr, J. R., Bone, J. T., Tinsley, I. J., Weswig, P. H., Yamamoto, R. S. (1967). Selenium in rats. II. Histopathology. In *Selenium in Biomedicine*, Muth, O. H. (ed.). AVI Westport, Conn., p. 153.

Horvath, P. M., Ip, C. (1983). Synergistic effect of vitamin E and selenium in the chemoprevention of mammary carcinogenesis in rats. *Cancer Res. 43*:5335.

Hughes, D. A., Bjeldanes, L. F. (1983). Influence of selenium-supplemented torula yeast diets on liver-mediated mutagenicity of aflatoxin B_1. J. Food Sci. 48:759.

Ip, C. (1985). Attenuation of the anticarcinogenic selenium by vitamin E deficiency. *Cancer Lett. 2*:

Ip, C. (1981a). Factors influencing the anticarcinogenic efficacy of selenium in dimethylbenz(a)anthracene-induced mammary tumorigenesis in rats. *Cancer Res. 41*:2683.

Ip, C. (1981b). Modification of mammary carcinogenesis and tissue peroxidation by selenium deficiency and dietary fat. *Nutr. Cancer 2*:136.

Ip, C. (1981c). Prophylaxis of mammary neoplasia by selenium supplementation in the initiation and promotion phases of chemical carcinogenesis. *Cancer Res. 41*:4386.

Ip, C., Daniel, F. B. (1985). Effects of selenium of 7,12-dimethylbenz[a] anthracene-induced mammary carcinogenesis and DNA adduct formation. *Cancer Res. 45*:62.

Ip, C., Ip, M. M. (1981). Chemoprevention of mammary tumorigenesis by a combined regimen of selenium and vitamin A. *Carcinogenesis 2*:915.

Ip, C., Sinha, D. (1981a). Anticarcinogenic effect of selenium in rats treated with dimethylbenz(a)anthracene and fed different levels and types of fat. *Carcinogenesis 2*:435.

Ip, C., Sinha, D. K. (1981b). Enhancement of mammary tumorigenesis by dietary selenium deficiency in rats fed a high polyunsaturated fat intake. *Cancer Res. 41*:31.

Ip, C., Ip, M. M., Kim, U. (1981). Dietary selenium intake and growth of the MT-W9B transplantable rat mammary tumor. *Cancer Lett. 14*:101.

Jacobs, M. (1977). Inhibitory effects of selenium on 1,2-dimethylhydrazine and methylazoxymethanol colon carcinogenesis. Correlative studies on selenium effects on the mutagenicity and sister chromatid exchange rates of selected carcinogens. *Cancer 40*:2557.

Jacobs, M. M. (1983). Selenium inhibition of 1,2-dimethylhydrazine-induced colon carcinogenesis. *Cancer Res. 43*:1646.

Jacobs, M. M., Forst, C. F., Beams, F. A. (1981). Biochemical and clinical effects of selenium on dimethylhydrazine-induced colon cancer in rats. *Cancer Res. 41*:4458.

Jacobs, M. M., Jansson, B., Griffin, A. C. (1977a). Inhibitory effects of selenium on 1,2-dimethylhydrazine and methylazoxymethanol acetate induction of colon tumors. *Cancer Lett. 2*:133.

Jacobs, M. M., Matney, J. S., Griffin, A. C. (1977b). Inhibitory effects of selenium on the mutagenicity of 2-acetylaminofluorene (AAF) and AAF derivatives. *Cancer Lett. 2*:319.

Jansson, B., Jacobs, M. M., Griffen, A. C. (1978). Gastrointestinal cancer: Epidemiologic and experimental studies. *Adv. Exp. Med. Biol. 91*:305.

Johnston, W. K. (1974). *Effect of selenium on chemical carcinogenicity in the rat.* M. S. thesis, Oregon State Univ., Corvallis, Oregon, 88 pp.

Kallistratos, G., Evangelou, A., Seferiadis, K., Vezyraki, P., Barboutis, K. (1985). Selenium and haemodialysis: Serum selenium levels in healthy persons, non-cancer and cancer patients with chronic renal failure. *Nephron 41*:217.

Kauppila, A., Sundstrom, H., Korpela, H., Viinikka, L., Yrjanheikki, E. (1984). Serum selenium and gynecological cancer: effect of selenium supplementation on plasma malondialdehyde and serum glutathione peroxidase. In *Icosanoids and Cancer*, Thaler-Dao, H. (ed.). Raven Press, New York, p. 263.

Kobayashi, M., Kogata, M., Yamamura, M., Takada, H., Hioki, K., Yamamoto, M. (1986). Inhibitory effect of dietary selenium on carcinogenesis in rat glandular stomach induced by N-methyl-N′-nitro-N-nitrosoguanidine. *Cancer Res. 46*:2266.

Kok, F. J., De Bruijn, A. M., Hofman, A., Vermeeren, R., Valkenburg, H. A. (1987). Is serum selenium a risk factor for cancer in men only? *Am. J. Epidemiol. 125*:12.

Kubota, J., Allaway, W. H., Carter, D. L., Cary, E. E., Lazar, U. A. (1967). Selenium in corps in the United States in relation to selenium-responsive diseases of animals. *J. Agr. Food Chem. 15*:448.

Lane, H. W., Medina, D. (1985). Mode of action of selenium inhibition of 7,12-demethylbenz(a)anthracene-induced mouse mammary tumorigenesis. *J. Nat. Cancer Inst. 75*:675.

Lane, H. W., Butel, J. S., Medina, D. (1987). Selenium, lipid peroxidation and murine mammary tumorigenesis. In *Proceedings of the Third International Symposium on Selenium in Biology and Medicine*, Combs, G. F., Jr., Spallholz, J. E., Levander, O. A., Oldfield, J. E. (Eds.). AVI, Westport, Conn.

Le Boeuf, R. A., Hoekstra, W. G. (1985). Changes in cellular glutathione levels: possible relation to selenium-mediated anti-carcinogenesis. *Federation Proc. 44*:2563.

Le Boeuf, R. A., Hoekstra, W. G. (1983). Adaptive changes in hepatic glutathione metabolism in response to excess dietary selenium. *J. Nutr. 113*:845.

Le Boeuf, R. A., Laishes, B. A., Hoekstra, W. G. (1985). Effects of dietary selenium concentration on the development of enzyme-altered liver foci and hepatocellular carcinoma by diethylnitrosamine of N-acetylaminoflurene in rats. *Cancer Res. 45*:5489.

Marshall, M. V., Arnott, M. S., Jacobs, M. M., Griffin, A. C. (1979). Selenium effects on the carcinogenicity and metabolism of 2-acetylaminofluorene. *Cancer Lett. 7*:331.

Martin, S. E., Schillaci, M. (1984). Inhibitory effects of selenium on mutagenicity. *J. Agric. Food Chem. 32*:426.

Masiak, M., Herzyk, D. (1984). Behavior of microelements in lung cancer patients. *Fresenius Z. Anal. Chem. 317*:661.

Mason, T. J., McKay, F. W. (1975). *Atlas of Cancer Mortality for US Countries: 1950–1969*. Dept. of Health, Education and Welfare, Washington, D.C.

McConnell, K. P., Jager, R. M., Bland, K. I., Blotcky, A. J. (1980). The relationship of dietary selenium and breast cancer. *J. Surg. Oncol. 15*:67.

McConnell, K. P., Jager, R. M., Higgins, P. J., Blotcky, A. J. (1978). Serum selenium levels in patients with and without breast cancer. In *Nutrition and Cancer*, Van Eys, J., Seelig, M. S., Nichols, B. S. (Eds.). S. P. Medical and Scientific Books, New York, p. 145.

McConnell, K. P., Borghamer, W. L., Jr., Blotcky, A. J., Hurt, O. J. (1975). Selenium levels in human blood and tissues in health and in disease. *J. Nutr. 105*:1026.

Medina, D. (1986). Mechanisms of selenium inhibition of tumorigenesis. *J. Am. Coll. Toxicol. 5*:21.

Medina, D., Lane, H. W. (1983). Stage specificity of selenium-mediated inhibition of mouse mammary tumorigenesis. *Biol. Trace Elem. Res. 5*:297.

Medina, D., Shepard, F. S. (1984). Selenium inhibition of the neoplastic transformation in preneoplastic mammary cell populations. *Cancer Lett. 24*:227.

Medina, D., Shepard, F. (1981). Selenium-mediated inhibition of 7,12-dimethylbenz(a)anthracene-induced mouse mammary tumorigenesis. *Carcinogenesis 2*: 451.

Medina, D., Shepard, F. (1980). Selenium-mediated inhibition of mouse mammary tumorigenesis. *Cancer Lett. 8*:241.

Menkes, M. S., Comstock, G. W., Vuilleumier, J. P., Helsing, K. J., Rider, A. A., Brookmeyer, R. P. (1986). Serum beta-carotene, vitamins A and E, selenium, and the risk of lung cancer. *New Engl. J. Med. 315*:1250.

Milks, M. M., Wilt, S. R., Ali, I. I., Couri, D. (1985). The effects of selenium on the emergence of aflatoxin B_1-induced enzyme-altered foci in rat liver. *Fund. Appl. Toxicol. 5*:320.

Miller, L., Mills, B. J., Blotcky, A. J., Lincleman, R. D. (1983). Red blood cell and serum selenium concentrations as influenced by age and selected diseases. *J. Am. Coll. Nutr. 4*:331.

Milner, J' A. (1986). Selenium and carcinogenesis. *ACS Symp. Ser. 277*:267.

Milner, J. A. (1984). Selenium and the transplantable tumor. *J. Agric. Food Chem. 32*:436.

Milner, J. A., Hsu, C. Y. (1982). Inhibitory effects of selenium on the growth of L1210 leukemic cells. *Cancer Res. 41*:1652.

Nelson, A. A., Fitzhugh, O. G., Calvery, H. O. (1943). Liver tumors following cirrhosis caused by selenium in rat. *Cancer Res. 3*:230.

Nigro, N. D., Bull, A. W., Wilson, P. S., Souillier, B. K., Alousi, M. A. (1983). Combined inhibitors of carcinogenesis: Effects on azoxymethane-induced intestinal cancer in rats. *J. Nat. Cancer Inst. 69*:103.

O'Connor, T. P. (1985). *Effect of Dietary Intake of Fat, Protein and Selenium on the Development of L-Azaserine Induced Preneoplastic Lesions in Rat Pancreas*. Ph.D. Thesis, Cornell University, Ithaca, N.Y., 114 pp.

Olsson, U., Onfelt, A., Beije, B. (1984). Dietary selenium deficiency causes decreased N-oxygenation of N,N-diethylaniline and increased mutagenicity of dimethylnitrosamine in the isolated rat liver/cell culture system. *Mutation Res. 126*:73.

Patterson, E. L., Milstrey, R.,Stokstad, E. L. R. (1957). Effect of selenium in preventing exudative diathesis in chicks. *Proc. Soc. Exp. Biol. Med. 95*:617.

Peleg, I., Morris, S., Hames, C. G. (1985). Is selenium a risk factor for cancer? *Med. Oncol. Tumor Pharmacother. 2*:137.

Pence, B. C., Buddingh, F. (1985). Effect of selenium deficiency on 1,2-dimethylhydrazine-induced colon tumors in rats. *J. Nutr. 1196.*

Perchellet, J. P., Abney, N. L., Thomas, R. M., Guislain, Y. L., Perchellet, E. M. (1987). Effects of combined treatments with selenium, glutathione, and vitamin E on glutathione peroxidase activity, ornithine decarboxylase induction, and complete and multistage carcinogenesis in mouse skin. *Cancer Res. 47*: 477.

Poirier, K. A., Milner, J. A., (1983). Factors influencing the antitumorigenic properties of selenium in mice. *J. Nutr. 113*:2147.

Poirier, K. A., Milner, J. A. (1979). The effect of various seleno-compounds on Ehrlich ascites tumor cells. *Biol. Trace Elem. Res. 1*:25.

Reddy, B. S., Tanaka, T. (1986). Interactions of selenium deficiency, vitamin E, polyunsaturated fat and azoxymethane-induced colon carcinogenesis in male F344 rats. *J. Nat. Cancer Inst. 76*:1157.

Robinson, M. F., Godfrey, P. J., Thomson, C. D., Rea, H. M., van Rij, A. M. (1979). Blood selenium and glutathione peroxidase activity in normal subjects and in surgical patients with and without cancer in New Zealand. *Am. J. Clin. Nutr. 32*:1477.

Romano, F., Andreis, P. G., Marchesini, C., Paccagnella, L., Armato, U. (1986). Studies on the mechanisms by which tumor promoters stimulate the growth of primary neonatal rat hepatocytes. *Toxicol. Pathol. 14*:375.

Rotruck, J. T., Pope, A. L., Ganther, H. E., Swanson, A. B., Hafeman, D. G., Hoekstra, W. G. (1973). Selenium: Biochemical role as a component of glutathione perioxidase. *Science 179*:588.

Safer, B., Jagus, B., Crouch, D. (1980). Indirect inactivation of eukaryotic initiation factor 2 in reticulocyte lysates by selenite. *J. Biol. Chem. 255*:6913.

Salonen, J. T. (1986). Selenium and human cancer. *Ann. Clin. Res. 18*:18.

Salonen, J. T., Salonen, R., Lappetelainen, R., Maenpaa, P. H., Althan, G., Puska, P. (1985). Risk of cancer in relation to serum concentrations of selenium and vitamins A and E: Matched case-control analysis of prospective data. *Br. Med. J. 290*:417.

Salonen, J. T., Alfthan, G., Huttunen, J. K., Puska, P. (1984). Association between serum selenium and the risk of cancer. *Am. J. Epidemiol. 120*:342.

Schillaci, M., Martin, S. E., Milner, J. A. (1982). The effects of dietary selenium on the biotransformation of 7,12-dimethylbenz(a)anthracene. *Mutation Res. 101*:31.

Schober, S. E. (1986). Vitamin A, vitamin E, selenium and colon cancer. *Dissertation Abs. Int. B. 46*:3808.

Schrauzer, G. N., Schrauzer, T., Mead, S., Kvehn, K., Yamamoto, H., Arakl, E. (1987). Selenium in the blood of Japanese and American women with and without breast cancer and fibrocystic disease. In *Proceedings of the Third International Symposium on Selenium in Biology and Medicine*, Combs, G. F., Jr., Spallholz, J. E., Levander, O. A., Oldfield, J. E. (Eds.). AVI, Westport, Conn.

Schrauzer, G. N., Molenaar, T., Mead, S., Kuehn, K., Yamamoto, H., Araki, E. (1985). Selenium in the blood of Japanese and American women with and without breast cancer and fibrocystic disease. *Jap. J. Cancer Res. 76*:374.

Schrauzer, G. N., McGuinness, J. E., Kuehn, K. (1980a). Effects of temporary selenium supplementation on the genesis of spontaneous mammary tumors in inbred female C_3H mice/St mice. *Carcinogenesis 1*:199.

Schrauzer, G. N., McGuinness, J. E., Kuehn, K. (1980b). Effects of temporary selenium supplementation on the genesis of spontaneous mammary tumors in inbred female C3H/St mice. *Carcinogenesis 1*:199.

Schrauzer, G. N., White, D. A., Schnieder, C. J. (1977a). Cancer Mortality correlation studies. III. Statistical association with dietary selenium intakes. *Bioinorg. Chem. 7*:23.

Schrauzer, G. N., White, D. A., Schneider, C. J. (1977b). Cancer mortality correlation studies. IV. Associations with dietary intakes and blood levels of certain trace elements, notable Se-antagonists. *Bioinorg. Chem. 7*:35.

Schrauzer, G. N., White, D. A., Schneider, C. J. (1976). Inhibition of the genesis of spontaneous mammary tumors in inbred C_3H mice: effects of selenium and of selenium-antagonistic elements and their possible role in human breast cancer. *Bioinorg. Chem. 56*:265.

Schrauzer, G. N., Rhead, W. J., Evans, G. A. (1973). Selenium and cancer: chemical interpretation of a plasma "cancer test." *Bioinorg. Chem. 2*:329.

Schroeder, H. A., Mitchner, M. (1971). Selenium and tellurium in rats: effects on growth, survival and turmors. *J. Nutr. 101*:1531.

Schwarz, K., Foltz, C. M. (1957). Selenium as an integral part of factor 3 against dietary liver degeneration. *J. Am. Chem. Soc. 79*:3292.

Schwarz, K., Bieri, J. G., Briggs, G. M., Scott, M. L. (1957). Prevention of exudative diathesis in chicks by factor 3 and selenium. *Proc. Soc. Exp. Biol. Med. 95*:621.

Scott, M. L. (1973). The selenium disease. *J. Nutr. 103*:803.

Shamberger, R. J. (1970). Relationship of selenium to cancer. I. Inhibitory effect of selenium on carcinogenesis. *J. Nat. Cancer Inst. 44*:931.

Shamberger, R. J., Frost, D. V. (1969). Possible protective effect of selenium against human cancer. *Can. Med. Assn. J. 104*:82.

Shamberger, R. J., Willis, C. E. (1971). Selenium distribution of human cancer mortality. *CRC Crit. Rev. Clin. Lab Sci. 2*:211.

Shamberger, R. J., Corlett, C. L., Beaman, K. D., Kastan, B. L. (1979).Antioxidants reduce the mutagenic effect of malonaldehyde and beta-propiolactone. *Mutation Res. 66*:349.

Shamberger, R. J., Tytko, S. A., Willis, C. E. (1976). Antioxidants and cancer. Part VI. Selenium and age-adjusted human cancer mortality. *Arch. Environ. Hlth. 26*:231.

Shamberger, R. J., Tytko, S. A., Willis, C. E. (1974). Antioxidants and cancer. II. Selenium and human cancer mortality in the United States, Canada and New Zealand. *Trace Sub. Environ. Health.* 7:35.

Shamberger, K. J., Rukovena, E., Longfield, A. K., Tytko, S. A., Deodhar, S., Willis, C. E. (1973). Antioxidants and cancer. I. Selenium in the blood of normal and cancer patients. *J. Nat. Cancer Inst.* *50*:863.

Schultz, J. D., Leklem, J. E. (1983). Selenium status of vegetarians, nonvegetarians, and hormone-dependent cancer subjects. *Am. J. Clin. Nutr.* *37*:114.

Skaare, J. U., Nafstad, I. (1978). Interaction of vitamin E and selenium with the hepatotoxic agent dimethylnitrosamine. *Acta Pharmacol. Toxicol.* *43*:119.

Souillier, B. K., Wilson, P. S., Nigro, N. D. (1981). Effect of selenium on azoxymethane-induced intestinal cancer in rats fed high fat diet. *Cancer Lett.* *12*: 343.

Sullivan, J. F., Blotcky, A. J., Jetton, M. M., Hahn, H. K. J., Burch, R. E. Serum levels of selenium, calcium, copper, magnesium and zinc in various human diseases. *J. Nutr.* *19*:1432.

Sundstrom, H., Ylikorkala, O., Kauppila, A. (1986). Serum selenium and thromboxane in patients with gynaecological cancer. *Carcinogenesis* 7:1051.

Sundstrom, H., Korpela, H., Viinikka, L., Kauppila, A. (1984a). Serum selenium and glutathione peroxidase and plasma lipid peroxides in uterine, ovarian or vulvar cancer, and their responses to antioxidant in patients with ovarian cancer. *Cancer Lett.* *24*:1.

Sundstrom, H., Yrjankeikki, E., Kauppila, A. (1984b). Serum selenium in patients with ovarian cancer during and after therapy. *Carcinogenesis* *5*:731.

Tanaka, T., Reddy, B. S., El-Bayoumy, K. (1985). Inhibition by dietary organoselenium, *p*-methoxybenzeneselenol, of hepatocarcinogenesis induced by azoxymethane in rats. *Jap. J. Cancer Res.* *76*:462.

Teel, R. W., Kain, S. R. (1984). Selenium modified mutagenicity and metabolism of benzo(a)pyrene in an S9-dependent system. *Mutation Res.* *127*:9

Thompson, H. J. (1984). Selenium as an anticarcinogen. *J. Agric. Food Chem.* *32*:422.

Thompson, H. J., Becci, P. J. (1985). Selenium inhibition of N-methyl-N-nitrosourea-induced mammary carcinogenesis in the rat. *J. Nat. Cancer Inst.* *65*: 1299.

Thompson, H. J., Becci, P. J. (1979). Effect of graded dietary levels of selenium on tracheal carcinomas induced by 1-methyl-1-nitrosourea. *Cancer Lett.* 7: 215.

Thompson, J. N., Scott, M. L. (1970). Impaired lipid and vitamin E absorption related to atrophy of the pancreas in selenium-deficient chicks. *J. Nutr.* *100*: 797.

Thompson, H. J., Tagliaferro, A. R. (1980). Effect of selenium on 7,12-dimethylbenz(a)anthracene-induced mammary tumorigenesis. *Federation Proc.* *39*:1117 (abstract).

Thompson, H. J., Herbst, E. J., Meeker, L. D. (1986). Chemoprevention of mammary carcinogenesis: A comparative review of the efficacy of a polyamine antimetabolite, retinoids and selenium. *J. Nat. Cancer Inst.* 77:595.

Thompson, H. J., Meeker, L. D., Kokoska, S. (1984). Effect of an inorganic and organic form of dietary selenium on the promotional stage of mammary carcinogenesis in the rat. *Cancer Res. 44*:2803.

Thompson, H. J., Meeker, L. D., Becci, P. J., Kokoska, S. (1982). Effect on short-term feeding of sodium selenite on 7,12-dimethylbenz(a)anthracene-induced mammary carcinogenesis in the rat. *Cancer Res. 42*:4954.

Thompson, J., Meeker, L. D., Becci, P. J. (1981a). Effect of combined selenium and retinyl acetate treatment on mammary carcinogenesis. *Cancer Res. 41*: 1413.

Thompson, H. J., Soule, R. A., Becci, P. J. (1981b). Inhibition of mammary tumorigenesis by graded levels of selenium. *Federation Proc. 40*:929 (abstract).

Tinsley, I. J., Harr, J. R., Bone, J. F., Weswig, P. H., Yamamoto, R. S. (1967). Selenium toxicity in rats. I. Growth and longevity. In *Selenium in Biomedicine*, Muth, O. H. (ed.). AVI, Westport, Conn., p. 141.

Tsen, C. C., Tappel, A. L. (1958). Catalytic oxidation of glutathione and other sulfhydryl compounds by selenite. *J. Biol. Chem. 233*:1230.

Vernie, L. N. (1987). Inhibition of protein synthesis and anticarcinogenicity of selenium compounds. In *Proceedings of the Third International Symposium on Selenium in Biology and Medicine*, Combs, G. F., Jr., Spallholz, J. E., Levander, O. A., and Oldfield, J. E. (Eds.). AVI, Westport, Conn., p. 1074.

Vernie, L. N., DeVries, M., Beckhuijsen, C., DeGoeij, J. J. M., Zegers, C. (1983). Selenium levels in blood and plasma, and glutathione peroxidase activity in blood of breast cancer patients during adjuvant treatment with cyclophosphamide, methotrexate and 5-fluorouracil. *Cancer Lett. 18*:283.

Vernie, L. N., Hamburg, C. J., Bont, W. S. (1981). Inhibition of the growth of milignant mouse lymphoid cells by selenodiglutathione and selenocystine. *Cancer Lett. 14*:303.

Vernie, L. N., Collard, J. G., Eker, A. P. M., DeWildt, A., Wilders, I. T. (1980). Studies on the inhibition of protein synthesis by selenodiglutathione. *Biochem. J. 180*:213.

Vernie, L. N., Bont, W. S., Ginjaar, H. B., Emmelot, P. (1975). Elongation factor 2 as the target of the reaction product between sodium selenite and glutathione (GSSeSG) in the inhibiting of amino acid incorporation in vitro. *Biochim. Biophys. Acta 414*:283.

Vernie, L. N., Bont, W. S., Emmelot, P. (1974). Inhibition of in vitro amino acid incorporation by sodium selenite. *Biochem. 13*:337.

Volgarev, M. N., Tscherkes, L. A. (1967). Further studies in tissue changes associated with sodium selenate. In *Selenium in Biomedicine*, Muth, O. H. (Ed.). AVI, Westport, Conn., p. 179.

Walker, C. H., Klein, E. (1915). "Selenium"–its therapeutic value–especially in cancer. *Amer. Med.* (Aug.):628.

Watrach, A. M., Milner, J. A., Watrach, M. A. (1982). Effect of selenium on growth rate of canine mammary carcinoma cells in athymic nude mice. *Cancer Lett. 15*:137.

Watson, R. R., Leonard, T. K. (1986). Selenium and vitamins A, E, and C: nutrients with cancer prevention properties. *Persp. Pract. 86*:505.

Welsch, C. W., Goodrich-Smith, M., Brown, C. K., Greene, H. D., Hamel, E. J. (1981). Selenium and the genesis of murine mammary tumors. *Carcinogenesis 2*:519.

Willett, W. C., Stampfer, M. J. (1986). Selenium and human cancer. *Acta Physiol. Toxicol. 59*(suppl. 7):240.

Willett, W., Polk, B. F., Hames, C. (1983). Prediagnostic serum selenium and risk of cancer. *Lancet 8342*:130.

Wilt, S., Pereira, M., Couri, D. (1979). Selenium effect on initiation and promotion of tumors by benzo(a)pyrene and 12-O-tetradecanoylphorbol. *Amer. Assoc. Cancer Res. 20*:21.

Wortzman, M. S., Besbris, H. J., Cohen, A. M. (1980). Effect of dietary selenium on the interaction between 2-acetylaminofluorene and rat liver DNA in vivo. *Cancer Res. 40*:2670.

Yu, S. Y., Chu, Y. J., Gong, X. L., Hou, C., Li, W. G., Gong, H. M., Xie, J. R. (1985). Regional variation of cancer mortality incidence and its relation to selenium levels in China. *Biol. Trace Elem. Res. 7*:21.

Part Four

PLANNING, CONDUCT, AND INTERPRETATION OF CANCER PREVENTION TRIALS

15

Approach to Selection of Agents for Cancer Prevention Trials

THOMAS E. MOON
The University of Arizona Health Sciences Center, Tucson, Arizona

INTRODUCTION

The primary objective of cancer prevention research is to select agents that reduce the incidence of cancer. Stages in the selection of possible cancer-preventive agents have been defined but have not been fully validated. Evaluation and updating of the rationale and interrelationship between these stages can result in an effective and more efficient plan to select agents. A plan with several stages to select cancer-preventive agents is reviewed. The plan is based upon the integration of current understanding of therapeutic drug development, experimental carcinogenesis, and accumulating data from laboratory and human cancer prevention research. The integration of resources of the federal government, universities, and industry can produce the timely selection and application of cancer-preventive agents.

STAGES IN AGENT DEVELOPMENT

A detailed plan for the selection of cancer-preventive agents includes three interrelated components; laboratory or preclinical, observational epidemiology, and experimental epidemiology or human intervention trials (Carrese, 1967). Inclusion of all three components in a cancer research program has not been widely accomplished to date. For example, development of cancer treatments primarily emphasizes laboratory and clinical research, while cancer etiology commonly emphasizes observational epidemiology and laboratory research. The inclusion of all three components reflects the broad scientific requirements to successfully meet the objectives of cancer prevention research. An additional component that is essential to all aspects of cancer research is the development of and reliance on technology—cancer prevention being no exception.

The interrelationship between these three components has occurred only partially to date in cancer prevention research, as exemplified by the rationale for use of retinoids and β-carotene in current human intervention trials. Trials using vitamin A as the intervention have been primarily rationalized by preclinical and clinical therapeutic studies with mixed results from observational epidemiology studies. In contrast, trials evaluating β-carotene have been largely rationalized by dietary epidemiology studies with limited data from laboratory studies. Continued integration between all three components appears reasonable, but a specific integration plan needs further development to ensure feedback between all components and appropriate emphasis of the steps within each component. Increased emphasis on observational epidemiology research appears warranted, especially with regard to the role of foods in cancer prevention. The multiple preventive and carcinogenic agents simultaneously contained in foods, and thus made available to the human host, appear to require an increased emphasis on such human studies.

Lack of a validated plan for agent development reflects the relative newness of cancer prevention and the current lack of agents fully proven to prevent cancer in humans. Ongoing cancer prevention trials will provide data and insights to modify and begin to validate the current plan.

Development of cancer therapeutic agents provides a model for the development of cancer prevention agents. However, differences exist in the rationale and logistics between the development of cancer therapeutic and preventive agents. For example, the number of agents available for evaluation and the rationale to combine agents to carry out multifactorial studies may require modification in the model.

The history of cancer therapeutic agent development is impressive in many ways including its duration and magnitude. As many as 40,000 agents per year were screened between 1955-1975 for therapeutic potential (Zubrod, 1966). Since 1975, the number of agents screened has been reduced to 15,000 per year using revised criteria, which place increased emphasis on chemical and biological considerations. The criteria were based upon preclinical in vitro and in vivo experimental systems (DeVita, 1979). Four to eight agents per year commonly entered cancer clinical therapeutic trials, or less than one in 3,000 agents screened. During 1949-1978, an average of one agent per year was licensed for general medical use in the therapy of cancer. Selection of one agent licensed out of at least 15,000 agents screened per year, large expenditures of funds, a multistage process requiring long durations of time to develop and evaluate each agent appear to be standard for selecting cancer therapeutic agents.

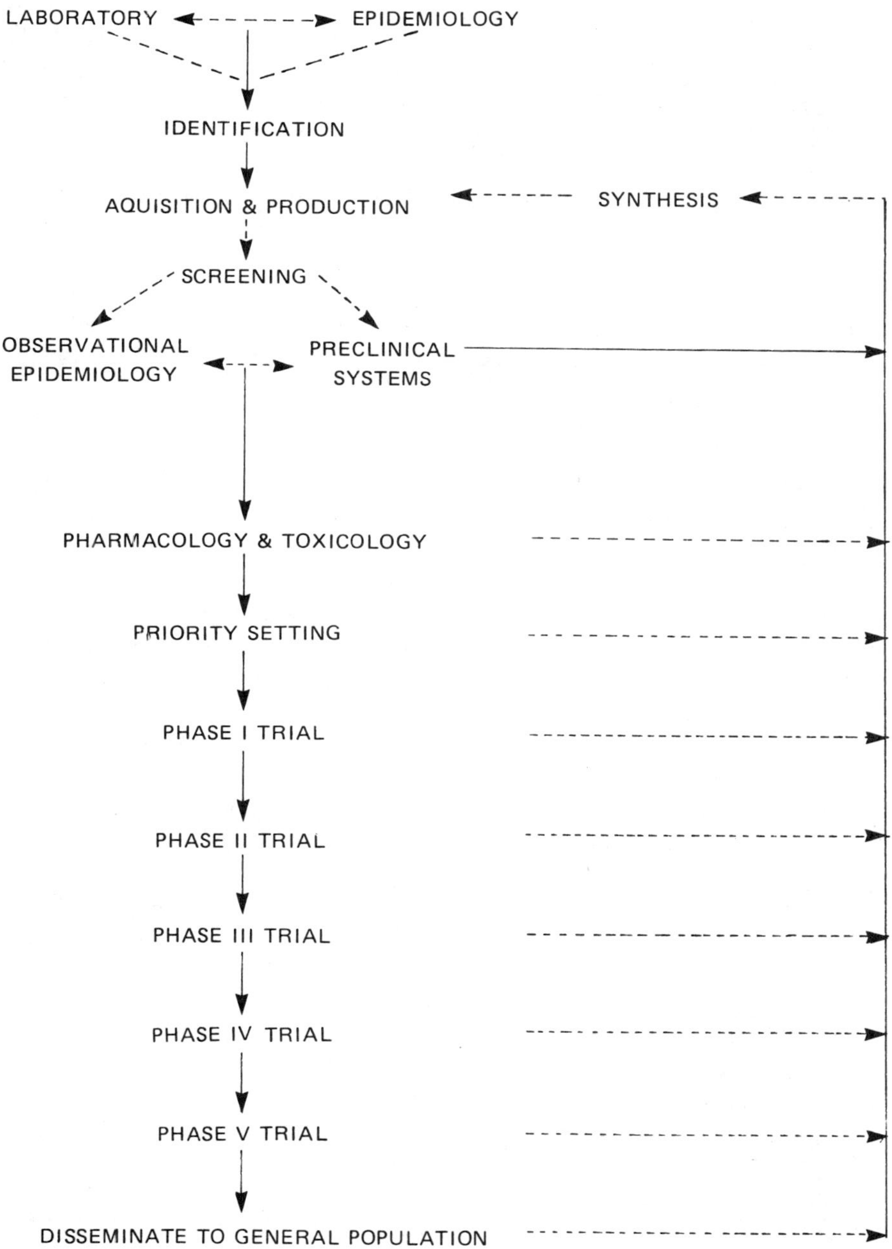

Fig. 1 Stages in agent development.

The stages of an integrated model for the selection of cancer-preventive agents are shown in Fig. 1. Selection begins with the identification and acquisition of agents. Production of sufficient amounts of the agent may be required to carry out toxicologic assessment. The next stage involves the screening for cancer-preventive activity of a new agent using an integrated approach that includes both preclinical and human studies. Studies in the pharmacology and toxicology stage are required to comply with Food and Drug Administration (FDA) regulations for obtaining an Investigational New Drug Application (INDA). Upon FDA approval for the INDA and priority setting, the human intervention trials of a new agent can proceed, following five phases: Phase I trials stressing pharmacology and toxicology considerations related to a range of doses of the agent; Phase II trials evaluating agent long-term safety and development of trial logistics; Phase III trials of efficacy comparing a new agent to placebo (or the standard cancer-preventive agent); Phase IV trials evaluating the efficacy of the agent in a defined population; and Phase V trials to evaluate the effectiveness of the agent in a defined community.

The proposed stages for the selection of cancer-preventive agents interrelate in a feedback loop. Such a feedback process would permit the evaluation of similar, natural or synthetic analogs that may have a different spectrum of efficacy, pharmacology, safety, or mechanism of action. This may be particularly important during this early period of cancer prevention research and selection of naturally occurring agents (such as vitamin A and carotenoids).

Adequate evaluation of each identified agent by systematically proceeding through every stage of the model (Fig. 1) is essential. Such a systematic procedure will not only accurately define the true efficacy and effectiveness of the agent but will also minimize inaccuracy of public information. The common public concept that everything causes cancer should not be replaced by false overexpectations that some agents can prevent all cancer or that increasing the dose of an individual agent will proportionally decrease the risk of cancer.

The model presented in Fig. 1 is similar to the stages used in the drug development program of the Division of Cancer Treatment, National Cancer Institute (NCI) (DeVita et al., 1979) and the plan proposed by the Division of Cancer Prevention and Control, NCI for the development of cancer-preventive agents (Boone, personal communication). Unlike the NCI plans, the model presented is not a linear array of preclinical and clinical studies but an integration of preclinical, observational epidemiology and human intervention studies. The full utilization of both observational epidemiology and preclinical studies to select agents could provide agents with better efficacy and specificity for different cancers and improved safety and understanding of the interrelationship of preventive and carcinogenic agents for human cancer.

IDENTIFICATION OF AGENTS

Review of available literature and reports on natural or synthetic agents provides a method to identify agents with some degree of cancer-preventive effect. Sources for review include in vitro and animal studies carried out by laboratory scientists, disease etiology studies carried out by epidemiologists and patient therapy studies carried out by clinical scientists. Each source provides a different set of experimental subjects, study methods, and insights into the carcinogenic process.

Approximately 600 compounds have been identified as having potential as cancer-preventive agents (Kelloff, personal communication). Table 1 lists the classes of these agents. Identified agents have been found to have some effect in reducing the risk of cancer in human epidemiology studies, animal models, or in vitro inhibition of transformation or mutagenesis.

Criteria useful in the selection of agents requires that studies include the quantity and duration of exposure of the agent and quantitative endpoints. Study methods must be carefully considered, including whether animal or human subjects were used, site of cancer, spontaneous or induced cancer, and related risk factors. A mechanism of action should be available. Use of tumor inhibition as the primary endpoint as contrasted to use of intermediate biochemical markers or precancerous lesions as endpoints needs further evaluation. Toxicologic evaluation in the experimental subjects must also be part of the selection criteria, including the type and severity of side effects.

The current state of knowledge has not provided sufficient scientific insights into the carcinogenic process or the development of cancer-preventive agents in order to determine the appropriate interrelationship and emphasis between in vitro, animal, epidemiologic, and clinical studies. Questions exist such as the adequacy of animal studies as the sole rationale to proceed to the next stage, and if

Table 1 Potential Chemopreventive Compounds

Antioxidants
Mixed Function Oxidase Modifiers
Ornithine Decarboxylase Inhibitors
Trace Minerals
Prostaglandin Synthesis Inhibitors
Retinoids
Pharmaceuticals

one confirmation is adequate in the same experimental model. Also, should consistency of results be required across experimental systems before proceeding?

AGENT ACQUISITION AND PRODUCTION

Acquisition of agents for screening may be obtained through voluntary submissions, solicitations, and specific requests to the pharmaceutical industry or individuals at universities. Availability of an agent is influenced by whether or not the agent is an experimental compound or licensed for use. Short- and long-term marketing considerations by the pharmaceutical industry and the agent's spectrum of indications may influence receptiveness to making the agent available for cancer prevention testing. The purity and stability of the agent, including related costs and who will bear such costs, before the agent is available for screening and in sufficient quantity and quality must also be considered. The formulation and production of an agent may require government support if availability is limited.

Industry can continue to play an important role to help expedite the development of potential cancer-preventive agents and their cost-sharing. Benefits from eventual marketing of proven agents will be largely realized by industry. An effective model is again provided by development of cancer therapy agents that has been impacted by the continuing involvement of industry.

Production and formulation is a critical step in the development of interventions because it facilitates the conduct of both toxicologic studies and intervention field trials. The investigator or the NCI must facilitate agent production for toxicologic studies and evaluation in humans. Efforts required to facilitate the production of an agent can be considerable. To date, agents have not been developed with primary emphasis on prevention of cancer but have been developed for other medical indications. Conflicts can occur when agents originally developed for other indications are considered for development as cancer prevention agents. The use of an agent for cancer prevention may result in different, often lower, doses but for longer durations of time and, thus, result in a differen spectrum of side effects in study subjects.

The relatively modest quantity of agent needed to carry out cancer prevention development, as compared to the full production runs for industrial marketing of an approved agent, requires careful planning to assure adequate and timely supply. The marketing potential anticipated by many pharmaceutical companies has resulted in increased availability of some potential cancer-preventive agents. However, the substantial commitment of resources required for the development of cancer-preventive agents, with principal support coming from the federal government, may reduce the number and timely evaluation of cancer prevention agents.

SCREENING OF AGENTS

The objective of screening is to evaluate potential agents for their degree and scope of inhibition of carcinogenesis. Agents screened would have some reported degree of cancer-preventive effect as discussed above. Screening of agents should follow a systematic evaluation plan including use of in vitro, in vivo, epidemiologic, and clinical studies. Apparent advantages and limitations of each type of study require additional understanding and interrelationship before an efficient evaluation plan is completed. A subsequent plan may place a different perspective than has been developed currently for the role and interrelationship of each type of study.

In vitro screening determines the degree and scope of inhibition or differentiation at the cellular level. These include transformations of genes, chromosomes, cells, and biochemical markers such as growth factors. Continuous animal and human cell lines, special cell cultures and organ cultures could provide a valuable screening resource (Yuspa et al., 1980; Colburn, 1982). Advantages of such in vitro systems include evaluation with different mechanisms of transformation, use of human cells where feasible, controlled laboratory experimental conditions, ease of quantification, sensitivity, plus time and cose efficiency.

Existing limitations of in vitro screening are their relevance to efficacy and safety in humans, primary use of fibroblast cell lines and not epithelial cells, plus inability to provide metabolic activation of the potential cancer-preventive agent.

In vivo screening of potential agents detects inhibition of carcinogenesis resulting from chemical initiators and promoters at specific concentrations and duration of exposure. The time to appearance of first tumor, number and size of tumors, inhibition in different animal models and different organ systems are used as criteria to evaluate efficacy (Huggins et al., 1964; Mirvich et al., 1975). Identified advantages of in vivo screening include use of whole animals, relative rapid tumor development when compared to spontaneous tumor models, controlled laboratory conditions, quantifiable endpoints, use of different mechanisms of carcinogenesis and inhibition, controlled timing and route of administration of both the carcinogen and the potential cancer-preventive agent, assessment of bioavailability, tissue distribution, metabolism, and toxicity. Animal tumor models of specific target tissues with importance to human cancer are most useful. These same animal tumor models have been extensively used in demonstrating carcinogenicity. Table 2 illustrates the in vitro screening approach considered by the National Cancer Institute (Boone, personal communication). Mice and rats are the in vivo models for which specific carcinogens are required to produce cancers in specific organs. For example, DMBA followed by TPA applied to mouse skin produce papillomas on the skin. In contrast, DMBA or NMU introduced in rats are specific to produce adenocarcinoma in mammary glands.

Table 2 Agent-Screening in vivo Models

Species	Organ	Carcinogen	Endpoint
Mouse	Skin	DMBA/TPA	Papilloma
	Lung	3-MCA	Squamous Cell and Adenocarcinoma
	Bladder	OH-BBN	Transitional Cell
	Connective Tissue	BALB 3T3	Fibrocarcinoma
Rats	Mammary	DMBA or NMU	Adenocarcinoma
	Colon	AOM	Adenocarcinoma

A criterion that requires tumor inhibition in more than one species and at multiple sites may be overly restrictive. Such a broad spectrum of effect need not be required as part of the in vivo criteria. Table 3 illustrates the critical choice of animal species, carcinogen, and tumor site in the screening of retinoids. Vitamin A and the synthetic retinoids represent related agents with similar structure that have been screened more extensively than other agents (Hill and Grubbs, 1982). Such extensive screening yields a spectrum of results on the

Table 3 Agent-Screening in vivo Retinoid Studies

Species	Site	Carcinogen	Agent	Effect
Mice				
CDI	Skin	DMBA/TPA	Retinyl palmitate	+
NMRI	Skin	BP	Retinyl palmitate	-
Rats				
Wistar-Lewis	Bladder	NMU	13cRA	+
Fisher	Bladder	FANFT	13cRA	-
Sprague-Dawley	Mammary	DMBA	Retinyl palmitate	-
Sprague-Dawley	Salivary gland	DMBA	Retinyl palmitate	+

+, Inhibition.
-, No inhibition.
Source: Modified from Hill and Grubbs (1982).

in vivo efficacy of retinoids. One view consistent with the data in Table 3 is that retinoids inhibit in vivo tumors in different species, using different carcinogens and different tumor organ sites. Such a view is consistent with retinoids having a broad spectrum of efficacy. Another view of the same data in Table 3 is that the efficacy of retinoids is not broad-based but depends upon the animal species, carcinogen, tumor site, and retinoid. The first row of Table 3 illustrates that skin tumors induced by DMBA/TPA in CDI mice are inhibited by retinyl palmitate. However, skin tumors produced by BP in NMIR mice are not inhibited by retinyl palmitate. Thus, inhibition of skin tumors appears to be dependent on the carcinogen and animal species. A similar variation in tumor inhibition using the synthetic retinoid 13-*cis* retinoic acid is observed for bladder tumors using different carcinogens in two different species of rat. In contrast, using the same carcinogen, DMBA, in the same rat species can produce mammary tumors or salivary gland tumors, depending upon the route of administration, and again shows differential tumor inhibition using retinyl palmitate. Based upon the in vivo retinoid screening data, the possibility of a false negative appears likely during the early screening of agents or as more data is collected using different species, carcinogens, and tumor sites.

The dose used to chemically induce tumors in animals may overwhelm the host's inhibitory capacity and thus differ from the human carcinogenic process. Also, tissue distribution of an agent and its metabolite may vary widely.

Quantifying tissue levels of β-carotene and vitamin A provides an example. Plasma β-carotene is dose dependent on dietary intake. In contrast, plasma retinol has been known for many years to be homeostatically controlled and is not dose dependent among individuals with a broad range of normal dietary intakes. Retinyl palmitate has been recently identified to vary by dietary dose in vivo and can serve as a marker of dietary intake of vitamin A (Peng et al., 1986). Data from Peng et al. (1986) shown in Table 4 illustrate the difference between use of plasma retinol and plasma retinyl palmitate as markers of vitamin A intake. Retinol has been shown to be quickly converted to retinyl esters, predominantly retinyl palmitate, during absorption into the gut. Thus, intake of retinyl palmitate is considered equivalent to intake of retinol. Table 4 shows that the choice of the biologic tissue impacts the understanding of the dose response effect of dietary vitamin A. Plasma retinol does not change while retinol levels in the liver, fat, and skin do show a dose-response effect. In contrast, plasma retinyl palmitate as well as retinyl palmitate levels in the liver, fat, and skin do change in a dose-dependent manner.

Human exposure to carcinogens in the environment and dietary agents in the foods consumed are of relatively low daily dose but persist throughout the lifetime of the host. Observational epidemiology studies provide a unique complement to laboratory studies for the screening of agents. Complete specificity is obtained by study of humans in a nonexperimental environment. Other ad-

Table 4 Retinol vs. Retinyl Palmitate Concentrations in Mouse Plasma and Tissues

	Group*	Plasma (μg/ml)	Fat (μg/g)	Liver (μg/g)	Skin (μg/g)
Retinol-	Control	0.27	0.29	27.60	0.10
	60 RP	0.37	1.90	28.20	0.68
	200 RP	0.36	4.63	32.44	2.46
	700/350 RP	0.35	4.56	57.39	3.18
Retinyl palmitates	Control	0.02	3.0	392	0.1
	60 RP	0.06	4.0	569	0.4
	200 RP	0.54	10.2	2056	2.0
	700/350 RP	1.41	9.0	2752	3.8

*, x10^3 IU Retinyl Palmitate/Kg diet

vantages include ability to quantify cancer-related events and improved understanding of the natural history of the events. Quantification of events would include the diagnosis of spontaneous cancer lesions, but in addition the diagnosis, progression, and regression of precancerous lesions. Also, biochemical markers of lesions would also receive better understanding as to their interrelationship to cancer-related lesions.

Disadvantages of epidemiologic studies used for screening the potential of agents include the long time interval to the diagnosis of a human cancer, limitations on the quantification of exposure to carcinogenic and preventive agents, and ability to isolate a single agent and its associated cancer risk.

Use of analytic (case-control and followup epidemiologic) studies with highly focused hypotheses can minimize these limitations. The hypotheses would focus on specific dietary agents, either naturally occurring or added during growth or processing of foods. The competition between cancer initiators, promoters, and preventive agents can be fully and simultaneously studied in humans. Such studies can evaluate the multiple mechanisms related to realistic timing, route of administration, and duration of exposure related to human carcinogenesis. For over 10 years, epidemiologic studies with focused hypotheses regarding carcinogenic agents have been key to the understanding of human carcinogenesis (Schottenfeld and Fraumeni, 1982). Examples of recent studies of dietary agents include fat and breast cancer plus fiber and colon cancer (Armstrong and Mann, 1984).

Continued evolution of epidemiology as a research discipline, improvements in the management of large volumes of multifactor data, better quantification of exposures of many specific dietary and other agents, and availability of multivariate statistical methods all provide the scientific and technological basis to carry out such focused epidemiologic studies (Beecher, 1985; Glass, 1986). Results of such studies will include specific quantitative measures of cancer risk reduction while simultaneously considering multiple other carcinogenic and preventive factors. Use of defined populations with ongoing surveillance provides study subjects that may be at high risk of cancer. Elevated risk of cancer may be related to a specific environmental exposure or a general condition such as older age.

Careful consideration of the etiology of human cancer and its relationship to in vivo models is critical in order to avoid a large false negative rate. Personal differences in dietary intake may be magnified by their differences in absorption, metabolism, and pharmacokinetics. Epidemiologic studies of human cancer avoid the extrapolation limitations of in vitro and in vivo studies but can only evaluate naturally occurring agents or agents added during food processing. This is not currently a substantial limitation as the number of such agents that may have potential cancer-preventive efficacy is large. The use of dietary intake methods to quantify exposure of the agent is applicable to many but not all occurring agents. For example, proformed vitamin A has been quantified to include all carotenoids, including α-, β-, and γ-carotene plus carotenoids with no vitamin A activity. The improved quantification of β-carotene and other carotenoids in fruits and vegetables provides the method to better evaluate the role of carotenoids as cancer-preventive agents (Chapter 8).

Screening of potential cancer therapeutic agents can also be carried out in the setting of clinical therapy of patients with cancer. Such studies provide a special opportunity to screen agents to evaluate, in humans, tumor inhibition in a dose-dependent manner, pharmacology, and safety. Recent examples include the evaluation of retinoids in the therapy of cancer patients with observed efficacy in patients with squamous cell cancers (Meyskens, 1986).

Another potentially important clinic population needing further evaluation is the use of patients with premalignant lesions as a study population for the screening of potential cancer-preventive agents. The potential role of such a patient population is discussed in the following section on phase II clinical trials.

PHARMACOLOGY AND TOXICOLOGY

Preclinical determination of an agent's safety in animals is required prior to initiation of human trials. Evaluation of an agent's toxicologic, pharmacokinetic, and pharmacodynamic profile is commonly carried out in rodents and dogs. The same animal models used for screening an agent's efficacy should be used to determine safety. Thus, screening for efficacy and safety can be carried out simultaneously in the same studies.

Animal models for efficacy and safety screening have been extensively used for development of therapeutic agents for the treatment of cancer and related diseases. Also, many of the same animal models have been used to screen for chemical carcinogenesis. Additional research is needed, however, to demonstrate the appropriate interpretation of animal models used to screen for safety and efficacy of potential cancer prevention agents. The toxicity from agents tolerated by human subjects participating in a cancer-prevention study is low compared to cancer patients receiving chemotherapy. This creates a critical difference in screening of cancer-preventive and therapeutic agents and the interpretation of animal models.

The design of animal safety studies must include short-term, lifetime, and multigeneration studies using a wide dose range of the agent. Teratogenicity and fetotoxicity are realistic concerns that must be evaluated. Acute, subchronic, and chronic endpoints should be used to screen the safety of agents. These endpoints require a wide spectrum of methods of determination that include gross necropsy, histopathology, clinical examination, plus plasma and tissue pharmacology. Studies simultaneously evaluating multiple cancer-preventive agents are also required.

Results from the screening stage of potential cancer-preventive agents must provide adequate assurance of efficacy and safety. Integration of information from both laboratory and focused epidemiology studies provide better insights into the efficacy and safety of an agent that is commonly available in the development of therapeutic drugs.

FDA APPROVAL

Animal toxicity studies are required to comply with Food and Drug Administration (FDA) regulations for obtaining acceptance of an Investigational New Drug application (INDA) to carry out initial human trials. The trials using currently available nutrients have required an INDA. For many of the agents currently used, investigators have cross-filed on existing INDs held by other investigators and pharmaceutal industries.

PRIORITY SETTING

Establishment of efficacy with a defined spectrum of toxicity is required of all potential cancer-preventive agents before being prioritized for entry into human intervention trials. Even if such information were available, added experience is needed to develop and evaluate an efficient strategy to prioritize agents for entry into human intervention trials. A list of considerations for the development of a strategy to prioritize agents includes: (1) degree of inhibition, (2) degree, type, duration, and reversibility of toxicity, (3) number of laboratory and epidemiology studies and their consistency, (4) number of studies by different investigators, (5) availability of the agent, (6) information on mechanism(s) of action, (7) where the agent inhibits the carcinogenic process, (8) spectrum of potential efficacy for common human cancers, (9) costs to begin human trials, (1) other agents competing for entry into intervention trials, (11) availability of appropriate study subjects, and (12) availability of funding for cancer prevention research.

Agents that have entered intervention trials have not competed to date for funds to enter intervention trials. Thus there is limited experience to calculate cost/benefit, risk/benefit, and feasibility/benefit ratios or other commonly used numerical strategy. One approach is to enter all possible agents with cancer-preventive potential into Phase I and Phase II intervention trials. This strategy would provide added data to prioritize which agents—and more relevant, which combinations of agents—to enter into Phase III trials.

PHASE I TRIAL

Human intervention trials provide the mechanism to carry out experimental studies that can provide evidence of cancer inhibition in humans that is unachievable by other studies. The design of intervention studies includes the assignment of the agent(s) to prospectively defined subjects and the control of risk factors. Phase I intervention trials provide the initial experimentation administration in humans of potential cancer-preventive agents. Agents commonly available in the diet or used as therapy must also complete this phase of evaluation.

Phase I trials have the objectives to evaluate agent "short-term" safety and pharmacology using several dose schedules. The results of phase I trials provide the safe starting dose range for the next evaluation phase. In addition, changes should be evaluated in possible biological markers of efficacy in the host.

If a recommended daily allowance (RDA) has been established for the agent, doses higher than the RDA should be evaluated for safety. The RDA was based upon a criteria to provide reasonable assurance that nutritional deficiencies will be avoided by most people. Doses higher than the RDA may be required to inhibit cancer or other chronic diseases.

Phase I trials can be carried out in either normal free-living volunteers or patients who are part of the clinical care system. Each type of subject offers complementary benefits. Normal free-living volunteers provide information on study objectives that can directly apply to a similar group of free-living subjects at risk of cancer. Patients with cancer may provide information on the spectrum and degree of toxicity observed from higher doses of the agent. The agent must offer acceptable therapeutic alternatives for the patient. Examples of patient groups treated and providing information to evaluate potential cancer prevention agents include acne patients, advanced cancer patients, and adjuvant (presumably disease-free from surgery or radiation therapy) cancer patients for the evaluation of retinoids. Xeroderma pigmentosa patients have provided information for the evaluation of β-carotene (Matthews-Roth, 1977; Meyskens, 1985).

Pharmacologic evaluation should consider both plasma and other tissue-specific levels of the agent. Continued development of analytic methods are required for assay of specific compounds and metabolites. The tissue distribution of the agent or its metabolites should be used to guide which cancer sites might provide an adequate evaluation of the efficacy of the agent in humans. Agents that are homeostatically controlled, such as retinol and calcium, should not be automatically excluded as potential cancer-preventive agents. As has been shown in adequately nourished subjects, pharmacologic dosing of retinol does increase the plasma levels of retinyl palmitate in a dose-response manner.

The duration of dosing prior to evaluation of plasma or other tissue concentration appears also to warrant careful consideration. Although the plasma level of the agent or its metabolite may be present and detectable within a short time after the subject is dosed with the agent, the availability of the agent in other tissues may vary widely with the duration of dosing. The example of linoleic acid in the dietary lipids of subjects who eat an adequate diet are notable. The reports indicate that up to three years may be required for the subcutaneous adipose tissue to reflect change in the level of linoleic acid in the dietary lipid (Mackie et al., 1987).

PHASE II TRIAL

Phase II intervention trials of potential cancer-preventive agents have a number of important objectives that differ from cancer therapeutic clinical trials. Reduction of risk of clinically diagnosed cancer is not easily estimated by phase II trials due to the low annual incidence of cancer and the long period of induction and promotion. Objectives of phase II trials that are important to the evaluation of intervention agents include identification of appropriate study populations, evaluation of recruitment strategies, compliance measurement and motivation, and evaluation of long-term safety. Identification of appropriate study populations for phase II and later stages depends on the mechanism of action of the potential cancer-preventive agent and where it inhibits the cancer initiation-promotion process. Agents that are thought to inhibit cancer initiation require a young population. In contrast, agents that inhibit late promotion stages of carcinogenesis may be applied to populations at high risk of cancer. High-risk populations have the potential of providing shorter study durations due to their shorter time to diagnosis of cancer. The level of effort and expense is high in identifying and maintaining followup on appropriate study populations. Phase II or III studies in progress will provide continued followup of their recruitment strategies and study populations in order to provide resources for future studies.

Persons with precancerous lesions provide an exceptional resource for the evaluation of new agents. These lesions may be self-identified by the person or health providers and provide an effective way for motivated persons to refer themselves for recruitment on a cancer prevention study. Many of these persons may not be part of an ongoing clinical care system and thus provide added opportunities for the evaluation of recruitment strategies. Lesions that bestow increased risk of cancer on their host include colon polyps, dysplasia of the cervix, dysplasia of the esophagus and head and neck, plus actinic keratoses and dysplasic nevi on the skin.

Intervention agents should be evaluated in humans with risk of the same type and location of cancer as identified in the preintervention phases. To carry out this extensive evaluation, establishment of a phase I cooperative group of institutions should be established to efficiently and effectively evaluate new intervention agents in a timely fashion. Institutions participating in this cooperative group should have the capability of performing pharmacologic and biochemical assays with the new agents.

PHASE III/IV/V TRIALS

Later phases of intervention evaluation, commonly referred to as phases III, IV, and V, attempt to establish the value of a new agent relative to a control agent (Greenwald et al., 1985). At the current time, placebo-controlled comparative intervention studies are required.

Phase III trials carry out the comparison in subjects that volunteer from a preselected group. Subjects from a specific clinic that have had a skin cancer removed and are thus at increased risk for the development of subsequent skin cancers provide one example of such a voluntary population at high risk of cancer. These subjects self-select themselves for participation in the intervention trials. Also, they are selected corresponding to which specific clinics are identified for recruitment of subjects.

A phase IV trial is similar to a phase III trial with the additional requirement that subject selection is from a defined population. An example is provided by selection of high risk of skin cancer subjects from all clinics from within a defined geographical region. The phase IV trial has the added requirement of a population base evaluation of the intervention. Phase III and IV trials have an emphasis on the measurement and motivation of intervention compliance with the intent towards evaluating intervention efficacy.

A Phase V trial evaluates the effectiveness of publicly encouraging use of the agent to lower risk of (specific) cancer. The intervention would be performed as part of the regular lifestyle of all members of a defined community. Endpoints for Phase V trials would include changes in community cancer incidence rates and level of compliance with recommended policy. Examples from the cardiovascular prevention literature provide optimism that Phase V cancer intervention trials are achievable (Fraser, 1986). Phase V cancer prevention trials have not been initiated.

ACKNOWLEDGMENT

The author thanks Lisa Brown for manuscript preparation.

REFERENCES

Armstron, B. K., Mann, J. J. (1986). Diet. In Vessey, M. P., Gray, M. (Eds.), *Cancer Risks and Prevention*. Oxford University Press, pp. 68–69.

Beecher, G. R. (1985). Progress in methods development and new nutrient data. Proceedings of 10th Nutrient Data Bank Conference, San Francisco, CA.

Carrese, L. M., Baker, E. G. (1967). The convergence technique: A method for the planning and programming of research efforts. *Management Science 13*(8):B420.

Colburn, N. H. (1982). The use of tumor promoter responsive cell lines to study preneoplastic progression. In Franks, L. M., Wigley, C. B. (Eds.), *Neoplastic Transformation in Differentiated Epithelial Cell Systems In Vitro*. New York, Academic Press.

DeVita, V. T., Oliverio, V. T., Muggia, F. M., et al. (1979). The drug development and clinical trials program of the Division of Cancer Treatment, National Cancer Institute. *Cancer Clinical Trials 2*:195–216.

Fraser, G. E. (1986). *Preventive Cardiology*. New York: Oxford University Press.

Glass, R. I. A.(1986). New prospects for epidemiologic investigations. *Science 234*:951–955.

Greenwald, P., Cullen, J. W. (1985). The new emphasis in cancer control. *JNCI 74*(3):543–551.

Hill, D. L., Grubbs, C. J. (1982). Retinoids as chemopreventive and anticancer agents in intact animals (Review). *Anticancer Res. 2*:111.

Huggins, C., Lorvaine, G., Fukunishi, R. (1964). Aromatic influences on the yield for mammary cancer following administration of 7,12-dimethylbenzaanthracene. *Proc. Natl. Acad. Sci. USA 51*:737–742.

Levine, N., Meyskens, F. L. (1980). Topical Vitamin-A and therapy for cutaneous metastatic melanoma. *Lancet 2*:224–226.

Mackie, B. S., Mackie, L. E., Curtin, L. D., Bourne, D. J. (1987). Melanoma and dietary lipids. *Nutrition and Cancer 9*:219–226.

Mathews-Roth, M. M., Pathak, M. A., Fitzpatrick, T. B., et al. (1977). Beta-carotene therapy for erythropoietic protoporphyria and other photosensitivity diseases. *Arch. Dermatol. 113*:1229–1232.

Meyskens, F. L., Goodman, G. E., Alberts, D. S. (1985). 13-cis Retinoic acid: Pharmalcology, toxicology and clinical applications for the prevention and treatment of human cancer. *CRC Crit. Rev. Hematol. Oncol. 3*:75–101.

Micozzi, M. S., Boone, C. W., Kelloff, G. J., et al. (1985). Chemoprevention of cancer: Implications for clinical Pharmacology. *J. Clin. Pharmacol. 25*:164–175.

Mirvish, S. S., Cardesa, C., Wallcove, L., et al. Induction of mouse lung adenomas by amines or ureas plus nitrite and by N-nitroso compounds: Effect of ascorbate, gallic acid, thiocyanate and caffeine. *JNCI*

Peng, Y. M., Alberts, D. S., Xu, M. J., et al. (1986). Effects of high dietary retinyl palmitate and selenium on tissue distribution of retinoids in mice exposed to tumor initiation and promotion. *J. Nutr. Growth and Cancer* :33–40.

Schottenfeld, D., Fraumini, J. F. (Eds.) (1982). *Cancer Epidemiology and Revention*. Philadelphia, W. B. Saunders.

Yuspa, S. H., Harris, C. C. (1982). Molecular and cellular basis of chemical carcinogenesis. In Schottenfeld, D., Fraumini, J. F. (Eds.), *Cancer Epidemiology and Prevention*. Philadelphia, W. B. Saunders, pp. 23–43.

Zubrod, C. G., Schepartz, S., Leiter, J., et al. (1966). The Chemotherapy Program of the National Cancer Institute: History, analysis and plans. *Cancer Chemother. Rep. 50*:349–540.

16
Design of Prevention Trials

STEVEN PIANTADOSI* and DAVID P. BYAR
National Cancer Institute, National Institutes of Health, Bethesda, Maryland

INTRODUCTION

There is a significant biometric aspect to virtually every problem faced by investigators who wish to develop and test measures to prevent disease. The optimal solution for the biometric problems that arise in the evaluation of the efficacy of cancer prevention strategies is usually directly related to the proper design and conduct of comparative clinical trials. The purpose of this chapter is to outline the important principles of clinical trial design that contribute to valid inferences about the comparison of various preventive measures and estimation of the magnitude of preventive effects. The methodology of clinical trials is not a new science, but its use in cancer prevention is relatively recent. Consequently, there is a limited amount of experience among cancer experts with the special problems of applying clinical trials methodology to assessing preventive measures. In writing this chapter, we have assumed that investigators have decided to evaluate one or more promising cancer prevention strategies and need an overview of the basic principles of clinical trial design. We shall also point out how the design issues for some prevention trials differ substantially from those encountered in trials designed to compare treatments. Other important issues in cancer prevention such as the scientific basis for designing treatments, actual conduct of trials, analysis of results, and interpretation are discussed in other chapters of this book.

It is an unfortunate fact that flaws in the design of biomedical studies almost never lend themselves to correction by virtuous analyses. While poorly done analyses can be corrected, flaws in design most likely would require repeating an entire time-consuming and costly study or, worse yet, having to live with un-

**Current affiliation*: The Johns Hopkins Oncology Center, Baltimore, Maryland

acceptable ambiguities in the results. Because of the expense, both human and monetary, of conducting prevention studies and the potential impact of applying incorrect conclusions to a population, cancer prevention studies must be designed very carefully.

Many strategies have been used by clinical investigators to obtain evidence about the relative effectiveness of medical therapies. These strategies fall into two main categories: observational studies and designed experiments. The strongest evidence favoring a particular hypothesis comes from independent verification of results of designed experiments by more than one investigator. The process of drawing inferences from such independent studies that test the same general hypothesis has been termed "overview." Cancer prevention, a young science with few study results, cannot yet expect to profit greatly from overviews. Not only are few results available, but repetition of similar studies is unlikely.

Observational studies are those studies in which the investigators do not have control over the method by which treatment (or exposure to risk factors) is assigned to each study subject. Since people obtain their medical treatments (or environmental exposures) in a nonrandom fashion, observational studies can only hypothetically control for known prognostic factors and cannot control at all for unknown factors which otherwise render comparisons of groups invalid. Consequently, such studies cannot provide conclusive evidence of a lack of bias when estimating treatment effects and are unsuitable for testing the small but important differences likely due to different prevention strategies. Thus, designed experiments, or more specifically clinical trials, are the best method for providing evidence about the relative efficacy of cancer prevention strategies. The focus in this chapter is on the design of cancer prevention clinical trials. Fundamentals of sound clinical trials such as randomization, adequate sample size and power, and appropriate trial architecture are emphasized, as are problems likely to complicate the process of design. For additional information regarding broad aspects of clinical trials, the reader is referred to more general discussions (Bull, 1959; Armitage, 1975; Peto et al., 1976, 1977; Freidman, Furberg, and DeMets, 1981; Simon, 1982; Office of Technology Assessment, 1983; Pocock, 1983; Shapiro and Louis, 1983; Buyse, Staquet, and Sylvester, 1984; Meinert, 1986).

GENERAL CONCEPTS

Types of Prevention Studies

The various types of cancer prevention studies can be classified by the stages in the process of carcinogenesis where the preventive measures are assumed to act. Although the precise mechanism and time course of carcinogenesis is unknown for any form of cancer, epidemiologic evidence suggests that the process may take a considerable period of time for some cancers. For example, age at menarche is a known risk factor for breast cancer, but breast cancer is relatively uncommon before age 30. Cigarette smoking may begin at age 20, but lung cancer due to smoking may not appear until many years later. Animal experiments have established that there are at least two stages in the process of carcinogenesis: initiation and promotion. Epidemiologic evidence concerning certain putative causes of cancer support this idea as well. For example, if smokers quit smoking, after a few years their excess risk of lung cancer is frozen, demonstrating that continued smoking is "promoting" carcinogenesis. If smoking only initiated cancer, then stopping smoking would carry no benefit. The next step after promotion is the appearance of preneoplastic or in situ lesions. Finally, some of these lesions progress to frank cancer that may be diagnosed by pathological examination of the tissue in question. This process is represented by the horizontal line in Fig. 1. The vertical line crossing the horizontal line at the right of the figure represents the point in time when a precancerous lesion has progressed sufficiently to be diagnosed as cancer. The arrows above the line indicate schematically the places along this continuous process where preventive measures might be postulated to have their effects. This suggested classification of types of cancer prevention trials was first proposed by Bertram, Kolonel, and Meyskens (1987).

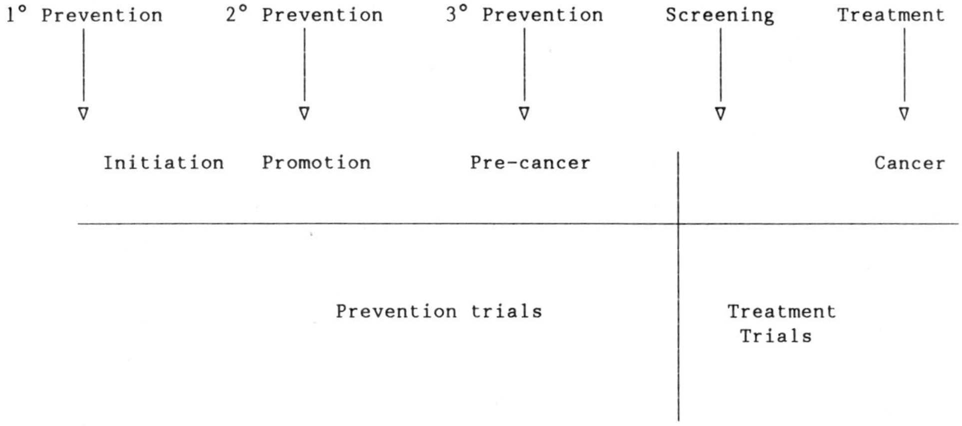

Figure 1 Schematic representation of carcinogenesis showing stages in the process where various preventive measures are presumed to act and where screening and treatment occur.

Primary prevention trials are designed to prevent initiation, and generally these trials would be expected to be the largest of all because the further we go to the left in the scheme of Fig. 1, the lower the risk of developing cancer. Examples of primary prevention might include discouraging teenagers from ever taking up tobacco use, the avoidance of sunlight or the use of blocking agents to prevent malignant melanoma and skin cancer, and possibly some dietary modifications. Secondary prevention attempts to remove or affect promoting factors. Examples might include smoking cessation, changes in diet, or the use of micronutrient or trace metal supplements. Tertiary prevention trials are those designed to test the effects of interventions on preneoplastic lesions such as leukoplakia in the mouth, cervical and esophageal dysplasia, or early skin cancers. Although studies of cancer screening are sometimes referred to as secondary prevention trials, this usage should be discouraged. They should simply be referred to as screening trials.

Phases or Research

Five phases of research in the context of cancer control have been discussed and can be applied directly to prevention. The types of studies are (I) hypothesis development, (II) methods development, (III) intervention trials, (IV) defined population studies, and (V) implementation (Greenwald and Cullen, 1985). In the pharmacologic or therapeutic model, only four phases of human studies are generally recognized by clinical investigators. These same phases apply conceptually to cancer prevention and can be extended to include an additional type of study (discussed below). The initial trials of pharmacologic agents in humans, phase I studies, are usually intended to obtain information on permissable doses and toxicity. This phase is relevant for cancer prevention using trace elements, drugs, or agents that could conceivably have toxicity but is not needed for studies testing the modification of lifestyle such as smoking cessation or dietary changes. In the pharmacological model, phase II studies attempt to estimate response rates when a chemotherapeutic agent is administered to subjects with various types of cancer. This phase of research generally applies only to tertiary cancer prevention studies where agents may be tried in small uncontrolled trials to determine whether or not they have any effect on preneoplastic lesions. The role of phase I and II studies in the process of evaluating some cancer-preventive strategies in humans has been supplemented by epidemiologic studies (e.g., the connection between certain cancers and dietary fat or the role of smoking as a cause of lung cancer). Phase III studies are generally designed to compare promising therapies to no treatment or a placebo, to standard treatment, or to each other. The methodology for designing and conducting phase III comparisons of cancer treatments translates directly to the issues in many cancer prevention trials. Phase IV studies are concerned primarily with long-term safety and efficacy (Food and Drug Administration, 1977). This idea is an important one to consider for the future of cancer prevention, since although most preventive agents are believed to have low toxicity, their administration to a large population will almost certainly result in some unanticipated effects in some subset of subjects. In cancer prevention and control, phase IV studies are termed "defined population studies" (Greenwald and Cullen, 1985) and are intended to measure the impact of an efficacious intervention in a defined population. Phase V studies apply interventions to a population at large and are intended to reduce cancer rates by a widespread application of proven methods.

Much attention has been devoted to the conduct of phase III studies, since they are usually very informative when properly done and are almost always very costly. In this chapter, we focus on the design of phase III studies because micronutrient interventions are currently being studied for efficacy. Only recently have major cancer prevention trials been planned and in only a few instances are early phase III results in humans available. In many ways, the methodological issues involved in designing these trials are quite similar to those for the more familiar cancer treatment trials. For example, the control of bias and adequate power against clinically important alternatives are clearly important in both types of studies. Many of the differences between the two type of trials relate to the vastly greater size and expense of prevention studies, which may be two orders of magnitude larger than those of treatment trials.

Differences Between Prevention and Treatment Trials

Some of the important respects in which prevention trials differ from treatment trials are listed in Table 1. The origin of ideas to be tested in treatment trials generally come from drug screening programs, basic research in surgery, radiation therapy, or immunology, or from animal experiments, but most ideas tested in cancer prevention arise from epidemiologic studies. These may be geographical comparisons or correlations, migrant studies, prospective follow-up studies, or case-control studies. Some ideas arise from animal experiments, but these studies are themselves often inspired by epidemiologic observations.

The kinds of interventions also differ between treatment and prevention trials. In treatment trials one is generally interested in chemotherapy, surgery, irradiation, or biological response modifiers, used singularly or in combination. All these treatments carry specific risks, which must be considered in the trial design. In prevention trials, the interventions are likely to be considerably less dangerous and quite different from those in treatment trials. For example, lifestyle changes such as smoking cessation, dietary alteration, or supplementation with micronutrients are more likely to be studied in prevention trials.

These differences in the kinds of interventions studied involve the participation of substantive experts from different areas. In treatment trials, the sub-

Table 1 Characteristics of Cancer Prevention Trials Compared to Cancer Treatment Trials

Characteristics	Phase III treatment trials	Phase III Primary and secondary prevention trials	Phase II and III tertiary prevention trials
1. Origin of ideas to be tested	• Drug screening • Basic research in surgery, radiation, and immunology • Animal experiments	• Epidemiologic studies • Animal experiments	• Epidemiologic studies • Animal experiments
2. Kind of interventions used	• Chemotherapy • Surgery • Surgery • Biologic response modifiers	• Lifestyle changes (e.g., smoking cessation, diet) • Micronutrients • Vitamins	• Micronutrients • Vitamins • Drugs
3. Kind of substantive expertise needed	• Oncologists • Surgeon • Radiotherapists • Immunotherapists	• Social psychologists • Nutrition experts	• Nutrition experts
4. Size	• Relatively small: 100-1,000 subjects per arm of study	• Large: thousands to millions of subjects per arm of study	• Small: 30-100 subjects per arm of study
5. Duration	• 3 months to 5 years	• 5-10 years	• 3 months to 2 years
6. Cost	• Hundreds of thousands of dollars	• Million to tens of millions of dollars	• Tens of thousands of dollars

stantive experts from different areas. In treatment trials, the substantive experts are likely to be oncologists, surgeons, radiotherapists, or immunotherapists, but in prevention trials they may be anthropologists, nutritional experts, social psychologists, and public health experts. Interventions to prevent cancer fall into two broad categories: avoidance and therapy or, as Peto has observed, things to be *proscribed* and things to be *prescribed* (Peto, personal communication, 1986).

The fourth way trials differ is in size. Treatment trials may be relatively small, that is, hundreds or thousands of patients per arm of the study, but primary and secondary prevention trials may involve thousands or even millions of subjects, the larger number corresponding to the cluster randomization of small cities as an extreme example. Tertiary prevention studies, to some extent playing the role of phase II studies in cancer prevention, may be quite small, involving only 30-100 subjects per arm of a typical study. The duration of treatment trials are frequently between three months and five years, but many primary and secondary prevention trials may require five to ten years of observation. Tertiary prevention trials can be quite short, typically in the range of three months to two years. Finally, a consequence of these differences is that the costs also differ. A typical treatment trial carried out by a cooperative group may cost hundreds of thousands of dollars, but primary and secondary prevention trials may cost millions or even tens of millions of dollars. Tertiary prevention trials can frequently be relatively inexpensive, costing merely tens of thousands of dollars for a single study. Although many exceptions can be found to the generalizations just presented, they are meant to provide a broad picture of the most typical and marked differences one might expect between prevention and treatment trials.

TERMINOLOGY

We have implicitly defined clinical trials in the introduction as planned experiments on human subjects. In practice, the term "clinical trial" is usually further qualified as randomized, controlled, double blind, or some combination. These terms imply that certain features to be discussed below have been incorporated into the study design. In order to discuss more precisely these and other aspects of trial design, we offer the following definitions or terms used in this chapter.

1. *Clinical trial*: A planned experiment in human subjects which attempts to provide information about feasibility, toxicity, or efficacy of an intervention or treatment.
2. *Design*: The process of or result of establishing the plan for a clinical trial which includes but is not limited to subject selection, control of bias, architecture, and sample size.

3. *Architecture*: The number of treatment arms and the allocation of treatments or interventions to the groups of a clinical trial.
4. *Sample size*: The number of subjects allocated to a trial.
5. *Bias*: Any differences between a true effect and the estimate of the true effect which cannot be attributed solely to chance.
6. *Randomization*: The process of assigning a subject to a treatment group entirely by chance.
7. *Null hypothesis*: The hypothesis of no difference between treatment or intervention effects.
8. *Alternative hypothesis*: A statement concerning the extent of difference(s) in the effect of two or more treatments or interventions as measured on some scale appropriate for the endpoint of interest.
9. *Size* (α-level): The probability of rejecting the null hypothesis when it is true, i.e., the probability of a type I error.
10. *Power*: The probability of rejecting the null hypothesis when an alternative hypothesis is assumed to be true. Power is one minus the probability, β, of a type II error.
11. *Protocol*: The written plan for the conduct of a clinical trial.
12. *Controls*: Generally, a group of subjects who receive no treatment or intervention, a placebo, or a standard therapy which is being compared to a new treatment or intervention.

These definitions are the same in the contexts of both prevention and treatment. The concept of trial architecture is termed "design" by some authors, but we have reserved the latter term for the broader aspects of trial planning.

IV. DESIGN PREREQUISITES

There are certain essentials in the design of good clinical studies, particularly phase III trials. These include an adequate demonstration of feasibility and a well-drafted study protocol. In the cancer treatment setting, phase II studies determine feasibility, but for primary and secondary prevention trials, a pilot study of another type may be necessary. The pilot study can aid in the determination of participation rates and thus can be valuable in the selection of trial architecture and study population. An example of such a pilot study is that conducted prior to the Physician's Health Study (Hennekens, 1984).

Another essential for good trial design is the study protocol. Many of the problems encountered in conducting clinical studies can be foreseen and avoided by carefully drafting the protocol. The protocol is the basic design blueprint for all aspects of the trial and should address specifically certain topics (see Table 2). The protocol is both a research plan and a patient management plan. Each section of the protocol must address both issues in a structured fashion. We now

Table 2 Important Protocol Contents

1.	Scientific rational
2.	Study objectives
3.	Selection of subjects
4.	Architecture
5.	Treatment of intervention Program
6.	Treating and reporting toxicity
7.	Collection of data
8.	Definition of endpoints
9.	Statistical considerations
10.	Informed consent
11.	References
12.	Data forms
13.	Study chairperson, list of investigators and institutions

discuss some specific features of those headings which are most relevant to the design of cancer prevention studies.

Objectives: Trial objectives should be relevant to the disease in question, e.g., the prevention of cancer incidence, and should be specific enough so as virtually to define the study endpoints and methods of evaluation. It is often said that approximate answers to the right questions are more useful than exact answers to the wrong questions. Following this dictum, objectives must be scientifically meaningful in addition to being attainable in practice. In reality, most studies will attempt to answer only one major question. Attempts to answer additional unplanned questions are frequently frustrated by inadequate statistical power, and reported significance levels from such analyses may be incorrect both because the questions may have been suggested by the data and because of the problem of multiple comparisons. In some cancer prevention trials, factorial designs might allow more than one question to be addressed in a single trial at only a modest increase in effort. Such designs are discussed in more detail below.

Subject Selection and Exclusion: Deciding which subjects to include in a trial is particularly important for cancer prevention studies as it can directly affect the generalizability of the results. It is a general principle in the therapeutic trials that patients should be excluded if the treatments under consideration pose additional risk to them. This principle is also important for cancer prevention trials because many strategies target healthy subjects, and even seemingly minor risks may have significant consequences in a large study population. While a study performed in a narrowly defined group of subjects may yield results that seem not be generalize clinically, they might more clearly answer a basic biological question because subjects have a more homogeneous prognosis and thus variability in responses will be reduced, increasing the statistical power to detect endpoint differences of any given size. If the result has basic biological implications, it will likely have wider applicability than just to the subjects studied. For example, a treatment that is shown to block promotion in heavy smokers could reasonably be expected to work in all smokers.

Another aspect of subject selection has importance for cancer prevention, namely that implied by noncompliance to assigned treatment or intervention. Subjects who are unlikely at the outset to complete the assigned therapy should generally be excluded. Subjects may fail to comply in treatment trials either because they are too well or too sick. In prevention studies, patients at higher or lower risk for the intended endpoint may fail to comply. For this reason, almost all clinical trial methodologists agree that analyses should be done according to treatment assigned (as opposed to treatment actually received), so as to minimize bias. Thus, subjects who fail to comply with the assigned treatment can dilute the comparison being made.

Endpoints: Cancer prevention endpoints are discussed in another chapter and are consequently only briefly mentioned here. Usually an implicit endpoint in cancer prevention is cancer incidence in population studies or diagnosis of cancer at the individual level. However, death due to cancer is an equally sensible endpoint and may be less subject to ascertainment bias. In tertiary prevention studies, regression of in situ cancer or other preneoplastic lesions may be appropriate endpoints. In studies designed to change risk factors already known or strongly believed to lead to cancer (e.g., smoking, diet), changes in these risk factors may serve as endpoints. In any case, endpoints must be meaningful, detectable, and clearly specified.

Study architecture: This is an interesting aspect of phase III cancer prevention studies and is an area in which such studies can differ from their therapeutic analogs. In particular, factorial designs are likely to be useful for prevention studies because of the need to evaluate multiple modalities such as vitamins, diet, and trace elements which can be administered simultaneously in their full dosages. Factorial designs are discussed below.

Treatment groups: The delineation of treatment groups also involves additional considerations in cancer prevention since the unit of intervention may be culturally or geographically defined groups of people rather than individuals. For example, planned smoking cessation intervention could lead to the random assignment of cities to two or more types of campaigns to stop smoking (as proposed in Community Intervention Trials for Smoking Cessation, 1986).

GENERAL METHODS FOR THE CONTROL OF BIAS

Bias is the bane of valid scientific inference. Cancer prevention studies are no different from their treatment analogs with regard to the desirability of bias control. Bias may affect inferences from a clinical study at the level of subject selection, treatment assignment, endpoint identification, or analysis. Statisticians have devoted a large amount of their collective effort to the elimination of bias in trial design and analysis while attempting to convince sometimes skeptical investigators that control of bias is an important goal. Historically, many important medical advances have been made without the need for the general methods of bias control discussed here (e.g., randomization and blinding). This is true because many therapeutic effects are large. For example, the efficacy of antibiotics and handwashing against infection and the role of cigarettes in causing lung cancer and cardiovascular disease were evident in spite of probable biases in the studies exposing them. However, the therapeutic efficacy of most cancer treatments and the hypothesized efficacy of most cancer prevention measures is not much larger than the biases that can enter poorly planned medical studies. Thus, the goal of reducing or eliminating bias is essential for accurately estimating treatment efficacy. Much has been written about the existence of various biases and the necessity of controlling them (e.g., Chalmers, 1983), so we will not discuss these general aspects further but proceed directly to a discussion of methods.

Concurrent Controls

In a planned clinical experiment, a group of subjects who receive either placebo therapy or the standard therapy are important as a basis for comparison. A controversial aspect of using a control group relates to using historical controls (i.e., a control group reported in a previous study) versus using concurrent controls. The motivation for using historical controls is twofold: there is no ethical dilemma when all subjects in a trial are given a promising therapy, and only one treatment must be evaluated resulting in greater efficiency (Gehan and Freireich, 1974). In practice, these advantages are usually outweighed by the greater advantages of a concurrent control group. In particular, although controls and treated subjects may not differ greatly with respect to known prognostic factors, only randomization (which implies concurrent controls) can assure comparability with respect to unknown factors as well. In addition, trends in medical care that are hard to quantify such as improving supportive therapy (fluids, antibiotics) make attributing differences solely to the new treatment a questionable practice unless controls are concurrent (Byar et al., 1976; Byar, 1980). The evaluation of cancer-preventive treatments illustrates another problem with historical controls: the incidence of the disease during the interval between the two groups may change appreciably due to factors that cannot be controlled in the comparison. This effect is illustrated by the changing pattern of cancer incidence in the United States that is not explained by age, sex, and race (Page and Asire, 1985). Thus, the use of concurrent controls is an important factor in the reduction of bias.

Randomization

Randomization is a cornerstone of bias reduction. As defined above, randomization guarantees that subjects in a clinical trial are assigned to treatment groups without bias and therefore allows treatment comparisons to estimate true differences in treatment efficacy. Such a guarantee enhances the credibility of the trial in the eyes of scientific investigators. Moreover, from a statistical point of view, randomization assures the correctness of the α-level (type I error). Although the intended probability of a type I error is controlled by the data analyst through the choice of statistical procedures, the true probability of this error may not be the value intended when randomization is not employed. Succinctly stated, randomization allows a statistical justification of the significance test.

A second justification for randomization is that it reduces the probability that treatment groups will differ with respect to important prognostic measures, both known and unknown. If the investigators have failed in their design or analysis to account completely for subject characteristics that strongly affect outcome, randomization assures that comparisons are nevertheless valid. Following Lachin (1982), the probability, p, that randomly chosen groups will differ by more than a specified amount can be calculated. If δ is the difference of the frequencies in the two groups, then the variance of δ based on binomial probabilities is $\sigma^2 = 2\theta(1 - \theta)/n$, where θ is the prevalence of the characteristic and n is the group size. Using the normal approximation to the binomial,

$$p = 2[1 - \Phi(\delta/\sigma)]$$

where Φ is the cumulative normal distribution function. For example, if a condition has a frequency of $\theta = 0.20$, then the probability of two randomly assigned groups of size $n = 100$ differing by more than $\pm\delta = 0.10$ is 0.08. Thus, even infrequently occurring factors are unlikely to be severely imbalanced in large groups.

A third reason for randomization is that it facilitates the use of blinding, which is another important bias-reducing technique discussed below. Although randomization may be performed without blinding, the two procedures can often be implemented simultaneously to reduce bias.

Some investigators have difficulty accepting the real and imagined ethical problems associated with the random assignment of subjects to treatment (Schafer, 1982). Physicians often feel that it is their responsibility to form opinions about the benefits of therapies, and coupled with their ethical role as advocates for the individual patient, the idea of assigning treatment to patients randomly is unacceptable. Indeed, it is true that much information about the possible efficacy of a new treatment is available before it is considered for human trials. However, in the face of considerable uncertainty that motivates a clinical trial, many physicians and patients do not perceive ethical difficulties with randomization. A recommendation to a patient based on substandard scientific evidence is presumably less ethical than randomization.

Unrestricted randomization is seldom used in clinical trials because some imbalances in treatment groups can occur. Rather, randomization is frequently "blocked," meaning that exact balance of treatment assignments is required at the end of predetermined groups or blocks of subjects. The size of the groups at which exact balance is achieved are multiples of the block size, and imbalances within a block never exceed one half the block size. Although this necessitates the nonrandom assignment of some of the subjects in a given block, provided the block size is large enough (e.g., eight subjects per block), the resulting treatment assignments are virtually random and never severely unbalanced. While smaller block sizes guarantee more perfect balance, they are also less random and allow the possibility that investigators will figure out the assignment scheme and select subjects preferentially for one or the other and thus introduce uncontrollable bias.

Another modification to pure randomization frequently used is stratification. Variables that influence response can be used to define strata, so that blocked randomization can be performed separately within each stratum. This porcedure ensures that treatment groups are comparable with respect to important prognostic factors and slightly increases statistical efficiency (Green and Byar, 1978; Palta, 1985). Among methodologists, the use of stratified randomization is not universally endorsed (Peto et al., 1976) since adjusted analyses can account for imbalances in important prognostic factors in the treatment groups. However, stratified randomization seems to have few serious drawbacks and is likely to make study results more convincing (Brown, 1980). Other methods besides randomization have been proposed for the allocation of treatments to subjects in a clinical trial. These methods generally involve stronger assumptions about the sequence of subject entry than does unrestricted, blocked, or stratified randomization (Taves, 1974). For example, if subjects are assumed to enter a study in a random fashion unrelated to prognosis, then certain deterministic allocation schemes would be statistically justifiable. However, most investigators prefer to have control over the process of randomization rather than leaving it to chance! These alternative methods have not yet been widely applied to cancer prevention (1979).

This discussion of randomization has pertained primarily to phase III studies since they attempt to assess treatment efficacy in a comparative setting. However, randomization may be used to control bias in phase II studies as well as in situations where several treatments are to be studied in the same population of subjects. Randomization of subjects to one of several protocols can be used to assure that systematic subject selection does not influence the observed rates. Thus, in the event of large observed differences, the most promising treatment can be selected for phase III investigations with less concern about bias.

Blinding

Blinding, or masking, refers to the situation in which subjects are unaware of which of two or more treatments they are receiving. The terminology is extended to "double blind" in those cases where the investigators are also blinded. In many situations, it is sensible for the trial monitoring committee to be blinded in addition to the subjects and investigators. This situation is termed "triple blinding" (Meinert, 1986) and allows any decisions about early termination, because of treatment differences or toxicity, to be made without regard for investigator bias. In addition, interim analyses by treatment groups, coded or otherwise, should not be available outside the monitoring committee since awareness of a treatment difference in any direction may influence investigators (O'Fallon, 1985). Blinding is particularly important in those situations where an endpoint requires subjective assessment by patients or investigators (e.g., certain toxicities or quality of life). For example, subjects and physicians who are aware of the treatment assignment might differentially report severity of symptoms according to their beliefs about the treatments. Subtler forms of bias could arise even when objective endpoints such as cancer incidence or death are used. The proper design of cancer prevention trials, as for all clinical trials, should include objectively defined endpoints, but blinding whenever possible is a sound practice.

Methods for employing blinding in a clinical trial are not usually complicated. They may be as simple as ensuring that medications given to all groups are identical in appearance and that those responsible for administering or distributing medication as well as the subjects are not aware of individual treatment assignments. For some cancer-preventive strategies such as dietary modification blinding is not possible. In this and similar cases, investigators must rely on the use of objectively determined endpoints to minimize bias.

SPECIAL DESIGNS APPROPRIATE FOR PREVENTION TRIALS

Factorial Designs

The term factorial design is used to describe an experiment where the effect of two or more factors, each having at least two levels so that differential effects can be observed, are studied simultaneously. The simplest such design is the 2 X 2 factorial, where the two levels of each factor might refer to the presence or absence of treatment A and the presence or absence of treatment B. Such a design is illustrated in Fig. 2. This design is in fact being used in the Physician's Health Study (Hennekens and Eberlein, 1985; Stampfer et al., 1985). The four treatment groups are; placebo + placebo, aspirin + placebo, placebo + β-carotene, and aspirin + β-carotene. In fact, the subjects take aspirin or aspirin placebo every other day and take β-carotene or β-carotene placebo on the intervening days. More complicated factorial designs result from studying more than two treatments or if any single treatment is given at more than two dosage levels. For example, a 2^3 factorial design would result from studying three treatments simultaneously and would involve eight treatment combinations: none of the treatments (or placebo for all three treatments), each treatment one at a time, all pairs of treatment, and finally all three treatments administered together. In the absence of important interactions between treatments, these designs can be quite efficient compared to studying each treatment separately.

For factorial designs studying four or more treatments, the number of treatment groups may become unmanageably large, posing logistical problems in drug formulation and distribution. An alternative approach is to use what are referred to as fractional factorial designs in which only certain of the 2^n possible treatment combination are studied. For example, if four treatments were under study, a half fractional factorial design would study only eight treatment combinations rather than the full 2^4 = 16. Exactly such a design is

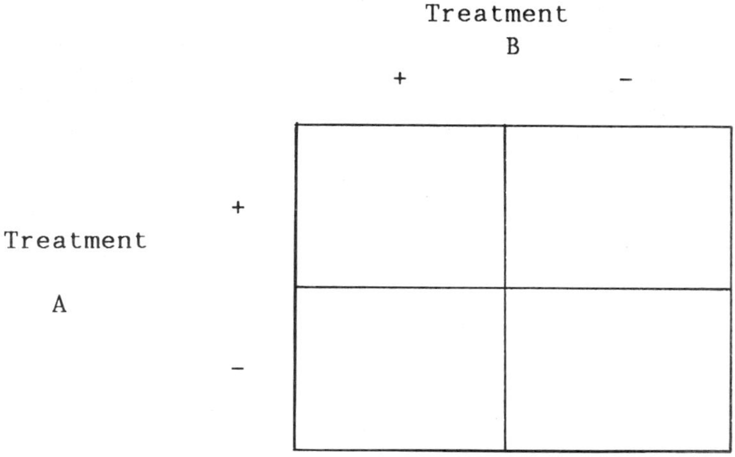

Figure 2 A 2 X 2 factorial design.

being used in an intervention study involving some 30,000 subjects in Linxian province in China in an attempt to prevent esophageal cancer (Blot and Li, 1985). In that part of north central China, as many as one in four persons in some communes dies of this neoplasm. In this study, each of the four factors is itself a combination of nutrients. In particular, factor A consists of retinol, β-carotene, and zinc, factor B of riboflavin and niacin, factor C of ascorbic acid and molybdenum, and factor D is vitamin E plus selenium. This list of vitamins and minerals is comprised of those for which there was some suspicion, usually based on biochemical evidence, of deficiency among the Linxian population.

Factorial designs should be considered whenever investigators are interested in studying more than one treatment and the treatments can be administered simultaneously at full dosage without prohibitive toxicity. It is generally considered desirable in addition that the actions of the treatment be different and that interactions between the treatments are likely to be unimportant. However, in situations where interactions are of special interest, factorial designs are also appropriate, although sample sizes must be increased relative to the design of trials simply aimed at detecting main effects of separate factors because the power of such trials to detect treatment interactions is reduced by the smaller number of subjects in each treatment group. Of course, separate trials for each treatment are of no value whatsoever in evaluating interactions.

We have written an article for the general medical audience explaining some of the features of factorial designs (Byar and Piantadosi, 1985). Stampfer et al. have discussed the 2 × 2 factorial design and its application in the aspirin β-carotene study alluded to above (Stampfer et al., 1985). Blot and Li, in discussing the nutrition intervention trials in Linxian province, have discussed fractional factorial designs and presented some interesting power calculations comparing the 2 × 2 factorial design with an alternate two-group design in which one group is given placebo and the other is given all four factors at once. In fact, they are using the two-group design in another smaller cancer prevention study in Linxian province targeting subjects who already have esophageal dysplasia. They note that in the presence of certain interactions the factorial design can be less powerful than the two-group design, but that the factorial design gives specific information about which factor(s) are responsible for any effects observed as well as information about interactions, neither of which are available in the alternative two-group design.

Cluster Randomization

As noted above in the section on randomization, in some instances it may be more efficient or more pertinent to randomize groups rather than individuals. Certain interventions such as a media campaign to discourage smoking may naturally target a population or group rather than an individual. Modification of diets for families or health education programs in factories provide other examples. Although the use of groups rather than individuals as the unit observation has been commonplace in fields such as educational evaluation, there are few examples in the medical area. However, a successful trial randomizing factories in Belgium to test measures for preventing coronary heart disease has been reported (Kornitzer et al., 1983), and the National Cancer Institute is planning to randomize 11 pairs of cities with populations between 50-150,000 to assess measures designed to encourage smoking cessation. We have heard of another trial being conducted in Russia to evaluate breast self-examination where the units of randomization are 32 polyclinics in Leningrad and 100 factories in Moscow.

In some situations cluster randomization may allow impressive reductions in costs compared to trials where individuals are randomized when that is a possibility. For example, if incidence of cancer were an endpoint, location of such randomized groups in areas already having incidence monitoring registries would provide a convenient method for determining the appropriate aggregate endpoints. Other economies might result from the ability to deliver the intervention more efficiently to groups rather than to individuals. Careful consideration should be given to using such innovative designs whenever possible instead of falling into the easy habit of considering intervention trials to be nothing more than very large treatment trials.

Case-Cohort Approach

Prentice has proposed a case-cohort design which may be used to save money in primary and secondary prevention studies (Prentice, 1986). He notes that because the rate of disease occurrence in such studies is typically quite low, much covariate information on disease-free subjects is largely redundant. Substantial costs in such studies might relate to performing biochemical measurements or hand-coding individual diet records for tens of thousands of subjects at baseline as well as throughout the duration of the trial in order to monitor compliance. He proposes instead that a random subcohort, possibly stratified, be identified at baseline. The biological samples or diet information, for example, would be collected for all subjects, but analysis of the samples or coding of the records would only be done for those in the random subcohort as well as for all cases as they develop. This approach is to be distinguished from the so-called synthetic retrospective study (Mantel, 1973; Liddell, McDonald, and Thomas, 1977), also called a "case-control within cohort design," in which controls are identified for each case retrospectively from among all subjects at risk when each case develops.

One problem with the synthetic retrospective study is that different controls need to be selected for each disease endpoint one wishes to analyze. Another difference is that the synthetic retrospective approach does not provide a basis for covariate monitoring during the course of followup as does the case-cohort approach. Finally, in a broad range of circumstances one might expect greater statistical efficiency from the case-cohort approach than from the synthetic retrospective approach because controls may properly serve as a member of the comparison group for cases occurring at various points in time.

Although this method is new and has not been used extensively to our knowlege, its distinct advantages recommend it as an important design to consider for large-scale cancer prevention studies. In fact, it was planned to use this approach in the Women's Health Trial, a secondary prevention trial intended to involve some 30,000 or more women at risk for breast cancer in which the intervention consists of eating a low fat diet. The principal method for monitoring the diet is the four-day food record compiled periodically by each participant. Substantial costs are involved in coding these records because even with computer-assisted coding scheme, about two hours of coder time is required for each subject's record. Adequate monitoring of compliance in groups can be obtained using only a 10% sample, although all participants would complete the diet records.

SAMPLE SIZE AND POWER

Introduction

A major component of any sample size estimate for a clinical trial is educated guesswork. This is true since the precise values for important parameters like event rates and accrual rates are not known beforehand. A second and equally important component in the process of trial design is a dialogue between the methodologist and the clinician which focuses on the smallest clinically important difference that the study intends to detect reliably. Inaccurate guesses for event rates could lead to underestimates of the sample size leading to low power. Similarly, poor understanding between the clinical and statistical investigators about the desirable magnitude of differences that can be detected as significant can also cause underestimates of the sample size and loss of power.

Many clinical trials employ sample sizes that are inadequate to meet reliably the objectives of the study (Freiman et al., 1978). In statistical terms, such trials have low power, that is, a high probability of type II error. It is also possible for even a properly designed trial to have incorrect significance levels or a high probability of type I error if inappropriate statistical methods are used in the analysis. However, improper analyses can be corrected, whereas inadequate sample sizes cannot and usually result in permanent ambiguity about negative findings.

If we assume, as is probably the case, the true cancer treatment advances are uncommon, then the majority of clinical trials are truly negative. However, because of the probability of a type I error, say $\alpha = 0.05$, some trials will incorrectly report a "significant" difference. Since many trials have insufficient power to distinguish treatment differences when they exist, many positive findings in the medical literature must be false positives. This effect can be quantified using Bayes theorem (Bayes, 1763; Kendall and Stuart, 1963), which, in this circumstance, relates the probability of a true treatment advance given a positive trial outcome to the probability of type I and type II errors. This discussion of the problem is somewhat simplistic since we assume a fixed probability of a true treatment effect when we should refer to a treatment effect of a certain size or greater. Furthermore, all trials will have a high power against some alternative, whereas we assume they have modest power against alternatives of importance. However, the simplified approach illustrates some points made by others (Peto et al., 1976; Pocock, 1982). Specifically, Bayes theorem states that

$$P(A|S) = \frac{P(S|A)P(A)}{P(S|A)P(A) + P(S|A^{-})P(A^{-})}$$

where the left-hand side is the probability of a true statement advance given a positive (significant) trial result, $P(S|A)$ is the probability of a positive trial result given that the treatment is truly better, $P(S|A^{-})$ is the probability of a positive trial result given that the treatment is ineffective, $P(A)$ is the unconditional probability of finding an effective treatment, and $P(A^{-}) = 1 - P(A)$. Substituting $\alpha = P(S|A^{-})$, $1 - \beta = P(S|A)$, and $\theta = P(A)$, we obtain

$$Pr(A|S) = (1 - \beta)\theta/((1 - \beta)\theta + \alpha(1 - \theta))$$

where $1 - \beta$ is the power of a trial. If we assume that the power of a trial is 0.5, $\alpha = 0.05$, and θ, the true probability of finding a treatment advance, is 0.10, then $P(A|S) = 0.53$, that is, almost half of reported positive results are false positives. However, if the power of the trials were 0.90, and all other parameters were the same, then $P(A|S) = 0.67$, a substantial increase, even if still somewhat unsettling. Even very high values for power are not sufficient to raise the true positive rate greatly unless θ can be increased also, for example, by extensive preliminary evaluation to raise the likelihood that those treatments tested in phase III trials are really beneficial. However, this latter strategy seems unlikely to be adopted since it could amount to repeated phase III testing. Thus, the only feasible option if we wish to avoid drawing incorrect conclusions too frequently is to design trials with high power.

It is probably not often sensible to design a clinical trial with a power less than 0.5, because this would mean that the probability of missing a clinically important difference would exceed that of finding it. From some viewpoints, low power trials can be justified (Baker and Heidenberger, 1987), but negative results remain uninterpretable. Apart from this issue, it is a waste of scientific resources to do inconclusive trials. A negative result in a trial with high power against an important clinical alternative is as informative as a positive result. Even ignoring the financial resources needed, cancer prevention trials will probably be lengthy studies with little hope of replication, and the consequences of incorrect conclusions will be magnified by the size of the populations to which positive or negative results will be applied. The significance level and power to employ in cancer prevention studies should depend upon the consequences of making type I and type II errors. When trying to prevent a common disease with relatively nontoxic agents such as vitamins, trace elements, or diet, the consequences of a type II error may greatly exceed those of a type I error. Thus, the customary 80 or 90% power and the 5% significance level may not be entirely appropriate for all cancer prevention studies. With these justifications for the proper design of such studies, we will discuss some of the important statistical considerations for determining sample size.

It is really only possible to design a trial with respect to a single endpoint, although investigators may have several questions in mind. Phase III clinical trials usually seek to compare either proportions of subjects meeting certain criteria (i.e., the probability of an event in a specified period of time) or the average time to the occurrence of an event (i.e., survival analysis). In cancer prevention trials where the incidence rate of cancer is relatively low in a healthy population, compared with, say, the death rate in subjects who already have the disease as in a therapeutic trial, the two approaches to sample size determination will yield similar results. However, both approaches are common and we will briefly discuss each.

Ideally, the sample size calculation should incorporate the same statistic that will eventually be used to test the data. However, some useful statistics lead to sample size equations which are too complicated to be of use. Consequently, sample sizes are often determined under the assumption of simpler parametric models and then verified to be approximately correct in more general settings. Sample sizes will also be affected by the decision to design for one-sided or two-sided hypothesis tests. One-sided tests require smaller sample sizes for a fixed significance level. Since the use of one-sided tests involves stronger assumptions about the treatments, two-sided tests should generally be employed unless the assumptions can be justified thoroughly. For example, a one-sided test might be appropriate for testing the effect of smoking cessation on lung cancer incidence but would not be appropriate when testing the effect of trace elements that could increase the incidence of some cancers.

Sample Size Calculation in Phase II Studies

Phase II studies in humans are generally noncomparative. Depending on the role of the phase II investigation in a larger scheme of research, different methods of estimating the required sample size may be used (Fleming, 1982; Whitehead, 1985, 1986; Herson and Carter, 1986). The simplified approach outlined here assumes that the goal of a phase II study is to estimate a response rate of some type in a population. In this case, sample size can be determined from the desired precision in the estimate of the response. For example, suppose the response of interest is the mean, μ, of some value in the population with a known variance σ^2. Then for large enough values of n, the total sample size, $\hat{\mu}$, the estimate of μ based on the sample is normally distributed with mean μ and variance σ^2/n. A 95% confidence limit on $\hat{\mu}$ is

$$\hat{\mu} \pm 1.96\sigma/\sqrt{n}$$

If a precision of $\pm x$ is desired in this confidence interval, the required sample size is

$$n = (1.96\sigma/x)^2$$

Frequently, we estimate the proportion of subjects who have a dichotomous response (e.g., regression by some criteria of a precancerous lesion). If the responses have a binomial distribution, the probability of a response is estimated by $p = r/n$, where r is the number responding out of n subjects, and the variance of p is $p(1 - p)/n$. Using the normal approximation to the binomial, we may substitute into the formula above to obtain

$$n = p(1 - p)(1.96/x)^2$$

The variance of p is largest for $p = 0.5$, and in the absence of knowledge about the true value of p, sample sizes based on $p = 0.5$ are slightly conservative but not very different for $0.2 \leqslant p \leqslant 0.8$. In circumstances where the normal approximation is not valid (e.g., extreme values for p), the sample size for proportions may be determined numerically from the binomial distribution.

Sample Size Calculation in Comparative Studies

For comparative cancer prevention trials, the difficult aspects of sample size determination arise early in the planning when one tries to estimate the event rates in the study population or, equivalently, when trying to identify a suitable study group based on expected event rates. The number or proability of events in the study population is a function of many factors including the length of accrual and followup, the baseline cancer or endpoint incidence, and the distribution of risk factors. In addition, in lengthy studies one must consider competing risks like death due to cardiovascular disease. Other complicating factors such as patient compliance and time-varying hazard rates must also be considered.

The discussion which follows temporarily neglects these considerations in order to present some useful and relatively simple formulas for sample size which are widely used. Following this, we discuss briefly some considerations in estimating event probabilities.

Continuous Response Measures

For comparing two normally distributed response variables r_1 and r_2, the usual test statistic is

$$Z = (r_1 - r_2)/\sqrt{\text{Var}(r_1 - r_2)}$$

If a response variable has means μ_1 and μ_2 in two groups and a common variance σ^2, then the sample means will have variance σ^2/n and

$$Z = \sqrt{n}(\hat{\mu}_1 - \hat{\mu}_2)/\sqrt{2}\sigma$$

where n is the sample size in each group. This statistic leads to a useful formula for sample size determination when comparing normally distributed responses,

$$n = 2(Z_\alpha + Z_\beta)^2\sigma^2/\delta^2 \tag{1}$$

where Z_α and Z_β are the standard normal quantiles for size and power, δ is the difference to detect with power $1 - \beta$, and n is the required sample size in each group (Snedecor and Cochran, 1980). Many equations for sample size determination are generalizations of this equation. For example, in comparative trials with time-to-event endpoints, a similar approach may be used. If event times are exponentially distributed and Δ is the hazard ratio, then the logarithm of Δ is approximately normally distributed with variance $\sigma^2 = 1/d_1 + 1/d_2$, where d_1 and d_2 are the numbers of events in the two groups. The equation analogous to (1) is

$$(1/d_1 + 1/d_2)^{-1} = (Z_\alpha + Z_\beta)^2/\log^2\Delta \tag{2}$$

When d_1 and d_2 are approximately equal, (2) becomes

$$n = 2(Z_\alpha + Z_\beta)^2/\log^2\Delta$$

which is a sample size formula due to George and Desu (1974). Equation (2) can be generalized to allow for both a followup period after accrual terminates and for loss to followup, as shown by Rubinstein, Gail, and Santner (1981). Under these additional assumptions, d_1 and d_2 can be replaced by their expectations to yield the sample size in one group

$$n_1 = \frac{(Z_\alpha + Z_\beta)^2}{\log^2\Delta} \sum_{i=1}^{2} (2(\lambda_i^*)^2/\lambda_i(1 + s))(\lambda_i^*T - e^{-\lambda_i^*\tau}(1 - e^{-\lambda_i^*T}))^{-1} \tag{3}$$

where λ_i denotes the event rate in group i, T the duration of subject accrual, τ the length of additional followup, and $\lambda_i^* = \lambda_i + \phi$ where ϕ is the loss to followup rate. Equation (3) is slightly more general than that presented in the reference, since it allows for differential allocation of subjects to the treatment groups where $s = n_2/n_1$. Although Equation (3) was derived under the assumption of exponential survival times, it results in sample sizes which are approximately valid for Weibull distributed survival times provided the shape parameter is between 0.3 and 3. In addition, although Equation (3) was derived using the "exponential maximum likelihood estimate" test, the sample sizes are approximately valid for the logrank test as well (Rubinstein, Gail, and Santner, 1981). There are also more direct methods for sample size using the logrank statistic (Freedman, 1982).

Dichotomous Response Measures

When event rates are low, there is little benefit to designing the trial in terms of time to event. In this situation, a dichotomous endpoint approach yields approximately the same results (Gail, 1985). Moreover, in some studies, the response of interest is the proportion of subjects in each group who have a dichotomous endpoint such as the occurrence or nonoccurrence of cancer in a 10-year period. Such endpoints are often called "t-year event rates," but actually are proportions rather than rates. Nevertheless, a frequently used test statistic for binary responses is

$$Z = (p_1 - p_2)(P(1 - P)(1/n_1 + 1/n_2))^{-1/2}$$

where p_1 and p_2 are the proportion responding in each group, n_1 and n_2 are the numbers of subjects in each group, and $P = (p_1 n_1 + p_2 n_2)/(n_1 + n_2)$. This statistic has the standard normal distribution for large values of n_1 and n_2. Sample size requirements for the comparison of two proportions using this test statistic have been derived by Fleiss (1981) and have been extended to unequal allocation of subjects to the treatment groups by Fleiss, Tytun, and Ury (1980). The formula is

$$n_1 = [Z_\alpha\sqrt{[(s + 1)P(1 - P)]} + Z_\beta\sqrt{[sp_1(1 - p_1) + p_2(1 - p_2)]}\,]^2/(s\delta^2) \qquad (4)$$

where s is the allocation ratio, $P = (p_1 + sp_2)/(s + 1)$, δ is the difference we wish to detect, and the other parameters are as above. This formula may be modified for relative risks instead of proportions and generalized to include equivalence type designs which attempt to show no difference between treatment groups. A thorough review of such formulae is given in Donner (1984). Provided that accrual is short compared to the followup period, this results in very similar sample sizes to Equation (2).

These sample size formulas quantify some important insights into trial design. First, the "information" in a trial is a function of the number of observed events rather than the total number of subjects studied. Applying this concept to cancer prevention trials we see that studies in high risk populations will have greater statistical power for a fixed total sample size. However, one must weigh the cost of finding and recruiting high risk subjects versus that of studying a larger sample of more easily obtained subjects. If the number of subjects is limited, power can be increased by extending the period of followup after accrual terminates so that events in the study population will continue to be observed. Although this approach prolongs the trial it may be the only way to correct for lower than planned accrual or event rates. This latter problem is common since subects enrolled in a clinical trial frequently have event rates lower than the target population.

Estimating Event Rates

As mentioned earlier, an essential prerequisite for sample size calculation is some estimate of expected event rates in the study population. This procedure can be complex since many factors must be considered. As an example, consider the hazard of developing cancer during a study of length d years. We denote the hazard by λ and it is a function of time, t, age at study entry, t_e, and possibly several other baseline factors denoted by the vector z. The risk of dying from a competing cause, denoted by γ, is also a function of t, t_e, and z. Similarly, the probability of developing cancer during the study, p, is a function of d, t_e, and z. The quantities p, λ, and γ can be related by the equation (Prentice and Self, 1986),

$$p(d,t_e,z) = \int_{t_e}^{t_e+d} \lambda(s;t_e,z) \exp[-\int_{t_e}^{s} (\lambda(u;t_e,z) + \gamma(u;t_e,z)du] ds$$

which states that for each time point, s, in the study, we estimate the probability of surviving the competing risk and developing cancer at s. Both probability distributions are assumed to be exponential. The determination of λ and γ to use in such an equation can be aided by a suitable analysis of observational studies. This formula could be generalized to allow for censoring.

Selecting a high risk population in which to conduct a trial requires screening a larger population for baseline prognostic factors. In cancer prevention, prognostic factors may be as simple as age since the incidence of many cancers increases rapidly with age, or more complicated such as the presence of biochemical markers or a history of factors associated with increased risk. In this regard, observaional studies may assist in identifying high risk populations in which to conduct prevention trials (Byar, 1984).

Sample Size Calculations for Cluster Randomization

If groups rather than individuals are randomized, the approaches to sample size calculation outlined above must be modified. Methods for doing so have outlined by Donner, Birkett, and Buck (1981) and are summarized here. Here again, we distinguish between continuous response measures and dichotomous endpoints.

Comparison of Means

We assume that each of two treatment groups consists of k subgroups of n individuals, and that a response variable in each group is normally distributed with an unknown common variance σ^2. The purpose of the study is to compare the underlying means of the two groups using the sample means, $\hat{\mu}_1$ and $\hat{\mu}_2$, computed in the usual fashion on the individuals. The variance of each mean is (Moser and Kalton, 1972)

$$\mathrm{Var}(\hat{\mu}_2) = \mathrm{Var}(\hat{\mu}_1) = \sigma^2(1 + (n - 1)\rho/nk$$

where ρ is the intraclass correlation. The quantity ρ is the ratio of the between group variance to the total variance and can be understood as the correlation between any randomly selected pair of responses within a subgroup. This formula reduces to the usual variance when n = 1. Using this expression, the variance of $\hat{\mu}_1 - \hat{\mu}_2$ can be calculated and substituted into the general sample size Equation (1) to obtain

$$n^* = 2(Z_\alpha + Z_\beta)^2\sigma^2(1 + (n - 2)\rho/\delta^2 \qquad (5)$$

where n* is the total size of each group and the other parameters are as above.

Comparison of Proportions

The sample size equation for the comparison of proportions is analogous to that for means. It depends upon a parameter κ which is a measure of intracluster dependence. When $\kappa = 0$, the members of a cluster are independent, and when $\kappa = 1$, the cluster behaves like a single individual (Cohen, 1960; Altham, 1976). The variance of the proportion responding in each group is

$$\mathrm{Var}(P) = P(1 - P)(1 + (n - 1)\kappa)/nk$$

where P is the overall proportion of responses in the study. Using this variance, tee sample size equation analogous to Equation (4) with equal group sizes becomes

$$n^* = (Z_\alpha + Z_\beta)^2(p_1(1 - p_1) + p_2(1 - p_2))(1 + (n - 1)\kappa)/(p_1 - p_2)^2 \qquad (6)$$

where n* is the sample size in each group.

Adjusting Sample Size for Complicating Factors

Real clinical trials differ from the idealizations on which sample size calculations are based in that almost invariably some factors reduce the ability to observe differences between groups. Such factors include censoring, subject noncompliance, pre-existing cases of disease when incidence is the endpoint, or delayed treatment effectiveness. Whenever possible, these effects should be anticipated and taken into account when estimating sample size or the power of the trial will be reduced. This is particularly important for cancer prevention trials (Moon, 1986).

In time-to-event studies, some subjects are lost to followup during the trial, and consequently their event times, (if events occurs) are not known (type I censoring). Instead, the subjects are known to be event-free up to the censoring time. Similarly, at the close of the study, some observations are censored (administrative or type II censoring) since the followup time is insufficient to observe all events. The effect of censoring is to reduce the amount of information. Thus, in time to event studies, censoring should be anticipated and the sample size should be estimated accordingly.

Another complication occurs when subjects allocated to a particular treatment fail to receive the intended treatment. The long duration of cancer prevention studies may increase problems with compliance. For example, in dietary modification studies, subjects may eventually adjust their prescribed diet because they have difficulty forming permanent new eating habits, or they may become aware of the risks of certain foods and avoid them. Such noncompliance dilutes any difference between treatment groups and therefore reduces statistical power. For example, suppose some fraction, f, of subjects in a treatment group with true response rate p_1 fail to comply with the regimen and consequently have responses, p_2, like the control group. The overall response rate in the treatment group is then

$$p^* = p_1(1 - f) + p_2 f$$

which is a weighted average of the two response rates. Consequently, the overall response rate in the treatment group will lie between the true response rates and the group differences will be diminished. Under this circumstance, the sample size is inflated by a factor of approximately $(1 - f)^2$ (Zelen, 1979). This is true because subjects must be analyzed as part of the treatment group to which they were originally randomized in order to avoid the potentially serious biases which can result if comparisons are made between groups selected, in part, by the subjects themselves or their physicians. A concise way of stating this is that clinical trials are tests of treatment policy rather than tests of the treatments themselves. The term "policy" indicates that investigators intend to administer treatments to groups of subjects but cannot guarantee that some factors will not interfere with completing therapy in particular cases.

In cancer prevention, the problem of pre-existing or prevalent cases causes similar effects (Patterson, 1987). If two treatment groups contain some subjects who will shortly develop cancer because, for example, they already had occult disease at the study outset, then the effect of prevention on the remaining subjects will be diluted by the prevalent cases. Among the subjects with occult cancers, the response rate is 1.0. Using the equation above where now f is the fraction of prevalent cases, the overall response rate in group 1 is

$$p_1^* = p_1(1 - f) + f$$

and similarly for group 2. Thus the difference in overall response rates between the two groups is reduced by the factor $1 - f$, that is $p_1^* - p_2^* = (p_1 - p_2)(1 - f)$. The effect on the estimate of relative risk, p_1^*/p_2^*, may be more serious. For example, suppose $f = 0.1$, $p_1 = 0.1$, and $p_2 = 0.2$. The $p_1^* - p_2^* = 0.09$ compared to $p_1 - p_2 = 0.1$. However, $p_1^*/p_2^* = 0.68$ compared to $p_1/p_2 = 0.5$.

Delayed treatment effectiveness means that the benefits of a new treatment take some time to be manifested in the recipients. In such a case, treatment and control groups may not differ during the early part of the study. The effect of this is to reduce the difference between groups throughout the study duration.

Accounting for these complications in the sample size and power estimates usually means more difficult mathematics and larger sample sizes. Equation (3) already accounts for the possibility of constant loss to followup and type II censoring. Other models have been proposed to address the issues of time-dependent event and dropout rates and noncompliance (Schork and Remington, 1967; Halperin et al., 1968; Wu, Fisher, and DeMets, 1980; Lachin, 1981). However, considerable information about the probable behavior of the subject population must be available to justify many strong assumptions. A reasonable and relatively simple approach is to use information about noncompliance to adjust the expected event rates (i.e., δ or p) and repeat the sample size or power calculation. Large changes in the answer should prompt investigation of alternative approaches. The power of a clinical trial as a function of either sample size or treatment difference is frequently relatively flat above 80-90%. Thus, modest misestimates of sample size because of these complications may not seriously affect power if it is high. However, the consequences of attenuated sample size or treatment difference in trials with low power (i.e., in the steep region of the power curve) are very severe.

A frequently overlooked but very flexible method for the statistical design of clinical trials is computer simulation. This method consists of simulating the responses of subjects in a clinical trial and analyzing the results with the intended statistic(s) (Halpern and Brown, 1975; Elashoff, 1986; Piantadosi, 1986). Since each simulated trial is based on the same hypothesized but known treatment difference, repetition of the "trials" allows power or, implicitly, sample size to be estimated. Simulation has several advantages over parametric or partially parametric design strategies. It allows the design to be made using in the analysis. More importantly, simulation has the potential to model nearly exactly the investigator's hypotheses about noncompliance, censoring and changes in the effectiveness of treatment over time. For example, the delay in onset of the effect of cancer prevention therapy can greatly affect required sample size. Simulation has the main disadvantage of requiring extensive computer resources, especially for the sample sizes likely to be needed in cancer prevention clinical trials. The need for such resources could be satisfied either by extremely fast mainframe computers or perhaps by small computers which can be dedicated to the calculations for a period of time. The simulation could also be hastened if the test statistic can be calculated from grouped data eliminating the need to stimulate each individual event (Baker and Heidenberger, 1987).

SUMMARY

We have attempted to outline the important features in the statistical design of cancer prevention trials. Primary, secondary, and tertiary cancer prevention studies have been distinguished. The design of primary and secondary cancer prevention clinical trials generally poses problems different from those in the usual treatment trials. In particular, cancer prevention studies are very large, expensive, and unlikely to be duplicated. Because of the impact of positive or negative results when applied to a large target population, investigators must be especially careful in the design of these trials to avoid biases and low statistical power. Because some cancer prevention studies may involve 5-10 years of follow-up, subject nocompliance may be an important issue. Tertiary prevention trials are essentially treatment trials in very early stages of cancer, and the familiar principles suitable for treatment trials may be used.

Some of the problems peculiar to cancer prevention studies can be minimized by special approaches such as factorial designs, cluster randomization, and case-cohort analysis. In spite of the differences between prevention and treatment trials, there are many similarities in the process of design. All types of trials share the need for clearly defined objectives, endpoints, and patient selection. Because only modest effects are expected from most preventive strategies, the control of bias in cancer prevention studies is as important as in treatment trials. Adequate sample size to ensure high power against meaningful clinical alternatives is a necessity in both types of studies, and consequently sample size estimation is similar. In many instances, sample size determination can be made from standard equations with suitable corrections for any complications which are anticipated. In other cases, more elaborate methods must be used because patient accrual, survival, or noncompliance may be more complicated. Simulation is a promising general method for dealing with these more complex situations.

ACKNOWLEDGMENT

The authors are grateful for comments from Dr. Mitchell Gail and the secretarial assistance of Jennifer Gaegler.

REFERENCES

Altham, P. M. E. (1976). Discrete variable analysis for individuals grouped into families. *Biometrika 63*: 263.

Armitage, P. (1975). *Sequential Medical Trials.* Thomas, Springfield, IL.

Baker, S. G., Heidenberger, K. (1987). A comparative decision-theoretic approach to selecting sample sizes for prevention trials. Unpublished manuscript.

Bayes, T. (1763). An essay towards solving a problem in the doctrine of chances. *Philos. Trans. R. Soc. Lond. 53*: 370.

Bertram, J. F., Kolonel, L. N., Meyskens, F. L. Jr. (1987). Strategies and rationale for chemoprevention of cancer in humans. *Cancer Research 47*, 3012-3031.

Blot, W. J., Li, J. Y. (1985). Some considerations in the design of a nutrition intervention trial in Linxian, People's Republic of China. NCI Monograph 69. Washington, D.C.: U. S. Government Printing Office.

Brown, B. W., Jr. (1980). Statistical controversies in the design of clinical trials. *Controlled Clin. Trials 1*: 13.

Buyse, M. E., Staquet, M. J., Sylvester, R. J. (1984). *Cancer Clinical Trials. Methods and Practice.* Oxford University Press, Oxford, 481 pp.

Byar, D. P. (1980). Why data bases should not replace randomized clinical trials. *Biometrics 36*: 337.

Byar, D. P. (1984). Sample size considerations for prevention studies. In *Chemoprevention Clinical Trials*, M. A. Sestili (Ed.). Washington, D. C. U.S. Government Printing Office. NIH Publication No. 85-2715.

Byar, D. P., Piantadosi, S. (1985). Factorial designs for randomized clinical trials. *Cancer Treat. Rep. 69*: 1055.

Byar, D. P., Simon, R. M., et al. (1976). Randomized clinical trials, perspectives on some recent ideas. *N. Engl. J. Med. 295*: 74.

Chalmers, T. C. (1983). The control of bias in clinical trials. In *Clinical Trials: Issues and Approaches*, S. H. Shapiro and T. A. Louis (Eds.). Marcel Dekker, New York, pp. 115-127.

Cohen, J. (1960). A coefficient of agreement for nominal scales. *Educ. Psychol. Measurement 37*: 37.

Community Intervention Trials for Smoking Cessation (1986). Study Protocol.

Donner, A. (1984). Approaches to sample size estimation in the design of clinical trials— a review. *Statistics in Medicine 3*: 199.

Donner, A., Birkett, N., Buck, C. (1981). Randomization by cluster. *Am. J. Epidemiol. 114*: 906.

Elashoff, R. M. (1986). Sample size in survival studies. Society for Clinical Trials: May 14, 1986. Quebec, Canada.

Fleiss, J. L. (1981). *Statistical Methods for Rates and Proportions.* Wiley, New York.

Fleiss, J. L., Tyrun, A., Ury,H. K. (1980). A simple approximation for calculating sample size for comparing independent proportions. *Biometrics 36*: 343.

Fleming, T. R. (1982). One-sample multiple testing procedure for phase II clinical trials. *Biometrics 38*: 143.

Food and Drug Administration (1977). *General Considerations for the Clinical Evaluation of Drugs.* Rockville, Maryland. Pub No. HEW(FDA) 77-3040.

Freedman, L. S. (1982). Tables of the number of patients required in clinical trials using a logrank test. *Statistics in Medicine 1*: 121.

Friedman, L. M., Furberg, C. D., DeMets, D. L. (1981). *Fundamentals of Clinical Trials.* John Wright, Boston.

Freiman, J. A., Chalmers, T. C., Smith, H., Jr., et al. (1978). The importance of beta, the type II error and sample size in the design and interpretation of the randomized controlled trial: survey of negative trials. *N. Engl. J. Med. 299*: 690.

Gail, M. H. (1985). Applicability of sample size calculations based on a comparison of proportions for use with the logrank test. *Controlled Clin. Trials 6*: 112.

Gehan, E. A., Freireich, E. J. (1974). Non-randomized controls in cancer clinical trials. *N. Engl. J. Med. 290*: 198.

George, S. L., Desu, M. M. (1974). Planning the size and duration of a clinical trial studying the time for come critical event. *J. Chronic Dis. 27*: 15.

Green, S. B., Byar, D. P. (1978). The effect of stratified randomization on size and power of statistical tests in clinical trials. *J. Chronic Dis. 31*: 445.

Greenwald, P., Cullen, J. W. (1985). The new emphasis in cancer control. *JNCI 74*: 543.

Halperin, M., Rogot, E., Gurian, J., Ederer, F. (1968). Sample sizes for medical trials with special reference to long-term therapy. *J. Chronic Dis. 21*: 13.

Halpern, J., Brown, B. W. (1975). A computer program for designing cancer clinical trials that allows arbitrary specification of survival functions and use of either the log rank or generalized Wilcoxon test. Stanford University Division of Biostatistics Technical Report No. 106, August, 1985.

Hennekens, C. H. (1984). Issues in the design and conduct of clinical trials. *JNCI 73*: 1473.

Hennekens, C. H., Eberlein, K. A., for the Physician's Health Study Research Group (1985). A randomized trial of aspirin and beta-carotene among U.S. physicians. *Prev. Med. 14*: 165.

Herson, J., Carter, S. K. (1986). Calibrated phase II clinical trials in oncology. *Statistics in Medicine 5*: 441.

Kendall, M. G., Stuart, A. (1973). *The Advanced Theory of Statistics.* Hafner Press, New York.

Kornitzer, M., DeBacker, G., Dramaix, M., Kittel, F., Thilly, C., Graffar, M., Vuylsteek, K. (1983). Belgian heart disease prevention project: incidence and mortality results. *Lancet* May 14: 1066.

Lachin, J. M. (1981). Introduction to sample size determination and power analysis for clinical trials. *Controlled Clin. Trials 2*: 93.
Lachin, J. M. (1982). Statistical elements of the randomized clinical trial. In *The Randomized Clinical Trial and Therapeutic Decisions*, N. Tygstrup, J. M. Lachin, and E. Juhl (Eds.). Marcel Dekker, New York.
Liddell, F. D. K., McDonald, J. C., Thomas, D. C. (1977). Methods for cohort analysis: appraisal by application to asbestos mining (with discussion). *J. R. Statist. Soc. A 140*: 469.
Mantel, N. (1973). Synthetic retrospective studies and related topics. *Biometrics. 29*: 479.
Meinert, C. L. (1986). *Clinical Trials*. Oxford University Press, Oxford.
Moon, T. E. (1986). Clinical trials of cancer prevention agents: true versus observed prevention effect. *Statistics in Medicine 5*: 435.
Moser, C. A., Kalton, G. (1972). *Survey Methods in Social Investigation*. Basic Books, New York.
O'Fallon, J. R. (1985). Policies for interim analysis and interim reporting of results. *Cancer Treatment Reports 69*: 1101.
Office of Technology Assessment, U.S. Congress (1983). *The Impact of Randomized Clinical Trials on Health Policy and Medical Practice: Background Paper*. Washington, D.C.: U.S. Government Printing Office, OTA-TP-H-22.
Page, H. S., Asire, A. J. (1985). *Cancer Rates and Risks*, 3rd Edition. Washinton, D. C. U.S. Government Printing Office. NIH Publication No. 85-691.
Palta, M. (1985). Investigating maximum power losses in survival studies with nonstratified randomization. *Biometrics 41*: 497.
Patterson, B. M. (1987). The impact of screening and eliminating pre-existing cases on sample size requirements for cancer prevention trials. *Controlled Clin. Trials 8*: 87-95.
Peto, R., Pike, M. C., Armitate, P., Breslow, N. E., Cox, D. R., Howard, S. V., Mantel, N., McPherson, K., Peto, J., Smith, P. G. (1976). Design and analysis of randomized clinical trials requiring prolonged observation of each patient: I. Introduction and design. *Br. J. Cancer 34*: 585.
Peto, R., Pike, M. C. Armitage, P., Breslow, N. E., Cox, D. R., Howard, S. V., Mantel, N., McPherson, K., Peto, J., Smith, P. G. (1977). Design and analysis of randomized clinical trials requiring prolonged observations of each patient: II. Analysis and examples. *Br. J. Cancer 35*: 1.
Piantadosi, S. (1986). Simulation for sample size in trials with arbitrary hazards. Society for Clinical Trials: May 14, 1986. Quebec, Canada.
Pocock, S. J. (1982). Statistical aspects of clinical trial design. *The Statistician 31*: 1.
Pocock, S. J. (1983). *Clinical Trials: A Practical Approach*. John Wiley & Sons, New York, 226 pp.
Prentice, R. L. (1986). A case-cohort design for epidemiologic cohort studies and disease prevention trials. *Biometrika 73*: 1.
Prentice, R., Self, S. (1986). Protocol for Women's Health Trial.

Rubinstein, L. V., Gail, M. H., Santner, T. J. (1981). Planning the duration of comparative clinical trials with loss to follow-up and a period of continued observation. *J. Chronic Dis. 34*: 469.

Schafer, A. (1982). The ethics of the randomized clinical trial. *N. Engl. J. Med. 307*: 719.

Schork, M. A., Remington, R. D. (1967). The determination of sample size in treatment-control comparisons for chronic disease studies in which drop-out or non-adherence is a problem. *J. Chronic Dis. 20*: 233.

Shapiro, S. H., Louis, T. A. (1983). *Clinical Trials: Issues and Approaches.* Marcel Dekker, New York.

Simon, R. (1979). Restricted randomization designs in clinical trials. *Biometrics 35*: 503.

Simon, R. M. (1982). Design and conduct of clinical trials. In *Cancer: Principles and Practice in Oncology*, V. T. DeVita, S. Hellman, and S. A. Rosenberg (Eds.). J. B. Lippincott Co., Philadelphia, pp. 198-225.

Snedecor, G. W., Cochran, W. G. (1980). *Statistical Methods.* Iowa State University Press, Ames, Iowa, pp. 83.

Stampfer, M. J., Burning, J. G., Willet, W., Rosner, B., Eberlein, K., Hennekens, C. H. (1985). The 2x2 factorial design: its application to a randomized trial of aspirin and carotene in U.S. physicians. *Statistics in Medicine 4*: 111.

Taves, D. R. (1974). A new method of assigning patients to treatment and control groups. *Clin. Pharmacol. Ther. 15*: 443.

Whitehead, J. (1985). Designing phase II studies in the context of a programme of clinical research. *Biometrics 41*: 373.

Whitehead, J. (1986). Sample sizes for phase II and phase III clinical trials: an integrated approach. *Statistics in Medicine 5*: 459.

Wu, M., Fisher, M., DeMets, D. (1980). Sample sizes for long term medical trials with time-dependent dropout and event rates. *Controlled Clin. Trials 1*: 109.

Zelen, M. (1979). A new design for randomized clinical trials. *N. Engl. J. Med. 300*: 1242.

17

Choice of Populations for Cancer Prevention Trials

MEIR J. STAMPFER, WALTER C. WILLETT, and
CHARLES H. HENNEKENS
Brigham and Women's Hospital, and Harvard Medical School, Boston, Massachusetts

INTRODUCTION

The population selected for a cancer prevention trial should be chosen to maximize the feasibility of recruitment and followup, the probability of compliance with all requirements of the trial, and the potential to provide meaningful results which are generalizable to a larger reference population. In this chapter, we discuss each of these aspects of population selection in detail, providing as a primary example our experience in the Physicians' Health Study. The Physicians' Health Study is a randomized, double-blind, placebo-controlled factorial trial of alternate-day aspirin (325 mg) in the reduction of total mortality and cardiovascular mortality, and β-carotene (50 mg every other day) in decreasing total cancer incidence. The trial is being conducted among 22,071 U.S. male physicians aged 40–85 (Stampfer et al., 1985a).

RECRUITMENT

Primary prevention trials for cancer generally require large numbers of subjects. Even if a high risk group is chosen, a sufficient sample size is needed to accumulate adequate endpoints to yield a meaningful result. Hence, such trials must be fairly simple and enroll subjects at low cost (Yusuf et al., 1984). Ease of recruitment is a critical issue. One common strategy is to relate recruitment to an employment group, which is the approach our research group successfully adopted in the Physicians' Health Study. This has also been applied to large-scale observational cohorts including the ongoing Nurses' Health Study (Stampfer et al.,

1985b) and the recently begun Health Professionals Followup Study. Another strategy used in secondary prevention is to institute the trial among patients at specific medical institutions. This approach, employed by Clark in his trial of selenium in recurrent skin cancer (Clark et al., 1985), has the advantage of facilitating both recruitment and followup. Other possibilities include large civic groups, clubs, or religious organizations. The Loma Linda, California, group invited a large number of Seventh Day Adventists to participate in a cohort study and was aided by the cooperation of church officials (Lemon et al., 1964). Similarly, Paffenbarger has studied college alumni (Paffenbarger et al., 1966). Another approach used for observational epidemiology is a geographically defined population such as Framingham, Massachusetts (Dawber, 1980). These approaches all offer similar advantages for ease of recruitment to a clinical trial of primary prevention.

COMPLIANCE

More important than ease of recruitment, however, is selecting a population that will comply with the requirements of the trial. Of necessity, most cancer prevention trials are long term. Hence, subjects must be prepared to maintain the treatment regimen for a long period, and therefore must be highly motivated. There are several ways to select good compliers and to maintain compliance in randomized subjects.

Run-in Period

In the Physicians' Health Study we instituted a run-in period before randomization. All subjects who were willing and eligible to participate were begun on active aspirin and β-carotene placebo for a several month period prior to randomization. In contrast to β-carotene, the action of aspirin is thought to be short term, and its effects disappear over a 10-day period as new platelets replace those inhibited by aspirin. Since the postulated beneficial effects are acute, we could use active aspirin to identify subjects who might subsequently withdraw from the trial because of perceived side-effects. β-Carotene is remarkably free of known adverse effects, so we could avoid its use in the run-in, thus preventing its accumulation in fat and other tissues in subjects before randomization. At the end of the run-in period, subjects were asked about their compliance and their willingness to participate fully in the trial during the subsequent several years. In our pilot studies, we found that the majority of dropouts ceased participation within the first few months of the trial. A run-in period of this duration might then be expected to identify and remove most of the potential dropouts prior to randomization. Use of the run-in period will reduce the total number of subjects, but by increasing the fraction who will remain with the trial until completion, the run-in may actually increase statistical power. The optimal final analysis, of course, must include all randomized participants, regardless of compliance. Those assigned to the treatment group who do not comply become similar to the control group in terms of treatment. Likewise, those assigned placebo who treat themselves become similar to the treatment group. Hence, any noncompliance tends to attenuate the observed effect attributable to the treatment. In the Physicians' Health Study, a highly compliant group of 22,071 participants yields greater statistical power to observe an effect if one is truly present than a trial of 33,224 which includes 11,153 noncompliant participants (Lang, 1986).

Selection of compliant participants by means of a run-in period will often prove useful, but the population selected initially should be intrinsically motivated to stay with the trial. The knowledge and interest of physicians probably made them easier to motivate than many other groups. However, one might easily conceive of groups, identified by their interest in health care or a desire to contribute to the health of the general public (demonstrated by supporting an altruistic organization), which would probably serve equally well in this regard. High risk groups might be motivated to compliance by fear of disease, but for the same reason they may fail to comply with any comparison regimen, particularly placebo, and may seek to obtain the experimental treatment outside the setting of the trial.

Self-Motivation and Self-Medication

The trial organizers should exert all possible efforts to maintain high compliance in all groups. In the Physicians' Health Study, the treatment regimen was planned so that subjects take just one pill per day. The pills are packaged in monthly calendar packs with each bubble numbered to correspond to the day of the month. This arrangement has proved quite helpful in increasing compliance. Participants are encouraged to integrate the pill taking into their daily routine by storing the calendar packs near their toothbrush, shaving gear, and the like. While frequent contact with participants can be helpful, the costs can be considerable.

Compliance with the trial implies more than simply continuing to take the experimental treatment. It also includes avoiding self-medication with the experimental treatment and complying with the requirement to report the occurrence of adverse effects and endpoints. These aspects of compliance will vary from trial to trial, depending in part on the nature of the intervention. A trial of liver cancer prevention using the hepatitis vaccine does not require sustained motivation of subjects. A trial of some experimental therapy not generally available will not have the problem of self-medication by those assigned to the placebo group. The Physicians' Health Study is testing two agents which are readily available to the participants and is therefore quite vulnerable to this potential problem. The promotion of β-carotene for cancer prevention and marked secular trend for micronutrient consumption can further accentuate this difficulty. So far, however, the problem has remained more potential than real. In selecting a population for a trial, one should choose a group likely to be resistant to these pressures if the agent to be tested is generally available.

Field Contact

A third element of compliance relates to the need for continued contact with the participants of the trial to fill out questionnaires and appear for examinations if necessary. The Physicians' Health Study is conducted entirely by mail, and their is virtually no personal contact between the investigators and participants. Therefore, there is great reliance on the participants to continue to fill out the questionnaires and to report accurately on side effects and endpoints. Because of their training, physicians may be well qualified to answer the medical questions. Nevertheless, it is still necessary to obtain medical records to confirm the self-reports and to apply uniform criteria. In general, for trials of this sort to succeed, the population selected must be one which will understand the need to maintain contact and to review medical records.

One advantage of professionals as subjects is that they tend to be geographically stable, and, because of their position in the community, they tend to be easier to trace than many other groups. In this trial, thus far, not a single participant has been lost to followup. Since most cancer prevention trials will require long-term followup, the choice of population should include ease of followup as an important consideration. Thus, for example, women will tend to be more difficult to follow than men due to name changes that may accompany changes in marital status, although this formerly common practice appears to be decreasing. Followup can be made much easier by collecting as many identifiers as possible at the outset of the trial. In the Physicians' Health Study, it has proven useful to have obtained both home and office telephone numbers, and the name and address of a contact person who is likely to always know the whereabouts of the participant. Asking for several such contacts may be useful. Knowledge of the social security number facilitates use of the National Death Index, though this is not a necessity (Stampfer et al., 1984). If the population chosen for a trial is one in which followup is likely to be difficult, one might consider requiring provision of these additional identifiers and contact individuals as a criterion for inclusion.

Another approach to facilitate followup is to conduct the trial among a population that is already under surveillance. Although all Americans are under surveillance for mortality via the National Death Index, it is more pertinent to consider surveillance for the endpoint of interest, cancer incidence. Thus, where possible, it might be advantageous to conduct a trial in a state or region with an ongoing comprehensive tumor registry.

STATISTICAL POWER

The ultimate goal of any trial of cancer prevention is to demonstrate a benefit of treatment or provide an informative null finding which is applicable to the broader target population. Such a result requires adequate statistical power, which in turn requires a sufficient number of endpoints. It is not reasonable to expect more than moderate (e.g., 30–50%) reductions in cancer incidence from dietary agents currently being considered. Hence, "sufficient" means a large number of endpoints. For example, in the Physicians' Health Study, we originally estimated that after an average of seven and one-half years of followup, we would have a probability of 92% to detect a difference of 20% in total cancer incidence between the β-carotene and placebo groups.

Sample Size Considerations

The choice of the population can greatly affect the expected number of endpoints. One approach, employed in the Physicians' Health Study, is to enroll a very large number of participants who are at usual risk for the disease. Actually, since physicians tend to smoke cigarettes less than the general population, they are at lower than average risk for cigarette-related cancer. Indeed it is often observed that individuals who volunteer for observational studies or clinical trials tend to be healthier than the general population. It is unclear how strong this "healthy volunteer effect" will prove to be for cancer, but organizers of trials should apply conservative estimates of expected numbers of endpoints based on general population rates.

High Risk Groups

A second approach, often used in cancer prevention trials, is to identify a high risk population. This has the important advantage of requiring fewer participants to yield a given number of endpoints but can raise some important difficulties. One, already discussed, is the possibility that randomized participants will seek treatment outside the trial. Another more important problem is that it may be difficult to apply the findings to the wider population. For example, if high risk subjects are chosen for a breast cancer prevention trial on the basis of a positive maternal and sibling history of the disease, many will have a strong genetic component. If the findings are positive, they might only be applicable for those with that particular genetic makeup. A null result might mean that the intervention was insufficient to overcome the strong propensity for the disease in the high risk group, but it still could have an impact in a population of average risk. If the

Table 1 Comparison of Statistical Power to Observe a Significant Difference (p_2 = 0.05) for a Hypothetical Trial of 10,000 Subjects, for Usual and High Risk Groups, Assuming that the Intervention Yields Either a Constant Rate Ratio or Constant Rate Difference

Risk group	Cumulative incidence rate	Statistical power
Assuming constant rate ratio:		
Usual risk		
control	0.004	
experimental	0.002	0.44
High risk		
control	0.020	
experimental	0.010	0.99
Assuming constant rate difference:		
Usual risk		
control	0.004	
experimental	0.002	0.44
High risk		
control	0.020	
experimental	0.018	0.11

high risk group is susceptible because of a deficiency of the intervention factor, a positive finding could not be applied to those at average risk who do not have such a deficiency. In many instances it may be necessary to conduct separate trials.

Although the high risk group will yield relatively more endpoints, this will not necessarily increase statistical power; in some instances power can be greatly impaired, as illustrated in Table 1. Use of the high risk group will increase power (compared to using a group at usual risk) under the assumption that the intervention yields a constant rate ratio (i.e., the effect of intervention, expressed as a rate ratio, would be the same in the low and high risk groups). However, if the intervention yields a constant rate difference, use of a high risk group can substantially decrease the power.

Selection of Endpoints

A third approach to increasing the number of endpoints is to monitor the emergence of precancerous lesions. This approach, employed by Stich and colleagues (Stich et al., 1984), among others, has several major strengths. Far fewer subjects are required, and often a result emerges much more rapidly. Also, some of the ethical dilemmas of a cancer prevention trial are avoided. The primary limitation, however, is that any effect on cancer can only be inferred. A null finding would by no means rule out an effect of cancer incidence by a promising agent, and though a positive finding would be encouraging, it would not confirm an anticancer effect. Such trials do provide useful information for guiding further research, and because of their economy and relatively rapid accumulation of endpoints, their use should be expanded. Choosing a population in which the incidence of precancerous lesions can be measured might be advantageous in many circumstances.

Regardless of which cancer, or precancer, endpoints are chosen for study, it is important to follow other events. Certainly one should always monitor mortality, and it is often useful to ascertain other adverse effects. For example, in a trial of a cholesterol-reducing agent for decreasing cardiovascular mortality, a finding that the benefits for coronary disease were accompanied by an excess of colon cancer were important in evaluating the risk to benefit ratio of that drug for use in the general population (Report from the Committee of Principal Investigators, 1978). A trial which relied solely upon, say, a tumor registry as a source of endpoint data would fail to observe an impact on other health outcomes.

The age structure of the population chosen for a trial will also have an impact on the number of endpoints. For most cancers, age itself is an important risk factor, and an older population can be considered a high risk group relative to a younger population. It is possible that the effect of a potential chemopreventive agent may differ in different age groups. One should bear in mind this uncertainty when choosing a population to study.

Treatment and Follow-Up Interval

Another area of uncertainty that affects the choice of population is the length of time that treatment must be given and followup maintained to observe a positive effect, or a null finding which is informative. The Physicans' Health Study was examined beyond its initial term, and nearly all participants agreed to continue active participation. Trial investigators should consider the possible need to extend the treatment period beyond that initially envisioned, and strive to choose a population which would accept such an extension. In many instances the followup interval will extend beyond the end of active treatment, particularly since followup, especially for fatal outcomes only, is generally far less expensive than continuing active treatment. For many trials, it will be useful to extend the followup for many years, well beyond the period of active treatment. Important unexpected findings could result. For example, when investigators of the Coronary Drug Project extended the followup to assess the incidence of cancer among those treated with cholesterol-lowering agents, not only were they able to demonstrate no such excess, but they also found a pronounced benefit of reduced mortality among those assigned to the niacin arm of the study (Coronary Drug Project Research Group, 1986). This clear benefit had not been apparent in the initial followup of the trial. Trial organizers should consider planning for such prolonged followup early in the design of the trial, and choose the population accordingly.

It is useful to distinguish between trials whose main goal is to test the efficacy of a cancer preventive agent and those that seek to demonstrate a program of cancer prevention in a population. Trials of efficacy may employ extraordinary efforts to gain high compliance, even if such measures could not be employed on a wide scale. Similarly, such trials may plan for a higher occurrence of adverse effects (presumably with subjects under close surveillance) than would be acceptable in the general population. Such a trial is more appropriate to a high risk group. The goals of a population cancer prevention trial are to evaluate a program that can readily be applied to the general population. In such a trial, a very high standard of the safety of the experimental agent is necessary. Simplicity of administration is also important. Although in practice many trials have elements of both, the conceptual distinction is still useful as it may help to guide in decision making. For example, in the Physicians' Health Study, we chose the 50-mg alternate-day dose of β-carotene partly because it was easy to administer and would be unlikely to unacceptably alter skin color (Willett et al., 1983). Both the efficacy trial and the demonstration program must have internal validity as the primary concern. However, generalizability is of greater concern in the demonstration program.

Generalizibility

The choice of the population bears directly on the issue of generalizability of the findings. Generalizability is a matter of judgment requiring consideration of the evidence from the trial, the characteristics of the population, and biological knowledge in general. A strict statistical approach of directly generalizing from a random sample to the population (as is done in a political poll) is almost never practical in medicine, and indeed is not necessary. We are constantly generalizing results across geographical, social, and temporal boundaries. For example, if individuals in the Framingham study with high blood pressure are at higher risk for stroke, we believe the same to be true of Oregonians. If a given drug for congestive heart failure is effective in France in 1983, we believe it will work in Germany in 1984. This belief is largely based on our knowledge that the causes and mechanisms underlying congestive heart failure are similar in those two situations. In contrast, however, if a particular diet reduces mortality in Sudan, we might hesitate to generalize the results to Japan, where dietary determinants of mortality are probably different. Where one draws the line is a matter of judgment. The choice of population in a trial clearly influences the ease of generalizability. As discussed above, if a high risk group is chosen, this may limit generalizability to the general population. Other population characteristics also have an influence. If a generally well-nourished group (like the physicians) is chosen, in the event of a null result, one cannot exclude an effect among a less well-nourished group. For example, if β-carotene intake has a threshold effect for cancer prevention and all the participants are already above that threshold because of good dietary practices, the effect will be missed.

A sound argument against generalizability of findings should be tested on known or suspected biological characterisitcs of the population which could plausibly influence the relationship between the intervention and disease occurrence. For example, we would not regard as a sound argument that results from the Physicians' Health Study could not be applied generally to U.S. males simply because physicians are different. Similarly, the fact that it is not a random sample or that good compliers were selected would not provide a basis for militating against generalizability unless a biologically based argument could be sustained. Thus, for example, although good compliers may be at lower risk for disease in general, if beta carotene protects good compliers relative to placebo, there is no reason to believe it would act otherwise for less compliant persons if they took it.

Although the ability to apply the results widely is advantageous, the dominant concern in a trial should be in obtaining internally valid results; that is, to reach a true answer to the research question posed in the population actually under study. It is fruitless to choose a population from which one can readily generalize the findings if in doing so one imperils the validity. By analogy, the laboratory scientist typically chooses an inbred strain of a single species to obtain valid data, and does not make a random selection from, say, all mammals.

In trials of cancer prevention, proper choice of the population is critical. Such a choice will have effects on the ease of recruitment and conduct of the trial, the validity of the findings, and the applicability of the results. Since these trials will typically be long term, the investigators will be forced to live with their choice for a long time. The suitability of any given population for a trial depends in part on the precise research question being addressed.

ACKNOWLEDGMENTS

Supported in part by grants from the National Institutes of Health (CA 42182, HL 34595, and CA 40360). Dr. Willett was supported by a Research Career Development Award from the National Heart, Lung, and Blood Institute (HL 01018).

REFERENCES

Clark, L., Graham, G., Bray, J. (1985). Nonmelanoma skin cancer and plasma selenium: a prospective study. *Am. J. Epidemiol. 122*:28 (abstract).

Coronary Drug Project Research Group. (1986). Fifteen-year mortality in Coronary Drug Project patients: long-term benefit with niacin. *J. Am. Coll. Cardiol. 8*:1245.

Dawber, T. R. (1980). *The Framingham Study: The Epidemiology of Atherosclerotic Disease*. Harvard University Press, Cambridge, MA.

Lang, J., for the Physicians' Health Study Research Group. (1986). The use of a run-in before randomization. *Controlled Clin. Trials* 7:242 (Abstract).

Lemon, F. R., Walden, R., Woods, R. W. (1964). Cancer of the lung and mouth in seventh-day adventists: preliminary report on a population study. *Cancer 17*:386.

Paffenbarger, R. S., Wolf, P., Notkin, J., Thorne, M. (1966). Chronic disease in former college students. I. Early precursors of fatal coronary heart disease. *Am. J. Epidemiol. 83*:314.

Report from the Committee of Principal Investigators. (1978). A cooperative trial in the primary prevention of ischemic heart disease using clofibrate. *Br. Heart J. 40*:1069.

Stampfer, M. J., Willett, W. C., Speizer, F. E., Dysert, D. C., Lipnick, R., Rosner, B., Hennekens, C. H. (1984). Test of the National Death Index. *Am. J. Epidemiol. 119*:837.

Stampfer, M. J., Buring, J., Willett, W., Rosner, B., Eberlein, K., Hennekens, C. H. (1985a). The 2x2 factorial design: its application to a randomized trial of aspirin and carotene among US physicians. *Stat. in Med. 4*:111.

Stampfer, M. J., Willett, W. C., Colditz, G. A., Rosner, B., Speizer, F. E., Hennekens, C. H. (1985b). A prospective study of postmenopausal therapy and coronary heart disease. *N. Engl. J. Med. 313*:1044.

Stich, H. F., Rosin, M. P., Vallejera, M. O. (1984). Reduction with vitamin A and beta-carotene administration of proportion of micronucleated mucosa cells in Asian betal nut and tobacco chewers. *Lancet 1*:1204.

Willett, W. C., Stampfer, M. J., Underwood, B. A., Taylor, J. O., Hennekens, C. H. (1983). Vitamins A, E and carotene: effects of supplementation on their plasma levels. *Am. J. Clin. Nutr. 38*:559.

Yusuf, S., Collins, R., Peto, R. (1984). Why do we need some large, simple randomized trials? *Stat. in Med. 3*:409.

18
The Effects of Subject Selection Factors in Cancer Prevention Trials

CURTIS J. METTLIN
Roswell Park Memorial Institute, Buffalo, New York

INTRODUCTION

The public health trial is regarded highly as a means for testing interventions thought effective in disease prevention. Part of the emphasis placed in clinical trial methodology on issues of diet and cancer may stem from the important contributions clinical trials have made in the realm of cancer therapy and experiments have made in basic research. The public health trial, however, is distinct from the randomized, double blind trial of drug efficacy. The public health trial may be more akin to the observational methodology of the epidemiologist as opposed to the experimental method of the laboratory scientist.

One of the reasons that public health trials generally are "quasi-" experimental rather than truly experimental is that participants in such trials usually are free-living persons who make their own choices about the manner and extent of their participation. This freedom to choose or decline participation is an important principle of the ethical conduct of human research but one which also has important implications for the validity of public health trials. Herein, the nature and possible significance of various subject selection factors in the conduct of human cancer prevention trials will be discussed. Because no large-scale cancer prevention trial has yet been brought to successful conclusion, the observations discussed will be derived mainly from preliminary studies and from experience in other realms of public health inquiry.

IMPORTANCE OF SELECTION FACTORS

The attributes of cancer which make trials concerning it susceptible to the effects of selection factors include cancer's relative rarity, the long interval over which carcinogenesis may occur, and the probable multifactorial nature of its causation. Cancer prevention trials can require (a) that large, unbinded, populations cooperate over long intervals, (b) that intervention groups willingly comply with changes in their lifestyles (which they may have been told may have no benefit to them), and (c) that persons allocated to control status accept not receiving the intervention (which they may have been told could have significant benefit for them). All of these factors may combine to render the trial methodology weaker when applied to cancer prevention than when employed for different purposes.

Many types of bias which are a function of selection and recruitment procedures have been examined in the methodological literature. The theoretical effects of selection factors on trial validity have been described in detail by Campbell and Stanley (1963). They classified effects according to whether they relate to the internal or external validity of the study. Internal validity concerns the question of whether study inferences will be correct for the population being studied, and external validity concerns whether study findings will be correct for other populations the study group is thought to represent.

Subject selection and recruitment may affect internal validity by populating the trial with persons who respond to influences other than the study intervention. For example, selecting only highly motivated individuals in order to ensure adherence to protocol may yield a study cohort who will respond to secular health trends contemporaneous to the trial. In recent coronary disease trials entire cohorts, intervention and control subjects, have responded to the general trend toward smoking cessation. This general preventive orientation may have mitigated against observation of the true effects of risk reduction interventions. In dietary trials for cancer prevention, a general tendency for the study subjects to adopt what are perceived as more "healthy" dietary habits during the study could similarly reduce the power to observe the effects of the study intervention.

External validity may be affected by populating the trial with individuals who are more or less likely to show the effects of intervention. For example, selecting only "high-risk" subjects in order to accelerate the accumulation of study endpoints jeopardizes the ability to generalize from the trial to the broader community of "average-risk" persons.

Feinstein and Horwitz (1979), commenting particularly on retrospective studies, mention both exclusion bias and susceptibility bias as potential risks. These biases are the result of arbitrarily restricting the range of characteristics which may be possessed by the treatment and control populations. For example, if an exposure or treatment in truth acts only upon precursor benign lesions in promoting disease, then selection of a study population without evidence of precursor states will ensure failure to detect the true effects. Conversely, supposing that a factor only is important when some other etiologic process does not operate, e.g., in the absence of precursor lesions, to especially recruit persons with precursor lesions similarly might yield a study biased toward no effect being observed.

Sackett (1979) has identified 22 different forms of bias that may result from the processes of specifying and selecting study populations. Many of these concern observational studies, but some are of particular relevance to the prevention trial and include:

1. *Popularity bias.* The tendency for some persons to prefer to participate in studies or projects examining a hypothesis which has been subject to publicity and public interest. The population recruited to study a fashionable hypothesis may differ from that which could be recruited to study a hypothesis of lesser public interest.
2. *Diagnostic suspicion bias.* The tendency for persons believed more likely potentially to be afflicted by a disease of interest to be recruited into a study of that disease. Such persons may not represent the broader populations to which one would wish to extrapolate.
3. *Diagnostic purity bias.* When populations are screened to eliminate preexisting incidences of the subject disease or co-morbidity which might affect participation, the population becomes unique from the broader community of mixed health status. When the selection process eliminates comorbidity which is integral to the etiologic process being studied, the risk of a false outcome is enhanced.
4. *Membership bias.* When populations are recruited from established social groupings such as clubs, associations, occupations or religious groups, factors coincidental to membership may confound extrapolation of findings. For example, studies among physicians must give due regard to the possibility that that group is exposed to a different mix of carcinogenic stimuli than the general population, e.g., experiencing a lower rate of exposure to cigarettes and possibly higher rates of exposure to potentially carcinogenic laboratory chemicals. The "healthy worker effect" (McMichael, 1976), wherein employed persons are known to reflect lower morbidity and mortality due to the selective influence of employment status, is a well-known bias occurring in occupational research. Where research subjects are recruited from health maintenance organizations or other health enrollment programs, a similar bias toward overrepresentation of persons receiving health counseling, early detection, and similar preventive health services may be suspected.

5. *Nonrespondent bias and volunteer bias.* Persons who cannot be recruited and those who join with little recruitment effort may differ with respect to important confounding factors. For example, in the Framingham cohort study of coronary disease risk factors, 31% of the invited participants refused invitation to clinical examination and 13% dropped out after an initial response. Further study of nonrespondents revealed that those who responded generally were healthier and experienced lower overall mortality than those who did not respond (Gordon et al., 1959).

TYPES OF SELECTION FACTORS

The potential sources of selection influences are as diverse as are their effects. Differential selection into study populations may be the result of investigator action, intended or not intended, as well as of self-selection by study subjects themselves. Study eligibility criteria defined by investigators may restrict participation according to health status, exposure to risk, and perceived likelihood of long-term compliance to study protocol. Very often, the focus of research is on so-called "high-risk" persons in the expectation that the high yield of findings in such groups will reduce the scale of effort required. However, Sondik and his colleagues (1974) have challenged the notion that such selection is necessarily beneficial to the efficiency of a trial. Some eligibility criteria, however, are essential to a study and are important to the rigor and feasibility of the trial. Such selection criteria typically are not troublesome since they are documented, uniformly applied, and introduced with forethought given to their consequences.

Investigators may influence selection in a number of ways that are not as well documented and produce results that are not as well accounted. For example, conducting recruitment through health care institutions and organizations may yield populations predominated by current and past users of the health care system. Recruiting populations in public settings in general may bias the population against large segments of the population who bear some social stigma such as drug use, alcoholism, or illegal residency status. Subject self-selection also may serve to facilitate the conduct of prevention trials. The volunteer bias discussed above may suggest that long-term intervention trials may be more populated by persons who evince enthusiasm for the research. This may result in better long-term adherence and the achievement of a greater difference in exposure to the intervention between the two groups.

RESEARCH ON SELECTION FACTORS

There is a body of literature on the influence of selection factors in true clinical trials such as are conducted to assess drug efficacy. Such factors as patient and physician preferences have been studied as they relate to referral and recruitment for trials of cancer chemotherapy (Barofsky and Sugarbaker, 1979; Cassileth et al., 1980; McCusker et al., 1982). For cancer prevention trials, however, these methodological inquiries are just now getting underway and the body of literature is relatively small.

Albanes and colleagues (1986) have studied the potential recruitment pattern for cancer prevention studies to be conducted among male cigarette smokers in Finland. They found that only 63% of invited eligible subjects aged 55-69 responded to the study invitation. In a group of 3393 persons with cytologically demonstrated esophageal dysplasia in Linxian, China, 93% were randomized to vitamin supplement intervention (Li et al., 1986). In contrast, only 61% of persons in the general population of Linxian responded to a similar invitation. These experiences may indicate the significance of individual perceived risk as a factor affecting self-selection for study participation.

Boyd and colleagues (1986) conducted a study to assess the feasibility of conducting a clinical trial of dietary fat reduction in patients with breast dysplasia and to assess compliance to a reduced fat diet. They found that 61% of those deemed eligible actually would agree to participate in the study. Their initial data did not analyze the characteristics which distinguished responders from nonresponders, and the level of bias introduced by subject self-selection is unknown. A more serious problem with respect to achieving an adequate number of participants arose from the high rate of dropouts initially encountered. This problem was to a large extent addressed by adopting a procedure of placing subjects on a trial protocol before randomization.

To investigate the potential for selection biases as they relate particularly to studies of diet and nutritional interventions for cancer prevention, we conducted a survey in a population of potential study participants at Roswell Park Memorial Institute. This study, the details of which have previously been reported, examined expressions of interest in participating in a study to examine an unspecified dietary change or use of vitamin supplements and cancer risk (Mettlin et al., 1985). Persons who had attended a cancer screening clinic at Roswell Park were asked to indicate whether they would be willing to participate in such a study. Additional information regarding the respondents' socio-demographic characteristics, health attitudes, and behaviors and other background characteristics also were assessed in the mailed questionnaire.

A total of 576 persons were surveyed. Of this total, 77% indicated some degree of interest in participating in the hypothetical study. The subjects were favorably inclined whether the study was of dietary change or vitamin supplementation. The findings indicated that those who were most interested in participating in cancer prevention research of this type were younger, had higher family incomes, were better educated, and had greater awareness of the possible link between diet and cancer. Among the subset of respondents who were cig-

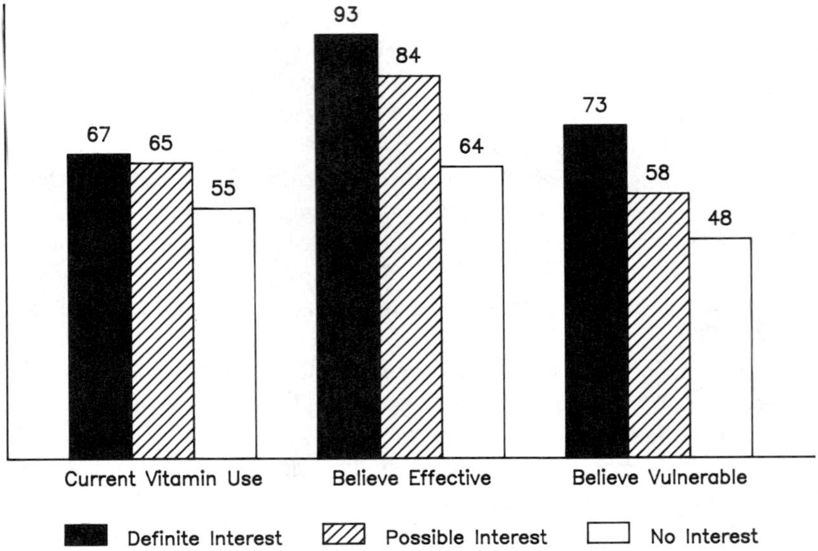

Figure 1 Percent of respondents with specific attitudes or traits among persons expressing different levels of interest in participating in a trial of dietary change for cancer prevention. Survey subjects were 575 well clients of the Roswell Park Prevention Detection Clinic.

arette smokers, those who desired to quit smoking and had previously attempted to quit were more likely to express interest in participating in the research compared to persons who did not express these traits.

The potential for bias in subject selection is illustrated further by the data in Fig. 1. We found that those most favorably disposed to participation are more likely to be regular vitamin users, to believe that cancer risk could be modified by diet, and to express greater concern about personal vulnerability to cancer. The greater belief in the efficacy of reducing cancer risk by dietary intervention among persons willing to participate was the greatest difference revealed in the survey. Interestingly, we did not find significant differences between subjects willing to participate in intervention research and those not willing with respect to reported frequency of consumption of fruits and vegetables.

Although the study we conducted was only of a hypothetical cancer prevention trial, the results did suggest a range of biases which may apply to an actual investigation. Firstly, the extent of interest in participation was remarkably high, with nearly three-fourths of respondents receptive to the prospect of participation. This enthusiastic response may be a function of the fact that study subjects were being recruited from a screening clinic population predisposed to cancer prevention activity. It also, however, may be a reflection of the popularity bias discussed above. The fact that persons most convinced that diet and vitamin interventions would affect risk is another indicator of the linkage between interest in the hypothesis and interest in participation.

Such attitudes predisposing to participation suggest that recruitment to cancer prevention trials may not be difficult, with large numbers of persons seeking to participate. This predisposition may, however, represent a risk to the research. Persons who already believe the validity of the hypothesis being investigated may act so as to confirm it by altering exposures to risk other than the study variable. It also raises the possibility that persons randomized to control group may adopt the intervention being studied outside the study protocol.

CONCLUSION

Although most public health policy decisions are made on the basis of other forms of evidence, the clinical trial is regarded as a superior source of knowledge about cause and effect in matters of human health. One reason the clinical trial is highly regarded is the extent to which this methodology mimics the experimental method of the laboratory scientist. Randomized controlled trials now are required in virtually all circumstances to establish the safety and efficacy of new drugs. When conducted properly, the clinical trial has a high degree of both internal and external validity. That is, the inferences about cause and effect are correct for the population actually studied, as well as for other groups represented by the study population.

So valuable has been the controlled clinical trial in the field of drug therapy that it is regarded by some as the standard of proof in the field of public health as well. While Snow's legendary removal of the handle of the Broad Street pump might be regarded as the first illustration of a public health study by planned intervention, there are many well-documented examples of community trials that have demonstrated the efficacy of disease control measures ranging from reduction of dental caries by water fluoridation to prevention of polio by vaccination.

In spite of the proven value of prevention trials in several realms, to date no intervention has been demonstrated by means of a controlled trial as effective or ineffective in preventing cancer. This may be the result of the fact that large-scale trials of cancer prevention only recently have been initiated. It also, however, may be the product of the great complexity attendant to the use of trial methodology in studying cancer prevention. The larger populations and the long observation periods required may make the cancer prevention trial susceptible to several sources of bias resulting from the selective participation by study subjects. Therefore, it is important that investigators using the trial methodology document the extent of subject self-selection in their studies and be attentive to its possible influence on inferences which may be derived from their data.

REFERENCES

Albanes, D., Virtamo, J., Rautalahti, M., Pikkarainen, J., Taylor, P. R., Greenwald, P., Heinonen, O. P. (1986). Pilot study: the U.S.–Finland lung cancer prevention trial. *J. Nutr. Growth and Cancer 3*:199.

Barofsky, I., Sugarbaker, P. H. (1979). Determinants of patient nonparticipation in randomized clinical trials for the treatment of sarcomas. *Cancer Clin Trials 2*:237.

Boyd, N. F., Cousins, M., Beaton, M., Han, L., McGuire, V. (1986). Methodological issues in clinical trials of dietary fat reduction in patients with breast dysplasia, in Ip, C., Birt, D., Rodgers, A., and Mettlin, C. (Eds.), *Dietary Fat and Cancer*. A. R. Liss, New York, pp. 117–126.

Campbell, D. T., Stanley, J. C. (1963). *Experimental and Quasi-experimental Designs for Research*. Rand McNally, Chicago.

Cassileth, B. R., Zupkis, R. V., Sutton-Smith, K., March, V. (1980). Information and participation preferences among cancer patients. *Ann. Int. Med. 92*: 832.

Feinstein, A. R., Horwitz, R. I. (1979). An algebraic analysis of biases due to exclusion, susceptibility, and protopathic prescription in case control research. *J. Chron. Dis. 34*:393.

Gordon, T., Moore, F. E., Shurtleff, D., Dawber, T. R. (1959). Some methodological problems in the long-term study of cardiovascular disease: observations on the Framingham study. *J. Chron. Dis. 10*:186.

Li, J. Y., Taylor, P. R., Li, G. Y., Blot, W. J., Yu, Y., Ershow, A. G., Sun, Y. H., Yang, C. S., Yang, Q., Tangea, J. A., Zheng, S. F., Greenwald, P., Cahill, J. (1986). Intervention studies in Linxian, China—an update. *J. Nutr. Growth and Cancer 3*:199.

McCusker, J., Wax, A., Bennett, J. M. (1982). Cancer patient accessions into clinical trials. *Am. J. Clin. Oncol. 5*:227.

McMichael, A. J. (1976). Standardized mortality ratios and the "healthy worker effect": scratching beneath the surface. *J. Occup. Med. 18*:165.

Mettlin, C., Cummings, K. M., Walsh, D. (1985). Risk factors and behavioral correlates of willingness to participate in cancer prevention trials. *Nutr. Cancer 7*:189.

Sackett, D. L. (1979). Bias in analytic research. *J. Chron. Dis. 32*:51.

Sondik, E. J., Brown, B. W., Jr., Silvers, A. (1974). High risk subjects and the cost of large field trials. *J. Chron. Dis. 27*:177.

19

Endpoint Identification: Selection and Ascertainment

BLOSSOM H. PATTERSON and STEVEN PIANTADOSI
National Cancer Institute, National Institutes of Health, Bethesda, Maryland

INTRODUCTION

The selection and ascertainment of endpoints play a central role in the design, conduct, and analysis of cancer prevention trials because the relevance and strength of inferences depend upon these two aspects of endpoint identification. The selection of endpoints is relevant to nearly every design consideration, although only a single protocol section is devoted to it. The methods, feasibility, and cost of ascertainment should be examined for each proposed endpoint during the design phase. This is especially important for prevention studies that require large numbers of subjects and are time consuming and costly to design and conduct.

The most basic observation in any clinical trial is a measurement of a response variable in a study subject, and endpoints are defined in terms of these measurements. An endpoint is a categorization of the individual subject's study measurements, or changes in those measurements, for the purpose of statistical analysis. The concept of an endpoint arises in two contexts, either in referencing a particular event (e.g., cancer occurrence), or as a population summary measure for the purposes of statistical design or analysis (e.g., five-year death rate). In this chapter we use the term endpoint primarily in the first context.

Cancer prevention involves studies in the broad areas of smoking, chemoprevention, diet, occupation, environment, and screening (Greenwald and Cullen, 1985). In this chapter we focus on the selection of meaningful study endpoints for prevention trials using micronutrients and on their subsequent ascertainment or identification. Five types of endpoints are relevant: (1) individual micronutrient status, (2) intermediate endpoints (preneoplastic lesions and biological markers), (3) cancer endpoints, (4) mortality endpoints and (5) toxicity endpoints. We begin by briefly reviewing general principles of endpoint selection, and then discuss the advantages, problems, and specific methods of acertainment for each of the above types of endpoints.

SELECTION OF ENDPOINTS

General Principles of Selection

The first step in endpoint selection is the specification of the questions the trial is designed to answer. The primary endpoint is determined by the question that the investigators are most interested in answering. Although a single hypothesis could be tested by observing any of several endpoints, a single endpoint should be selected to answer each question because it is almost always easier to interpret. In a chemoprevention trial, several questions may be of interest: Does the intervention change micronutrient blood or tissue levels? Does it affect incidence or time to occurrence of a preneoplastic condition or of the target cancer? Does it reduce cancer mortality? Each of these questions is addressed by a different endpoint.

Precision and Accuracy of Prevention Endpoints

Precision refers to the reproducibility of a measurement on the same specimen in the laboratory. It a measure of the variability in values obtained on repeat testing. Sources of variation include differences in the quality of equipment and in the skill and experience of those making the measurements, both within and between laboratories. Accuracy is determined by the correctness and lack of bias in the measurement. For example, consider a study having as an endpoint a preneoplastic lesion. A specimen from a study subject is an imperfect measurement of the endpoint because the biopsy may miss the dysplastic cells. Even when the technique is appropriate, the accuracy of a single measure can still be decreased by within-subject variability. When values fluctuate over time, as for example biological variables affected by cyclical patterns such as hormonal changes, a single measurement may not be a good approximation of the "true" value of the variable for an individual. In these cases, it may be sensible to define the "true" value as the average of several values.

The ability to detect treatment differences in a response variable is a function of precision and accuracy, as it is affected by the total variability in the responses. Total variability is the sum of three sources of error: laboratory error, within-subject error, and between-subject error (that due to subject-to-subject differences). If the first two sources of variability can be reduced, the ability to detect differences of a given size between treatment groups will increase.

Types of Endpoints

The goal of cancer prevention is the reduction of cancer incidence and mortality without unacceptable toxicity. Appropriate endpoints for chemoprevention studies are selected to measure one of three effects: micronutrient status, efficacy, and toxicity. We first discuss measures of micronutrient status, which can reflect both efficacy and toxicity. We then consider three types of endpoints that can be used to measure efficacy: effects on intermediate endpoints (preneoplastic lesions or biological markers), cancer incidence, and mortality. Finally, we briefly discuss toxicity endpoints.

Micronutrient Status

Implicit in the theory of preventing cancer by introducing micronutrients into the diet are the ideas that deficiencies in these substances may predispose toward the development of cancer and that dietary supplementation may correct deficiencies, leading to a decrease in cancer incidence. In general, exposure levels at which there are no overt health consequences, but at which there may be an elevated risk of cancer, are not known. The level of intake considered adequate for good nutrition may be different from that which is protective against cancer. In order to look for deficiencies and to determine the effect of supplementation, an appropriate index of micronutrient status must be determined, assay methods must be made available, and the "normal" concentration range of the micronutrient determined. We discuss these problems and issues and, where relevant, use the trace element selenium as an illustration.

An ideal index of micronutrient status should quantify an individual's exposure to a vitamin or trace element. However, available indices can typically measure the effects of exposure rather than the exposure itself. Analytical techniques include dietary assessment, functional biochemical and physiological measurements, and measures of levels in the blood, urine, and tissues for selenium, for example (Levander, 1985). Assessment of status by measuring dietary intake has many pitfalls which are discussed elsewhere in this volume. For example, dietary intake of selenium varies depending on foods consumed; in addition, the selenium content of a given food may itself vary. Functional biochemical and physiological measurements, when these have been identified, may be promising methods of measuring status. For selenium, activity of the selenium-dependent enzyme, glutathione peroxidase, is a possible measure of status. Blood levels have been used as an index of selenium status in humans (Willett et al., 1983). Different blood components may reflect different aspects of overall status; plasma and serum levels are short-term indicators of selenium status, while red cell levels can be used to monitor long-term status (Levander, 1986). A variety of tissues may be used in assessing selenium status (e.g., muscle tissue, hair, toenails). In Western countries, however, antidandruff shampoo containing selenium may contaminate hair samples. Assessment of urinary selenium excretion requires 24 hr samples because levels in random samples vary widely.

Assays are available for some vitamins and trace elements; Reynolds (1984) gives an overview of laboratory methods for monitoring levels of vitamins A and E (and related compounds), vitamins B_6 and B_{12}, ascorbic and folic acid, and selenium. All utilize blood or urine samples. However, adequate methods for measuring many potential preventive agents are not yet available (Micozzi et al., 1985).

Normal, deficient, and toxic levels have been determined for some vitamins and trace elements. However, when designing a study, it is important to have measurements of levels in the target population because these may differ from levels reported in the literature.

When supplementation is undertaken, it is important to measure micronutrient status during the trial. If the agent is effective or toxic, the time to event and the associated blood or tissue levels are important endpoints. It should be emphasized that levels of some substances (e.g., possibly vitamin A compounds) may be under active physiological control, so that attempts to raise them without causing excessive toxicity may be futile. However, increased consumption of some such substances might result in increased tissue levels or increased amounts of active metabolites. In such a case, serum levels would not be a sensible endpoint, but the tissue levels or measures of some related compounds might.

The impact of micronutrient supplementation depends on the body's handling of the agent. Single-dose kinetic tracer studies can provide information on the absorption, excretion, and storage in various body pools for vitamins and trace elements. Kinetic models can be used to predict micronutrient levels in various body pools after long-term supplementation. This information can be valuable in predicting the length of time that supplementation must be continued before reaching steady state (i.e., when the state in which the amount of agent excreted equals that ingested) and in estimating the associated total body load.

The most relevant micronutrient levels may be those in the tissues from which the target cancer arises; levels in body pools that can be readily sampled (e.g., blood) may not accurately reflect these levels. In some cases, kinetic models may be used to predict levels in tissues of greatest interest.

Intermediate Endpoints

Intermediate endpoints are changes, conditions, or events that are on the pathway to malignancy and consequently may predict the later occurrence of cancer. Intermediate endpoints possibly useful for chemoprevention trials include a variety of precancerous conditions and tumor markers. The association between such endpoints and the "final" endpoint, invasive cancer, is imperfect and generally not well known. There will practically never be a one-to-one correspondence between observation of either of these types of endpoints and the subsequent development of invasive cancer. Some preneoplastic and perhaps some neoplastic conditions may disappear or revert to normal regardless of treatment. Others never progress or may never be diagnosed.

The use of intermediate endpoints offers advantages over the use of invasive cancer endpoints, as discussed by Micozzi et al. (1985). These include shorter followup time and, when all the subjects have the precursor condition or marker, a smaller sample size. Limitations include the unavailability of reliable methods of measuring some precursor lesions and markers and the lack of knowledge about their relationship to the eventual development of frank cancer. Therefore, the use of such endpoints will depend in part on the underlying model of cancer development assumed for the particular site.

Preneoplastic conditions For the purposes of this chapter, we define a preneoplastic condition as any change in normal conditions that may be associated with the (future) development of cancer (Stout, 1932). Factors associated with an increased risk of cancer can be categorized on a continuum from risk factors, which are not necessarily in the direct chain of transformation from normal to malignant to noninvasive cancer. Preneoplastic conditions, being intermediate transformations, are frequently reversible. For example, current understanding about the pathogenesis of uterine cervical carcinoma indicates that sexual promiscuity may be a risk factor, whereas severe cervical dysplasia is a preneoplastic condition, and carcinoma in situ is the noninvasive state mentioned above.

The strong association between cancer and preneoplastic conditions indicates that the latter can be sensible endpoints for clinical studies because interventions which favorably affect precursors may prevent cancer. For the purposes of cancer prevention, a preneoplastic condition is not necessarily restricted to the tissue of tumor origin. For example, changes in serum or tissue levels of β-carotene or certain trace elements could meet the criteria for a preneoplastic conditioning provided the association between such occurrences and neoplasia is well established. In keeping with initiator-promoter theories of carcinogenesis, preneoplastic conditions may result from either the initiation of cancer (e.g., changes in cell kinetics or DNA synthesis) or from the promotion of preclinical cancers which would regress without promotion. The manifestation of these changes may be either morphological, physiological, or both.

Preneoplastic changes are detectable in many organs that are frequent sites of human malignancy. For example, the uterine cervix, oral mucosa, large bowel, esophagus, skin, and stomach are sites in which well-defined cellular atypia frequently precedes the manifestation of invasive cancer. The typical pathological change in preneoplastic cells is dysplasia, i.e., abnormal development, which implies a progression beyond simple cellular abnormality or metaplasia. We briefly discuss some of these cancer sites as a means of illustrating the important features of preneoplastic endpoint identification for cancer prevention. A more detailed treatment of these and other cancers is given in Correa (1982).

Uterine cervix. The epithelial cells of the cervix can undergo transformation in several stages: inflammation, reserve cell hyperplasia, squamous metaplasia, mild, moderate, or severe dysplasia, and carcinoma in situ. The evidence from screening and epidemiologic studies suggests a progression through these various stages to carcinoma in situ. Regression of the milder forms of dysplasia is common, with less tendency for more severe forms of dysplasia to regress. There is evidence that cervical screening has resulted in a decline in incidence and mortality which has not been accompanied by a decline in the rate of carcinoma in situ (Correa, 1982). This suggests that a successful reduction in the occurrence of preneoplastic endpoints might not result in fewer cases of invasive cancer. On the other hand, in populations with extensive screening programs, most cases of invasive cancers are found in women who were not screened (Johannsen, Giersson, and Day, 1978). A preneoplastic endpoint such as severe dysplasia could, in principle, be used in a randomized clinical trial because the criteria for its determination are firmly established, as is the apparent progression through dysplasia to invasive cancer. Thus, apart from the ethical issues that can arise in studying interventions in this population, these preneoplastic lesions are sensible endpoints.

Miller (1985b) discusses a problem arising from incomplete information on the natural history of cervical cancer. Two types of cancer of the cervix have been postulated: one in which the preclinical stage is slowly progressive and contrbutes little to eventual mortality, and one in which the preclinical stage is rapidly progressive and has a high probability of becoming invasive cancer and ending in death (Bailar, 1961; Ashley, 1966; Pedersen, Hoeg, and Kolstad, 1971). If a high proportion of lesions identified by screening fall in the first class, then a large effort is required to identify those women who have a high probability of developing progressive disease. Miller suggests that screening programs may be concentrating on women at lowest risk of developing invasive cancer, while missing some at highest risk. Among screen-detected cancers, there will typically be an overrepresentation of slow-growing tumors, a phenomenon referred to as length-biased sampling (Connor and Prorok, 1987). If length-biased sampling occurs in the recruiting process for a chemoprevention trial in which entry criteria require that subjects have a preneoplastic lesion, individuals with slowly progressive lesions are more likely to be accrued into the trial than those with more rapidly progressing lesions. As a result, the intervention would not be tested on persons at highest risk of developing or dying from the target cancer.

Gastric carcinoma. Metaplasia of the gastric mucosa is associated with gastric carcinoma (Imai, Kubo, and Watanabe, 1971). Gastric mucosal changes can progress from chronic atrophic gastritis, through intestinal metaplasia, to epithelial dysplasia. Extensive precursor lesions are associated with superficial carcinoma, which may remain noninvasive for many years. There are certain dietary factors that appear to be related to the development of these precursor lesions.

Because individuals with dysplasia are thought to be at high risk of developing carcinoma and the histological manifestations of gastric dysplasia are clear, these precursor lesions may also be sensible endpoints for prevention strategies.

Colon carcinoma. The adenomatous polyp is thought to be the precursor lesion for colonic carcinoma based on epidemiologic and experimental evidence (Morson, 1974). Followup studies suggest that the resection of adenomatous polyps prevents colon cancer. However, as Morrison (1985) points out, these studies were improperly analyzed, and no conclusion can be drawn about the efficacy of resection in preventing cancer. It remains an open question whether polyps are indeed precursor lesions, or whether instead they may be a disease condition which coexists with colon cancer. These lesions, however, meet the important criteria of objectivity for good endpoints because there would be general agreement among examiners about their presence. The elimination of adenomatous polyps by whatever means (e.g., excision or dietary prevention) may be a sensible cancer prevention strategy while the occurrence of the polyps themselves are at present the best preneoplastic endpoints available for colon cancer.

Skin. Precursors of skin cancer are focal hyperkeratosis and dysplasia, usually secondary to excessive solar radiation exposure. Although these lesions are common, they meet the already delineated criteria for preneoplastic endpoints. Thus, a possible clinical trial using sunscreen to prevent basal cell skin cancer might have hyperkeratoses as an endpoint. Study of the preneoplastic condition called the dysplastic nevus syndrome (Greene and Fraumeni, 1979; Elder et al., 1980) has helped our understanding of the role of ultraviolet radiation in the development of melanotic skin cancer.

We have omitted detailed discussion of some other cancer sites for which plausible precursor conditions exist. In particular, mouth, esophagus, and bladder cancers are examples. Leukoplakia, esophageal dysplasia, and bladder polyps are each sufficiently well associated with the development of cancer in the respective organ that they might be sensible prevention endpoints.

Biological markers Biochemical and biological tumor markers are associated with the presence of cancer. Under some circumstances, changes or elevations in their levels may be useful in chemoprevention studies. Kobayashi (1987) lists three problems associated with these markers: (1) there may be lack of sensitivity, (2) known tumor markers are not released into the blood in the early stages of cancer, and (3) it is difficult to detect tumor-specific markers in early cancer, while it is relatively easy to detect tumor-associated markers. Markers such as carcinoembryonic antigen, α-fetoprotein, and human chorionic gonadotropin have been used for cancer screening but are sometimes believed to lack high enough specificity and sensitivity for early cancer prevention (Herberman, 1983). However, these and other markers have been studied prospectively and found to be of some value for cancer screening (Pluygers, 1986; Pluygers et al., 1986). Thus, the possibility exists that these or similar tumor markers will be useful endpoints for cancer prevention strategies. An important question to consider in this regard is whether the particular biochemical markers are elevated in the preneoplastic phase or are produced by an already established cancer.

Cancer Incidence

A cancer endpoint is either the occurrence or recurrence of a specified cancer in a study subject, or the time to such an event. Cancer endpoints are the most sensible and important endpoints in chemoprevention studies because they are unambiguous and readily interpretable. However, passive followup techniques cannot be used to ascertain these events, a problem to be discussed later. Except possibly in studies in which subjects are health professionals, medical personnel are required to identify cancers. Especially in large trials, this can be expensive and require a large study staff.

The specificity with which the cancer endpoint is defined will be dictated by what is known about the action of the intervention. A preventive agent may be thought to show promise against all cancers, in which case the primary endpoint would be "any cancer." Total cancer incidence is a primary endpoint in a randomized trial of β-carotene among U.S. physicians (Hennekens and Eberlein, 1985). More typically, interventions are targeted at specific sites or at a histologic subset of tumors occurring at a given site.

Mortality

Mortality endpoints include fact of death, time to death, and cause of death. Specific cause of death categories that may be important in the assessment of the efficacy and possibly the toxicity of an intervention include deaths for cancer of a specific site, deaths from all neoplasms, death from causes consistent with observed or suspected side effects, and deaths from all causes.

The death certificate provides space for both antecedent and contributory causes of death. The *Physician's Handbook* (U.S. Department of Health and Human Services, 1978) contains instructions for physicians on the registration of deaths. Part I of the cause of death statement gives immediate and antecedent causes. The underlying cause of death is the condition that started the sequence of events between normal health and the immediate cause of death. Space is provided for recording the interval between the onset and death for the immediate cause, the antecedent condition(s) (if any), and the underlying cause. Part II records other significant conditions that may have contributed to death but were not related to the immediate cause. Numerous studies on the quality of medical certifications reported on death certificates suggest that the quality varies by cause of death and characteristics of the decedent (National Center for Health Statistics, 1982).

Wong et al. (1978) suggest a method for forming a matrix of primary by contributory causes to give an overall picture of mortality patterns. Their method is useful for comparing disease combination in two groups. This technique can be used to identify disease combinations and make comparisons of the members within the groups with a given primary cause and with contributory causes.

In addition to cause of death information, the death certificate also provides demographic information helpful in verifying that the study subject and the decedent are the same individual. The death certificate also gives the name of the hospital or institution (or other location) where the death occurred, the name and address of the certifying physician and of the attending physician (if different from the certifier), and an indication of whether an autopsy was performed. These can be useful in cases where the investigator seeks additional information on the subject's medical history from hospital records or from the subject's personal physician.

Cause of death information on the death certificates may be supplemented by a review, by the investigator, of each death. Information on underlying causes and recent hospitalizations might be included in such a review.

A major disadvantage of the use of mortality endpoints is the length of time that must elapse for most prevention trials before sufficient numbers of deaths can be observed. In contrast to most cancer therapy trials in which patients have short survival times, subjects in cancer prevention trials are healthy, and many are young, having a long life expectancy. Unlike preneoplastic and neoplastic endpoints, which require active followup, an advantage is that some mortality information can be obtained by passive followup. In a later section, we discuss methods of ascertaining survival status.

Toxicity

Toxicity endpoints address the types, severity, and duration of adverse effects of the agent and are measured over the entire course of the trial. Little is known about the incidence rates of adverse reactions to the prolonged use of many proposed chemopreventive agents. For example, knowledge of the side effects of synthetic retinoids is based on acute or subacute exposures, and the effects of chronic exposures in humans are not known (Meyskens, 1984). Safety factors, including both short- and long-term adverse effects, are of paramount importance in prevention trials because the study populations are usually healthy, even in those cases where high risk individuals are being studied (Sestili, 1984). The degree of toxicity which is considered acceptable may vary with the population at risk, however. Close, centralized monitoring for adverse effects can help identify problems early.

ASCERTAINMENT OF ENDPOINTS

Followup for endpoint ascertainment can be either active or passive. Active followup involves contact with the study subjects, while passive followup encompasses a variety of indirect methods of determining subject status. Micronutrient status, toxicity, intermediate, and cancer endpoints typically must be determined directly by the study personnel. Survival status can be obtained either directly, by contacting study subjects or their physicians, or indirectly, through searches of mortality files and other records. In countries or regions of the United States with tumor registries, cancer endpoints may be determined by linking study and registry records; in general, summary statistics are returned.

In some situations, endpoints can be reported by study subjects. The Physicians' Health Study is a trial conducted entirely by mail in which the 22,071 study subjects are U.S. physicians. Health status is self-reported on questionnaires at six months and then at annual intervals. The research group conducting the trial believes the level of ascertainment and documentation of endpoints will be greatly enhanced because of the very accurate self-reporting of symptoms and medical conditions by the participants and the availability of unusually complete medical records on physicians (Hennekens and Eberlein, 1985). However, self-reporting would not be expected to be as accurate in studies involving the general population.

Screening to Detect Endpoints

Virtually all cancer prevention trials must include some sort of screening component in order to ascertain micronutrient status, intermediate endpoints, and cancer endpoints. In many cases, screening is necessary to establish a baseline against which to measure a later outcome. Screening has been defined as the examination of asymptomatic people in order to classify them as likely, or unlikely, to have the disease in question (Morrison, 1985). We extend this definition to include examination for precursor lesions and biological markers. Further, we conceive of a screening component in a very broad sense as encompassing any method (e.g., physical exam, questionnaire, collection of biological specimens) used by study personnel to ascertain a nonsurvival endpoint. Subjects may be screened before randomization and at intervals while on study, and as they go off study. In this section, we discuss reasons for including a screening component in a trial, characteristics of screening tests, and, finally, screening procedures.

There are several reasons for determining the baseline value of a variable prior to randomization. Eligibility criteria may be linked to the outcome measure in studies using micronutrient and intermediate endpoints. Persons defined to be at high risk because of very low levels of a micronutrient might be sought for studies in which both the prevention effect and the effect on body status of supplementation are being tested. Some trials using preneoplastic or tumor marker endpoints similarly may require subjects with a lesion or abnormal marker level. Changes are determined from measurements at the beginning, possibly during, and at the end of the trial.

Screening may also be undertaken when the study endpoint is the development of a preneoplastic lesion or of a cancer. Subjects may be screened prior to randomization to identify people with preexisting (but undiagnosed) disease. In prevention trials with these endpoints, the hypothesis of interest is whether an intervention is effective in preventing cancer (or a precursor) in a population consisting of persons without any evidence of disease. In practice, however, it is only possible to observe the incidence of cancer (or a precursor) in a mixed population, those who are initially disease-free and those who entered the trial with existing (but undiagnosed) disease. Patterson (1987) shows that the presence of the latter in the study group will result in an underestimate of the true intervention effect unless sample size is increased to take into account anticipated preexisting cases. The number and impact of preexisting cases on sample size may be diminished by excluding from the trial those with screen-detectable disease.

Subjects may also be screened periodically during the trial in those cases in which a screen exists, in order to detect early disease. "Pseudo-disease," defined by Morrison (1985) as a lesion that does not cause symptoms but appears serious pathologically, can be a problem in prevention trials as it is in screening studies. Pseudo-disease is discovered as a result of screening, and would not otherwise become known. The mental anguish and unnecessary treatment of persons with this nonprogressive disease have been discussed in the screening literature. As an alternative to screening, endpoint determination may depend on the appearance of clinical symptoms. However, periodic screening may be done throughout some studies because it may be unethical not to screen subjects at high risk of developing cancer.

To avoid bias, it is essential that followup be the same in both the treatment and control groups. This may be especially difficult in trials in which the treatment group is seen more frequently than the control group. The protocol should define closely what is to be considered an incident cancer, and events confirmed by independent review.

Characteristics of Screening Tests

Performance characteristics of screening tests are discussed in Habbema and van Oortmarssen (1982). The quality of a screening test is based on its ability to

Table 1 Classification of Screening Test Results

	Disease		
Screen	+	-	
+	TP	FP	TP + FP
-	FN	TN	FN + TN
	TP + FP + FN + TN		

TP = True Positives
FP = False Positives
FN - False Negatives
TN = True Negatives

$$\text{Sensitivity} = \frac{TP}{TP + FN}$$

$$\text{Specificity} = \frac{TN}{FP + TN}$$

$$\text{Predictive Value of a Positive Test Result} = \frac{TP}{TP + FP}$$

$$\text{Predictive Value of a Negative Test Result} = \frac{TN}{TN + FN}$$

classify correctly those tested as having or not having the disease. Screening test results can be classified according to Table 1. Sensitivity is the probability that a person with the disease will have a positive test result, and specificity is the probability that a person without the disease will have a negative test result. The predictive value of a test is the probability that the test result is correct, i.e., that it accurately reflects an individual's disease state. The predictive value depends on disease prevalence; as prevalence decreases, the predictive value of a positive test decreases, while that of a negative test improves. Estimates of a test's sensitivity and specificity vary with the population being tested. For example, mammography is more sensitive among postmenopausal women than among younger women with denser breasts (Strax, 1985). The International Union Against Cancer recommends that when a screening test is to be used in a study, its sensitivity and specificity be evaluated and stated and that a quality control program be in place to ensure that the stated levels are attained and maintained (Miller, 1978).

Screening Procedures

Some screening procedures present problems when there is a lack of experience in screening for the particular marker or lesion under study. Laboratory procedures may have to be developed and documented for collecting, storing, and processing the specimens. In those cases where an assay must be developed, the methodology should be worked out before the trial, so that the minimum quantity of a specimen necessary is known, and its collection feasible. In addition, the stability of the substance of interest (e.g., biological markers, micronutrients, trace elements) in the specimen should be determined under routine handling procedures. For example, when the levels of micronutrients in plasma are to be measured, their stability under conditions of freezing and thawing should be investigated.

Interpreting the specimen can present special problems for intermediate endpoints because there may be uncertainty as to what constitutes an abnormality. Classification systems exist only for a few preneoplastic lesions.

Diagnostic followup is an ethical requirement for programs involving screening, and essential to the complete and accurate ascertainment of endpoints (Friedman, 1985). It may be necessary to educate both trial subjects and the community of medical practitioners as to the approaches which should be followed in the event of an abnormal finding (Miller, 1985a). Miller notes that those identified as having an abnormal lesion will not automatically comply with recommendations for its treatment. In the initial phases of many breast cancer screening programs, it has been necessary to demonstrate the importance of these abnormalities to the community of medical practitioners and to convince them that they should be treated seriously (Miller and Bulbrook, 1982). Miller notes that this is one of the problems that arises from the fact that the biological features, natural history, and other characteristics of some of the lesions identified in a screening program may be in doubt. Similar problems can be expected to arise in the assessment of preneoplastic lesions in chemoprevention trials.

Ascertainment of Mortality Endpoints

General Principles of Ascertainment

The survival status of all subjects should be determined, both during the study and after active followup has terminated, to avoid possible bias in the study results. Gail (1985) discusses the potential impact of "controllable" losses to followup on the interpretation of clinical trial data. Controllable losses are those subjects lost to followup for whom, in principle, it is possible to retrieve survival information by further investigation. If the subjects lost from the intervention group are not comparable to those lost from the placebo control group, a bias may be introduced and an erroneous conclusion drawn about the intervention's efficacy. Bias can also be introduced if either deaths or survival are unevenly reported; this can happen after active followup has terminated. Because of long latency periods, prevention trials with cancer endpoints may include a period of passive followup. If survival is reported more thoroughly than deaths after active followup has ended, survival curves will be biased upward; if deaths are preferentially reported, the bias will be downward. In order to avoid this type of bias in studies where survival in the various study arms will be compared, a cut-off date must be chosen and subjects dying after that date counted as alive in the analysis. The cut-off date is the last time at which information is available on the vital status of almost all subjects.

Methods of Ascertainment

The investigator usually requires an indication of whether the study subject is alive or dead; if dead, date of death, and cause of death. Active followup allows the investigator to establish that an individual is alive on a certain date. Passive followup techniques are best suited to discovering deaths because they provide information on possible decedents by name. Based on this information, estimates of the numbers alive can be made.

We discuss three methods of ascertaining vital status. These are tools for passive followup and involve investigator-initiated searches of files. They are the Social Security Administration (SSA) files, the National Death Index (NDI), and credit bureau files. There are other resources, for example, State vital statistics records.

Searches of the SSA files and the NDI are most useful for ascertaining mortality for individual study subjects. Both are national in scale. SSA files are limited to information on those in the Social Security system, while the NDI contains information on all deaths since 1979. Credit bureau files contain data on individuals involved in any kinds of financial transactions, and are usually regional in coverage. They provide a means of inferring that particular study subjects were alive on a certain date.

All of these tools operate by record linkage. It is important to determine before the trial begins what information is necessary to use these files effectively and to plan to collect and verify the required data. Data should be supplemented and corrected while subjects are being actively followed.

Social Security file searches* To initiate a search of the Social Security files, the investigator requests a health and mortality study, indicating the anticipated number of records to be submitted, and giving a brief description of the study and the study population. The minimum data required for a search are Social Security number (SSN) and surname. Files searched include the Summary Earnings Record file and the Master Beneficiary Record file. Deaths are entered within three to six months, but there is a two-year lag time in updating other information (e.g., that on the living) in these files, so a researcher planning to use this resource should choose the cut-off date selected for purposes of data analysis accordingly.

The researcher receives the results of the search in about three to four months. Mortality information for each possible decedent includes SSN, other surnames on record, and either the city and state in which a claim for survivor's benefits was filed, or state of last known residence. In addition, the SSA returns a count of those in the "assumed living" category. This count is based on a search of files of current wage earners subject to Social Security deductions and of recipients of retirement benefits. The investigator also receives lists of mismatches (the SSN and first six letters of the surname don't match those in the SSA files), nonexistent SSN (the SSN provided has not been issued, indicating a recording or keying error), and status unknown. This last category includes those not falling in any of the above categories, for example, wage earners not subject to SSA deductions and persons not gainfully employed.

An estimate of the proportion surviving can sometimes be made by adding together the counts in the "assumed living" and the "status unknown" categories. However, there are some caveats. The "assumed living" category may include persons who are deceased, but whose deaths did not get recorded in the SSA files. The "status unknown" category similarly may include persons who are deceased and would not be expected to be in the Social Security files. A second caveat is that, in some instances, the SSN in the SSA files and that given to an investigator may not belong to the same person. For example, a woman who does not have her own SSN may use that of her husband. If he is deceased, his death will be identified. Conversely, if she has died and he has not, her death will not be identified.

The National Death Index The NDI is a central, computerized index of death record information compiled from magnetic tapes submitted to the National Center for Health Statistics (NCHS) by the state vital statistics offices. This computer file contains a standard set of identifying information for each person dying in the United States, Puerto Rico, or the Virgin Islands, beginning

---

*This information is based on conversations with employees of the Social Security Administration.

Table 2 Data to Be Submitted by NDI Users

Items Used in Searching the NDI file	
	First name
	Last name
	Middle initial
	Father's surname (for females)
	Social Security number
	Month, day, and year of birth
	Sex
Items Used in Assessing the Quality of Each Match	
	State of birth
	State of residence (last known)
	Race
	Marital status
	Age at death (actual or estimated)

with 1979. The NDI was established to assist medical and health investigators in determining whether persons in their studies may have died and, if so, to provide the names of the states in which the deaths occurred and the corresponding death certificate numbers. Cause of death information must be obtained from the death certificates; it is not in the NDI file.

As a tool for followup, the NDI can be especially useful for cancer prevention trials that involve large numbers of persons, long time periods, or many geographic areas. In most cases, subjects will be healthy, mobile, and many will be young, necessitating extended periods of followup.

We summarize the steps involved in using the NDI. A more detailed discussion is given by Patterson and Bilgrad (1986). The investigator's first objective is to ensure the collection of all the NDI data items: those used in searching the NDI file and those used in assessing the quality of the resulting matches (Table 2). The minimum data required for a search of the NDI are either first name and last name and either SSN or month and year of birth.

To arrange for a search, the investigator submits a "National Death Index Application Form" to the NCHS.* It is reviewed within two to three months. If approved, the investigator submits a data file containing subject names and related data to the NCHS. The file may be on magnetic tape conforming to NCHS coding and formatting specifications (given in the *NDI User's Manual,* National

*Division of Vital Statistics, National Center for Health Statistics, 3700 East-West Highway, Room 1-44, Hyattsville, MD 20782.

USER REQUEST RECORD (POSSIBLE MATCHES = 4) NDI APPL NO 842899 CONTROL NO 4507

POSSIBLE DECEDENT NAME	FATHERS SURNAME	SOC SEC NO	BIRTH DATE MO	DY	YR	AGE	SEX	RACE	MS	SOR	SOB	USER DATA
REGINA HANES		114576493	12	10	18	-	F	-	M	PA	LA	011580

POSSIBLE NDI RECORD MATCHES (IN RANKED ORDER)

	STATE OF DEATH		CERT NUMBER	DATE OF DEATH	NAME F	M	L	FATHERS SURNAME	LN/ FS	SOC SEC NO	BIRTH DATE MO	DY	YR	AGE	SEX	RACE	MS	SOR	SOB
*	PENNSYLVANIA		861098	02-01-81	X	B	X	-		XXXXXXXXX	X	X	X	-	X	-	X	X	X
	LOUISIANA		421304	07-07-80	X		X	-		--XXXXX-X	X		+01	-	X	-	X		X
	LOUISIANA	A	421304	07-07-80	I	B	X	-		--XXXXX-X	X		+01	-	X	-	X		X
	INDIANA		698637	03-21-79	X		N	-	N	---X--X--	X	X	-05	-	X	-	?		

Column heading abbreviations:

LN/FS = Last name on user record compared to father's surname on NDI record.

MS = Marital status

SOR = State of residence

SOB = State of birth

Symbols used within the table:

* = *All* items provided on user record matched exactly with items on NDI record.

X = User data item and NDI data item matched exactly.

Blank = User data item and NDI data item did not match.

\- = Data item not provided by user. For SSN: specific digits did not match. For LN/FS: comparison was not attempted.

? = Insufficient information on NDI record.

A = Alias name on NDI record.

I = Only first initial of first name matched.

N = Names matched only on NYSIIS phonetic codes.

B = Middle initials not provided on either record. This occurrence is treated as a match on middle initial.

+01 = Birth year on the NDI record is one year more than the year on the user record.

-05 = Birth year on the NDI record is five years less than the year on the user record.

Fig. 1 NDI Retrieval Report. (From Division of Vital Statistics, National Center for Health Statistics.)

Center for Health Statistics, 1981), or, for requests of 300 or fewer user records, on NCHS coding sheets. The user receives the results of the search within three weeks. All of the user's data are returned to him. The NCHS retains no copies; it is required by law to maintain the confidentiality of identifiable data.

The user receives (on magnetic tape and/or on computer printout) the Retrieval Report, which contains a listing of his records that matched one or more NDI records. An example of a hypothetical Retrieval Report for one user record is shown in Fig. 1. The user's data are printed under "User Request Record." Possible NDI record matches are listed hierarchically, beginning with the NDI record that had agreements (denoted 'X') on the greatest number of data items. For each match, the state of death, date of death, and death certificate number are given. The investigator also receives death certificate request forms which group all of the possible NDI record matches by state of death. The user checks off the certificates in which he is interested and sends the forms and payments to the respective states.

The effectiveness of the matching process is dependent on the completeness and quality of both the state death certificate information and the data submitted by the user, the effectiveness of the NDI matching criteria, and the ability of the user to assess the quality of the resulting matches. The completeness and quality of data items in the NDI are thought to be high. The user can improve the accuracy of his data by verification of key punching and computerized edits. Errors should be corrected and missing data obtained while subjects are being actively followed. This is important if any type of record linkage is anticipated as, for example, follow-back studies of physicians' or hospital records.

The effectiveness of the matching criteria is reflected in the percentage of true matches (NDI records correctly linked to user records), false matches (NDI records incorrectly linked to user records), and nonmatches (persons in the user's file are deceased, but not linked to corresponding NDI records). The user can include test records in his submission and use search results for these records to estimate match rates for his submission. A sample of known decendents can be used to estimate the true match rate, and a sample of persons not in the NDI files (e.g., persons who died before 1979, or persons known to be alive) can be used to estimate the number of false positives. True match rates have ranged from 92 to 98% in studies that included Social Security numbers for most subjects. The number of false matches depends on the number of years of deaths searched. Most false matches can be easily eliminated by visual inspection. For large studies, computer processing of results may be necessary.

Credit bureau files A search of credit bureau files may be undertaken to try to locate subjects not located by other methods. These files contain transaction dates for many financial activities and are constantly updated. If a study subject is paying bills, it is likely that there will be a transaction date for him in the file, and it may be inferred that he was alive on that date. For each subject the investigator provides name, city, and state of residence (at a minimum) as well as other demographic information such as SSN and date of birth. For any matches, the credit bureau typically returns the date of last transaction and an indication of which of the data items in their file matched those furnished by the investigator. By law, the fact and source of any inquiry regarding a credit file must be recorded in that file, and, if no file exists, one must be created. Therefore, it is important that the investigator request the date of the most recent genuine transaction, such as payment of a credit card bill, in order to avoid getting the date of last inquiry. When a subject is deceased, and his spouse maintains credit in his name, as is often the case among older individuals, an erroneous conclusion regarding survival status can be drawn.

CONCLUSIONS

We have discussed a variety of endpoints that may be appropriate for cancer chemoprevention trials. The use of micronutrient, intermediate, cancer, and mortality endpoints each has particular benefits and shortcomings. The study protocol should specify the particular endpoint selected to answer each study question and describe the methods by which it will be ascertained. The protocol is particularly important because the choice of endpoint will influence many aspects of study design, such as trial duration and sample size. The inferences made from trial results are no better than the quality of the underlying data, which in turn depends on accurate and thorough ascertainment of the selected endpoint in the study population. Incomplete ascertainment can lead to biased results.

The use of intermediate endpoints for cancer prevention offers several advantages. The time required until endpoints can be observed depends on the lag time to treatment efficacy, not on the latent period of a given cancer. Consequently, the study results could be available in a matter of a few years and might benefit the general population sooner. In those situations where all subjects have the precursor lesion or marker, an endpoint could be observed in each. Required sample size in such a high risk group could be much smaller than in trials with cancer endpoints. However, such trials provide information only on the fate of the precursor endpoint. Only a larger study with a cancer endpoint can determine whether the intervention actually prevented either the target cancer or cancer morbidity and mortality.

Some biochemical markers offer promise because they may be easy to access on a population scale. However, the temporal sequence of marker appearance relative to cancer appearance must be firmly established before such markers can be used as prevention endpoints.

In situations where intermediate endpoints do not exist, are unreliable, or are too difficult to assess, a cancer endpoint must be used. Especially in the case of large trials, mortality endpoints should also be included in the study design in order to determine whether an intervention that decreased cancer incidence also decreased cancer mortality. Long-term followup, extending beyond a study's intended duration, may be important when trying to answer some study questions. Survival and cause-of-death information permit examination of mortality patterns among study participants to investigate the possibility that an intervention is associated with long-term toxicities or morbidities.

We have outlined several options for endpoint ascertainment. The reliability of study results rests on the completeness and accuracy of ascertainment. Planned active followup is the most accurate, complete, and costliest option but may be optimal for ascertaining micronutrient, intermediate, and cancer endpoints. In some instances, endpoints can be reported by study subjects. More often, they must be ascertained through some sort of screening procedure. In this case, the screening component in a prevention trial will be similar in many respects to that in screening trials. Of central importance are the screening test and associated laboratory tests. We stress the importance of stringent quality control at every step: the collection, processing, and interpretation of the specimens, reporting the findings, and in the subsequent followup of subjects with positive results.

Full and accurate ascertainment of deaths is crucial to the avoidance of bias in the study results. In circumstances where passive followup is necessary, three methods could be useful: searches of the Social Security files, the National Death Index (NDI), and searches of credit bureau files. Results of a search of the Social Security Administration files include an estimate of the numbers of those "assumed living," and searches of credit bureau files can provide, for those subjects found in their files, a date on which it can be assumed the subject was living. The NDI files contain information on virtually all deaths occurring in the United States since 1979 and offer an efficient method of ascertaining mortality even many years after the study's end.

REFERENCES

Ashley, D. J. B. (1966). Evidence for the existence of two forms of cervical carcinoma. *J. Obstet. Gynaecol. Br. Commonw. 73*:382.

Bailar, J. C. (1961). Uterine cancer in Connecticut: late deaths among 5-year survivors. *JNCI 27*:239.

Connor, R. J., and Prorok, P. C. Issues in the conduct and analysis of randomized trials in cancer screening (submitted for publication).

Correa, P. (1982). Morphology and natural history of precursor lesions. In *Cancer Epidemiology and Prevention*, D. Schottenfeld and J. F. Fraumeni (Eds.). W. B. Saunders, Philadelphia, pp. 90–115.

Elder, D. E., Goldman, L. I., Goldman, S. G., Greene, M. H., Clark, W. J., Jr. (1980). The dysplastic nevus syndrome—a phenotypic association of sporadic cutaneous melanoma. *Cancer 46*:1787.

Friedman, G. D. (1985). Application of screening, including multiphasic screening, to target populations. In *Screening for Cancer*, A. B. Miller (Ed.). Academic Press, New York, pp. 69–83.

Gail, M. H. (1985). Eligibility exclusions, losses to follow-up, removal of randomized patients, and uncounted events in cancer clinical trials. *Cancer Treat. Rep. 69*:1107.

Greene, M. H., Fraumeni, J. F., Jr. (1979). The hereditary variant of malignant melanoma. In *Human Malignant Melanoma*, W. H. Clark, L. I. Goldman, and M. J. Mastangelo (Eds.). Grune and Stratton, New York, pp. 139–166.

Greenwald, P., Cullen, J. W. (1985). The new emphasis in cancer control. *JNCI 74*:543.

Habbema, J. D. F., van Oortmarssen, M. (1982). Performance characteristics of screening tests. *Clinics in Lab. Med. 2*:639.

Hennekens, C. H., Eberlein, K. (1985). A randomized trial of aspirin and β-carotene among U.S. physicians. *Prev. Med. 14*:165.

Herberman, R. B. (1983). Uses and limitations of tumor markers. In *Oncodevelopmental Markers*, F. Witt (Ed.). Academic Press, New York, pp. 409–418.

Imai, T., Kubo, T., Watanabe, H. (1971). Chronic gastritis in Japanese with reference to high incidence of gastric carcinoma. *JNCI 47*:179.

Johannsen, G., Geirsson, G., Day, N. (1978). The effect of mass screening in Iceland, 1965–74, on the incidence and mortality of cervical carcinoma. *Intl. J. Cancer 21*:418.

Kobayashi, T. (1987). Correlation between tumor markers and tumor size. *Cancer Det. Prev. 10*:81.

Levander, O. A. (1985). Considerations on the assessment of selenium status. *Federation Proc. 44*:2579.

Levander, O. A. (1986). The need for measures of selenium status. *J. Amer. Coll. Toxicol. 5*:37.

Meyskens, F. L., Jr. (1984). Laboratory monitoring for vitamin A and the retinoids in chemoprevention trials. In *Chemoprevention Clinical Trials: Problems and Solutions*, M. A. Sestili (Ed.). NIH Publication No. 85-2715, pp. 93–95.

Micozzi, M. S., Boone, C. W., Kelloff, G. J., Tangrea, J. A., Helzlsouer, K. J., Taylor, P. R. (1985). Chemoprevention of cancer: Implications for clinical pharmacology. *J. Clin. Pharmacol. 25*:164.

Miller, A. B. (Ed.) (1978). Summary and general recommendations. In *Screening for Cancer*, vol. 40, UICC Tech. Rep. Ser., Int. Union Against Cancer, Geneva, pp. 334–338.

Miller, A. B. (1985a). Principles of screening and of the evaluation of screening programs. In *Screening for Cancer*, A. B. Miller (Ed.). Academic Press, New York, pp. 3–24.

Miller, A. B. (1985b). Screening for cancer of the cervix. In *Screening for Cancer*, A. B. Miller (Ed.). Academic Press, New York, pp. 295–323.
Miller, A. B., Bulbrook, R. D. (1982). Screening, detection and diagnosis of breast cancer. *Lancet 1*:1109.
Morrison, A. S. (1985). *Screening in Chronic Disease*. Oxford University Press, New York.
Morson, B. (1974). The polyp-cancer sequence in the large bowel. *Proc. Roy. Soc. Med. 67*:451.
National Cancer Center for Health Statistics (1981). *User's Manual: The National Death Index*. U.S. Government Printing Office, Washington, D.C., DHHS Publication No. (PHS)81-1148.
National Center for Health Statistics (1982). Annotated Bibliography of Cause-of-Death Validation Studies: 1958–1980. U.S. Government Printing Office, Washington, D.C. DHHS publication No. (PHS)82-1363.
Patterson, B. H. (1987). The impact of screening and eliminating prevalent cases on sample size requirements for cancer prevention trials. *Control. Clin. Trials 8*:87.
Patterson, B. H., Bilgrad, R. (1986). Use of the National Death Index in cancer studies. *JNCI 77*:877.
Pedersen, E., Hoeg, K., Kolstad, P. (1971). Mass screening for cancer of the uterine cervix in Ostfold County, Norway: An experiment. Second report of the Norwegian Cancer Society. *Acta Obstet. Gynaecol. Scand.* Suppl. 11.
Pluygers, E. P. (1986). Tumor markers for cancer detection II. *Cancer Det. Prev. 9*:505.
Pluygers, E. P., Beauduin, M. P., Baldewyers, P. E., Burion, J. A. (1986). Tumor markers for cancer detection I. *Cancer Det. Prev. 9*:495.
Reynolds, R. D. (1984). Laboratory monitoring for nutritional status. In *Chemoprevention Clinical Trials: Problems and Solutions*, M. A. Sestile (Ed.). NIH Publication No. 85-2715, Washington, D.C., pp. 119–122.
Sestili, M. A. (1984). Safety considerations in the conduct of chemoprevention trials. In *Chemoprevention Clinical Trials: Problems and Solutions*, M. A. Sestili (Ed.). NIH Publication No. 85-2715, Washington, D.C., pp. 83–86.
Stout, A. P. (1932). *Human Cancer*. Lea & Febiger, Philadelphia, p. 18.
Strax, P. (1985). Mammography. In *Screening for Cancer*, A. B. Miller (Ed.). Academic Press, New York, pp. 141–161.
U.S. Department of Health and Human Services (1978). *Physician's Handbook on Medical Certification: Death, Birth, Fetal Death*. U.S. Government Printing Office, Washington, D.C., DHHS Publication No. (PHS)81-1108.
Willett, W. C., Polk, B. F., Morris, J. S., Stampfer, M. J., Pressel, S., Rosner, B., Taylor, J. O., Schneider, K., Hames, C. G. (1983). Prediagnostic serum selenium and risk of cancer. *Lancet II*:130.
Wong, O., Rockette, H. E., Redmond, C. K., Heid, M. (1978). Evaluation of multiple causes of death in occupational mortality studies. *J. Chron. Dis. 31*:183.

20

Practical Aspects of Cancer Prevention Trials

MARGUERITE M. STEVENS, E. ROBERT GREENBERG, and JOHN A. BARON
Dartmouth Medical School, Hanover, New Hampshire

The randomized clinical trial is an elegant and simple concept. In theory an investigator has only to identify a study group, choose an intervention and control, and wait until enough outcome events have occurred. Then the analysis is simply a comparison of the rate of events in the treated and control groups. In practice, however, clinical trials are rarely so simple. They require years to plan and complete, and they consume vast amounts of money and personal effort. Some practical aspects of cancer prevention trials merit special attention, beyond that pertaining to clinical trials in general. In this chapter we examine the special requirements for cancer prevention trials, noting the practical difficulties in these studies and describing possible solutions to study management problems.

Clinical trials of cancer prevention (in contrast to screening) are a recent undertaking (Greenwald and Sondik, 1986), and to our knowledge, none of any size has yet been completed. It is difficult, therefore, to judge and impossible to know which strategies will be more or less likely to yield success in carrying out these studies. There are available to investigators, however, several helpful texts on clinical trials (Tygstrup et al., 1982; Shapiro and Louis, 1983; Meinart, 1986) and the National Cancer Institute has published a monograph detailing some of the initial experiences with cancer prevention studies in particular (Sestili and Dell, 1984). Our own approach is based partly on these publications and partly on our experiences while conducting two multicenter studies of cancer prevention. One study is a randomized trial of β-carotene (50 mg) or placebo in over 1800 persons at high risk for nonmelanoma skin cancer. The other study, also a randomized trial, uses a 2 × 2 factorial design to test the efficacy of β-carotene

(30 mg) or of vitamin C (1 g) and vitamin E (400 mg) in combination. The subjects for this second study are persons who recently had a neoplastic polyp removed from the large bowel and are thought to be at higher risk of developing new polyps. In carrying out these studies we have gained some insights which may prove useful to investigators engaged in similar chemoprevention trials.

GENERAL CONSIDERATIONS

Studies of cancer-preventive strategies will usually need to be large clinical trials, both because the study outcomes will be relatively rare and because the probable effects of the intervention will be modest at best. The reason that study outcomes will be rare (except in studies of special high-risk groups) is that cancers occur in the general population at a rate of only three or four per thousand per year. Even among the most elderly, who are at highest risk of cancer, the disease is diagnosed in less than three per hundred each year (Young et al.). For studies of cancers of any specific site, the rate of occurrence will be one or two orders of magnitude lower than for cancer of all sites. Thus, enormous sample sizes are necessary. The reason to anticipate only a small treatment effect is that acceptable interventions must be remarkably free of toxic side effects (Greenberg et al., 1985), and we should not generally expect a very safe agent to be also very effective, as evident from pharmacology. Even a moderate reduction in cancer risk, if applicable to a large population, would be of enormous public importance, however, and investigators should not be deterred from studying interventions that show relatively weak effects in laboratory or epidemiological studies (Weinstein, 1983). But the small treatment effect will only be demonstrable in a large clinical study.

The need for a large sample size often requires that the study be a collaborative multicenter endeavor, which entails administrative complexity. Also, an unusually great proportion of the investigators' efforts will have to be directed toward identifying and enrolling adequate numbers of eligible and cooperative participants. These aspects of the trial create unavoidable costs, and, more importantly, they impose special requirements on the investigators with regard to patient recruitment and coordination of study centers. Using a simple protocol, but one written in great detail, will facilitate administration and lessen costs (Yusuf et al., 1984).

Another important feature of many cancer prevention clinical trials is that the participants are generally not ill, i.e., they suffer no noticeable discomfort or disability, even though they may be at high risk of developing cancer. In recruiting subjects and in maintaining their cooperation, the study investigators must approach these persons differently from patients who are not well. Someone who feels fine may be less inclined to enroll in a medical trial, and once enrolled may be more inclined to drop out. If an illness or symptom develops during the study, he or she may fault the study intervention. On the other hand, if she or he remains well, enthusiasm for taking pills, answering questionnaires, and attending clinics may be rapidly lost. For these reasons the cancer prevention trial should be as unobtrusive to the participant as possible. The intervention should be simple, easy to follow, and virtually free of unpleasant side effects. The study followup plan should make as few demands as possible on the participants, preferably requiring no more clinic visits than their usual medical care. These points cannot be overemphasized, for shortfalls in subject accrual and lack of adherence to the study intervention by randomized subjects can have devastating effects on study power and validity (Peto et al., 1976; Ellenberg, 1984; Moon, 1986).

A final general point about cancer prevention trials is that they often involve a treatment or intervention which is readily available to the public. Subjects randomized to the control group can easily adopt interventions such as dietary modification, smoking cessation, or a nutritional supplement. In our own two clinical trials the study agents, β-carotene and vitamins C and E, are easily bought in any pharmacy or health food store. In fact, in the midst of our studies, advertisements in popular magazines appeared in which the potential value of β-carotene in health was presented. This promotion may affect the cooperation of potential and randomized participants. A difficult problem occurs when a substance may be widely recommended to the public on the basis of a prudent assessment of available data but for purposes other than those under investigation. There is, therefore, a concern in many cancer prevention studies that the control group will, in fact, be partially treated, as has occurred in at least one study of heart disease prevention (Multiple Risk Factor, 1982).

POPULATION SELECTION AND ACCRUAL

The principal factors in choosing a population for study are discussed elsewhere in this text (Chapter 17). Briefly, the process involves achieving a balance. First, we would like to study people with a relatively high risk of cancer, so that the study sample can be kept to a manageable size. Against this must be balanced our desire that the results be applicable to the majority of people, whose risk is not greatly elevated. Second, we should only enroll subjects who are likely to cooperate fully with the study protocol. The difficulty is that these people are also more likely to follow a healthy lifestyle on their own (by not smoking, for example), and may thus be at lower than average risk for cancer. In striking these balances, we should always opt for a choice that favors study validity and power rather than study generalizability. It is better, for example, to study a group which is highly cooperative, though atypical of the general population, than to study a representative but uncooperative group, for we first must know whether the intervention is effective before asking whether it is broadly acceptable.

The practical problems of accrual become apparent once the trial actually begins. To assemble a study population of sufficient size can require a high level of effort. If the goal is to enroll persons with an ordinary risk of cancer, the number of potential study subjects is vast indeed. The investigator can then afford to choose carefully, enrolling only those most highly motivated, and still reach the very large sample size required (tens of thousands). The work in this type of study will include substantial clerical effort, mailing and receiving (or not receiving) consent forms and questionnaires for as many as five or ten potential subjects for every one who eventually is randomized. If the study involves patients with a preneoplastic condition or those who are otherwise at high risk, the investigator will have a much smaller pool of potential subjects from which to recruit. In this situation, the number of persons eligible for study who eventually enroll may prove to be far less than initially estimated, possibly leading to a shortfall in study accrual.

Doctors tend to overestimate the numbers of patients they can enter into a clinical trial (Collins et al., 1984). In our study of skin cancer prevention, for example, some dermatologists forecast the number of potential subjects by counting their annual number of office visits for treatment of skin cancer. Once study enrollment began, it became apparent that some patients had several office visits each year, so there were fewer patients than visits. Furthermore, some of the skin cancer patients could not be located, and others were too ill or frail to survive the expected five years of observation. Patients such as these should not be enrolled in a cancer prevention trial, for study power will fall if many of them die or drop out early in the trial. This occurs partly from a drop in sample size but, more importantly, because the intervention will probably not achieve full efficacy until a year or more after its initiation, and the population followed in the later years will contribute more useful information about treatment differences. We also learned that even among patients eligible for participation in our trials, about half were not interested in enrolling, and others were thought by the study staff to be unlikely to adhere to the experimental regimen. In the skin cancer study, during chart review, about 40% of previous skin cancer patients did not meet the eligibility requirements of age and good health. Of the remaining patients who were chart eligible, 19% could not be contacted, 17% did not wish to participate, and 3% proved to be poor candidates for randomization during a placebo run-in trial. Thus, fewer than 35% of patients who might have been enrolled actually were randomized.

In planning our studies, we decided on stringent eligibility criteria, which included requirements that the patients be healthy and free of disabling cardiovas-

Table 1 Desirable Characteristics for Potential Study Subjects

Good Health
Expected to survive the long followup period
Able to make clinic visits
Not overwhelmed by requirements to take other meds
Likely to cooperate
Socially connected:
Live with spouse or family
Unlikely to leave the area
Understands study purpose and requirements
Altruistic motives
Willing to forego the intervention
Will not take vitamins or alter diet on his own
Willing to chance receiving placebo

cular disease. The investigators in the skin cancer study debated whether to relax these requirements because of a possible shortfall in accrual. In retrospect, they were wise to maintain the strict criteria for study entry, since the most frequent reason for stopping capsules after randomization has been the occurrence of serious illness unrelated to the study agents. Another advantage has been the relatively small number of deaths among study participants, in part due to this policy of excluding patients with serious illnesses.

The use of a placebo control can give rise to other problems in accrual. A major reason for refusals in both our studies was patients' concerns about getting sufficient vitamins, for many potential subjects did not believe that they could obtain adequate nutrition from dietary sources alone. They were willing to be in the study only if we would guarantee their receiving the active agent or if they could continue to take their own vitamins. Since we did not allow either option, these patients were not randomized. We discovered that many people firmly believe that cancer can be prevented by taking vitamins. For vitamin-conscious subjects who were eager to cooperate with the study protocol, we suggested two high quality B-complex vitamin preparations which do not contain the study agents. Another possible solution would be to use a very low dose vitamin supplement as the control, so that both the treated and control groups would get at least some supplemental vitamins.

The above considerations have allowed us to develop a mental profile of the ideal candidate for the chemoprevention study. In *evaluating* patients for possible study enrollement we try to *assess* them in these critical regards: (1) general health, (2) anticipated cooperation, and (3) willingness to be "untreated" (Table

1). Our first concern is that the person be well enough to meet the study requirements for clinic followup visits, capsule taking, and questionnaire completion. The study physicians and clinical coordinators jointly make this determination, and they exclude anyone whose longevity seems limited or who appears unlikely to cope well with the study regimen. We secondly assess whether the person is likely to cooperate in a long-term study. We seek people who are socially connected as shown by their living arrangements and membership in religious and social organizations. It is important that they see themselves as attached to their local community and do not expect to move from the area in the foreseeable future. They should be able to understand the reason for the clinical trial and should be unhesitatingly willing to follow the requirements for visits, blood drawing, etc. We also look for people whose motives are altruistic, that is, they want to participate for the good of others rather than to improve their own health. Third, we try to be certain that the potential subject is willing to forgo the study intervention. They must realize that for each agent there is a 50:50 chance that they will receive the placebo version. They must be overtly willing to take placebo and not to take vitamins proscribed by the study.

Our principal approach to ensuring adequate accrual has been to collaborate with other clinical centers. The burden in obtaining eligible, cooperative subjects is thus spread out over several medical research institutions. Furthermore, each collaborating clinical center may draw on different patient sources, including university hospitals, Veterans Administration hospitals, military hospitals, and private practices. Using several clinical centers with multiple sources within them creates organizational complexities and potential problems with quality control (Ederer, 1975), but there also are advantages. Besides enlarging the pool of potential participants for the study, the involvement of multiple collaborating investigators helps to ensure a broad representation of different clinical and scientific viewpoints during the planning, conduct, and analysis of the study.

MAINTAINING COOPERATION

In any cancer prevention study, treated subjects who do not take their capsules will resemble the control subjects with regard to study outcomes, and they will thereby reduce the distinction between treated and control groups. In our cancer prevention trials, control subjects who obtain and take β-carotene, vitamin C, or vitamin E would have a similar effect of reducing the treatment difference. Thus, lack of adherence to the treatment protocol causes a potentially devastating loss of study power, in addition to producing an underestimate of the effect of the intervention. To avoid the undesirable result of inconclusive or misleading findings, the investigators must conduct their study in a way that will maintain the cooperation of participants.

In our trials, the capsules are large and the observation period long. The participants in general do not have symptoms to motivate them to take their capsules and to come for examinations. We can hope that the study is doing them some good, perhaps by ensuring adequate medical surveillance for new cancers; nonetheless some come to see their participation as possibly harmful to their health. Subjects seem to be especially liable to become uncooperative if they continue to manifest endpoints. Some participants who developed a new skin cancer, for example, concluded that the intervention was therefore not effective and possibly dangerous for them. Others came to believe that they were taking placebo and had to be persuaded that they should not buy β-carotene on their own, lest they confuse the study results. Subjects who already believed in the efficacy of vitamin supplements but agreed to stop taking them so that they could participate in the clinical trial were another group who tended to worry about how the study affected their health. They thought that their previous vitamin supplements protected them from acute illnesses, like colds and influenza, or that vitamins alleviated the symptoms of age or chronic illness. As soon as they became ill again, some of them responded by wanting to stop the study capsules and return to their previous vitamin supplements.

Another impetus for participants' stopping study agents comes from the informed consent document. In ours we are required to list all the symptoms even loosely associated with the study agents. This without doubt sensitizes study participants to these symptoms and leads them to conclude that the capsules cause any listed symptom which they eventually experience. Also, it is difficult to convince someone that respiratory infections and other minor illnesses are not related to the capsules, especially if he or she develops a new problem. We have been told by subjects, for example, that the β-carotene (or placebo) has caused bronchitis and even an ingrown toenail, two problems almost certainly unrelated to this study agent.

The elderly seem to be at particularly high risk for noncompliance in following the study plan. In a clinical trial involving subjects with precancerous lesions, such as colorectal polyps, or those who are otherwise at high risk of cancer, the pool of potential subjects will include a large number of older adults. Our policy in the two cancer-preventive trials has been to enroll persons up to age 80 if they are in good health and able to attend the study clinical appointments. Older participants, however, tend to have chronic illnesses requiring medication, and we did not fully foresee the effect this would have on their adherence to treatment. When a new illness occurs and more medicines must be added, the study capsules may drop to a low priority. Subjects often feel overwhelmed by illness and unable to cope with taking another pill or attending another clinic visit. Furthermore, physical slowness and fear of falling in the elderly may cause them to miss study appointments in the morning or during bad weather. Some older subjects have retired and moved to milder climates where we have no clinical centers.

Table 2 Mechanisms for Ensuring Aherence to Treatment

Screen carefully before enrollment
Doctor and study coordinator evaluate candidate
Subjects not enrolled if hesitant about joining
Use placebo initiation trial
Subject must take at least 80% of prescribed agent
Allows subjects to drop out before randomization
Maintain frequent contact
Staff use telephone and mail contact between clinic visits
In person visits with coordinatory and/or doctor occur at least yearly
Each contact is used to reinforce cooperation
Emphasize allegiance to the study
Reinforce altruistic motivation
Do not emphasize interest in the study agent or intervention

While we predicted mortality and incapacitating illness relatively accurately, we did not fully anticipate the fall in cooperation due to the gradual deterioration of health or the changes in lifestyle which come with advancing age.

Maintaining the enthusiasm of participants requires special effort, and there is no single or easy approach. We attempt to ensure adherence to the study regimen by several mechanisms (Table 2). First, before entering the study, all potential subjects are assessed for compliance by both a study coordinator and a physician. Patients are not enrolled if they seem hesitant to participate, or if the study staff has serious doubts about their future cooperation. Second, before randomization, every patient must successfully complete a trial period during which she or he is given the placebo pills (or capsules). Patients who fail to take at least 80% of the pills during this time are not randomized. In our skin cancer prevention study, we used a one-month placebo trial and just over 8% of enrolled patients were dropped before randomization. In the first two months after randomization there were further dropouts, however, and we now believe that a one-month trial is too brief. In the later polyp prevention study we opted for a three-month placebo trial, and we seem to have fewer early dropouts after randomization. Third, we try to maintain frequent personal and mail contact with participants. We send questionnaires to subjects (and often phone them) every three to four months, and we see them at regular clinic visits. With every contact, including the initial one, we emphasize the length of time they will be studied, the fact that the study is double-blinded, and the importance of regular capsule taking and examinations. We explain to them that they and we will not know whether the intervention works until the study has been completed and that there is little information we can give them in the meantime. This may all be clear at the initial visit and at the end of the placebo trial period, but, nevertheless, over time subjects often forget or become discouraged or bored. They need reminders and they need encouragement. Fourth, we try to foster allegiance to the clinical trial rather than to the active agent under study. Focusing on the agent may just encourage the subject to obtain the substance on his or her own. We emphasize that the participant is helping to advance medical knowledge, and we downplay the possible health benefits of being in the study. This approach appeals to a surprising number of participants, many of whom are retired but want to remain useful and involved in their later years. Others, particularly at Veterans Administration Hospitals, are genuinely grateful for the free medical care they have received over the years and are eager for the opportunity to "repay" in this way.

We believe that the key to good cooperation is the attitude and activity of the clinical study coordinator. A coordinator who makes contact regularly and enthusiastically, and who is both familiar with and supportive of the study, is tremendously effective. This kind of coordinator knows all the study participants well and can tailor encouragement and support to them individually. Sometimes what is needed is help getting through an administrative maze in scheduling check-ups at a large hospital. Sometimes, for a lonely patient, it is a sympathetic ear during a phone call. Most of our coordinators have developed, and have shared with each other, some wonderful, personal techniques. These include sending birthday cards to participants and having a surprise gift (such as a packet of home-made brownies) waiting after each annual examination.

The coordinating center offers other reinforcements to cooperating study participants. For each cancer prevention trial we have a booklet which describes the trial and gives definitions in question-and-answer style; for example, "What is a placebo?" "What is an informed consent?" The booklet also outlines the subject's study obligations, lists the names and telephone numbers of local study staff, and has space for jotting down questions and concerns. Annually we send out a newsletter, addressing topics suggested by study coordinators and subjects. We also arrange to send each year a token of recognition for participation, such as a certificate, a letter of appreciation, or even a rose (which was our most popular gift).

Since study coordinators give much of themselves to the study, especially by supporting and encouraging patients, they need recognition similar to that given the co-investigators. We therefore have a yearly study coordinators' meeting, with an agenda set by them and with time for them to discuss their successes and frustrations. They attend with enthusiasm and share knowledge and techniques generously. Similar meetings are useful for the investigators associated with the study. Maintaining *their* motivation is also important, especially since the structure of the trials may work against this. The large numbers of co-investigators and the long time required for a trial do not lead to individual fame or the publications on which academic success is often based. Like the study subjects, the investigators too must be motivated largely by altruism.

AGENT HANDLING

A large-scale nutritional supplement trial carried out at multiple centers involves special problems in agent distribution. The investigators need to project their requirements for agents well in advance and should order materials in bulk. We package our agents in calendar packs, which require considerably more space than the materials alone. Actual accrual may not follow projections, so careful records are important and adjustments must be made periodically, based on patient enrollment figures, available storage space and agent shelf life. In our experience no clinical center has much space for storing packaged drugs. We have therefore set aside a separate room in the coordinating center where we store boxes of calendar packs under specific temperature, light, safety, and access conditions. Our own space requirements are moderate. Consider, however, the storage space needed for a large trial of a fiber supplement packaged as a snack food. Every day each person would take three snack packets weighing about 35 g and occupying about 300 cc in volume. Allowing an additional 50% for packing space, a three months' supply of packages for one person would occupy a 0.5-meter-square box. A study involving 10,000 participants might require storage area equal to a very large house.

Another factor to consider is the effect of packaging on subject adherence, on blinding, and on agent shelf life. We have found that subjects seem to be more reliable in taking medicines supplied in calendar packs rather than in bottles. This type of packaging costs one or two dollars more per patient-month, and these costs should be included in the initial budget estimate. Calendar packs also require more storage space and more careful handling in distribution, since they are somewhat fragile. We use tinted calendar packs to deter study staff from looking for subtle differences between active/placebo agents, even though the agents are manufactured to be identical in appearance. Lastly, the storage life of an agent may be influenced by its packaging. The "blisters" in calendar packs allow some movement of air and moisture, which may lead to deterioration of capsules and pills stored for long periods. Our agents are shipped in bulk from the manufacturer to a pharmaceutical packaging firm, which stores them under optimal conditions of temperature, humidity, and darkness. This firm then makes up calendar packs several times a year as we need them and ships the calendar packs to our coordinating center for interim storage and distribution to the clinical centers.

Our agents are FDA-controlled substances (despite their widespread availability over the counter), and the Investigational New Drug permit requires close monitoring of drug-handling procedures. The FDA requires us to describe, in the operations manual for each project, how the drugs are received, stored, distributed, and destroyed. The most efficient and effective distribution to subjects in our trials is by the clinical study coordinators rather than the hospital pharmacies. There is considerable paperwork in keeping track of the drugs as they are sent from manufacturer, to packager, to coordinating center storage, to shippers, to the clinical center, and lastly to the subject. In our experience preparing a routine shipment of a four months' supply of drugs for distribution to 400 people requires 10 person-hours, plus an additional 10 hours for paperwork. We have also found it necessary to honor requests for additional special shipments of study agents required by losses in shipment or special subject needs such as long periods of travel.

ASSESSING ENDPOINTS

In a cancer prevention study the goal of which is the avoidance of clinically evident cancers or cancer death, the recognition of the study endpoint is relatively straightforward. For the most part, invasive cancers result in a histological (or cytological) confirmation of the diagnosis. Aggressive detection efforts such as mammographic screening might result in biased recognition of disease if unequally applied to treatment and control groups, however, this is not likely to occur in a double-blind clinical trial. A more serious problem arises when the endpoints of a prevention study are precancerous or subclinical lesions. In these trials there are a number of issues that must be addressed if endpoints are to be measured completely and consistently across the study.

The first issue is definition. Every study endpoint must be defined so that staff at the clinical centers know exactly which lesions to count and measure. This may involve biopsies, in which event specified slides should be prepared. To be sure that endpoints are not being missed, the investigators need to seek slides and pathology reports both for the specific diagnoses of interest, and also for a list of related diagnoses which might mimic the condition under study. For example, in the skin cancer prevention trial the coordinating center pathologist reviews all slides which the clinical center pathologist diagnosed as melanoma, basal cell carcinoma, baso-squamous carcinoma, squamous cell carcinoma, keratoacanthoma, and Bowen's disease (or squamous cell carcinoma in situ). In addition, the coordinating center pathologist reviews slides for every skin lesion that was clinically suspected of being cancer. We obtain lists of all other skin lesions removed and request slides of any which may be appropriate for review. Thus far the coordinating center pathologist has reviewed slides from over 800 skin lesions. About 40% of these were not diagnosed as cancer by the local dermatopathologist, but the slides were obtained and reviewed anyway to lessen the chances of missing a cancer endpoint.

The second issue is confirming every endpoint of interest. Many practitioners are not in the habit of obtaining a biopsy of all skin cancers or premalignant lesions, but, for study purposes, everything clinically suspicious of cancer *must* be biopsied. For example, some dermatologists' usual practice when confronted with a patient having multiple basal cell skin cancers is to biopsy one and destroy the others by cautery. To participate in the skin cancer prevention trial, these physicians agreed to biopsy all these tumors and to send one slide of each to the coordinating center. (The study pays for the additional pathology costs in these instances.) Likewise, in the polyp prevention study, all polyps must be submitted for pathology review, and none is destroyed by cautery.

Close surveillance of the subjects is necessary to capture all desired endpoints. Some patients in the skin cancer prevention study are occasionally treated by physicians who are not associated with the study. We must largely depend on subject recall to identify any skin cancer taken off by nonstudy doctors; these are then followed up by contacting the doctor and obtaining slides. In the skin cancer prevention study we have at times identified skin cancers by reviewing pathology records for subjects who did not recall having anything removed from their skin. To the extent this is possible, study staff should monitor medical records and pathology logs to ensure that important outcomes are all counted.

Obtaining pathology slides from multiple laboratories, many of them unfamiliar with our clinical trials, involves careful organization, tracking, transport, and return of slides. The post office or other carriers lose and break some slides, so we cannot use an only copy, and they must be packaged carefully. A few laboratories are willing to provide recuts free; from others we must purchase recuts, while still others will give us an original slide on short-term loan. We find that locating pathology slides, obtaining them, keeping records, shipping, and returning them is one of the most time-consuming jobs a coordinator has after patient accrual. Processing slides is also time consuming at the coordinating center, and many hours must be allotted for it.

A last consideration with endpoints is who determines the final diagnosis. In the design of any trial there must be a clear, final assessment of whether an endpoint has occurred. One can choose to accept the opinions of the many different pathologists at the clinical centers or of one pathologist engaged by the coordinating center specifically to review material and to determine diagnoses in the trial. In some trials the investigators submit a percentage of slides for a second reading to ascertain the level of interreader agreement. In the skin cancer prevention study we have retained a separate pathologist to give third readings of slides only in cases of disagreement between the clinical center pathologist and the coordinating center pathologist. Thus far, we have found excellent agreement between the clinical center and coordinating center diagnoses, and only about 5% of slides must be submitted for a third opinion.

MONITORING SIDE EFFECTS AND DEATHS

In the current cancer prevention clinical trials involving micronutrients, the investigators are using agents chosen partly on the basis of their lack of apparent toxicity. Many of the agents can be purchased without prescription and in identical formula to the capsules in our trials. We must not forget, however, that these substances have never been taken by great numbers of people in large doses for long periods of time in a controlled setting. It is possible that we may find previously unrecognized side effects or, perhaps more likely, we may be able to document the relative safety of the agents.

We have tried to minimize the possibility of severe side effects by excluding persons who are more likely to experience toxicity and those in whom toxicity poses severe risks. For instance, no woman with childbearing potential is eligible to participate in our trials because there are unconfirmed reports of fetal toxicity with β-carotene. We have also implemented procedures which permit rapid detection of toxicity if it occurs. There are three types of procedure. First, subjects complete questionnaires on a regular schedule, every few months. These questionnaires ask about changes in health, symptoms, and hospitalizations. Every positive response generates a telephone call from the clinical center coordinator to determine the nature and severity of problems. We obtain the discharge diagnoses for all hospitalizations, and we encourage subjects to call us collect or to send in prepaid postcards if they have any troublesome symptoms between questionnaires.

Second, whether a subject wants to stop taking the agent because he has symptoms, or whether a doctor suggests stopping the study agent, the physician co-investigator completes a toxicity evaluation form designed to assess the likelihood that a given incident is truly a drug-related problem. In cases of suspected toxicity, we usually institute a stop and restart trial of the capsules to help us assess whether the symptoms were related to taking the study agent.

Third, we review all deaths occurring among randomized subjects, regardless of whether they were still taking their capsules in the months before death. The clinical center's staff notify the coordinating center by phone as soon as they learn of a death, and they report the initial assessment of the cause of death. We later obtain a death certificate from the state office of vital records. Since the death certificate usually takes several months to arrive, the coordinator's immediate report is important for monitoring toxicity.

The clinical center coordinators try, at least yearly, to contact patients who have dropped out of the study. We have discovered how important it is to keep tracing information. Subjects move and may not file changes of address. They may get unlisted telephone numbers, or share a residence and not maintain a telephone in a name we know. To ensure keeping in contact, the investigators should obtain names, addresses, and telephone numbers of relatives, doctors, and friends for all newly enrolled study participants. Invariably, a small number of participants drop completely from sight and cannot be located even to determine whether they are alive. At the end of our studies we will submit a list of the names and other identifying data for these lost patients to the National Center for Health Statistics' National Death Index (NDI). The NDI will attempt to match persons on our list with their list of all deaths in the United States. The match is made principally on the basis of name, sex, parents' surnames, date and place of birth, and social security number (Curb et al., 1985). Prevention trial investigators who hope to use the NDI should collect these data at the outset from all enrolled patients.

Within the coordinating center one of us (JB) has been assigned to review all reports of side effects or death. When deemed necessary he can break the treatment code and "unblind" himself. The overall responsibility for the assessment of safety is assigned to a safety and data monitoring committee in both studies. These committees are each composed of three individuals who are otherwise unconnected with the clinical trials or the participating investigators. Each committee is chaired by a biostatistician with extensive experience in clinical trials. The committees periodically review unblinded data on illnesses, symptoms, and deaths among study participants, and in future they will review data on drug efficacy within the studies. Lastly, all reports of death or serious illnesses associated with the study agent must be sent to the Food and Drug Administration for review as a condition of the Investigational New Drug permit.

SPECIMEN PROCUREMENT

The collection and analysis of blood, tissue, and other specimens will be prominent activities in many prevention studies. Our own trials involve analysis of blood specimens at the coordinating center to determine β-carotene, retinol, and tocopherol. We also plan to examine a subset of bloods for zinc, iron, calcium, selenium, and other minerals. Obtaining high quality plasma and sera for these analyses requires substantial effort beforehand, since the specimens are drawn in 27 different clinical laboratories, each associated with one of 10 clinical centers. Although we provided explicit protocols, as well as special mineral-free vacutainer tubes, and storage and shipping containers, some clinical center staff lacked sufficient technical training for our laboratory work and had difficulty carrying out the procedures. For example, we have received serum when plasma was specified and vice versa. Other problems have included sending wrong, broken, leaking, or improperly labeled tubes. We have also been sent tubes on wet ice and one shipment of tubes that had been left on a loading dock in Phoenix, Arizona, for three summer days. The solution has been to provide the laboratories and study coordinators with detailed guidelines and examples of both "how to" and "how not to" carry out each step. We also encourage direct telephone communication with our laboratory staff for every question, no matter how small.

DATA MANAGEMENT AND QUALITY

The practical issues of data collection, processing, and management in a cancer prevention trial are similar to those for clinical trials in general. An extensive description of data management techniques has been published, so we will address this topic only briefly. In essence, the goal is to obtain high quality data; the problem is to develop mechanisms by which this can be achieved without extraordinary cost. There is no way to pay for enough data management personnel to do all we might wish to have done. Compromises must be accepted and there are steps to take at the beginning of a trial to ensure regular receipt of high quality data.

A detailed protocol is essential to data quality. For example, before any subjects are enrolled, clinical center staff must be absolutely clear about what to do if the randomization code on a particular subject is broken at the clinical center. Likewise, the coordinating center must know in advance how to monitor whether subjects actually got the treatment to which they were randomized. In a good protocol there are few options undiscussed. The protocol should state what constitute major and minor protocol violations, such as failure to implement procedures. Regular tallying and publishing of violations can help in the assessment of data quality and staff performance.

All data generated at the clinical sites must be transmitted to the data processing site. Organizing, copying, and shipping paper is an unappealing aspect of a study coordinator's job, and we try to make this task less onerous by providing monthly reminders and maintaining regular shipping schedules. Some clinical trials involve data entry at the clinic using microcomputers. This obviates the need to copy and send paper records since magnetic disks or phone lines can be used. We have not tried this, although other investigators have with some success. In our trials, drug receipt cards are sent to the coordinating center once a week; these let us know which subjects have actually received their own capsules. The drug receipt cards also trigger our data system to arrange for the next drug shipment. Toxicity evaluation reports are sent upon completion of the evaluation. All other regularly generated data are sent no later than 30 days

Data Collection Points	Data wanted	Instrument/Procedure	Disposition of Data
Roser of potential participants	Name, date of birth or social security number	Local record	DDCC
Subjects identified as nonparticipant	Reasons for nonparticipation	Nonparticipation form	DDCC
Intake appointment	Consent for participation	Informed consent	1 copy to patient 1 copy to clinical center
	Background information	Intake questionnaire	Keep in clinical center until patient is either randomized or declared nonparticipant, then to DDCC.*
	Medical information	Physician's assessment	Keep in clinical center until patient is either randomized or declared nonparticipant, then to DDCC.*
	Documentation of status	Drug receipt card	Send ASAP to DDCC.* 1 copy at clinical center
One month appointment	Compliance and toxicity	Interval questionnaire	DDCC
	Toxicity symptoms and resolution	Toxicity evaluation form	Keep 1 month in clinical center for completion, then send to DDCC.*
	Laboratory determinations	Laboratory form	DDCC, when requested
		Blood sample	DDCC, when requested
	Safety monitoring	Capsule in sealed, labelled envelope	Keep at clinical center
	Documentation of status	Drug receipt card	Send ASAP to DDCC. 1 copy at clinical center
Four- and eight-month appointments	Compliance and toxicity	Interval questionnaire	DDCC
	Toxicity symptoms and resolution	Toxicity evaluation form	Keep 1 month in clinical center for completion, then send to DDCC.
	Laboratory determinations	Laboratory form	DDCC, when requested
		Blood sample	DDCC, when requested

	Safety monitoring	Capsule in sealed, labeled envelope	Keep at clinical center
	Documentation of status	Drug receipt card	Send ASAP to DDCC 1 copy at clinical center
Annual appointment	Compliance and toxicity	Interval questionnaire	DDCC
	Toxicity symptoms and resolution	Toxicity evaluation form	Keep 1 month in clinical center for completion, then send to DDCC
	Medical information	Physician's form	DDCC
	Laboratory determination	Laboratory form	DDCC, when requested
		Blood sample	DDCC, when requested
	Safety monitoring	Capsule in sealed, labeled envelope	Keep at clinical center
	Documentation of status	Drug receipt card	Send ASAP to DDCC
Response to toxicity complaint	Toxicity symptoms and resolution	Toxicity evaluation form	Keep 1 month in clinical center for completion, then send to DDCC.*
Death	Causes	Uncertified copy of death certificate	DDCC
		Death certificate report form	DDCC
Noncompliance	Reasons	Exit form	DDCC

Please note: The original of the study instrument should be sent to the coordinating center. A copy should be kept in the clinical center.

*DDCC = Dartmouth Data Coordinating Center.

Fig. 1 Data Collection Points.

after the subject contact. We have shipping logs to accompany all data. On these, the shipped forms are entered by study identification numbers, so that both the clinical center and data processing staff will have good records of which data forms have been sent or received.

COORDINATION

Sometimes the management of a multicenter clinical trial appears to be more of a commerical venture than a scientific study. Collaborative studies are complex and costly and they benefit from well-trained administrators. The investigators must deal effectively with issues of budgeting, organization, and personnel management. For example, it is important to have detailed guidelines and job descriptions for co-investigators, other physicians, and study coordinators at the clinical centers and at the coordinating center. In our trials the staff at the coordinating center have clearly defined responsibilities for administration, clinical issues, component coordination, and data processing.

We now see the role of the clinical center coordinator as the key to getting work done. This one person must oversee the day-to-day work and is the first line of response for problems, be they concerns of patients or questions from the coordinating center. This job seems to carry with it a high risk of "burnout," and we have had several changes in personnel. To ease the coordinator's job the study investigators should develop a study coordinator's handbook, or manual of operations, which goes beyond guidelines and rules and gives detailed descriptions of (1) how to recruit, (2) how to get good service from medical records departments, laboratories, and pathology departments, (3) how to recognize side effects, and (4) how to schedule appointments within the protocol time specifications.

It is especially important for the clinical center coordinators to have a detailed protocol, which foresees the many variations, aberrations, and idiosyncrasies of human nature and which provides them with guidelines and solutions for all situations. The goal is for all study subjects to progress through the trial in an identical way. Assuring this is a big task, since at a minimum one must keep track of the disease endpoints, toxicity, and patient adherence; the implementation of prevention trials therefore generates many study instruments. Despite our avowed interest in simplicity and our constant vigilance to limit paperwork, one of our clinical trials requires 12 kinds of forms, the other, 14. In addition to forms, subjects have annual meetings with clinical study coordinators or physicians and there are interval telephone contacts between patients and coordinators. As an example, we include a data collection schedule from one of our trials (Fig. 1). The protocol must specify what to do when subjects transfer their medical care to physicians who are not part of the study staff, when subjects must temporarily stop taking capsules for any reason, when randomized subjects do not fully participate, and when other unexpected happenings occur. Lastly, the protocol should lead to the development of a procedure manual which describes, in exacting detail, every step of the study, including how to complete the forms, how to ship specimens, etc. With some foresight and a great deal of good fortune, the protocol and procedure manual will require only minimal updating once the study is in progress.

Before the study actually begins, the investigators should meet to review the results of any pilot tests of study instruments and to approve the final study plan and protocol. The cancer prevention trial will require years to reach a definite conclusion, and in the collaborative study the credit (or blame) for the end result must rightfully be shared among the collaborating investigators. It is important that they all be involved as colleagues during the planning phases, so that they may work as colleagues during the implementation of the study. Collaborative clinical trials are not the way to seek quick fame or wealth, and there is no place in them for the overlarge ego. The group of investigators must work together, in complete cooperation, and it is the job of the coordinating center to ensure that this occurs.

SUMMARY

In this chapter we have stressed that cancer prevention trials may appear simple and elegant at the outset, and perhaps even when completed, but while in progress they are not only expensive and time consuming, but fraught with complexities and some unique problems. If investigators rigorously follow guidelines for conducting clinical trials and anticipate problems, however, they can conduct prevention trials that have strong potential for providing solid answers about cancer prevention.

The first key element is meticulous and detailed planning, including close attention to personnel requirements, before subject accrual begins. The investigators must develop strategies for selecting a population, accruing patients, and maintaining cooperation. The most important subsequent concern is to ensure adequate study power, and this requires enrollment of enough subjects, maintaining their adherence to therapy, and obtaining complete and accurate follow-up of endpoints. Other considerations, while secondary, are also important; there must be plans for handling agents, monitoring side effects and deaths, procuring specimens, and managing data. If the investigators can develop the right strategies and implement them through a clear, detailed protocol, the trial will have the best chance to succeed.

REFERENCES

Collins, J. F., Williford, W. O., Weiss, D. G., Bingham, S. F., Klett, C. J. (1984). Planning patient recruitment: Fantasy and reality. *Statistics in Medicine 3*: 435.

Curb, J. D., Ford, C. E., Pressel, S., Palmer, M., Babcock, C., Hawkins, C. M. (1985). Ascertainment of vital status through the National Death Index and the Social Security Administration. *Am. J. Epidemiol. 121*:754.

Ederer, F. (1975). Practical problems in collaborative clinical trials. *Am. J. Epidemiol. 102*:111.

Ellenberg, S. S. (1984). Randomized designs in comparative clinical trials. *N. Engl. J. Med. 210*:1404.

Greenberg, E. R., Beck, R., Baron, J. (1985). Carotenoids in prevention of cancer. In *Retinoids: New Trends in Research and Therapy*, J. H. Sauret (Ed.). S. Karger, Basel.

Greenwald, P., Sondik, E. (1986). Diet and chemoprevention in NCI's research strategy to achieve national cancer control objectives. *Ann. Rev. Public Health 7*:267.

Meinart, C. L. (1986). *Clinical Trials: Design, Conduct, and Analysis*. New York: Oxford University Press.

Moon, T. E. (1986). Clinical trials of cancer prevention agents: true versus observed prevention effect. *Statistics in Medicine 5*:435.

Multiple Risk Factor Intervention Trial Research Group. (1982). Multiple Risk Factor Intervention Trial: risk factor changes and mortality results. *JAMA 248*:1465.

Peto, R., Pike, M. C., Armitage, P., Breslow, N. E., Cox, D. R., Howard, S. V., Mantel, N., McPherson, K., Peto, J., Smith, P. G. (1976). Design and analysis of randomized clinical trials requiring prolonged observations of each patient: I. Introduction and design. *Br. J. Cancer 34*:585.

Sestili, M. A., Dell, J. G. (Eds.). (1984). *Chemoprevention Clinical Trials: Problems and Solutions*. Department of Health and Human Services, Bethesda, Md. NIH Publications No. 85-2715.

Shapiro, S. H., Louis, T. A. (Eds.). (1983). *Clinical Trials: Issues and Approaches*. Marcel Dekker, Inc., New York.

Tygstrup, N., Lachin, J. M., Juhl, E. (Eds.). (1982). *The Randomized Clinical Trial and Therapeutic Decisions*. Marcel Dekker, Inc., New York.

Weinstein, M. C. (1983). Cost-effective priorities for cancer prevention. *Science 221*:17.

Young, J. L., Percy, C., Asire, A. (Eds.). Surveillance Epidemiology and End Results: Incidence and Mortality Data, 1973–1977. National Cancer Institute Monograph #57.

Yusuf, S., Collins, R., Peto, R. (1984). Why do we need some large, simple randomized trials? *Statistics in Medicine 3*:409.

21
Data and Safety Monitoring

DAVID L. DeMETS
University of Wisconsin, Madison, Wisconsin

INTRODUCTION

In the informed consent process for clinical trials, the concept is at least implicit, if not explicit, that a study will not continue any longer than necessary to achieve the objectives. Specifically, it will not continue if the intervention being studied demonstrates sufficient harm or risk relative to the potential benefit. This issue is especially compelling for cancer prevention trials where the subjects are relatively healthy individuals who are at higher risk for cancer than the general population. Thus, for groups conducting cancer prevention trials, it is imperative that the results of the trial be monitored in an ongoing fashion to assure that the trial is being properly conducted and will produce valid results, that the intervention has not already proven to be beneficial, and that the risk benefit ratio is still favorable. This dimension of ongoing data monitoring is in contrast to the classical laboratory situation where the experiment is designed, the data collected, and results analyzed at the conclusion of the project. The monitoring of a cancer prevention trial is a complex process. Many issues must be considered simultaneously, and statistical approaches must be utilized to accommodate the repeated analyses of interim results. These topics will be discussed in further detail in this chapter.

AREAS MONITORED

Just as there are many components that must be considered in the design of a cancer prevention trial, there are many aspects in the conduct that also must be monitored to assure the best possible study. These aspects range from subject recruitment and baseline evaluation to their safety and followup evaluation. In addition, we want the subjects and health professionals to follow the protocol as closely as possible. We also need the data to be as complete and as accurate as feasible. Therefore, we will consider some of the areas that must be monitored to produce a successful cancer prevention trial.

Recruitment

Obviously, no trial can be successful if it does not recruit the number of patients required by the design or at least a reasonable approximation to that goal. To date, most cancer clinical trials have been of a therapeutic nature, i.e., treating patients who have already been diagnosed with cancer. Prevention trials differ from therapeutic trials in that subjects usually have not, as yet, been diagnosed with cancer, even though they may be at "high" risk. This usually means that investigators must seek participants beyond their own clinic, such as individuals who live in the surrounding community. As described by Friedman, Furberg, and DeMets (1985), recruitment of subjects in this setting is a very challenging task. Without careful monitoring of recruitment, the trial may fall behind in its schedule. This lag can cause serious scientific and fiscal problems.

Investigators are typically enthusiastic at the start of a prevention trial about their ability to recruit the specific number of subjects required by protocol. During the course of the protocol design, a number of inclusion and exclusion criteria are decided upon. These criteria reduce the number of subjects who might be eligible to participate. Some individuals may choose not to participate after they appreciate the nature of the trial and what is required of them. Physicians may not choose to enter a subject for various medical reasons. Recruitment for cancer prevention trials also depends on the aggressiveness of the publicity or outreach in the community. Experience from prevention trials in other disease areas suggest that 10 to 20 individuals must be screened for every subject randomized into the trial. This level of effort is often not fully appreciated at the start of prevention trials.

Many prevention trials have as a primary outcome the time to some event such as death, a cause-specific death, or some nonfatal event such as the first diagnosis of cancer. Thus, the time the subject is exposed to the intervention being evaluated is an important part of the design of the trial. Since most clinical trials recruit patients over a long period of time or in a staggered fashion, subjects recruited at the beginning will contribute more person years of exposure to the intervention than those entered later in the trial. Falling behind in recruitment and then catching up in the last days of the entry period does not provide the trial with the same amount of information as a uniform rate of recruitment. This delay may reduce the power of the trial to detect meaningful differences.

Table 1 Recruitment Status

Time (wk)	Clinic 1 Goal	Clinic 1 Attained	Clinic 1 %	Clinic 2 Goal	Clinic 2 Attained	Clinic 2 %	Total Goal	Total Attained	Total %
10	100	100	100	100	0	0	200	100	50
20	200	200	100	200	50	25	400	250	62
30	300	300	100	300	150	50	600	450	75
40	400	400	100	400	300	75	800	700	87
50	500	500	100	500	500	100	1,000	1,000	100

For these reasons, recruitment must be monitored in an ongoing fashion for the trial as a whole and for each participating clinic. Goals should be set for each clinic for various time points. One technique, described in Friedman, Furberg, and DeMets (1985), is to tabulate or plot the cumulative number of subjects over time by site and by study goal. This is shown for a hypothetical case in Table 1. In this example, Clinic 1 attained its goal while Clinic 2 fell substantially behind. Even though Clinic 2 eventually caught up, the trial lost power because subjects were treated and followed for fewer weeks. If all sites fall behind, then serious consideration must be given to the feasibility of the trial as currently designed. Relaxing eligibility criteria is one possible solution, but this usually will not solve the recruitment problem completely.

Eligibility

The protocol usually details the qualifications for a subject to be eligible for a prevention trial. Whether patients who are actually randomized to a trial meet those criteria is an important consideration. May et al. (1981) assert that all subjects who are entered or randomized into a clinical trial must be accounted for in the analysis. If entered subjects can be withdrawn from the analysis because they are later deemed ineligible, the results of the trial may be biased. On particular reason for potential bias is that the eligibility might be reevaluated if the outcome of the subject was not favorable. If the reevaluation was different between treatment groups, more subjects at higher (or lower) risk would be removed from one group than the other, thus creating a biased comparison. Since all subjects must be accounted for in the analysis, then having subjects who are "ineligible" causes a problem. No resolution will be totally satisfactory and, therefore, the number of such cases should be kept to a minimum. If the number is small, their impact on the results should not be dramatic. Analysis should, at a minimum, be done both with and without the "ineligibles."

One reason sometimes given for ineligible subjects being randomized involves a clerical error in obtaining baseline determinations. Another reason is that results had to be obtained from some central laboratory and the subject was entered before the results were confirmed. The registration/randomization process itself must have enough built-in double checks such that the number of ineligible subjects will be very small.

A large number of "ineligible" subjects randomized at a particular site may be a sign of other problems. The investigator may be having trouble in recruiting and is entering subjects who are on the borderline of the eligibility criteria. It also may be a sign of operational difficulties at the site itself. Staff may not understand the protocol eligibility criteria or may be having difficulty in performing some of the measurements required for entry. In any case, the monitoring system should alert the trial leadership that such a situation exists and steps should be taken to correct the problem as soon as possible.

Baseline Variables

In addition to determining trial eligibility, baseline variables are obtained for several other reasons. One reason is that we must be able to describe to the medical community the type of individual that was studied in order to interpret and generalize the final results. Baseline variables are also used for stratification in the analyses. They may be especially important in isolating which subjects are at risk for a particular toxicity.

Another reason is to be able to monitor the randomization process itself. While this hopefully should never be a problem, there have been instances where the randomization process was violated. In one case, this violation was discovered by noting that a particular clinic had an unusual imbalance in the baseline characteristics, more than would be expected by chance alone.

Monitoring the quality of baseline data can provide some indication of what quality will most likely be received from future followup examinations. It is much easier to correct problems before they exist too long than to discover them later when they cannot be straightened out.

If recruitment is a problem in a trial, then an up-to-date assessment of the patients in the trial is helpful in judging whether altering the eligibility criteria would aid the recruitment. For example, if the baseline distribution of age is skewed towards the lower end of the criteria, lowering the age cut-off might allow more subjects to participate. In practice, however, minor adjustments to entry criteria do not lead to large increases in recruitment.

Compliance to Protocol

The ability to detect whether a new cancer prevention strategy can alter an identified outcome depends in part on the degree to which patients comply with the protocol. If only one-half of the patients adhere to the intervention, then the power of the trial is also reduced. While we may intend to have good compliance for our intervention, subjects in prevention trials are relatively free to comply as they wish.

Some noncompliance can be allowed for in the design of the trial. Lachin (1981) describes a simple model for increasing sample size during the design phase to accommodate noncompliance. If R denotes the fraction of individuals in the intervention group who are dropping out of the program, then the sample size must be increased by a factor of $1/(1 - R)^2$. For example, if 0.25 do not comply, then the study size must be increased by almost 80 percent. Wu, Fisher, and DeMets (1980) provide more elaborate models for noncompliance adjustments, which were developed for prevention trials in general.

Withdrawal of subjects from the analysis for noncompliance is not acceptable because this will bias the comparison of intervention with a control, an issue discussed by May et al. (1981) as well as by investigators of the Coronary Drug Project Research Group (1980). In this latter case, subjects on placebo who compiled had a more favorable response than those placebo subjects who do not comply. We must analyze all subjects who are randomized, regardless of their compliance, since compliance itself is an outcome.

Since noncompliance may reduce the power of the study, the data monitoring system must be able to measure the degree of poor adherence. While some noncompliance is inevitable, there may also be possibilities to minimize this if detected early enough. Noncompliance late in the trial has less impact on the power loss than noncompliance early in the trial. Thus, it is important to measure the degree of noncompliance as soon as possible.

Investigators may have difficulty with a particular drug dose level or nutritional intervention. A particular diet may be hard to stick with, but there may be alternative foods that would be acceptable. Prevention trials often involve a behavioral modification, and the noncompliance may be due to the noneffectiveness of the behavior modification strategy being used. Comparison of noncompliance across sites is a good way of determining if the noncompliance is a studywide issue or isolated to a particular investigator. Not all investigators may be equally motivated or able to take on the tremendous challenge of getting all these relatively healthy subjects to substantially modify their behavior. Without the investigators' best effort, the compliance may not be what it should or could be.

Satisfactory measures of compliance are not always available. For drug studies, pill counts or tracers detected in the urine or serum are often used with some degree of success. If a diet modification is being tested, dietary recalls may be used to evaluate intake. Surrogate measures, such as nutritional components detectable in the serum, may also be possible. Indirect measures of compliance include monitoring how well patients attend clinic visits and how complete the data collection is. It is unlikely that any one strategy will be sufficient to assess compliance. More than one method should be used in order to get some sense of the adherence level.

Primary and Secondary Outcome Variables

One major focus for data monitoring is the primary and secondary outcome variables. The ideal situation is for a prevention trial to have a single or primary outcome variable which determines the success of the intervention strategy being studied. Often this is the time to the occurrence of some event, such as incidence of cancer or death due to cancer. Even if death due to cancer is the primary outcome, disease-free survival may be a "secondary" outcome of interest. Other biochemical or biological markers may be of interest as well. Another aspect may be measures of the subject's quality of life. Prevention tirals often have more than one dimension, even if a primary outcome is clearly identified. Monitoring the intervention is, therefore, more complex than observing a single variable.

As indicated earlier, there is an implicit, if not explicit, assumption that a trial will not continue unnecessarily if interim results already establish that the intervention is successful. However, even if intervention is looking favorable with regard to the overall comparison on the primary variable, secondary variables may have a different trend which does not favor the new intervention. Another case might be where the overall trend is favorable but not consistent across important subgroups such as sex or age categories, thereby making it difficult to interpret or generalize the results.

One would like to have consistency in the outcome variables, even though the primary outcome should be given the most weight. If some consistency is not observed, the monitoring process may not be able to come to a conclusion for early termination. At a minimum, the decision will not be easy and may even be controversial. Factors to be considered in such decisions are discussed later.

The primary outcome and safety measures at a minimum will be carefully examined periodically during the course of a trial. Repeated testing of these data increases the chance of a false positive result unless precautions are taken in the interpretation of interim results. Statistical procedures are available to aid in this interpretation and are described later.

Safety Variables

A second major focus of data monitoring is the issue of safety and toxicity. In order to fully evaluate the risk-benefit ratio of any new intervention, the potential harm must be thoroughly examined. In contrast to the primary or secondary outcome, where ideally a few variables are identified, numerous variables can and must be monitored for evidence of adverse effects. Moreover, some of the measures can be objective (such as blood chemistries, chest X-rays, and body temperature) and others (such as physical complaints) may be quite subjective. In some instances, grading schemes for toxicity (such as the one used by the Eastern Cooperative Oncology Group) offer a systematic scoring system.

One important task is to define the most anticipated adverse effects carefully. Part of the definition should consider whether the outcome can be ascertained equally in both the intervention and the control group. Often prevention trials involve behavior modification, which may result in more frequent contact with the intervention group. If this is the case, there is a greater opportunity to learn about adverse or safety problems with that group. Comparisons with the control group could easily be misleading. The data monitoring system must be careful to avoid this situation if possible or at least be cautious in interpreting the results of such comparisons. One solution is to require that toxicity be recorded only at common points in time to avoide ascertainment bias.

Subjects in the control group may develop symptoms or complaints. This was seen, for example, in a cardiovascular prevention trial which compared aspirin versus placebo for reducing cardiovascular death in men at high risk (Aspirin Myocardial Infarction Study Group, 1980). In this trial, 2 to 3% of the subjects in the placebo group complained of ulcer symptoms. Furthermore, the rate of complaints increased with time. In another trial (Beta Blocker Heart Attack Trial, 1982), two-thirds of placebo subjects complained of shortness of breath, while only 6% did so at baseline. Thus, we must interpret adverse effects of any new intervention in context of a control group.

Rare but serious adverse effects will not be observed very frequently in most prevention trials, despite their large size. Thus, adverse effects, which might be a real safety issue, could be overlooked or not easily evaluated. It is not easy to determine how long one must observe subjects to be convinced that the intervention is reasonably safe. Since the intervention might be used on a large number of relatively healthy individuals, this is a real dilemma. The National Death Index allows for long-term monitoring of mortality, but this is an extreme index of possible adverse effects.

The number of statistical tests can be as large as the number of variables being monitored. Some statistical tests will be significant by chance alone, and performing large numbers of them only increases the chances of a false positive. Thus, some conservative interpretation is required. However, if the approach were used that multiplies the observed p-value by the number of variables tested and requires this value to be smaller than a traditional 0.05 significance level, the chance for a true adverse effect to be declared significant is very remote. Safety variables are measured repeatedly, as is the primary outcome variable, making the chance of a false positive even grater. Statistical methods discussed later, for controlling the false positive error rate for a single variable tested repeatedly do not, as yet, adjust for the testing of several variables. The evaluation of adverse effects must be judged in the context of the severity, the pattern across several toxicity measures, and knowledge about the biological aspects as well as the level of the "nominal" significance level.

Historically, however, clinical trials have not been major contributors to our knowledge of rare adverse effects, according to a review by Temple, Jones, and Crout (1979). The major reasons are that the duration of followup is too short or the number of patients too small. Even in prevention trials, several thousand subjects might be exposed only for a few years–not enought to detect rare adverse events. In addition, subjects who are likely to be high risk candidates for adverse effects are often excluded deliberately by the entry criteria.

Despite the problems with adequately assessing the potential adverse effects of a new cancer prevention strategy, subject safety must be carefully monitored, taking into consideration the issues raised. It is important to prevent healthy subjects in a prevention trial from unnecessary or unreasonable risk. To achieve this, the data collection and reporting system must be brought up to date on a relatively frequent basis.

Data Quality

A formal periodic review of the quality of data should be part of the data monitoring. The quality of a trial is a function of the quality of the data. Minimizing poor quality data starts with well-designed and field-tested forms, proper training of clinic staff, an operations manual with precise definitions, and a system for rapidly processing forms and entering data. Even with these systems in place, a surveillance process must be installed.

During the progress of a trial, data forms should be monitored for completeness and timeliness. If feasible, a small percent of randomly selected forms should be audited against source documents to check for the accuracy of the data. An unusually high number of incomplete or tardy forms, relative to other clinics, may be a signal of operational problems within that clinic. The number of clinic visits missed by subjects also indicates the quality of the clinic operations which, in turn, indicates the quality of the data from that site.

If central laboratories are used to obtain standardized data, an external surveillance system should be established to ensure consistency and promptness of results. One method for checking the accuracy and reproducibility of a laboratory's common results is to submit identical but masked samples for analysis. Delayed reports can signal more serious problems. In a recent prevention trial, a high quality research laboratory was observed to be falling behind in data submission and then in the completeness of forms as well. A site visit revealed that the research laboratory was not prepared to process the high volume of specimens required by a prevention trial, even though their scientific credentials were outstanding. After a site visit, another laboratory was selected which could handle the volume required. Because the data monitoring system was in place, the problem was identified early enough such that the trial was not jeopardized.

MONITORING COMMITTEE AND THE DECISION PROCESS

A very large number of elements of a prevention trial must be carefully monitored in an ongoing and timely manner. Since the outcome variables and issues raised frequently involve several disciplines, a data monitoring committee is often constituted. No one individual is likely to have sufficient expertise in all of the areas to be able to do the monitoring adequately.

Shaw and Chalmers (1970) argue that the individual investigator taking care of the subjects and attempting to evaluate them in an unbiased manner should not be aware of any trends in the data. Furthermore, if randomization is still ongoing, knowledge of interim results with respect to primary, secondary, and adverse effects can place the investigator in an awkward position in recruiting additional subjects. Presumably, the investigator must remain neutral as to the benefits of the new intervention in order to randomize a subject to either intervention or control. For these reasons, the members of the data monitoring committee are often independent of the study.

The data monitoring committee should have as members physicians knowledgeable about the intervention being evaluated, statisticians with clinical trials expertise, epidemiologists, and often a subject advocate or an ethicist. This committee must meet periodically, typically once or twice a year, and evaluate the risk-benefit ratio for continuing the trial. It must survey the quality of the trial in all of its dimensions discussed previously. The interaction of the committee members is crucial for the monitoring process to be successful. Stopping a trial ahead of schedule under such circumstances may serve only to add confusion to the scientific and medical issues. While no two trials will provide the same scenario, terminating a trial early is not a simple process. DeMets (1984) reviewed the experiences of several published trials which were recently completed, confirming the fact that early termination is complicated and requires that several factors be considered simultaneously before a decision can be reached.

Friedman, Furberg, and DeMets (1985) describe some of these decision factors. First, we must be sure that the observed differences are not due to some imbalance in prognostic factors, even if the study was randomized. We need to be sure that there is no bias in the ascertainment of the outcome variables, especially if the study was not masked. Prevention trials often have a behavioral modification component which may result in the experimental group receiving more contact and, thus, the chance for more "observation." We also want to assess the impact of missing data on the conclusions. One of the most important considerations is that of internal consistency across the various outcome measures, across relevant subgroups, and over the participating clinical centers. Some degree of consistency in results on these factors adds confidence to the decision making. Consistency of results to external information should also be discussed. Finally, the objective of a clinical trial is to obtain results that will be convincing to some segment of the medical community. If results from a trial terminated early will not be convincing, then that decision may jeopardize the entire effort and the contribution of the subjects who participated.

Some clinical trials, such as the cardiovascular trial conducted by the Beta Blocker Heart Attack Trial Research Group (1982), were successfully terminated early with the results being easily accepted. As reviewed by Kolata (1979), the termination of the University Group Diabetes Project for issues relating to toxicity was controversial for several years. Because of the tremendous responsibility that must be borne by the data monitoring committee, a multidisciplinary membership is very helpful if not a requirement.

As a final point, some trials may be considered for early termination not because of evidence for early benefit or toxicity but rather because there is no trend at all. If the study has little chance of ever obtaining a conclusive result, then, for ethical as well as financial reasons, the trial may be terminated early. This is an issue especially relevant to prevention trials, where lifestyle modifications are often employed and there is uncertainty as to how long it takes for these modifications to have an impact on the risk of cancer. When the Coronary Drug Project Research Group (1975) reported on the nicotinic acid treatment arm, there initially was no difference in total mortality compared to placebo, although the nicotinic acid group had fewer myocardial infarctions. However, using the National Death Index, subsequent followup on the cohort in 1985 (see Canner, 1985) indicated a significant difference in mortality favoring treatment. The issues of when to "give up" on a prevention trial is very complex and no simple solution can be presented. Rather, each study must be discussed in its own context, carefully weighing the costs, risks, and benefits.

STATISTICAL ISSUES

As discussed, there are many ethical, scientific and statistical issues in the monitoring of a prevention trial. One statistical aspect that must be considered is how to perform the monitoring for the primary and secondary outcomes as well as toxicity. This issue will be reviewed in this section.

Repeated Significance Testing

As already described, clinical trials usually have several variables which are being measured. Statistical testing on several variables is a common problem in medical research, sometimes referred to as the multiple testing problem. Another related problem in clinical trials is the repeated significance testing of the same variable at various points in time during the course of the study. While this repeated testing is necessary to comply with the ethical requirements, the impact is to increase the chances of finding false positive results, that is, claiming that the treatment is effective when in actuality it is not. This is a well-known problem and has been studied extensively. Classical sequential designs have been described by Wald (1947) and by Armitage (1975). However, despite the theoretical appeal of the classical sequential designs, these solutions have not been widely used in medical trials.

While classical solutions are not utilized, one cannot ignore the repeated testing problem. Armitage, McPherson, and Rowe (1969) computed the increase in the false positive rate or type I error. If we tested a single variable only once at the 5 percent significance level using the critical values of ±1.96, then we would have a 5 percent chance of claiming treatment differences incorrectly. If we tested the same variable twice, each time using ±1.96 as the critical value, then the actual false positive error rate is approximately 8 percent. If this is done 5 or 10 times, the error rate is about 15 or 20%, respectively. Clearly, these are not acceptable false positive error rates, particularly for studies as important and far reaching as cancer prevention trials.

Historically, statisticians have relied upon conservative interpretation of interim analyses to avoid or minimize the risk of increased type I error. While these methods were somewhat "ad hoc" in nature, they formed the basis for the development of procedures which were more formal and more accurately controlled the type I error. Even though these methods assume that only one variable is being monitored, they can serve as useful guides in the interpretation of interim analyses. An overview of this development may be found in articles by DeMets and Lan (1984) and by Gail (1984). A brief outline of some of the results is presented in the next two sections.

Group Sequential Designs

One general solution to the repeated significance testing problem is referred to as group sequential procedures. The term "group" refers to the fact that interim analyses are usually done after a new group of subjects have been entered or an additional number of events have been observed. This is in contrast to the classical sequential methods which compare treatments after each new subject or event has been observed. All of the group sequential procedures adjust the critical value used at each interim analysis to obtain an overall prespecified type I error. Each method uses a different algorithm or theoretical model for obtaining the critical values.

One of the first and simplest methods was proposed by Haybittle (1971) and promoted by Peto et al. (1976). The procedure requires that no interim analysis be considered sufficient for early termination unless the statistical test statistic is larger than 3.0 or perhaps 3.5. This strategy is so conservative that any adjustment to the final scheduled analysis would be minimal and thus ignored if the number of interim analyses is not too large. Using final critical values of ± 1.96 would give a type I error close to, but not exactly, 5% for a two-sided test. Fleming, O'Brien, and Harrington (1984) have extended this strategy to compute critical values which would produce an exact prespecified type I error.

An alternative strategy to the Haybittle-Peto boundary values is due to Pocock (1977). In this model, the same critical value is used at each analysis and is computed in order to produce the desired type I error. The theoretical model for the Pocock procedure is more formal than the simple Haybittle-Peto method and is based on the method used by Armitage, McPherson, and Rowe (1969). It requires that the number of interim analyses to be performed be specified in advance. It also requires that the number of subjects or events be equal between analyses, although the method is not especially sensitive to this assumption according to DeMets and Gail (1985). If, for example, we were to design our prevention trial for four interim analyses and the scheduled final analysis with a desired type I error of 5% (two-sided), then the critical value for the test statistic would be 2.413. This value would be used at each analysis. An observed test statistic larger than 2.413 might be considered evidence for a careful evaluation of early termination. Otherwise, we would continue the trial unless this were the scheduled termination of the trial.

A third group sequential method was developed by O'Brien and Fleming (1979) and is based on the same statistical model as that of Pocock. The difference is in the critical values that are proposed. Instead of using constant critical values for all analyses, the O'Brien-Fleming procedure adjusts the critical value as the trial progresses. Starting with a large conservative critical value, it is decreased with each analysis to a final value which is close to the "nominal" value. To use the same example as described above, the critical values for the five scheduled analyses would be 4.56, 3.23, 2.63, 2.28, and 2.04, respectively. Other group sequential boundaries have been described by Whitehead and Stratton (1983) and Whitehead (1982).

These procedures are members of a large class of group sequential procedures developed by Lan and DeMets (1983). In their model, the requirements for a prescribed number of interim analyses and for approximately equal number of subjects or events between analyses have been removed. Instead, their method

Table 2 Group Sequential Boundaries for Five Analyses (n = 5) and Two-Sided Significance Level of 0.05

	Critical values for Test Statistic for 3		
Analysis	Haybittle-Peto	Pocock	O'Brien-Fleming
1	±3.0	±2.413	±4.56
2	±3.0	±2.413	±3.23
3	±3.0	±2.413	±2.63
4	±3.0	±2.413	±2.28
5	±2.0	±2.413	±2.04

requires that the total amount of information to be obtained is specified in advance. Their model allows critical values to be generated at arbitrary points during the trial. Models can be specified which produce Pocock and O'Brien-Fleming type critical values.

There are advantages to the three types of models described above in detail. The critical values for the example described are summarized in Table 2 for these three group sequential procedures. The Haybittle-Peto method is simple and does not require the number of analyses to be specified, nor does it require equal numbers of new observations. It does, however, have a very conservative interpretation of interim results, even the last one prior to the scheduled final analysis. Thus, it does not allow much opportunity for early stopping. The Pocock method is not quite so conservative and thus allows for an earlier stopping time. It does, however, require a larger critical value at the last scheduled analysis (e.g., 2.413) than the two other methods. In order to compensate for this and maintaine the same level of power in the design, a larger sample size must be proposed. The O'Brien-Fleming critical values, in a sense, provide a compromise between the other two. Early in the trial, the values are very conservative but the criteria are relaxed or decreased as the trial continues. It provides the opportunity for early stopping, although very early stopping is less likely to occur. It does not demand an increase in sample size since the final critical value is not substantially increased. For prevention trials where the outcome is often long-term followup for some event, the Haybittle-Peto or O'Brien-Fleming methods might be more suitable than the Pocock method.

If prevention trials do utilize time to some event, such as a cancer death or first diagnosis of cancer, then lifetable methods (such as the log rank test) would be utilized in the analyses. The group sequention methods described are applicable to this setting as well. The justification is provided in work by Tsiatis (1981, 1982) and by DeMets and Gail (1985).

Recent work has also established how to compute significance levels using group sequential methods (see Fairbanks and Madsen, 1982). Their method is based on the Armitage, McPherson, and Rowe (1969) model used to generate the critical value. The probability of obtaining a more extreme result than the one observed is computed, given that the previous critical values were not exceeded. This probability is added to the probability of crossing each preceding boundary to obtain the overall p-value.

Confidence intervals can also be computed for the group sequential methods using work by Tsiatis, Rosner, and Mehta (1984) or, for the more general Lan-DeMets method, in work by Kim and DeMets (1985). For the O'Brien-Fleming type critical values, the adjustments to the naive confidence intervals are modest using these approaches. Jennison and Turnbull (1984) have also urged that confidence intervals, adjusted for the repeated testing, be formally utilized in the monitoring process. If the confidence interval contains estimates of treatment differences which are of no medical interest, then we should continue the trial to rule these out. If the interval does not include such outcomes, then early termination should be considered.

In general, group sequential designs such as those described provide reasonable solutions to the repeated testing problem. They have been utilized in a number of non-cancer trials and are currently being utilized in ongoing cancer prevention trials.

Curtailed Sampling

Often during the monitoring process the question arises as to whether the interim trends are such that the results at the scheduled conclusion of the trial are already determined or nearly so. For example, the intervention group might have substantially fewer deaths than the control group at an interim evaluation. We might ask if the results are so overwhelming that it would be difficult, if not impossible, for the intervention superiority to cease. A contrasting example might be that there is no difference at all in the number of deaths, or there may even be slightly more deaths in the intervention group. The question in this case is whether it is possible, realistically, for the intervention group to recover and be significantly superior to the control group at the end of the trial. These two scenarios represent the issue considered in the method of curtailed sampling.

If absolute certainty in the ultimate outcome is required, the process is often described as deterministic curtailed sampling or just curtailed sampling. However, if the requirement of certainty is relaxed to highly probable, then the procedure is referred to as stochastic curtailed sampling or conditional power. The theoretical basis for this approach was established by Lan, Simon, and Halperin (1982), although the method was being used in practice much earlier in the 1970s by investigators such as the Coronary Drug Project Research Group (1981).

The computational aspects of this procedure are simple in concept, although they may be somewhat complicated for some applications. The task is to compute the probability that the final test statistic will fall into the region which rejects the null hypothesis (e.g., greater than ± 1.96), given the current value of the statistic and assuming the true value of the treatment difference to be in effect for the remainder of the study. If the current trend favors the intervention, we would compute the probability γ_0 that the intervention is superior assuming that the null hypothesis is true (that is, there is no treatment difference). We might interpret a large value of γ_0 as saying that we have a very good chance of rejecting the null hypothesis at the end of the trial. If this is the case, we might consider not continuing the trial to the end. The question is how large the value of γ_0 should be to make this decision. The results of Lan, Simon, and Halperin (1982) indicate that the actual type I error rate will be no more than the value of the "nominal" significance level (alpha) divided by γ_0 (e.g., $0.05/\gamma_0$). For this case, if the value of γ_0 is 0.80, the actual type I error is bounded by 0.063. For a γ_0 of 0.85, the error is 0.059. These results suggest values of γ_0 greater than 0.85 would be adequate to indicate that the study was essentially over. An example of this situation has been described by DeMets et al. (1984) for a cardiovascular trial.

The situation where no trend or a slightly harmful effect is observed is more complicated. Here the probability of the final test statistic being in the rejection region, given the current statistic, is computed under the proposed alternative hypotheses. If this probability, denoted as γ_1, is very small for a series of "reasonable" alternatives, we may believe that the intervention cannot recover sufficiently to be declared superior to the control. Again, the results of Lan, Simon, and Halperin (1982) indicate that the actual type II error or false negative rate will be at most the value of the "nominal" type II error divided by $(1-\gamma_1)$. This result provides the monitoring group with a guide as to how much of a risk is being taken by not continuing the trial.

The stochastic curtailed procedure is being utilized in some cancer therapeutic trials. For prevention trials, this procedure must be used very conservatively. How long is required for a cancer prevention strategy to take effect is not likely to be well known. Terminating too quickly could deny some intervention strategies a chance to be successful.

Stochastic curtailment has been extended by Spiegelhalter, Freedman, and Blackburn (1986) using a Bayesian modification. Their approach utilizes a prior distribution on the alternative hypotheses and obtains a predictive power of obtaining a positive result.

Early Redesign

Occasionally, in the monitoring of a clinical trial, it becomes evident that the assumptions used in the design are not at all close to what is being observed. One common situation is that the event rate is less than predicted, thus making it more difficult to detect treatment differences or to rule them out. When this situation arises, the monitoring group has three basic options: (1) continue on to almost certain doom, (2) quit, or (3) make a design modification, if possible, which will place the study back on track. If the third alternative seems feasible, then it should be quickly and carefully explored. In addition, if recruitment is still ongoing, it might be feasible to randomize additional patients. If that is not possible, perhaps a longer followup period might be planned for. Another consideration might be to define a new outcome variable which has a higher event rate. For example, instead of just considering the time to a cancer death, we might define a new outcome as time to a cancer death or the first diagnosis of cancer.

Whether or not a redesign is feasible, part of the responsibility of the data monitoring activity is to evaluate the validity of the design assumptions and, thus, the ultimate success of the trial. Stochastic curtailed sampling will aid to some extent by indicating for the alternative assumed how much the power will be decreased, given the reduced event rate. However, stochastic curtailed sampling usually does not give strong evidence for a decision until the second half of a trial, and the redesign should take place well before that.

CONCLUSIONS

Data monitoring is required for all medical trials for ethical and scientific reasons. This responsibility is complex and often dealt with best by a small independent committee with a multidisciplinary membership. Many different dimensions of a trial must be reviewed periodically, typically every six months, in order to meet these obligations. Due to these repeated evaluations, special statistical methods must be employed to keep false positive error rates at acceptable levels. These methods are simple to use and have been employed in a number of trials. However, these methods are guidelines and not absolute rules, due to the complexity of prevention trials.

REFERENCES

Armitage, P. (1975). *Sequential Medical Trials*, second edition. John Wiley and Sons, New York.

Armitage, P., McPherson, C. K., Rowe, B. C. (1969). Repeated significance tests on accumulating data. *Journal of the Royal Statistical Society* Series A 132:235.

Aspirin Myocardial Infarction Study Research Group. (1980). A randomized, controlled trial of aspirin in persons recovered from myocardial infarction. *JAMA 243*:661.

Beta-Blocker Heart Attack Study Group. (1982). The Beta-Blocker Heart Attack Trial—A randomized trial of propranolol in patients with acute myocardial infarction. I. Mortality results. *JAMA 247*:1707.

Canner, P. L. (1983). Monitoring of the data for evidence of adverse or beneficial treatment effects. *Controlled Clinical Trials 4*:467.

Canner, P. L. (1985). Mortality in Coronary Drug Project patients during a nine year post-treatment period (abstract). *J.A.C.C.*, 5:442.

Coronary Drug Project Research Group. (1975). Clofibrate and niacin in coronary heart disease. *JAMA 231*:360.

Coronary Drug Project Research Group. (1980). Influence of adherence to treatment and response of cholesterol on mortality in the Coronary Drug Project. *NEJM 303*:1038.

Coronary Drug Project Research Group. (1981). Practical aspects of decision making in clinical trials: The Coronary Drug Project as a case study. *Controlled Clinical Trials 1*:363.

DeMets, D. (1984). Stopping guidelines versus stopping rules: A practitioner's point of view. *Communications in Statistics—Theory and Methods 13*(19): 2395.

DeMets, D. L., Gail, M. H. (1985). Use of logrank tests and group sequential methods at fixed calendar times. *Biometrics* (December).

DeMets, D., Lan, G. (1984). An overview of sequential methods and their application in clinical trials. *Communications in Statistics—Theory and Methods 13*(19):2315.

DeMets, D., Hardy, R., Friedman, L., Lan, G. (1984). Statistical aspects of early termination in the Beta-Blocker Heart Attack Trial. *Controlled Clinical Trials 5*:362.

Fairbanks, K., Madsen, R. (1982). P values for tests using a repeated significance test design. *Biometrika 69*:69.

Fleming, T. R., O'Brien, P. C., Harrington, D. P. (1984). Designs for group sequential tests. *Controlled Clinical Trials 5*:348.

Friedman, L. M., Furberg, C. D., DeMets, D. L. (1985). *Fundamentals of Clinical Trials*, second edition. PSG Publishing Co., Inc., Littleton, Mass.

Gail, M. (1984). Nonparametric proposals for monitoring comparative survival studies. In *Handbook of Statistics*, Vol. IV, P. R. Krishnaiah (Ed.). North Holland Publishing, Amsterdam.

Haybittle, J. L. (1971). Repeated assessment of results in clinical trials of cancer treatment. *British J. Radiol. 44*:793.

Jennison, C., Turnbull, B. W. (1984). Repeated confidence intervals for group sequential clinical trials. *Controlled Clinical Trials 5*:33.

Kim, K., DeMets, D. L. (1985). Estimation following group sequential tests in clinical trials. *University of Wisconsin Clinical Cancer Center Biostatistics Technical Report*, No. 32.

Kolata, B. G. (1979). Controversy over study of diabetes drugs continues for nearly a decade. *Science 203*:986.

Lachin, J. M. (1981). Introduction to sample size determination and power analysis for clinical trials. *Controlled Clinical Trials 2*:93.

Lan, K. K. G., DeMets, D. L. (1983). Discrete sequential boundaries for clinical trials. *Biometrika 70*:659.

Lan, K. K. G., Simon, R., Halperin, M. (1982). Stochastically curtailed tests in long-term clinical trials. *Communications in Statistics* C(Sequential Analysis) 1:207.

May, G. S., DeMets, D. L., Friedman, L. M., et al. (1981). The randomized clinical trial: Bias in analysis. *Circulation 64*:669.

O'Brien, P. C., Fleming, T. R. (1979). A multiple testing procedure for clinical trials. *Biometrics 35*:549.

Peto, R., Pike, M. C., Armitage, P., et al. (1976). Design and analysis of randomized clinical trials requiring prolonged observations of each patient. I. Introduction and design. *British J. Cancer 34*:585.

Pocock, S. J. (1977). Group sequential methods in the design and analysis of clinical trials. *Biometrika 64*:191.

Pocock, S. J. (1983). *Clinical Trials: A Practical Approach*. John Wiley and Sons, New York.

Shaw, L. W., Chalmers, T. C. (1970). Ethics in cooperative clinical trials. *Ann. N.Y. Acad. Sci. 169*:487.

Spiegelhalter, D. J., Freedman, L. S., Blackburn, P. R. (1986). Monitoring clinical trials: Conditional or predictive power? *Controlled Clinical Trials 7*:8.

Temple, R. J., Jones, J. K., Crout, J. R. (1979). Adverse effects of newly marketed drugs (editorial). *NEJM 300*:1046.

Tsiatis, A. A. (1981). The asymptomatic joint distribution of the efficient scores tests for the proportional hazards model calculated over time. *Biometrika 68*: 311.

Tsiatis, A. A. (1982). Repeated significance testing for a general class of statistics used in censored survival analysis. *J. Am. Stat. Assoc. 77*:855.

Tsiatis, A. A., Rosnar, G. L., Mehta, G. R. (1984). Eacxt confidence intervals following a group sequential test. *Biometrics 40*:497.

Wald, A. (1947). *Sequential Analysis*. John Wiley and Sons, New York.

Whitehead, J. (1982). *The Design and Analysis of Sequential Clinical Trials*. Ellis Harwood, Chichester.

Whitehead, J., Stratton, I. (1983). Group sequential clinical trials with triangular continuation regions. *Biometrics 39*:227.

Wu, M., Fisher, M., DeMets, D. (1980). Sample sizes for long-term medical trials with time-dependent droupout and event rates. *Controlled Clinical Trials 1*: 109.

22

Aspects of the Analysis and Reporting of Prevention Trials

ROSS L. PRENTICE and STEVEN G. SELF
Division of Public Health Sciences, Fred Hutchinson Cancer Research Center, Seattle, Washington

INTRODUCTION

This chapter discusses data analysis procedures that are pertinent to the monitoring and evaluation of disease prevention trials. The preferred choice of test statistic to compare intervention and control groups arises directly from the anticipated form of the primary endpoint relative risk function for intervention versus control subjects. Explanatory data analyses may require specialized methods corresponding to sampling procedures that are intended to reduce trial cost. It is argued that relative risk regression models provide a natural unifying framework for addressing these topics and for the reporting of trial results. The use of relative risk regression methods for basic trial comparisons, and for more general analyses, is described. The importance of reporting trial results in a manner that relates to epidemiologic or other data that may have motivated the trial, particularly if the trial turns out to be negative, is discussed.

This presentation is intended to apply not only to cancer prevention trials but also to other individually randomized nutritional and lifestyle interventions and to chronic diseases other than cancer.

As background for a discussion of data analysis procedures for primary prevention trials, it seems pertinent to emphasize some of the key differences between prevention trials and, say, cancer therapy trials. In fact, while there is much to be learned from a rich history of experiences with therapeutic clinical trials, the presumption that therapeutic trial procedures apply more or less directly to prevention trials needs to be systematically challenged and reevaluated in order that appropriately specialized and efficient prevention trial procedures may be developed.

A major difference between the two types of trials concerns the comparative infrequency of primary endpoint events in disease prevention trials. For example, in spite of the prevalence of coronary heart disease (CHD) in the United States, and in spite of the fact that study subjects were selected to be in the upper 15% in respect to anticipated CHD risk, only about 2% of randomized men experienced the primary endpoint–CHD mortality–during the course of the multiple risk factor intervention trial (MRFIT Research Group, 1982). Similarly, a Women's Health Trial (WHT) is currently underway to determine whether a low fat diet can reduce breast cancer incidence among women at "increased" risk for this disease. The anticipated breast cancer incidence in the control group is less than 0.5% per year. Note that it is the infrequency of disease events that causes the case-control design, rather than the cohort design, to be the mainstay for most cancer epidemiology.

A second feature of disease prevention trials in the comparatively long period of time, as measured from the beginning of intervention, that may be necessary before a discernable reduction in disease risk can be expected to occur. Lengthy study durations, measured in years rather than months, as is typical for cancer therapy trials, are necessary in part because of the infrequency of endpoint events, but a more fundamental issue concerns the anticipated biological effects of intervention activities. For example, MRFIT men would presumably have experienced many years of hypertension, unfavorable lipid profiles, or cigarette smoking habits prior to the beginning of intervention activities. Intuitively, the resulting arterial changes can be expected to reverse only gradually as a function of the duration of intervention on these risk factors, and complete reversal may never occur. Similarly in the WHT, the hypothesized role for dietary fat in breast cancer is primarily as a promoter of previously initiated cells (e.g., Hopkins et al., 1981; Cohen, 1986). Recent carcinogenesis concepts (e.g., Moolgavkar and Knudson, 1981) then suggest that any breast cancer benefit of a low fat diet would be achieved gradually and approximately linearly as a function of years of intervention. Similar promotional mechanisms have been postulated for putative protective effects of selected micronutrients in relation to cancer incidence (e.g., Micozzi et al., 1985). In contrast, cancer therapeutic strategies typically involve removal or eradication of cancerous tissue as completely as possible during a treatment period of at most a few weeks duration. Corresponding therapeutic benefits, in terms of relapse rates or disease rates, may correspondingly be much reduced soon after the initiation of treatment.

The two features mentioned above combine to indicate that primary prevention trials will typically need to be quite large. For example, MRFIT randomized 12,866 men and followed them for an average of more than seven years in order to yield the 2% coronary heart disease mortality previously mentioned. The current WHT design calls for randomization of 32,000 women with an average of 8.5 years of followup. In contrast, most cancer therapy trials randomize at most a few hundred patients. Some other distinctions between therapeutic and prevention trials also contribute to differential trial sizes. Prevention trial subjects are usually free-living, ostensibly healthy, volunteers. Hence there may be limited ability to ensure, or even to measure, compliance to a prescribed intervention program. Also, a long trial duration provides opportunity for noteworthy drift in control group risk factor levels, either on the basis of trial participation or because of secular trends outside the control of trial investigators. Futhermore, prevention trials must emphasize safety at the risk of losing efficacy in view of the usual absence of a clinical care context and of the apparent disease-free status of study subjects. A therapeutic trial among seriously ill patients, on the other hand, may be able to risk toxicity in order to achieve efficacy.

In summary, prevention trials typically require large numbers of subjects to be followed for substantial periods of time, resulting in very substantial costs. Specialized design, conduct, and analysis procedures may correspondingly be required in order to ensure trial efficiency.

ASPECTS OF TRIAL PLANNING THAT AFFECT DATA ANALYSIS PROCEDURES

The prevention trial costs alluded to above place a special emphasis on careful trial planning. An informed specification on key trial design assumptions may require the synthesis and analysis of data from a variety of sources. Often the most critical design assumption concerns the hypothesized ratio of endpoint event rates between intervention and control subjects. This assumption may be combined with assumptions concerning disease rates in the absence of intervention, compliance rates, and competing risk mortality rates in order to establish the necessary sample size to meet certain statistical significance level and power criteria. Such synthesis and analysis of available data may well play a valuable role in defining cost-effective trial eligibility criteria and in identifying efficient recruitment strategies. A relative risk regression framework will often be natural and convenient for both trial planning and analysis.

The design of MRFIT (1977) relied heavily on the experience of the Framingham cohort. An odds ratio model that is multiplicative in diastolic blood pressure, serum cholesterol, and cigarette smoking history was used to define risk factor configurations that identified men in the top 10 or 15% in terms of estimated risk of CHD mortality for the age range in question. This odds ratio model also provided estimated CHD mortality rates for control group subjects, in the absence of control group drift in the three risk factors, upon taking suitable account of the regression to the mean that arises from measurement error in the screening of risk factors. The Framingham data could also have been used in the specification of the ratio of intervention to control group CHD mortality rates. Instead, the relative risk function for fully compliant intervention versus control subjects was evidently simply assumed to drop lineraly from unity at randomization to 0.65 by the end of three years of intervention and subsequently to remain flat for the trial duration. Some simple complicance assumptions then allowed the calculation of the sample size previously mentioned. The "linear with break point" form of the relative risk is pertinent to the desirable form of the test statistic for the basic trial comparison. A relative risk function that is multiplicative in baseline risk factors may be convenient, for example, in relating the magnitude of any intervention benefit to baseline measurements.

A rather detailed design exercise was carried out in planning the WHT. Some aspects of this exercise will be outlined here in order to motivate the statistical test that will be used to perform the basic trial comparison. A full account of the WHT design will be presented for publication elsewhere. Raw data from the Cancer and Steroid Hormone Study, a large breast cancer case-control study, and from the Breast Cancer Detection and Demonstration Program were combined with age-specific breast cancer incidence rates from the national Surveillance, Epidemiology and End Results (SEER) program to estimate baseline breast cancer rates corresponding to possible risk factor eligibility criteria. This led to the selection of one or more classical breast cancer risk factors along with estimated dietary percent calories from fat above the median as the eligibility criteria that would be practical when considering both trial sample size and subject recruitment. Risk factor frequencies from a survey of women in a large health maintenance organization in Seattle were also used in the estimation of baseline breast cancer rates and trial eligibility rates. The basic intervention versus control relative risk assumption was framed in terms of the ratio of breast cancer rates for a woman with a baseline 40% calories from fat diet, who drops to and maintains a 20% calories from fat diet throughout the entire trial period, versus a woman staying with a baseline 40% calories from fat diet. This relative risk function was postulated to drop linearly from unity at randomization to 0.5 by the end of a 10-year trial period. The terminal value of 0.5 was based primarily on international correlation data. A simple linear regression analysis of age-standardized breast cancer incidence from a range of countries having adequate cancer registries (Gray et al., 1979) versus per capita food disappearance rates data (FAO, 1971) yields an approximate linear relationship between breast cancer incidence and percent calories as fat, with a relative risk of about 0.5 corresponding to 20% versus 40% calories from fat. This relative risk of 0.5 may then be a tentative estimate of the breast cancer reduction that would follow from a 20% versus a 40% lifetime percent calories from fat diet. That such a lifetime benefit should be achievable by as few as 10 years was examined in relation to the breast cancer experience of migrant populations. Data from Polish migrants to the United States (Staszewski and Haenszel, 1965) and Italian migrants to Australia (personal communication, Dr. Tony McMichael) appear to support a rather complete adaptation of breast cancer rates within the first generation and perhaps even within the first decade after migration. Data from Japanese migrants to the United States (Beull, 1973) appear to adapt more slowly, perhaps because of a more gradual acculturation. An approximate linear dependence of relative risk as a function of time from the beginning of intervention is supported, for example, by the two-stage carcinogenesis model of Moolgavkar and Knudson (1981), with dietary fat playing a promotional role. This model also suggests an independence of the dietary fat relative risk on the levels of other baseline risk factors.

Ordinarily the results of analytic epidemiologic studies would play a central role in specification of the relative risk for a 20% versus 40% lifetime percent calories from fat diet. Such studies within North American populations, however, pertain to a rather narrow range of percent calories from fat that does not extend below 30%, and individual dietary fat intakes are estimated with substantial measurement error using standard dietary assessment instruments. These two features imply that one can only expect about a 10% higher breast cancer incidence for U.S. women above versus below the median in estimated dietary percent calories from fat. Such a small differential may well be dominated by the biases that may attend case-control or cohort studies. Even in the absence of such biases observational studies would need to be considerably larger than those conducted to date in order to detect such a small effect with reasonable power. Furthermore, the results of U.S. case-control and cohort studies of most rigorous design appear to be heterogeneous and, if combined, yield a broad confidence interval on the relative risk that includes both the value (1.1) projected from the international data and the value (1.0) that reflects no association between dietary fat and breast cancer (Prentice et al., 1988). For these reasons the analytic epidemiologic data were not helpful in a specification of the basic trial relative risk assumption.

The WHT trial design assumptions lead to an overall intervention versus control group relative risk function that decreases approximately linearly as a function of time from the beginning of intervention. For reasons described below this function suggests a test statisitc for the basic trial comparison that is a weighted sum across breast cancer incidence times of the observed minus conditionally expected numbers of breast cancers in the intervention (or control) group with weights that are simply equal to the time from randomization. Such a test weights heavily the disease events occurring toward the end of the trial, while virtually ignoring those occurring soon after randomization.

A later section will provide a more general discussion of the choice of test statistic for the primary trial comparison in relation to the trial design assumptions.

ASPECTS OF TRIAL CONDUCT THAT AFFECT DATA ANALYSIS PROCEDURES

Two distinct aspects of trial conduct will be discussed in this section: the first concerns sampling procedures, in relation to the processing of covariate data, that may effect valuable cost savings. The second concerns the monitoring of trial endpoints toward modification of trial procedures, including the possibilities of early stoppage. Both aspects have some implications for data analysis and trial reporting.

Disease prevention trials typically include the periodic collection of data and specimens from all study subjects. For example, questionnaires and blood or other body specimens may be collected at baseline aand periodically thereafter. These materials are used to monitor the safety of intervention programs and the achievement of intervention goals; to attempt to "explain" differences in end-point rates between intervention and control subjects; to identify any subsets of subjects with unusual intervention versus control disease experience; and to examine epidemiologic or biochemical issues quite apart from the basic trial comparison. The fact that prevention trials typically involve large cohorts with infrequent endpoint events implies that much of the expensive coding and analysis of these materials, collectively referred to as covariate data, can be avoided with little loss in respect to the uses listed above. In particular, monitoring for compliance, or for the achievement of intervention goals more generally, can typically be conducted with adequate precision by analyzing covariate data on a small fraction of the entire trial cohort. The same statement can be made in respect to the safety monitoring of intervention and control subjects on a group basis, though if individual safety monitoring is necessary there will, of course, be no alternative to processing of certain covariate data on all relevant subjects. For the other purposes mentioned above, namely explanatory analyses, interaction analyses, and ancillary study analyses, appropriate relative risk regression analysis procedures have recently been developed that allow either a random subcohort or matched control samples to provide a comparison group for subjects developing primary endpoint events during followup. These procedures can be applied, often with nearly full efficiency relative to full-cohort analysis, while requiring the processing of raw covariate data on only a small fraction, e.g., 10-20% of the cohort.

In the WHT, principal covariates derive from baseline and biennial four-day food records and blood samples and a series of pre- and postrandomization questionnaires ascertaining the frequency of deitary intakes and breast cancer risk factors. The hand-coding of the food records for linkage to a nutritional database and the analysis of blood samples in respect to plasma cholesterol and other concentrations would constitute a quite substantial cost if carried out for the entire trial cohort. Instead, a 10% random subcohort is selected for covariate data analysis on an ongoing basis, while the analysis of stored covariate information will take place following diagnosis for all subjects experiencing endpoint events. About 3% of WHT subjects are expected to develop breast cancer duirng trial followup. It follows that a 10% subcohort will lead to explanatory relative risk analyses with efficiency in the vicinity of 75% relative to a full-cohort analysis, while there is, of course, no loss of efficiency for the basic trial comparison. Clinic personnel are blinded as to the identity of the 10% subcohort in order to avoid any differential intervention or followup activities among subcohort subjects.

Though we will not go into detail here, the manner in which disease events are monitored in prevention trials also has some implications for data analysis and reporting. Specifically, periodic formal comparisons among disease rates in intervention or control groups, with the possibility of early trial termination if a sufficient differential exists, requires testing procedures that acknowledge the sequential aspects of the significance testing. For example, the WHT is planned with formal tests at the end of trial years 5, 7, and 10 (the planned termination), with corresponding significance levels of 0.005, 0.006, and 0.046, respectively, in order to yield an overall significance level of 0.05 (see Fleming et al., 1984). Sequential stopping procedures also have implications for the interpretation of explanatory data analyses and even for analyses based on secondary endpoints (e.g., Whitehead, 1986). Early stopping considerations may also involve stochastic curtailed testing procedures (e.g., Halperin et al., 1982; Lan et al., 1982), whereby one calculates the probability that the test statistic at the subsequent time of planned termination will exceed its critical value, or the probability that it will fail to exceed the critical value, given the accumulated data and given appropriate disease rate projections. If either of these probabilities is sufficiently large, there may be a basis to consider early trial termination. The WHT monitoring plan calls for an annual update and projection of trial design assumptions in respect to subject accrual, compliance, and eligibility risk factor distribution, followed by a recalculation of the basic trial power. If the projected power drops below 50% remedial actions, including the possibility of early trial termination, will be initiated.

There would appear to be motivation in the prevential trial context for developing testing procedures that formally acknowledge the possibility of extending the trial followup period if suggestive, but not definitive, disease incidence differentials arise at the planned termination. Prevention trials will often be designed with sample sizes that are as small as can be justified, under design assumptions that may tend to be optimistic or, at least, tenuous. Trial power can be expected to be quite sensitive to followup duration, particularly if the intervention versus control relative risk function decreases monotonically with followup. Our group in Seattle is currently considering the operating characteristics of α-level tests that involve testing at a level slightly less than α at the planned termination, with continued followup and retesting if the statistic at planned termination is not significant but has marginal significance level near α (e.g., less than 10% for a 5% level test). See Brookmeyer and Self (1985) and Andersen (1987) for related methods for assessing the value of continued follow-up for estimation or testing given interim trial results.

Generally speaking data analysis methods, other than for the basic test itself, are not well developed in the presence of the type of sequential endpoint monitoring that may affect trial duration.

METHODS FOR DATA ANALYSIS AND REPORTING

Relative Risk Regression Methods

Relative risk (RR) regression methods provide a natural and comprehensive framework for disease rate comparison and analysis in prevention trial settings. RR regression models focus on the ratio of disease intensity (hazard) rates between intervention and control groups, or on the ratio of hazard rates to a standard hazard rate more generally, while avoiding unnecessary modeling restrictions on other aspects of the hazard rate model.

In order to be more specific, let t denote time from randomization in an individually randomized disesase prevention trial, while z distinguishes a control ($z = 0$) and an intervention group ($z = 1$). Let $\lambda(t;z)$ denote the instantaneous disease rate (hazard rate) at time t in randomization group z. The relative risk for the intervention versus the control group of time t from randomization is defined as

$$RR(t) = \frac{\lambda(t;0)}{\lambda(t;1)}$$

An RR regression model would specify a parametric form for RR(t), such as $RR(t) = \theta$, which requires hazard rates to be proportional, or $RR(t) = 1 + t\beta$, which allows the relative risk to linearly increase or decrease from unity as a function of time from randomization.

Relative risk models may be extended from this simple two-sample problem to quite general regression problems that may include covariates that are evolving stochastically over the trial followup. Let z(u) be a vector of covariate measurements for a subject at time (from randomization) u, while $Z(t) = [z(u), 0 \leqslant u < t]$ represents the subject's covariate history prior to time t. This history may include baseline risk factor levels and intervention group assignment as part of z(0), as well as postrandomization measurements at followup time u in z(u). Let $Z_0(t) = [z_0(u); 0 \leqslant u < t]$ denote a certain "standard" covariate history prior to time t. The relative risk (process) at time t can then be defined as

$$RR[Z(t);t] = \frac{\lambda[t;Z(t)]}{\lambda[t;Z_0(t)]}$$

The ratio of the hazard rate process corresponding to a general covariate history Z(t) to that for the standard history. A relative risk regression model (e.g., Cox, 1972; Kalbfleisch and Prentice, 1980; Prentice and Farewell, 1986) then involves a parametric specification of the RR process without any restriction on the baseline hazard rate $\lambda_0(\cdot)$. Specifically, one may suppose

$$RR[Z(t);t] = r[x(t)\beta]$$

where $r(\cdot)$ is a fixed function, standardized so that $r(0) = 1$, for example, $r(\cdot) = \exp(\cdot)$ or $r(\cdot) = 1 + (\cdot)$, and $x(t) = [x_1(t), \cdots, x_p(t)]$ is a regression *p*-vector defined as an appropriate function of Z(t) and t with $x_0(t) = (0, \cdots, 0)$ corresponding to $Z_0(t)$, while $\beta^T = (\beta_1, \cdots, \beta_p)$ is a corresponding relative risk parameter to be estimated. Upon denoting $\lambda_0(t) = \lambda[t;Z_0(t)]$, the RR regression model can be written in a standard form as

$$\lambda[t;Z(t)] = \lambda_0(t)r[x(t)\beta] \tag{1}$$

Under standard independent disease time and independent censorship assumptions (e.g., Self and Prentice, 1982), the relative risk regression parameter β can be estimated from data on a cohort of size n using the partial likelihood (Cox, 1975) function

$$L(\beta) = \prod_{i=1}^{n} \left[\frac{r[x_i(t_i)\beta]}{\sum_{\ell=1}^{n} Y_\ell(t_i) r[x_\ell(t_i)\beta]} \right]^{\delta_i} \tag{2}$$

where t_i is the time of disease occurrence ($\delta_i = 1$) or terminal right censorship ($\delta_i = 0$) for the ith individual in the cohort, while $Y_\ell(t)$ indicates whether [$Y_\ell(t) = 1$] or not [$Y_\ell(t) = 0$] the ℓth subject is "at risk" (i.e., alive under active follow-up) for an observable disease occurrence at time t. It has been shown (e.g., Andersen and Gill, 1982; Prentice and Self, 1983) that Equation (2) can be manipulated as if it were an ordinary likelihood function as far as asymptotic likelihood inference is concerned. Asymptotic distributional results for the maximum partial likelihood estimate ($\hat{\beta}$) can be expected to provide reasonable approximations with a moderate number of disease events under the exponential relative risk form $r(\cdot) = \exp(\cdot)$. Likelihood ratio procedures or score procedures using an appropriate "expected" variance estimator, but not asymptotic distributinal approximations for $\hat{\beta}$ itself, can be advocated for other relative risk forms, such as the linear form $r(\cdot) = 1 + (\cdot)$ (e.g., Prentice and Mason, 1986). Equation (2) can accommodate a moderate degree of disease time grouping without incurring noteworthy bias in the estimation of β. As an extreme special case, the disease time information may be grouped over the entire trial followup period in which case, if the fraction of the cohort experiencing disease is small (e.g., <0.10), estimation based on Equation (2) will yield results in close agreement to those from a binary logistic regression analysis with odds ratio function $r[x(t)\beta]$. Relative to such a binary logistic analysis, estimation based on Equation (2) has the advantage of being able to appropriately acknowledge different potential followup periods among study subjects, to acknowledge dropouts and deaths due to competing risks and, perhaps more importantly, Equation (2) allows the regression vector to include postrandomization covariate measurements while a binary logistic analysis does not provide a conceptual framework for such inclusion. A useful generalization of Equation (1) allows the baseline hazard rate $\lambda_0(\cdot)$ to be allowed to differ arbitrarily among a fixed number of strata in which case the partial likelihood becomes a product of terms (2) over strata. Stratum assignments for a subject may even be allowed to vary over the trial followup course, a valuable feature if individual study subjects are followed for the occurrence of more than one disease event (e.g., Prentice et al., 1981). A consistent estimator of the cumulative baseline hazard rate $\Lambda_0(t) = \int_0^t \lambda_0(u)du$ is given by

$$\hat{\Lambda}_0(t) = \sum_{i=1}^{n} \delta_i I(t_i \leqslant t) \left[\sum_{\ell=1}^{n} Y_\ell(t_i) r[x_\ell(t_i)\hat{\beta}] \right]^{-1} \tag{3}$$

where $I(t_i \leqslant t)$ takes value one if the failure ($\delta_i = 1$) or censoring ($\delta_i = 0$) time t_i for the ith subject is equal or less than t, and value zero otherwise.

Choice of Test Statistic for Basic Trial Comparisons and Methods for Explanatory Analyses

The score statistic $U(\beta_0) = \partial \log L(\beta_0)/\partial\beta_0$ provides a natural approach to testing the hypothesis $\beta = \beta_0$ within the model (1). Consider the special case of testing the null hypothesis $\beta = 0$ for an intervention (z = 1) versus a control (z = 0) group without other covariates. The modeled regression variable may be specified as the scalar $x(t) = zg(t)$ where $g(\cdot)$ is a fixed function, such as $g(t) \equiv 1$ or $g(t) = t$, that determines the hazard ratio form as a function of time from randomization. The corresponding score statistic is proportional to

$$\sum_{i=1}^{n} \delta_i g(t_i)[z_i - n_1(t_i)n(t_i)^{-1}] \tag{3}$$

where $n(t)$ and $n_1(t)$ are, respectively, the total number of subjects, and the number of intervention subjects at risk at time t. This statistic is, in fact, the weighted sum over distinct disease incidence times of the observed minus conditionally expected number of disease events in the intervention group, with weight g(t) at followup time t. This test is readily generalized for the comparison of more than two groups.

The WHT design specifies a hazard ratio for the target 20% calories from fat diet that decreased linearly in time relative to a typical 40% calories from fat diet. The breast cancer relative risk in the intervention versus control group is expected to be approximately linearly decreasing from an initial value of unity even after allowing for an anticipated lack of compliance to intervention goals and anticipated control group drift. Hence the test statistic above, based on $r(u) = 1 + u$ and $g(t) = t$, will be nearly optional under trial design assumptions and has been adopted as a test statistic for trial monitoring and reporting. The manner in which it will be used for possible early trial termination was mentioned in the preceding section.

Aside from possible slight influences of the sequential monitoring on interpretation, the RR regression formulation of the preceding subsection and the corresponding partial likelihood function (2) can be used for a broad range of analyses beyond the basic test for differences in disease rates between intervention and control groups. For example, the regression vector x(t) can be extended to include baseline disease risk factors to ensure that baseline heterogeneity in risk does not affect the interpretation of the basic trial comparison. Product terms between baseline risk factor indicators and intervention versus control group indicator variables allow one to study dependence of the magnitude of any intervention effect on such factors. The inclusion of postrandomization measurements, such as serum nutrient levels in a cancer prevention or dietary intervention trial, in the modeled regression variable allows one to attempt to "explain" any difference between intervention and control disease rates in terms of biological or other "markers" and hence gain some insight into the mechanism of any intervention effect on disease rates. The RR regression approach also allows an exploration of the dependence of relative risk on a subject's preceding intervention history (e.g., time since beginning of intervention, degree of compliance) yielding possible further insights into intervention efficacy. Finally the same RR regression approach is well suited to a whole range of ancillary observational studies which examine the relationship between epidemiologic, biochemical, or other measurements and disease events, often carried out separately for control and intervention groups. Formal recognition of random measurement errors (e.g., Prentice, 1982) in certain covariate histories (e.g., most dietary intakes) will be essential to the proper interpretation of these explanatory and ancillary analyses.

As mentioned previously the processing of the raw materials for explanatory analyses and for ancillary studies will often be inappropriately costly if carried out on the entire trial cohort. The next subsection outlines estimation in the RR regression model (1) under so-called case-cohort and synthetic case-control sampling procedures.

Data Analyses Following Case-Cohort or Case-Control Sampling

The case-cohort approach (Prentice, 1986) to the processing of prospectively collected raw materials to determine individual covariate histories Z(t) involves the selection of a random subcohort $C \subset [1, \cdots, n]$ of the entire cohort. Covariate data processing, such as the hand-coding of diet records, the biochemical analysis of blood samples, and even the processing of questionnaire information then takes place only for subcohort subjects and for subjects developing trial endpoint events. The relative risk parameter β in the RR regression model (1) can be estimated under case-cohort sampling by using the "pseudolikelihood" function

$$\tilde{L}(\beta) = \prod_{i=1}^{n} \left[\frac{r[x_i(t_i)\beta]}{\sum_{\ell \in \tilde{R}(t_i)} Y_\ell(t_i) r[x_\ell(t_i)\beta]} \right]^{\delta_i} \tag{4}$$

which is identical to (2) except that the ith determinator summation is restricted to $\tilde{R}(t_i) = C \cup [i]$, the union of the subcohort and the ith subject. The maximum pseudolikelihood estimator $\tilde{\beta}$ quite generally has an asymptotic normal distribution with mean β (Self and Prentice, 1988), and an appropriate variance estimator is available (Prentice, 1986). Unlike the partial likelihood (2), the contributions to the score statistic $\tilde{U}(\beta) = \partial \log \tilde{L}(\beta)/\partial\beta$ from distinct disease incidence times are not statistically uncorrelated so that a specialized variance estimator for $U(\beta)$ and for $\tilde{\beta}$ is required. The cumulative baseline hazard function can be estimated under case-cohort sampling using

$$\hat{\Lambda}_0(t) = mn^{-1} \sum_{i=1}^{n} \delta_i I(t_i \leqslant t) \left[\sum_{\ell \in C} Y_\ell(t_i) r[x_\ell(t_i)\beta] \right]^{-1} \tag{5}$$

where m is the size of the subcohort.

Quality control considerations may require the storage of certain subcohort covariate materials for concurrent analysis with corresponding materials on cases; that is, on individuals developing disease events.

An alternate procedure for estimation in (1) while sampling within a trial cohort involves the matching of each subject developing an endpoint disease to one or more subjects without disease at the time of disease occurrence (e.g., Liddell et al., 1977; Breslow et al., 1983). Provided matched controls are selected independently with replacement at distinct disease occurrence times, estimate of β can be based on a likelihood function that is formally identical to (4) but with $\tilde{R}(t_i)$ consisting only of any case ($\delta_i = 1$) and its corresponding matched controls at t_i. In fact, $\tilde{L}(\beta)$ has a partial likelihood interpretation in this circumstance (Oakes, 1981) and so may be manipulated as an ordinary likelihood function for asymptotic inference on β.

The case-cohort approach would appear to possess a number of advantages relative to this "synthetic case-control" approach in the prevention trial setting. The subcohort, in the case-cohort approach, provides a natural mechanism for assessing the achievement of intervention goals and for the identification of adverse effects on a groupwise basis; the subcohort provides a natural "comparison group" for a range of disease endpoints, whereas, strictly, the matched case-control appoach requires a distinct set of controls for each disease; the case-cohort approach allows esimation of the cumulative baseline failure rate, via (5), whereas no comparable estimator has been proposed under the case-control sampling. Finally, the case-cohort approach appears to often have somewhat better efficiency properties for a given expected number of subjects requiring covariate data analysis than does the case-control approach (e.g., Self and Prentice, 1988) owing to the strict alignment of a given control to only the case (or cases) to which it happens to be matched in the case-control analysis. Either approach will typically give rise to near full efficiency, relative to the full-cohort analysis based on (2), if the ratio of disease-free to diseased individuals exceeds five (i.e., efficiency about 90% or greater). However, the comparative efficiency of the two sampling procedures is a rather complicated function of the structure of the data and model, and the case-control approach will, in some circumstances, have an efficiency advantage if the subcohort is sparse at the times of occurrence of many cases. Study of the comparative efficiency of the case-cohort approach to that of a cross-sectional case-control approach based on a grouping of the disease occurrence data would appear to be worthwhile.

As mentioned previously, a 10% subcohort, the identity of which is blinded to clinic personnel, is being implemented in the WHT. Virtually all trial materials will be processed on an ongoing basis only for the subcohort, with little impact on the efficiency of explanatory or ancillary studies and, of course, with no impact on the primary test (3), since intervention group assignment is available for all subjects.

Interpretation and Reporting of Negative Trials

The manner of interpreting and reporting nonsignificant test results seems particularly important in the prevention trial context. Substantial costs and logistical challenges will sometimes lead to sample sizes that, though large, are considerably too small to allow a powerful test under defensible design assumptions. There may be quite limited data pertinent to the specification of key design assumptions. For example, adequate data on compliance rates may often be unavailable at the time of trial design. Similarly, there may be little direct information to allow an informed assumption concerning the time course of any disease reduction following the initiation of intervention activities. These considerations suggest considerable caution in interpreting a negative test at trial termination as supportive of the null hypothesis of no intervention effect on diseases rates. Rather it will be important to report a range of intervention versus control group differences that are consistent with available data and to intrepret such differences, if possible, in relation to intervention effects that may have been anticipated in view, for example, of prior epidemiologic studies.

The RR regression methods described above provide a method of quantitatively summarizing intervention versus control group hazard ratios that are consistent with the data. For example, one may report an estimated hazard ratio $\hat{\theta} = e^{\hat{\beta}}$ and a corresponding confidence interval (θ_1, θ_2) which can be assumed to include unity in the circumstance of a negative test result, but will also include values (e.g., θ_1) which may differ enough from unity to show that practically important intervention effects are consistent with the data in spite of the negative test. A more refined approach would present an estimated relative risk function over the trial followup period along with corresponding confidence bands. See also Hauck and Anderson (1986) for a proposal for presenting such information using equivalence testing methods.

Unfortunately, a quantitative presentation of the magnitude of intervention versus control group differences that are consistent with the data will often not be highly insightful in the absence of a framework for anticipating such magnitude. For example, suppose the WHT were to yield a summary intervention versus control breast cancer relative risk estimate of 0.90. The corresponding 95% confidence interval would have expected value approximately equal to (0.80, 1.02) and the corresponding test statistic can be expected to be nonsignificant at the 5% level. How should this result be interpreted? On the one hand, the fact that the confidence interval barely exceeds unity suggests that there is a suggestion of an intervention effect. On the other hand the proximity of the point estimate to unity and the rather narrow confidence interval could easily be interpreted as providing strong evidence that any dietary fat effect must be small and practically unimportant. Such an interpretation would be premature in the absence of further analysis, however, since a small differential in fat intakes in the two groups, for example, can by itself imply a relative risk close to unity, even if dietary fat has the previously mentioned strong relationship to breast cancer incidence suggested by the international correlation data. In fact, the series of design assumptions employed in the WHT leads to a projected summary relative risk of about 0.84 taking the international correlations at face value, so that the confidence interval mentioned above could be interpreted as indicating a reasonable correspondence between trial results and the international data in spite of the negative test. More constructively a recalculation of the projected summary relative risk under a face value interpretation of the international correlation data could be carried out that would make use of trial data on intervention compliance rates and control group drift, on followup durations, and on overall trial breast cancer incidence. Such a summary relative risk could then be examined in relation to the observed relative risk point estimate and confidence interval in order to assess rather directly the quantitative agreement between the association suggested by international correlation data that motivated the WHT and the observed trial results. This type of presentation could also be carried out for specific subsets of the trial followup period.

Disease prevention trials may often be preceded by observational studies with predictor variables that correspond to the factors targeted for intervention in a prevention trial. An attempt to relate trial results to results that would be anticipated if such observational studies provided unconfounded estimates of the association of interest would seem to be a valuable aspect of trial interpretation and reporting, particularly if the basic trial test results are negative.

An Additional Data Analysis Problem

The above presentation points to a few topics in the analysis of individually randomized trials that merit further study. Disease prevention trials of lifestyle interventions may in some circumstances be more efficient if groups rather than single individuals comprise the basic unit of randomization. Data analysis methods that acknowledge the correlations induced by the group randomization are currently not well developed. Procedures that would allow comparison of the efficiency of individual versus group randomization at the design stage particularly merit further study.

ACKNOWLEGMENTS

This work was supported by grants GM-24472, CA-38526, and CA-34847. Helpful input on the part of colleagues participating in the WHT is also acknowledged.

REFERENCES

Andersen, P. K. (1987). Conditional power calculations as an aid in the decision whether to continue a clinical trial. *Controlled Clin. Trials 8*:67.

Andersen, P. K., Gill, R. D. (1982). Cox's regression model for counting processes: A large sample study. *Ann. Statist. 10*:1100.

Breslow, N. E., Lubin, J. H., Marek, P., Langholz, B. (1983). Multiplicative models and cohort analysis. *J. Am. Statist. Assoc. 78*:1.

Brookmeyer, R., Self, S. G. (1985). The effect of additional followup and accrual on survival time data. *Biometrics 41*:129.

Buell, P. (1973). Changing incidence of breast cancer in Japanese American women. *J. Natl. Cancer Inst. 51*:1479.

Cohen, L.A. (1986). Dietary fat and mammary cancer. In *Diet, Nutrition and Cancer: A Critical Evaluation*, vol. 1, *Macronutrients and Cancer*, B. S. Reddy and L. A. Cohen (Eds.). CRC Press, Boca Raton, Fla., pp. 78-100.

Cox, D. R. (1972). Regression models and life tables (with discussion). *J. R. Statist. Soc. B 34*:187.

Cox, D. R. (1975). Partial likelihood. *Biometria 62*:269.

Food and Agricultural Organization (FAO) of the United Nations (1971). *Food Balance Sheets, 1964-1966 Averages*. FAO, Rome.

Fleming, T. R., Harrington, D. P., O'Brien, P. C. (1984). Design of group sequential tests. *Controlled Clin. Trials 5*:348.

Gray, G. E., Pike, M. C., Henderson, B. E. (1979). Breast cancer incidence and mortality rates in different countries in relation to known risk factors and dietary practices. *Br. J. Cancer 39*:1.

Halperin, M., Lan K. K. G., Ware, J. H., Johnson, N. J., Demets, D. L. (1982). An aid to data monitoring in long-term clinical trials. *Controlled Clin. Trials 3*:311.

Hauck, W. W., Anderson, S. (1986). A proposal for interpreting and reporting negative studies. *Statist. Med. 5*:203.

Hopkins, G. J., Kennedy, T. G., Carroll, K. K. (1981). Polyunsaturated fatty acids as promoters of mammary carcinogenesis induced in Sprague-Dawley rats by 7,12-dimethylbenzanthracene. *J. Natl. Cancer Inst. 66*:517.

Kalbfleisch, J. D., Prentice, R. L. (1980). *The Statistical Analysis of Failure Time Data*. Wiley, New York.

Lan, K. K. G., Simon, R., Halperin, M. (1982). Stochastically curtailed testing in long-term clinical trials. *Com. Stat. C 1*:207.

Liddell, F. D. K., McDonald, J. C., Thomas, D. C. (1977). Methods for cohort analysis: Appraisal by application to asbestos mining (with discussion). *J. R. Statist. Soc. A 140*:469.

Micozzi, M. S., Boone, C. W., Kelloff, G. J., Tangrea, J. A. Helzlsouer, K. J., Taylor, P. R. (1985). *J. Clin. Pharmacol. 25*:164.

Moolgavkar, S. H., Knudson, A. G. (1981). Mutation and cancer: A model for human carcinogenesis. *J. Natl. Cancer Inst. 66*:1037.

Multiple Risk Factor Intervention Trial (MRFIT) Group (1977). Statistical design considerations in the NHLI Multiple Risk Factor Intervention Trial (MRFIT). *J. Chron. Dis. 30*:261.

Multiple Risk Factor Intervention Trial (MRFIT) Research Group (1982). Multiple Risk Factor Intervention Trial: Risk factor changes and mortality results. *J. Amer. Med. Assoc. 248*:1465.

Oakes, D. (1981). Survival times: Aspects of partial likelihood. *Int. Statist. Rev. 49*:235.

Prentice, R. L., Williams, B. J., Peterson, A. V. (1981). On the regression analysis of multivariate failure time data. *Biometrika 68*:373.

Prentice, R. L. (1982). Covariate measurement errors and parameter estimation in Cox's failure time regression model. *Biometrika 69*:331.

Prentice, R. L. and Self, S. G. (1983). Asymptotic distribution theory for Cox-type regression models with general relative risk form. *Ann. Statist. 11*:804.
Prentice, R. L. (1986). A case-cohort design for epidemiologic cohort studies and disease prevention trials. *Biometrika 73*:1.
Prentice, R. L., Farewell, V. T. (1986). Relative risk and odds ratio regression. *Ann. Rev. Public Health* 7:35.
Prentice, R. L., Mason, M. W. (1986). On the application of linear relative risk models. *Biometrics 42*:109.
Prentice, R. L., Sullivan, M., Self, S.G. (1988). Dietary fat and breast cancer: An assessment of the epidemiologic literature in relation to the design of the Women's Health Trial. Submitted for publication.
Self, S. G., Prentice, R. L. (1982). Commentary on Andersen and Gill's "Cox's Regression Model for Counting Processes: A large sample study." *Ann. Statist. 10*:1121.
Self, S. G., Prentice, R. L. (1988). Asymptotic distribution theory and efficiency results for case-cohort studies. *Ann. Statist 16*:64.
Staszewski, J., Haenszel, W. (1965). Cancer mortality among Polish-born in the United States. *J. Natl. Cancer Inst. 35*:291.
Whitehead, J. (1986). Supplementary analysis at the conclusion of a sequential clinical trial. *Biometrics 42*:461.

23

Future Strategies for Cancer Prevention Trials

FRANK L. MEYSKENS, Jr.
The University of Arizona College of Medicine, Tucson, Arizona

Where are we?

Any attempt to gaze into the crystal ball should necessarily be built on past and current observations, experiences, and, whenever possible, data. The interpretation of apparent nutritional associations and cancer incidence from established epidemiologic techniques has provided a signpost but not definite proof for causality. Laboratory studies of dietary micronutrients have been comparatively few with investigators emphasizing powerful pharmacologic agents that produce irrefutable effects. Analysis of available data for both dietary micronutrients and drugs, however, leads to the same general conclusion: the process of carcinogenesis can be inhibited, but the response is carcinogen, anticarcinogen, dose, tissue, and most importantly, species specific. The inconclusive observations provided by epidemiologic and laboratory studies affirm the proposition that only intervention trials may conclusively resolve the role of dietary micronutrients in cancer prevention.

The type of trials that have emanated from these initial considerations needs further viewing. Early on there was considerable interest in developing true dietary interventions in which the entire diet would be changed using behavior-altering techniques. However, for a variety of reasons, including most notably the failure of such proposals to survive scientific peer review, the approach was redirected to examine the role of individual micronutrients in controlled "public health" influence in the design of the early trials, with an insistence on the "lowest dose possible" of the intervention agent. A summary of these ongoing trials has recently been published (Bertram et al., 1987). The majority of the investigations use either β-carotene or retinol as the intervention agent, although ascorbic acid, α-tocopherol, folic acid, riboflavin, selenium, and calcium are used in some trials.

What are the advantages to the way in which the field of dietary intervention for cancer prevention has developed to date?

Dietary intervention for cancer prevention is currently highlighted by relatively well-defined trials which use low doses of single micronutrients. This approach appeals to the conservative clinical scientist, only somewhat to the public health-oriented individual, but even less to the biologically oriented clinician. However, few side effects will be seen and if a trial were strongly positive, widespread adoption may be feasible since "pill taking" is common in our society.

What are the disadvantages to the current approach?

The dose-reponse curve for micronutrients to produce a cancer-preventive effect is unknown. The assumption has been made that doses of a vitamin or mineral which define the recommended daily allowance for preventing nutritional deficiency are somehow closely related to the effect of a micronutrient as an inhibitor of carcinogenesis. This supposition may well not be true, particularly since effective doses of micronutrients in animal experiments to prevent cancer are invariably high. In these early clinical trials the worst outcome to be expected might be completely negative results with no difference in cancer incidence between intervention and placebo groups. Such a result would have a significant palling effect on further exploration of micronutrients as cancer prevention agents.

As the trials utilize highly defined groups of individuals and agents, generalizability might be difficult.

Where then should be our major new or redefined direction(s)?

I propose that the following areas should each be explored in depth to maximize the likelihood that the role of micronutrients in cancer prevention will be properly understood:

1. More clear definition of the genotypic contribution of the human host to cancer risk.
2. Increased understanding of the natural history of human cancer and the attendant phenotypic stresses which promote the process of carcinogenesis or cause preneoplasias to progress.
3. Increased biological, biochemical and pharmacologic understanding of how micronutrients work.
4. Development of intermediate endpoints or proxies for cancer or cancer risk.

5. Second generation trials based on the results from the initial studies.
6. A better laboratory or epidemiologic understanding of the interaction of multiple micronutrients as preventive agents.
7. A unified dietary approach to cancer prevention.

What are some of the major scientific features which need to be known to understand the interaction of dietary micronutrients with the carcinogenesis process?

Experiments of nature such as xeroderma pigmentosum, Bloom's syndrome, and many others (Chapanti and German, 1985) established the general principle that intrinsic genetic changes can predispose to subsequent cancer development. More recent studies have localized the alteration to specific DNA sequences (oncogenes), retinoblastoma and neuroblastoma, perhaps being the best studied to date. New advances in biotechnology have allowed the characterization of the genome via the use of restriction fragment length polymorphism (RFLP). Using this technique, case-control studies have demonstrated a marked increase in risk for certain cancers based on RFLP patterns (Lidereau et al., 1986). These results raise the possibility that individual cancer risk can be related to the genetic constitution of an individual. Enormous experimental possibilities and profound ethical responsibilities flow from such a concept. We may well be able to select individuals based on their genetic pattern as subjects for dietary micronutrient intervention studies such that the risk of transformation to a certain malignancy is accurately known. Consequently, the number of subjects required for a trial will be markedly reduced, the need for a control group may be obviated, and the results will be generalizable to the population at actual rather than at estimated risk.

A great deal has been learned about the effect of exogenous risk factors for certain types of cancer. Smoking and lung cancer and ultraviolet radiation and skin cancer are two well-known examples. Less is known for inhibitors of carcinogenesis, but recent data documenting the marked decrease of ovarian and endometrial cancer in women taking birth control pills is noteworthy (Lee et al., 1987). Advances in cell and molecular biology have established the association of viruses with hepatoma, cervical cancer (and dysplasia), and other malignancies and alterations in the genetic material demonstrated. How do micronutrients interact with critical phenotypic stress such as physical, chemical, hormonal, and viral agents? Indeed, very little is known.

An increased understanding of the biological, biochemical, and pharmacological mechanisms of how micronutrients work is needed. Extensive chemical manipulation of the vitamin A molecule has clearly shown that biochemical and pharmacological properties can be changed and end biological effect improved. Limited studies also show that the chemical forms of selenium and α-tocopherol are critical to function. Can we build a better preventive agent by chemical manipulation to selenium, vitamin E, and other micronutrients? We do not know.

Particularly important in the design of prevention trials is the pharmacologic properties of micronutrients. One woud think that the characteristics of distribution of micronutrients in the human body would have been well studied. Surprisingly, this assumption is not true. Retinoids have been modified so that certain of the compounds are preferentially distributed to breast, liver, or skin (Lippman et al., 1987). Can similar chemical manipulations lead to preferential distribution of other micronutrients. We do not know.

To better understand and study the process of carcinogenesis in humans, advances in the biology or biochemistry of markers of early disease will need to be developed. Optimally, damaged cells should be detected soon after insult. The measurement of specified DNA-adducts by immunochemical means may well provide a critical early indication. Studies of the interaction of "anti-initiators" (such as β-carotene) at this earliest stage of DNA alteration are badly needed. At the macroscopic level, proliferative or preneoplastic lesions such as dysplastic cells (cervical, oral cavity, bladder) or polyps (colon, bladder) provide an easily measurable proxy for cancer development, as well as a rich source of tissue for laboratory and clinical study of micronutrient effects. There is, however, a wide distance between DNA-adduct formation and preneoplasia; and the development of intermediate biochemical markers will also be important.

An alternative approach to monitoring the carcinogenesis process is the measurement of noncellular and, consequently, indirect elements which are affected by, or serve as a marker for, a carcinogen. Changes in bile acid concentrations, mutagen content, or bacterial type or capacity in the large bowel in response to phenoytypic stress (fat, fiber) represent the best studied indicators (Reddy et al., 1987). Little is known about the effect of extracellular products on other tissues and their use as indicators of micronutrient effect.

What can we learn from current intervention trials in our planning for second-generation studies?

Experience and results from laboratory and epidemiologic investigations and cancer prevention trials indicate the following:

1. A logical approach to the use of micronutrients (and other compounds) for cancer prevention trials must be developed.
2. The use of multiple micronutrients in one arm of a trial should be continued.
3. Testing of a unified dietary approach to cancer prevention should be undertaken.

4. Further research in the design and analysis of prevention trials should be undertaken.

The choice of micronutrients for cancer prevention studies has to date largely occurred in the absence of complete or critical data. I propose that optimally the following should be demonstrated before use of a micronutrient in a randomized phase III intervention trial:

1. Epidemiologic evidence for a favorable association of a micronutrient with cancer incidence. At least two positive case-control studies or one follow-up investigation involving the relevant target organ should be available. Evidence of a dose-response effect between micronutrient intake and cancer rate should be evident, or if unavailable, an odds ratio of greater than 2.0 should be measurable.
2. Favorable effects of the micronutrient on in vitro biochemical parameters at reasonable concentrations. Alteration of activity in the appropriate direction of ornithine decarboxycylase, protein kinase C, cyclic AMP, or production of growth factors are examples of such markers. Many others exist.
3. Activity of the micronutrient in at least two separate prevention animal model systems. Preferably the two systems should utilize either different tissues or species as the indicator lesion or host. A dose-response effect should be evident for either (preferably both) the carcinogen or the inhibitor. An effect should be evident at pharmacologically achievable doses of the micronutrient.
4. Presence of the micronutrient in the relevant tissue in humans. Pharmacologic monitoring of micronutrients in either serum or tissue (very rare) has been surprisingly casual to date, with our knowledge limited to a few reported trials with certain retinoids. Demonstration of the presence of a micronutrient (or a predicted effect of the compound) in target tissue would seem a minimum criteria.
5. Evidence of no, little, or well-defined side effects in humans. At least one-year trials of the micronutrient(s) at the projected phase III dose should be undertaken. The subjects can be either normal volunteers, individuals at high risk for cancer, or patients with easily monitored preneoplasias. The definition of an acceptable toxicity will require careful consideration of the risk group being studied.
6. Regulatory approval of the use of the micronutrient. Two major problems have existed to date: (a) nonavailability of an IND for many micronutrients. Since most of these compounds are in the public domain, obtaining regulatory approval has been vexing; (b) some pharmaceutical companies have occasionally been considered in their participation, largely due to the potential liability in such trials, and the National Cancer Institute has as-

sumed responsibility. With all good intentions, a federal Safety and Protocol Committee has been created. However, the result has been confusion and disagreement between investigator and NCI program staff about responsibilities and other issues, a secondary level of peer review, and hence interminable delay in trial implementation. Improvement in this review system is very much needed.

Mechanistic considerations and limited laboratory and epidemiologic studies suggest that micronutrients might be more effective as preventive agents if used in combination. One can make many a priori arguments for such an approach, but I would maintain that utilization of combinations should be subject to the same level of scrutiny as for the development of single micronutrients outlined above. The history of medical therapeutics supports the use of agents in combinations to achieve increased effectiveness, but several dramatic examples caution against automatic acceptance of combinations based on single agent data.

Changes in many aspects of the diet may be required to effect a long-lasting alteration in the phenotypic environment. The public has become enamored of a lifestyle characterized by high physical activity and a low fat, high fiber, high vegetable diet. Adoption of this general approach as a secular trend may well impact on the incidence of cancer and possibly obscure results of ongoing or future trials. Formal testing of such a generic approach is well worth considering, although implementation would require substantial resources and a broad societal effort.

Consideration of the design and analysis of cancer prevention trials with micronutrients has presented formidable difficulties and hence new opportunities. We should use lessons from both clinical trials and public health approaches, but as Byar and Piantadosi, Prentice and Self point out in this volume, new approaches need to be developed to deal with the issues raised by these unique and new types of intervention trials.

REFERENCES

Bertram, J. S., Kolonel, L. N., Meyskens, F. L., Jr. (1987). Rational and strategies for chemoprevention of cancer in humans. *Cancer Res. 47*:3012.

Chaganti, R. S. K., German, J. L, (1985). *Genetics in Clinical Oncology*. Oxfor University Press, New York.

Lee, N. C., Wingo, P. A., Gwinn, M. D., Rubin, G. L., Kendrick, J. S., Webster, L. A., Ory, H. W. (1987). The reduction in risk of ovarian cancer associated with oral-contraceptive use. *N. Engl. J. Med. 316(11)*:650.

Lidereau, R., Escot, C., Theillet, C., Champeme, M. H., Brunet, M., Gest, J., Callahan, R. (1986). High frequency of rare alleles of the human c-Ha-ras-1 proto-oncogene in breast cancer patients. *J. Natl. Cancer Inst.* 77(93):697.

Lippman, S., Kessler, J., Meyskens, F. L., Jr. (1987). Retinoids as preventive and therapeutic anticancer agents. *Cancer Treat. Rep. 71*:3012.

Reddy, B. S., Sharma, C., Simin, B., Engle, A., Laakso, K., Puska, P., Korpela, R. (1987). Metabolic epidemiology of colon cancer: effects of dietary fiber on fecal mutagens and bile acids in healthy subjects. *Cancer Res. 47*:644.

Index